YOUR BABY'S FIRST YEAR

Tanya Altmann, MD, FAAP

Editor in Chief

Pediatrician and Founder, Calabasas Pediatrics Wellness Center

Calabasas, California

Adjunct Clinical Professor at Children's Hospital Los Angeles and Keck School of Medicine, Los Angeles, California

BANTAM
NEW YORK

A note about revisions: Every effort is made to keep *Your Baby's First Year* consistent with the most recent advice and information available from the American Academy of Pediatrics. In addition to major revisions identified as "Revised Editions" and "Sixth Edition," the text has been updated as necessary for each additional printing listed below.

As of the time of initial publication, the URLs displayed in this book link or refer to existing websites on the internet. Penguin Random House LLC is not responsible for, and should not be deemed to endorse or recommend, any website other than its own or any content available on the internet (including without limitation at any website, blog page, or information page) that is not created by Penguin Random House.

AAP disclosures: Dr. Tanya Altmann has disclosed a financial relationship as a consultant with Bubs Australia, Sydney office, and with Ember Mug. Any other disclosures were reviewed and determined not relevant to the work related to *Your Baby's First Year.* Disclosures are reviewed and mitigated through a Conflict of Interest process that consists of reviewing pertinent information, which is then used to decide what action is required to maintain content integrity. There may be instances where no action is necessary. This process has been approved by the AAP Board of Directors.

Bantam Books
An imprint of Random House
A division of Penguin Random House LLC
1745 Broadway, New York, NY 10019
randomhousebooks.com

2025 Bantam Books Mass Market Edition

Originally published in the United States in hardcover in 1991 and in revised paperback editions in 1993, 1998, 2004, 2009, 2014, and 2020 by Bantam Books, an imprint of Random House, a division of Penguin Random House LLC.

ISBN 978-0-593-98387-4

Cover design: Ruby Levesque

Printed in the United States of America

2nd Printing

Bantam Books mass market edition: September 2025

The authorized representative in the EU for product safety and compliance is Penguin Random House Ireland, Morrison Chambers, 32 Nassau Street, Dublin D02 YH68, Ireland, https://eu-contact.penguin.ie.

YOUR BABY'S FIRST YEAR

This invaluable volume was prepared under the editorial direction of distinguished pediatricians Tanya Altmann, MD, FAAP, and David L. Hill, MD, FAAP, and draws on the contributions and practical wisdom of more than 100 pediatric experts. Written in a warm, accessible style and illustrated with helpful drawings and diagrams, this book gives you the information you need to safeguard your baby's most precious asset: their health.

In *Your Baby's First Year* you'll find:

- A month-by-month guide to your baby's first year that lets you know what to expect in terms of growth, behavior, and development
- Health Watch features that alert you to potential medical problems at each stage
- Safety Check reminders for home, outdoors, and car travel
- A discussion of family issues—from grandparents and siblings to single parenting and stepfamilies

Plus reliable information on:

- Nutrition, with advice on breastfeeding and bottle-feeding, and when to introduce solid foods
- All common infectious diseases, from chickenpox and measles to flu and ear infections
- Developmental disabilities, such as congenital abnormalities, cerebral palsy, hearing loss, autism, and intellectual disability
- Skin problems, from birthmarks to sunburn
- Emergencies, including bites, poisoning, choking, and CPR
- Feeding and nutrition
- Car safety seats
- Sleep habits and challenges

ADDITIONAL PARENTING BOOKS FROM THE AMERICAN ACADEMY OF PEDIATRICS

Baby and Toddler Basics: Expert Answers to Parents' Top 150 Questions

The Baby Bonding Book: Connecting With Your Newborn

Baby Leads the Way: An Evidence-Based Guide to Introducing Solid Foods

The CALM Baby Method: Solutions for Fussy Days and Sleepless Nights

Caring for Your Baby and Young Child: Birth to Age 5

Heading Home with Your Newborn: From Birth to Reality

High Five Discipline: Positive Parenting for Happy, Healthy, Well-Behaved Kids

Lighthouse Parenting: Raising Your Child With Loving Guidance for a Lifelong Bond

The New Baby Blueprint: Caring for You and Your Little One

My Child Is Sick! Expert Advice for Managing Common Illnesses and Injuries

New Mother's Guide to Breastfeeding

Raising an Organized Child: 5 Steps to Boost Independence, Ease Frustration, and Promote Confidence

Raising Twins: Parenting Multiples from Pregnancy Through the School Years

Retro Baby: Timeless Activities to Boost Development—Without All the Gear!

Retro Toddler: More Than 100 Old-School Activities to Boost Development

Return to You: A Postpartum Plan for New Moms

Understanding the NICU: What Parents of Preemies and Other Hospitalized Newborns Need to Know

To find additional AAP books for parents, visit aap.org/shopaap-for-parents, amazon.com/americanacademyofpediatrics, or your favorite bookseller or library.

healthychildren.org

Powered by pediatricians. Trusted by parents.

from the American Academy of Pediatrics

REVIEWERS AND CONTRIBUTORS

Editor in Chief
Tanya Altmann, MD, FAAP

Associate Medical Editor
David L. Hill, MD, FAAP

Founding Editor Emeritus
Steven P. Shelov, MD, MS, FAAP

Associate Medical Editor Emeritus
Robert E. Hannemann, MD, FAAP

AAP Board of Directors Reviewer
Martha C. Middlemist, MD, FAAP

American Academy of Pediatrics
CEO/Executive Vice President
Mark Del Monte, JD

Vice President, Publishing
Mark T. Grimes

Senior Editor, Consumer Publishing
Kathryn Sparks

Editor, Consumer Publishing
Holly Kaminski

Editorial Assistant, Publishing
Grace Klooster

American Academy of Pediatrics Reviewers and Contributors

Committee on Drugs

Committee on Fetus and Newborn

Committee on Infectious Diseases

Committee on Nutrition

Committee on Pediatric AIDS

Committee on Pediatric Emergency Medicine

Committee on Psychosocial Aspects of Child and Family Health

Committee on Substance Use and Prevention

Council on Child Abuse and Neglect

Council on Children and Disasters

Council on Children with Disabilities

Council on Communications and Media

Council on Community Pediatrics

Council on Early Childhood

Council on Environmental Health and Climate Change

Council on Foster Care, Adoption, and Kinship Care

Council on Genetics

Council on Injury, Violence, and Poison Prevention

Family Partnerships Network

Section on Administration and Practice Management

Section on Allergy and Immunology

Section on Breastfeeding

Section on Cardiology and Cardiac Surgery

Section on Child Death Review and Prevention

Section on Clinical Pharmacology and Therapeutics

Section on Critical Care

Section on Dermatology

Section on Developmental and Behavioral Pediatrics

Section on Emergency Medicine

Section on Endocrinology

Section on Epidemiology, Public Health, and Evidence

Section on Gastroenterology, Hepatology, and Nutrition

Section on Hematology/Oncology

Section on Home Care

Section on Hospital Medicine

Section on Infectious Diseases

Section on Lesbian, Gay, Bisexual, and Transgender Health and Wellness

Section on Nephrology

Section on Neurological Surgery

Section on Neurology

Section on Obesity

Section on Ophthalmology

Section on Oral Health

Section on Orthopedics

Section on Otolaryngology—Head and Neck Surgery

Section on Pediatric Pulmonology and Sleep Medicine

Section on Plastic Surgery

Section on Rheumatology

Section on Surgery

Section on Uniformed Services

Section on Urology

Subcommittee on Bronchiolitis

Subcommittee on Children and Adolescents with Attention Deficit Hyperactivity Disorder

Subcommittee on Febrile Infants

Subcommittee on Hyperbilirubinemia

Subcommittee on the Management of Infantile Hemangioma

Subcommittee on Screening and Management of High Blood Pressure in Children

Subcommittee on Type 2 Diabetes

Subcommittee on Urinary Tract Infection

Task Force on SIDS

ACKNOWLEDGMENTS

We thank Founding Editor Emeritus Steven P. Shelov, MD, MS, FAAP; Associate Medical Editor Emeritus Robert E. Hannemann, MD, FAAP; and the countless contributors and reviewers for their work on the first seven editions of *Caring for Your Baby and Young Child*. Special thanks to Marc Weissbluth, MD, FAAP, for his review and consultation on the chapter "Your Child's Sleep."

Illustrators:

Wendy Wray/Morgan Gaynin, Inc.
Alex Grey
Anthony Alex Letourneau

PLEASE NOTE

The information contained in this book is intended to complement, not substitute for, the advice of your child's pediatrician. Before starting any medical treatment or medical program, you should consult with your child's pediatrician, who can discuss your child's individual needs and counsel you about symptoms and treatment. If you have questions regarding how the information in this book applies to your child, speak to your child's pediatrician.

Products mentioned in this book are for informational purposes only. Inclusion in this publication does not constitute or imply a guarantee or an endorsement by the American Academy of Pediatrics.

The information and advice in this book applies to all sexes and genders; however, for easier reading, pronouns such as "they" are used in this publication. Best efforts were made to use people-first language, and as such, certain phrasing may not read as familiar. For example, "an overweight child" now reads as "a child with overweight" or "a child has overweight."

• • •

The American Academy of Pediatrics constantly monitors new scientific evidence and makes appropriate adjustments in its recommendations. For example, future research and the development of new childhood vaccines may alter the regimen for the administration of existing vaccines. Therefore, the schedule for immunizations outlined in this book is subject to change. These and other potential situations serve to emphasize the importance of always checking with your child's pediatrician for the latest information concerning the health of your child. For additional information on caring for your child and their health and well-being, visit HealthyChildren.org.

DIVERSITY, EQUITY, AND INCLUSION STATEMENT

The AAP is committed to principles of diversity, equity, and inclusion in its publishing program. Editorial boards, author selections, and author transitions (publication succession plans) should be designed to include diverse voices that reflect society as a whole. Editor and author teams are encouraged to actively seek out diverse authors and reviewers at all stages of the editorial process. Publishing staff are committed to promoting diversity, equity, and inclusion in all aspects of publication writing, review, and production.

This book is dedicated to all the people who recognize that children are our greatest inspiration in the present and our greatest hope for the future.

CONTENTS

INTRODUCTION xxi

PART 1

1. **Delivery and the First Moments** 3
   - Routine Vaginal Delivery 3
   - Birth by Cesarean Section 6
   - Delivery Room Procedures Following a Normal Vaginal Birth 8
   - Leaving the Delivery Area 10
2. **Your Newborn's First Days** 13
   - In the First Days 14
   - If Your Baby Is Premature 21
   - How Your Newborn Behaves 29
   - Going Home 31
   - Parenting 33
   - Health Watch 40
3. **Feeding Your Baby** 46
   - Breastfeeding 49
   - Bottle-Feeding 80
   - Supplementation for Breastfed and Bottle-Fed Infants 94
   - Burping, Hiccups, and Spitting Up 95
4. **Basic Infant Care** 101
   - Day to Day 102
   - Your Baby's Basic Healthcare 127
5. **Your Baby's First Month** 131
   - Growth and Development 131
   - Basic Care 150
   - Health Watch 158
   - Safety Check 163
6. **Your Baby at 2 Months** 167
   - Growth and Development 168
   - Basic Care 179
   - Health Watch 185
   - Immunization Update 186
   - Safety Check 186
7. **Your Baby at 4 Months** 188
   - Growth and Development 189
   - Basic Care 199
   - Health Watch 202
   - Immunization Update 204
   - Safety Check 204
8. **Your Baby at 6 Months** 206
   - Growth and Development 207
   - Basic Care 213
   - Health Watch 222
   - Immunization Update 225
   - Safety Check 225
9. **Your Baby at 9 Months** 226
   - Growth and Development 227

Basic Care 248
Behavior 255
Immunization Update 259
Safety Check 260

10. **Childcare** 263
What to Look for in a Care Provider 263
Choices in Care 265
Building a Relationship with Your Child's Care Providers 279
Resolving Conflicts 281
What to Do When Your Child Is Sick 282
Controlling Infectious Diseases 284
Preventing Injuries and Promoting Car Safety 289
Caring for Babies with Special Healthcare Needs 291

11. **Keeping Your Child Safe** 297
Why Children Get Injured 297
Safety Inside Your Home 300
Baby Equipment 313
Safety Outside the Home 321
In the Community and Neighborhood 342

PART 2

12. **Abdominal/Gastrointestinal Tract** 347
Abdominal Pain 348
Celiac Disease 350
Constipation 352
Diarrhea 354
Food Poisoning and Food Contamination 361
Hepatitis 368
Inguinal Hernia 372
Umbilical Hernia 373
Communicating Hydrocele 374
Malabsorption 375
Vomiting 377

13. **Asthma and Allergies** 382
Asthma 382
Eczema 392
Food Allergy 395
Nasal Allergy/Allergic Rhinitis 399
Hives/Urticaria 402
Insect Bites and Stings 404

14. **Chest and Lungs** 408
Bronchiolitis 408
Cystic Fibrosis 411
Cough 413
Croup 416
Influenza (Flu) 418
Pneumonia 421
Tuberculosis 424
Whooping Cough (Pertussis) 427

15. **Chronic Health Conditions** 430
Coping with Chronic (Long-Term) Health Problems 430
Receiving the Diagnosis of a Chronic Condition in Your Child 431
Navigating the Healthcare System 433
Getting Help for Your Child 435

16. **Developmental Disabilities** 438
Autism Spectrum Disorder 440

Cerebral Palsy 443
Congenital Abnormalities 449
Hearing Loss (Hearing Impairment) 458
Intellectual Development Disorder 464

17. Ears, Nose, and Throat 468
Colds/Upper Respiratory Infections 468
Middle Ear Infections 471
Herpes Simplex 478
Sore Throat (Strep Throat, Tonsillitis) 480

18. Emergencies 484
Bites 487
Burns 490
Cardiopulmonary Resuscitation (CPR) and Mouth-to-Mouth Resuscitation 493
Choking 494
Cuts and Scrapes 497
Dental Trauma 501
Drowning 501
Electric Shock 503
Fingertip Injuries 505
Firearms 506
Fractures/Broken Bones 508
Head Injury/Concussion 511
Poisoning 513

19. Environmental Health 520
Air Pollution 520
Asbestos 521
Carbon Monoxide 522
Drinking Water 524
Fish 529
Lead Poisoning 530
Pesticides/Herbicides 536
Radon 537
Smoke Exposure 537

20. Eyes 541
Vision Screening Recommendations 542
Amblyopia 544
Cataracts 544
Eye Infections 545
Eye Injuries 546
Eyelid Problems 549
Strabismus 550
Tear (or Lacrimal) Production Problems 552
Vision Difficulties Requiring Corrective Lenses 553

21. Family Issues 555
Adoption 555
Child Abuse and Neglect 556
Separation and Divorce 560
Sibling Rivalry 561
Single-Parent Families 564
Stepfamilies 567
Twins and Other Multiples 567

22. Fever 572
Treating a Febrile Seizure (Convulsion) 573
What Type of Thermometer Is Best? 574
When to Call the Pediatrician 575
Home Treatment 577

23. Genital and Urinary Systems 581
Blood in the Urine (Hematuria) 581
Circumcision 583
Hydronephrosis 583
Hypospadias and Chordee 584
Labial Adhesions 585
Meatal Stenosis 587
Posterior Urethral Valve 587

Testicular Torsion 589
Undescended Testicles (Cryptorchidism) 590
Urinary Tract Infections 591

24. Head, Neck, and Nervous System 595
Head Tilt (Torticollis) 595
Meningitis 597
Mumps 600
Seizures, Convulsions, and Epilepsy 602

25. Heart and Blood 605
Anemia 605
Arrhythmias 608
Heart Murmur 611
Kawasaki Disease 613
Sickle Cell Disease 616

26. Immunizations 620
Important and Safe 620
What Shots Does Your Child Need? 623

27. Media 631
Development and Learning 631
Sleep 633

28. Musculoskeletal Problems 635
Arthritis 635
Bowlegs and Knock-Knees 638
Elbow Injuries 638
Flat Feet/Fallen Arches 640
Limp 641
Pigeon Toes (Intoeing) 643

29. Skin 647
Birthmarks and Hemangiomas 647
Chickenpox (Varicella) 650
Cradle Cap and Seborrheic Dermatitis 653
Fifth Disease (Erythema Infectiosum) 654
Hair Loss (Alopecia) 655
Impetigo 656
Measles 657
Molluscum Contagiosum 660
Mosquito-Borne Illnesses (Zika and West Nile) 660
MRSA Infections 664
Ringworm (Tinea) 665
Roseola Infantum 666
Rubella (German Measles) 667
Scabies 669
Scarlet Fever 671
Sunburn 672

30. Your Child's Sleep 675
How Much Sleep Does My Child Need? 675
Sleep Routines and Dealing with Crying 678
Sharing the Bedtime Routine 680
Parent Sleep Deprivation 680
Implementing a Sleep Plan 680
Daytime Nap Evolution 684
Getting the Most Out of Sleep 685
Dealing with Other Sleep Concerns 688
Putting Sleep in Perspective 688

Appendix 691

Index 707

INTRODUCTION

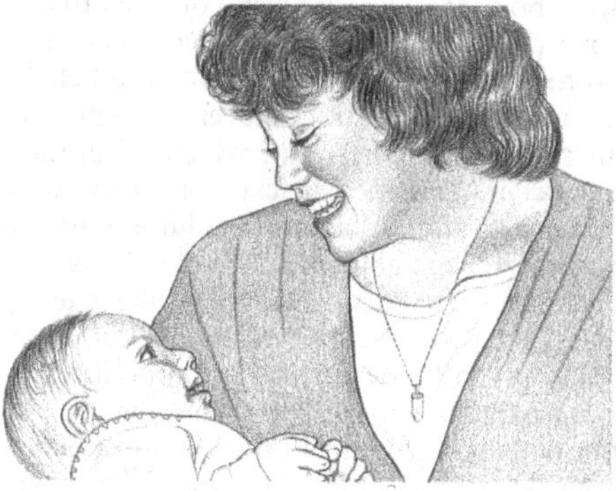

Congratulations! You are likely reading this book because you are pregnant, or have a newborn, or care for a child under the age of 1 year old. No matter what the reason, this book will provide you with everything you need to know to raise a healthy, happy, and resilient child. Whether you choose to read it from cover to cover, read the chapter for your baby's current age to discover what they will be doing next month, or just flip to the specific symptoms, illness, or issue that your baby has, you will find a wealth of information vetted by an organization comprised of more than 67,000 pediatricians. That's a lot of brainpower and advice!

Most of your newborn's needs are the same as generations ago, while others have changed due to modern-day busy lifestyles. Babies always need love, nutritious food, good health, secure surroundings, skills to build self-esteem and resilience, and plenty of one-on-one time together with you reading books and having fun. They don't need distractions or electronics.

For you, becoming a parent is one of the greatest gifts, and you will learn, grow, and smile every day in ways you didn't even know were possible. There will be good days and some not-so-good days, but that's normal life. Don't beat yourself up if the diaper doesn't get put on correctly or if you're late getting out the door with baby in tow. As long as everyone is safe and healthy, take each day in stride and enjoy every minute that you can.

It's also important to know when you need to ask for help. If you're overtired or overstressed, ask your partner, a relative, or a friend to lend a hand. Whether you need help breastfeeding or cooking, you can't do it all every day, and that's okay. Reach out to your support team, which should also include your pediatrician. Your pediatrician can help advise you on feeding, sleeping, and behavior in addition to seeing your child for complete well-child exams and sick visits.

The days and years pass quickly, so take a few photos or journal along the way, because before you know it your baby will be going off to kindergarten! In the following chapters, you will learn about caring for your newborn and young child, from helping with nutrition, sleep, and behavior to fevers, tummyaches, and other illness symptoms or concerns that come up along the way. Of course, if you have any questions about what you have read, have a specific concern, or are worried about anything, please contact your pediatrician. After all, that is what we are here for, even in the middle of the night!

PART 1

CHAPTER 1

DELIVERY AND THE FIRST MOMENTS

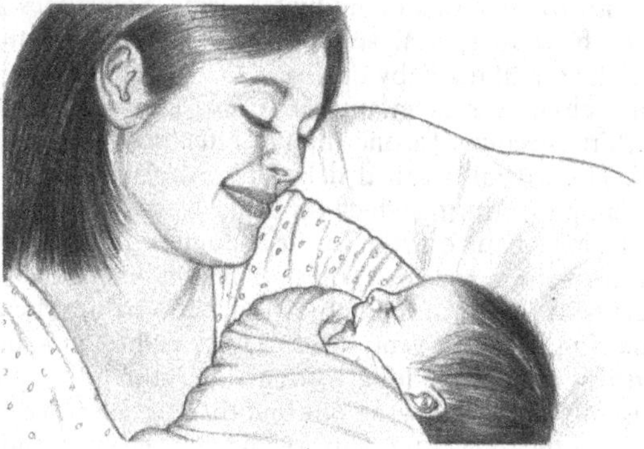

It's hard to imagine any life event that matches childbirth for the anticipation, excitement, and anxiety involved. It's inevitable that you will enter into this moment with expectations from stories, books, television, movies, and even your own prior experiences. It is also inevitable that each birth will be unique, and that no one can predict exactly what will happen.

Routine Vaginal Delivery

In the weeks leading up to the birth of your baby, you'll probably feel some apprehension along with your excitement. Then, usually between the thirty-seventh and forty-second week, you'll go into labor. Although no one knows for certain what triggers this process, shifts in hormone levels appear to play a role. Your amniotic sac may rupture on its own, or your doctor or midwife will do it (commonly referred to as "breaking your water") at some point before delivery. As you proceed through labor, your uterus will contract rhythmically, or squeeze, which moves your baby down the birth canal. At the same time, these contractions will completely efface, or thin, and then dilate, or open, your cervix to about 10 centimeters (4 in.).

In a routine vaginal delivery, your first view of your child may be the top, or crown, of their head, which may be seen in a mirror if you choose. After delivery of the head, there is usually one last pause before the push that sends your baby's body into the doctor's or midwife's arms. Sometimes a vacuum or forceps, special supplies used by obstetricians, are used to help pull the baby out.

For well-appearing infants, it is now common to wait at least thirty seconds to one minute after delivery to cut the umbilical cord (also called delayed cord clamping or timed cord clamping), during which time the obstetrician or midwife may place the baby on your lower abdomen. Once the pulsing in the cord stops, the cord will be clamped and cut (there are no nerves in the cord; the baby will feel no pain). The clamp remains in place for twenty-four to forty-eight hours, or until the cord is dry and no longer bleeds. The stump that remains will usually fall off between one and three weeks after birth.

Most of the time, after delivery and delayed cord clamping, your baby will be placed directly on your chest, belly down, for skin-to-skin care. Your provider will dry your baby, put a hat on your baby, and cover your baby with a warm blanket while your newborn settles on your chest. This first hour of skin-to-skin contact allows you and your baby to get to know each other and has other important health benefits. Sometimes babies need to be evaluated and brought to a warmer immediately after birth. If that happens, when your infant is stabilized they can be brought to you for skin-to-skin care.

Even if you've seen pictures of newborns, you're bound to be amazed by the first sight of your own. When your newborn's eyes open, they will meet yours with curiosity. All the activity of birth may make your baby alert and responsive to your touch, voice, and warmth. Take advantage of this attentiveness, which may last for a few hours. Watch how the baby moves toward your breast, seeking that first feeding. These moments are magical for you and your baby. They should be allowed to happen. Attendants should not wash you or the baby or otherwise interfere. The smell and feel of you at that moment will guide the newborn to their first feeding. As with many birth parents, you may find that putting your baby to your breast creates an intense emotional bond between you and your newborn.

Fresh from birth, your baby may be covered with a white cheesy substance called vernix. This protective coating is produced toward the end of pregnancy by the sebaceous (oil-producing) glands in your baby's skin. Your newborn may also be wet with amniotic fluid. If there was tearing of tissue in the vaginal area, you may see some blood on the baby's skin. Your newborn's skin, especially on the face, may be quite wrinkled from the wetness and pressure of birth.

NURSING AFTER DELIVERY

We recommend that you plan to breastfeed your baby. Today, most hospitals encourage breastfeeding within the first hour following routine delivery, while the baby is held skin-to-skin, unless the baby is having difficulty breathing or other medical problems, which may require monitoring. (See *pages 9–10* for detailed information on Apgar scoring.)

Breastfeeding right away benefits the mother by causing the uterus to contract, reducing the amount of uterine bleeding, and it benefits the newborn by giving protection against infections. (The same hormone that stimulates the milk ejection reflex, or let-down response, triggers uterine contractions.)

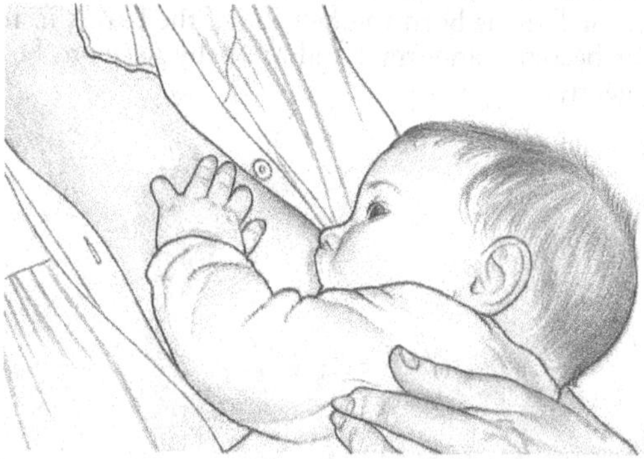

The first hour or so after birth is the ideal time to begin breastfeeding. Your baby is alert and eager. When put to the breast, your baby may first lick it. Then, with a little help, your newborn may latch on to the areola (not the nipple) and suck vigorously for several minutes. If you wait until later, your newborn may be sleepier and have more difficulty latching effectively.

For the first two to five days after delivery, your body produces colostrum, a thin, yellowish fluid that contains protein and antibodies that protect your baby from infection. Colostrum provides all the nutrients and fluids your baby needs in those first few days after birth. (For a complete discussion of breastfeeding, see *Chapter 3*, Feeding Your Baby.) Many hospitals have lactation consultants (professional experts to help mothers with breastfeeding); ask for their help if you are having any difficulty in establishing successful breastfeeding, especially if this is your first baby.

Birth by Cesarean Section

There are many reasons why your baby may need to be delivered by Cesarean section (C-section), a surgery where an incision is made in the abdomen and uterus to birth the baby. Delivery by Cesarean section is more common if the birth mother had a previous C-section, if the baby is in a breech (head-up) position, if the cervix does not adequately dilate, if the obstetrician feels that the mother's or baby's health might suffer if the baby is born vaginally, or if the baby's heart rate slows or becomes abnormal and the baby needs to be delivered urgently.

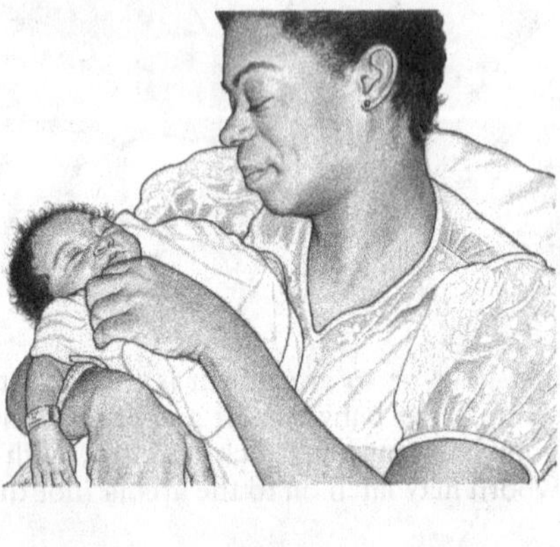

The birth experience with a C-section is different from that of a vaginal delivery. Typically, the entire operation takes no more than an hour, and depending on the circumstances, labor may not be experienced. Another important difference is that medication may be needed to numb the spinal nerves of the mother from the waist down prior to surgery. Rarely, general anesthesia may need to be used. In some cases, these medications may slightly affect mom and baby, but your obstetrician and anesthesiologist can discuss all this with you.

Even with a C-section delivery, as long as the baby is healthy and stable, immediate skin-to-skin care is still encouraged for bonding and breastfeeding if desired.

BONDING

If you deliver without complications, you'll be able to spend the first hour or so with your newborn. Because babies are usually alert and very responsive during this time, researchers have labeled this the sensitive period.

The first exchanges of eye contact, sounds, and touches between the two of you are all part of a bonding process, which helps lay the foundation for your relationship as parent and child. Although it will take months to learn your child's temperament and personality, many of the core emotions you feel may begin to develop immediately after birth.

It's also quite normal if you do not immediately have tremendously warm feelings for your baby. Labor is a demanding experience, and your first reaction may well be a sense of relief that it's over. If you're exhausted and emotionally drained, you may simply want to rest. Give yourself some time, until the strain of labor fades, and then request your baby. Bonding has no time limit.

Also, if your baby is taken immediately to the nursery for medical attention, or if you were sedated during delivery, or if you didn't give birth to your child, don't despair. You needn't worry your relationship might be harmed because bonding didn't occur in this first hour. You can love your baby just as much, even if you couldn't watch their birth or hold them immediately afterward. Your baby will also be just as loving and connected to you.

Delivery Room Procedures Following a Normal Vaginal Birth

Your baby should be placed skin-to-skin after birth if possible, and Apgar scores can be assigned while you hold your baby. It is important when parent and baby are healthy and stable to maximize skin-to-skin procedures as much as possible during the first hours after delivery. Skin-to-skin contact can help stabilize a newborn's blood sugar concentrations and body temperature. It can also help prevent hypothermia (decreased body temperature), decrease crying, and provide stable blood flow and breathing, especially for late preterm newborns. For the mother, skin-to-skin contact decreases maternal stress and may help reduce postpartum hemorrhage.

After about an hour, your baby will be weighed, measured, and examined. Your newborn will be given a dose of vitamin K to help with normal blood clotting. Because during the birthing process bacteria can infect a baby's eyes, your baby will be given an antibiotic eye ointment (erythromycin eye ointment is commonly used) to prevent a potentially serious eye infection from occurring.

You and your baby will receive matching bracelet or anklet labels to identify that this is your newborn, and they will be checked frequently during your hospital stay.

Depending on the hospital routine, the umbilical cord stump may be dried and cleaned and your baby may be given their first bath. All medically stable newborns weighing at least 4 pounds 6½ ounces (2 kg) should receive their first dose of hepatitis B vaccine within twenty-four hours after birth. You will need to sign a consent form for the vaccine to be given.

VITAMIN K

Vitamin K plays a critical role in preventing serious, life-threatening bleeding in your newborn. Newborns often do not have enough vitamin K in their bodies because they lack the bacteria that help make this nutrient. All newborns should receive an injection of 0.5 to 1 mg of vitamin K shortly after birth. Those who don't receive this injection are at greater risk of bleeding in various parts of the body and brain. Rarely, such bleeding can result in brain damage or death and can occur as late as two to six months after delivery. Vitamin K has been used for a long time and is proven to be safe and effective.

APGAR SCORES

As soon as your baby is born, a member of the birth team will set a timer for one minute and another for five minutes to give your baby's first tests, called Apgars.

The Apgar scoring helps the physician to estimate your baby's general condition at birth. It measures your baby's heart rate, breathing, muscle tone, reflex response, and color at one minute after birth and at five-minute intervals if the scores are low. It cannot predict how your baby will develop, nor does it indicate intelligence or personality. However, it alerts your baby's care providers to evaluate the need for assistance as your baby adapts to the new environment.

Each characteristic is scored, 2 points for each category if all is completely well. For example, if your newborn has a heart rate of more than 100 beats per minute, cries lustily, moves actively, and grimaces or otherwise responds to rubbing and stimulation by the hospital providers, but is blue, their one-minute Apgar score would be 8 (with 2 points off because they are blue and not pink). Most newborn infants have Apgar scores greater than 7. Because hands and feet remain blue until babies are quite warm, few score a perfect 10.

If your baby is having difficulty breathing, moving, or crying at birth, hospital providers specially trained in evaluation and resuscitation of newborns will evaluate and treat the baby accordingly. This may include drying the baby vigorously and/or using a special mask over the nose and mouth attached to a bag to give breaths of air or oxygen, called positive pressure ventilation. This intervention usually leads to improvements in breathing, movement, and color. If these strategies do not help, a tube can be placed into their airway (the windpipe, or trachea, which goes into their lungs) to help breathing by pushing air and oxygen directly into the lungs. Also, fluids and medications may have to be administered through the umbilical cord vein to strengthen their heartbeat if needed. Your baby may be taken to the special-care nursery or neonatal intensive care unit (NICU) for observation or more intensive medical attention.

APGAR SCORING SYSTEM			
Score	**0**	**1**	**2**
Heart rate	Absent	Less than 100 beats per minute	More than 100 beats per minute
Respiration	Absent	Slow, irregular; weak cry	Good; strong cry
Muscle tone	Limp	Some flexing of arms and legs	Active motion
Reflex*	Absent	Grimace	Grimace and cough or sneeze
Color	Blue or pale	Pink body; blue hands and feet	Completely pink

* Reflex is assessed by gently placing a catheter or bulb syringe in the infant's nose and watching their response of sneezing or crying.

Lastly and importantly, both you and a support person of your choosing will receive matching labels bearing the newborn's name. After you verify the accuracy, these labels will be attached to your wrist, the wrist of your partner or other person of your choosing, and your baby's wrist (and often the baby's ankle as well). Each time the baby is taken from or returned to you while in the hospital, the nurse will check these bracelets. Many hospitals also footprint newborns as an added precaution and attach a small security device to the baby's ankle.

Leaving the Delivery Area

If you delivered in a birthing room or alternative birth center, you probably won't be moved right away. But if you delivered in a conventional delivery room, you'll be taken to a recovery area, where you can be watched for any issues such as excessive bleeding. Unless your infant requires urgent medical attention, ask to not be separated from your infant. Your infant should receive their first medical examination by your side. This exam will measure the baby's vital signs: temperature, respiration, and pulse rate. The examiner will check your baby from head to toe, paying specific attention to their color, activity level, and breathing pattern. If vitamin K and antibiotic eye ointment were not given earlier, they will be administered now. The first bath should be delayed twelve to twenty-four hours to help with breastfeeding and bonding. Depending on your baby's gestational age, the season, and whether you received immunization for respiratory syncytial virus (RSV) during pregnancy, your baby may receive an immunization before leaving the hospital or at your pediatrician's office. This shot will help prevent RSV, a serious respiratory virus that can lead to hospitalization and life-threatening illness in infants who contract it.

NEWBORN SCREENING TESTS

Shortly after birth, and before being discharged, your baby will be given a number of screening tests to detect a variety of birth defects (e.g., blood spot test for genetic disease or low thyroid hormone, pulse oximetry screening test to detect selected heart diseases, and newborn hearing screen). These tests are designed for early detection of rare diseases to enable their prompt treatment, prevent disabilities, and sometimes save lives. While laws mandate some tests, tests performed may differ from state to state (and change periodically). Before your baby is born, talk to your pediatrician about which screening tests your baby will undergo, including benefits and risks, and whether consent is necessary. Ask when test results will be available and what the results mean, especially if they are out of the normal range; this may not necessarily indicate a congenital condition (birth defect) or genetic disease, so inquire if retesting will be done.

Should I Store My Newborn's Cord Blood?

Umbilical cord blood has been used successfully to treat a number of genetic, blood, and cancer conditions in children, such as leukemia and immune disorders. Some parents choose to store their baby's cord blood for possible future use. However, there are no accurate statistics on the likelihood of children someday needing their own stored cells. The American Academy of Pediatrics discourages storing cord blood at private banks for later personal or family use as a general "insurance policy." Rather, they encourage families to donate their newborn's cord blood, which is normally discarded at birth, to cord blood banks (if accessible in their area) for other individuals in need. (You should be aware, though, that your baby's donated cord blood would not be available as a personal stem cell source if your baby needs it later in life.)

Before your baby is born, you and your partner should discuss with your obstetrician and/or pediatrician the pros and cons of storing your child's cord blood. You may need to register for cord blood collection, pay, order the storage kit, and sign a consent form prior to the onset of labor. Some states now mandate that obstetricians and pediatricians discuss cord blood collection with their patients.

Keep in mind that because cord blood is collected from the cut umbilical cord after the baby is born and the umbilical cord is clamped and cut, it does not affect the baby or the birth experience. The cord blood stem cell collection process should not alter the routine practice for the timing of umbilical cord clamping.

Once the cord blood is collected, it is typed and screened for infectious diseases and hereditary hematologic diseases. If the donation meets all the required standards, it will be cryogenically stored for potential transplantation if a match is found, or it might be used for quality improvement and research.

CHAPTER 2

YOUR NEWBORN'S FIRST DAYS

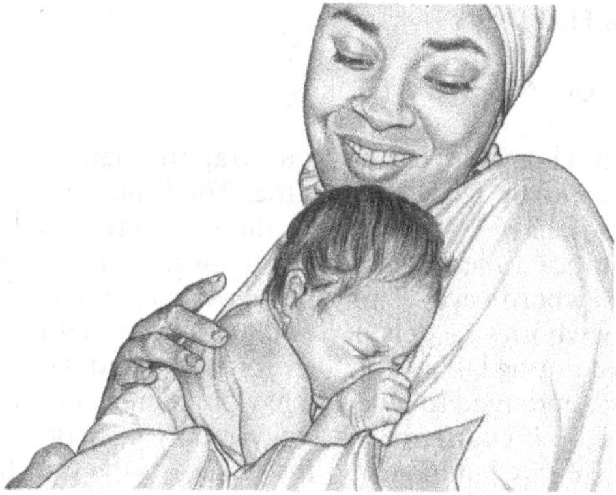

Whether you are having your own or you are adopting, fostering, or providing kinship care for a newborn, you've spent months waiting and preparing to welcome this new little human. Your baby is uniquely special—unlike anyone else. You'll see a unique personality emerging from the very start. If you are parenting a baby born to someone else, you'll marvel at this unique personality just like every other new parent.

Some babies waste no time protesting wet diapers from day one and complain loudly until they are changed, fed, and rocked back to sleep. Infants who behave like this not only tend to spend more time awake than other babies, but also may cry and eat more. Other newborns won't seem to notice when their diapers are dirty and may be more likely to object to an exposed bottom during changes. These babies tend to sleep more and eat less frequently than their more sensitive counterparts. These kinds of differences are normal and can serve as hints of your child's personality.

Some parents say that after their baby's spending so many months in the womb, it is difficult to view them as a separate human being, with thoughts, emotions, and desires of their own. Making this adjustment and respecting their baby's individuality, however, are important parts of being a parent. If parents identify their baby's uniqueness, they'll have a much easier time accepting the person their baby will become in the years ahead.

In the First Days

How Your Newborn Looks

As you relax with your baby, unwrap the blankets and examine your baby from head to toe. You'll notice many details that may have escaped you in the moments after birth. You may notice a blood-red spot in the whites of one or both of your newborn's eyes. This spot, as well as the general puffiness of a newborn's face, is most commonly caused by pressures exerted during labor. Although you might find them a bit worrisome, both tend to fade in a few days, much like a bruise on your skin. If your baby was delivered by C-section, they may not have this puffiness and the whites of the eyes likely will not have any red spots.

At birth your baby's skin will seem very delicate. Whether your baby is born early, late, or on time, peeling skin is normal and usually requires no treatment. All babies, including those with a dark-skinned heritage, have lighter-appearing skin at birth. This gradually darkens as they become older.

As you examine your baby's shoulders and back, you may notice fine hair, called lanugo. This hair is produced toward the end of pregnancy; however, it's usually shed before birth or soon thereafter. If your baby was born before their due date, they are more likely to still have this hair, and it may take a couple of weeks to disappear.

You also may notice various spots and marks on your baby's skin. Some, like those appearing around the diaper edges, may be due to pressure. Mottled or blotchy-looking patches are commonly caused by exposure to cool air and will disappear quickly with warming up. If you find scratches, particularly on your baby's face, it's a good reminder it's time to trim your baby's fingernails. For some new parents this can be a nerve-racking task, but using a nail file can be less stressful than traditional clippers.

The following are the most common skin markings in newborns.

Salmon-Colored Patches, or "Stork Bites." Distributed over areas where a stork supposedly would carry a baby in its beak, "stork bites" are patches, light to deep pink in color, most commonly located on the bridge of the nose, lower forehead, upper eyelids, back of the head, and/or the neck. They are the most common birthmark, especially in light-skinned babies. Also called angel kisses, they typically fade over the first few months to years but may become apparent later in life with flushing.

Dermal Melanocytosis Spots. These birthmarks vary considerably in size, but all are flat areas of skin containing extra pigment, causing a brown, gray, or even blue (like a bruise) appearance. Most often located on the back or buttocks, these spots are very common, especially in dark-skinned babies. They usually disappear before school age and are of no medical significance.

Pustular Melanosis. These are small blisters that typically appear at birth, then peel and dry up within a couple of days, leaving dark spots like freckles that usually disappear over several weeks. Some newborns may have only the spots, indicating they had the rash before birth. While pustular melanosis is common (particularly in babies with darker skin) and is a harmless newborn rash, it is always important to have all blister-like rashes evaluated by your baby's doctor to rule out infection.

Milia. These tiny white bumps or yellow spots are found on the cheeks, on the chin, or across the tip of the nose, and are caused by skin gland secretion. This common newborn rash generally disappears on its own within the first two to three weeks after birth.

Miliaria. Often referred to as heat rash or prickly heat, miliaria most often occurs in hot, humid climates or when babies are too bundled up. The rash can contain tiny sweat blisters and/or small red bumps. It shows up most often in skin folds and covered areas, and usually goes away within a few days.

Erythema Toxicum. This rash can look concerning but is common and usually appears within the first few days after birth.

It consists of multiple red splotches with yellowish white bumps in the center, which come and go days after birth and completely resolve in a week or so.

Capillary Hemangiomas. These raised red spots are caused by a strawberry-like collection of blood vessels in the skin. For the first week or so, they may appear white or pale, then turn red and raised later. While they often enlarge during the first year, most shrink and many disappear by school age. Depending on the spots' location and size, your baby's doctor or a dermatologist may want to treat them.

Port-Wine Stains. These large, flat, and irregularly shaped dark red or purple areas are caused by extra blood vessels under the skin. Port-wine stains are usually located on the face or neck but, unlike hemangiomas, don't disappear without treatment. These birthmarks can be treated, sometimes with laser surgery, by either a plastic surgeon or a pediatric dermatologist. (See also Birthmarks and Hemangiomas, *page 647*.)

When born, babies may have an elongated shape to their head, and may also have scalp swelling in the area pushed out first during birth. If you press gently on this area, your finger may even leave a small indentation. This swelling (called caput) is not serious and should disappear in a few days.

Sometimes there may be swelling under a newborn's scalp, present on one or both sides, which is firm or springs right back after it is gently pressed. This type of swelling is likely a cephalohematoma and is caused by pressure on the head when compressed against the maternal pelvis during labor or pressure from forceps or a vacuum extractor used to assist birth. While not serious, it represents some bleeding along the outer side of the skull bones (not inside the brain) and usually takes six to ten weeks to disappear. As the blood gets reabsorbed, the area may occasionally get hard and calcified and the swelling may take longer to go away.

All babies have two soft spots, or fontanelles, on the head. These are the areas where the immature bones of the skull that are similar to pieces of a puzzle are still growing together. The larger opening is toward the front; a smaller one is at the back. Parents needn't be afraid to touch these areas gently, as there is a thick, durable membrane that protects the brain.

Babies are born with hair, but the amount, texture, and

color vary from one newborn to another. Most, if not all, "baby hair" falls out during the first six months and is replaced by mature hair. The color and texture of the mature hair may be different from the hair the baby was born with.

In the first few weeks following birth, babies can be affected by the hormones they were exposed to during pregnancy. As a result, babies' breasts may be enlarged temporarily and might even secrete a few drops of milk. This is normal. It may occur in all babies, regardless of their sex, and normally lasts less than a week, although it can last longer. It is best not to press or squeeze a baby's breast, since this won't reduce swelling and could cause irritation and infection (mastitis). In infant girls, there could be a discharge from the vagina, often white mucus, though sometimes it may be bloody. Although disconcerting to new parents, this so-called pseudo-menses is harmless.

Your baby's abdomen may seem prominent, and you may even notice a small area that seems to bulge during crying spells. This bulge is called a hernia. Small hernias are most commonly seen around the umbilical cord (belly button) but may also appear in a line down the center of the abdomen. (For more information, see Umbilical Hernia, *page 373*.)

The genitals of newborn babies can be reddish and seem large for bodies so small. The scrotum of a baby may be small and smooth, or it might be large and wrinkled. The testicles can appear to move in and out of the scrotum, and sometimes will move as far up as the base of the penis or even to the crease between the thigh and belly. As long as the testicles are located in the scrotum most of the time, the fact that they move around is normal.

Sometimes you'll notice a buildup of fluid in a sac called a hydrocele (see *page 374*) inside the scrotum. This buildup will shrink gradually without treatment over several months as the fluid is reabsorbed by the body. A bulge in the groin or scrotal sac in boys is often due to an inguinal hernia (see *page 372*) and is frequently seen in premature infants. It usually appears a few weeks after birth and may get bigger with crying or straining. If it cannot be pushed all the way back in, contact your baby's pediatrician or take your baby to the emergency department because the hernia can be "strangulated" (twisted around the blood vessel), requiring surgery. On rare occasions, in a boy the testicular area becomes red and swollen and the infant appears to be in pain (crying incessantly) due to a condition called testicular torsion (see *page 589*). This is an emergency and requires immediate surgery, and the baby should be taken to the emergency room.

In boys, at birth the foreskin is attached to the head, or glans, of the penis, and cannot be pushed back as it can in older children and adults. There is a small opening at the tip through which urine flows. If the baby is circumcised, the connections between the foreskin and the glans are separated and the foreskin is removed, leaving the head of the penis visible. Without a circumcision, the foreskin will separate from the glans naturally during the first few years. (For a detailed description, see Circumcision, *page 583*.)

CARE OF THE PENIS

Circumcised Penis. The circumcision procedure usually will be performed in the hospital prior to discharge, but it may be done after discharge during the first weeks at the discretion of your pediatrician (see Circumcision, *page 583*). Ritual circumcisions for religious reasons are usually performed in the second week. After the procedure, a light dressing with petroleum jelly may be placed over the head of the penis. Some pediatricians recommend keeping a clean dressing over the area until the penis is fully healed, while others advise leaving it off. The important thing is to keep the area clean. If stool gets on the penis, wipe it gently with soap and water.

The tip of the penis may look red for the first few days, and you may notice a yellow secretion. Both indicate that the area is healing normally. The redness and secretion disappear gradually within a week. If the redness persists or there is swelling or crusted yellow sores, there may be an infection. This does not happen often, but if you suspect an infection, consult your pediatrician.

After the circumcision has healed, usually the penis requires no additional care. Occasionally a small piece of foreskin remains. You may pull back this skin gently each time the baby is bathed so long as it retracts easily. Examine the groove around the head of the penis and make sure it's clean.

If circumcision is desired but is not performed within the baby's first two weeks (perhaps for medical reasons), it is usually put off for several weeks or months. The follow-up care is the same whenever it is done. Should circumcision become necessary after the newborn period, general anesthesia is often used, and it is a more formal surgical procedure with control of bleeding and suturing of skin edges.

Uncircumcised Penis. In the first few months, you should simply clean and bathe your baby's uncircumcised penis with soap and water, like the rest of the diaper area. Initially, the foreskin is connected by tissue to the glans, or head, of the penis, so you shouldn't try to retract it. No cleansing with cotton swabs or antiseptics is necessary.

The doctor will tell you when the foreskin has separated and can be retracted safely. This will not be for several months or years and should never be forced; if you force the foreskin to retract before it is ready, you could cause painful bleeding and tears in the skin. After natural separation occurs, retract the foreskin regularly to gently cleanse the end of the penis.

As your baby gets older, you'll need to teach them what they must do in order to urinate and wash the penis. Teach your child to clean the foreskin by:

- Gently pulling it back away from the head of the penis
- Rinsing the head of the penis and inside fold of the foreskin with soap and warm water
- Pulling the foreskin back over the head of the penis

Your Baby's Birth Weight and Measurements

What makes a baby big or small? The following are some of the most common causes.

Large Babies. A baby may be born large for a number of reasons, including:

- Being born to large biological parents
- Excessive weight gain in the mother during pregnancy
- A pregnancy that lasts longer than forty-two weeks
- Overstimulation of the fetus's growth in the uterus
- Fetal chromosomal abnormalities
- Diabetes in the mother before or during pregnancy
- The mother having birthed other children (often each baby weighs more than the one before)

Large babies may have metabolic abnormalities (such as low blood sugar and calcium), traumatic birth injuries, higher hemoglobin levels, jaundice, or various birth defects. Almost one-third of large babies initially have feeding difficulties. Your pediatrician will keep a close watch on these issues.

Small Babies. A baby may be born small for a number of reasons, including:

- Being born early (preterm)
- Being born to small biological parents
- Fetal chromosomal abnormalities
- Inadequate weight gain by the mother in pregnancy
- The mother's chronic diseases, such as high blood pressure, heart disease, or kidney disease
- Placental issues
- The mother's substance use (including alcohol and tobacco) during pregnancy

A small baby may need to have temperature, blood glucose, and red cell count (hemoglobin level) closely monitored. After birth, the pediatrician will thoroughly evaluate a small infant and decide when they are ready to go home.

To compare your baby's measurements with those of other babies born after the same length of pregnancy, your pediatrician will use growth charts (see the Appendix, *pages 699–702*.)

As illustrated in the first two growth charts, 80 out of 100 babies born at forty weeks of pregnancy (full term) weigh between 5 pounds 11½ ounces (2.6 kg) and 8 pounds 5¾ ounces (3.8 kg). This is a healthy average. Those above the 90th percentile are considered large, those below the 10th percentile small. Keep in mind that these early weight designations (large or small) do not predict a child's size as an adult, but they do help determine whether your baby needs extra attention during the first few days after birth. Head circumference and length will also be measured and compared to growth charts.

At every physical exam, the pediatrician will measure the baby's length, weight, and head circumference and will plot them on growth charts similar to the ones in the Appendix, *pages 699–702*. In a healthy, well-nourished infant, these three measurements should increase at a predictable rate. Any interruption in this rate can help the doctor detect and address any feeding, developmental, or medical issues. It is important to note that early infant weight loss in the first forty-eight to seventy-two hours may be caused by the mother getting fluids during the birthing process and is common with prolonged labor or C-section births. The fluid shift that happens during this time may be misinterpreted as a feeding issue or inadequate milk supply.

If Your Baby Is Premature

Premature birth occurs in about 10 percent of pregnancies in the United States. Almost 60 percent of twins, triplets, and other multiple deliveries result in preterm births. A birth is considered preterm when a baby is born before completing thirty-seven weeks of pregnancy. Other categories of newborns include late preterm (thirty-four to thirty-six weeks), moderately preterm (thirty-two to thirty-six weeks), very preterm (less than thirty-two weeks), and extremely preterm (less than twenty-eight weeks).

If your baby is born prematurely, they may neither look nor behave like a full-term infant. While the average full-term newborn weighs about 7 pounds (3.17 kg), a premature newborn might weigh 5 pounds (2.26 kg) or even considerably less. Moderately to late preterm (those born before thirty-seven weeks' gestation) and very preterm infants (those born before thirty-two weeks) often require medical care in the neonatal intensive care unit or special-care nursery because they are not fully developed at birth. All extremely preterm infants (those born before twenty-eight weeks) require medical care in the neonatal intensive care unit or special-care nursery. The length of time they require care varies tremendously, but often they need to be hospitalized until their approximate due date or until they can maintain temperature, tolerate feedings, and gain weight. Preterm infants can have a variety of short- and long-term medical problems.

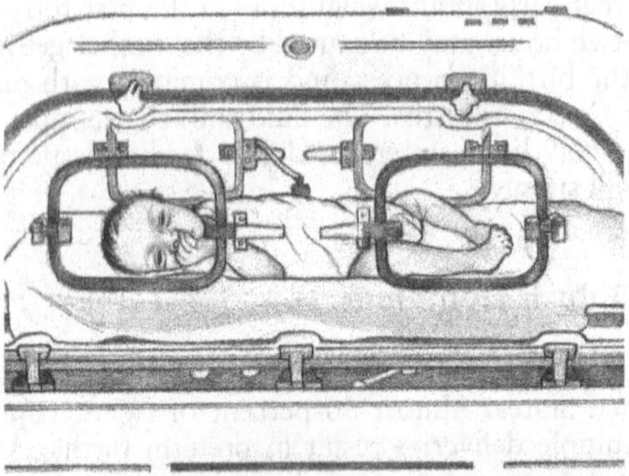

Your premature baby will be placed immediately after birth in an enclosed bed to keep them warm.

The earlier your baby arrives, the smaller they will be, the larger their head will seem in relation to their body, and the less fat they will have. With so little fat, their skin will seem thinner and more transparent, allowing the blood vessels beneath to show. They also may have fine hair, called lanugo, on their back and shoulders. Their features will appear sharper and less rounded than they would if born at term, and they may not have any of the white, cheesy vernix that would otherwise protect their skin at term birth.

Due to having less fat, your premature baby may get cold at the usual room temperatures, which can be prevented by skin-to-skin contact with you or your partner and may require blankets. Immediately after birth, your baby may be placed in an incubator (often called an Isolette) or under a special heating device called a radiant warmer. Here the temperature can be adjusted as needed. Your baby will be moved to a special-care nursery, often called a neonatal intensive care unit (NICU). Some hospitals may have a special room for you and the baby in the NICU where you or your partner can stay to facilitate skin-to-skin care and breastfeeding. In other NICUs, you will be able to join your baby there once you are medically stable. Special-care nurseries feature equipment and specially trained staff to assist in the care of preterm or ill newborns.

You may also notice that your premature baby will cry only softly, if at all, and may have trouble breathing because their respiratory system is still immature. If your baby comes more than two months early, breathing difficulties can cause serious health problems. Doctors will keep your baby under close observation, watching breathing and heart rate with a cardiorespiratory monitor. Babies who need help breathing may be assisted by a ventilator (breathing machine) or breathing assistance techniques like high-flow nasal cannula (HFNC) or continuous positive airway pressure (CPAP). As important as this care is for your baby's survival, the move to the special-care nursery may be stressful for you and your family. Although with all the health worries you may miss the experience of holding, breastfeeding, and bonding with your baby after delivery, your baby's nurse and physician will facilitate these activities as soon as the baby is stable.

Baby blues and postpartum depression occur more frequently when the baby must stay in the NICU. In the first few days, with the adjustment to your baby's stay in the hospital, you may experience temporary baby blues.

To help ease the transition, ask your nurse to let you see your baby as soon as possible after delivery, and become as active as you can in their care. Spend as much time in the special-care nursery as your condition—and your baby's condition—permits. Your special-care nursery will encourage you to do skin-to-skin as soon as your baby's medical needs allow. Also important in keeping postpartum depression at bay are eating healthy, sleeping (try to sleep between pumping sessions, even during the day), exercising when feeling well enough, and getting support from friends and family. If after a few weeks you still feel depressed, talk to the NICU social worker for a referral to a counselor or doctor.

You can also feed your baby as soon as your doctor says it's okay. The nurses will instruct you on either breastfeeding or bottle-feeding techniques and expressing your milk, whichever is appropriate for the baby's needs and your desires. Premature babies often require special feeding techniques or tube feeding. When your baby is taking feedings, breast milk offers the best nutrition and provides antibodies and other substances that enhance immune response and help resist infection. Breast milk holds special advantages for premature infants, one of which is preventing a complication called necrotizing enterocolitis (NEC; see *page 28*). If it's too difficult for your premature baby to nurse, you can pump breast milk for feeding through a feeding tube or bottle. Ask your nurse or lactation consultant for help in pumping your milk by hand and with a breast pump. It is important to initiate pumping as soon as possible after delivery and to continue pumping every two to three hours, or eight times per day, to keep up your milk supply. Your colostrum, the yellowish liquid that comes in at first, may not come in for a few days. Do not get discouraged. If you are able to breastfeed, it will come in. Once breastfeeding directly, your baby should nurse frequently to increase your milk supply. Even so, mothers of premature babies sometimes continue pumping in addition to frequent breastfeeding to maintain a good milk supply. If your own milk is not available, pasteurized donor breast milk is also available specifically for preterm infants depending on your hospital's policy. Donated breast milk does not provide the fullest protection against illnesses, since it must be heat-treated (pasteurized) to destroy any potentially dangerous bacteria, viruses, or other infectious particles, but it does still provide immune benefits and many other nutrients that are absent in formula feeds. Your physician and nutritionist may suggest fortifying the milk with additives to provide extra calories if your baby is not gaining weight adequately. For very or extremely premature infants, it is important to keep pumping and use donor breast milk only as a bridge until your breast milk comes in.

Using breast milk (also known as human milk) that has not been pasteurized or purchasing milk from an unknown source does pose potential risks of infection for the infant. In addition, the donor may not have pumped or stored the milk under the most hygienic conditions. Milk purchased over the internet has been shown to be contaminated with bacteria, altered with other milk or formula, or not kept frozen throughout the shipping process. This milk should not be fed to infants.

When a premature baby is in the NICU, kangaroo care is a way to bond with your baby. Both the mother of the premature baby and the mother's partner can put the naked (except for a diaper) baby skin-to-skin on their bare chest with a blanket to cover the baby. The baby will stay warm, and the parent and infant can bond. Kangaroo care has been determined to keep the baby's breathing and heart rate more regular, allow better sleep, keep the baby calmer (crying less), and improve weight gain for the baby. Kangarooing usually feels good for the parents and may increase production of breast milk for the mother.

HEALTH ISSUES OF PREMATURE BABIES

Because premature babies are born before they are physically ready to leave the womb, they often have health problems due to immature organs or the treatment necessary in the NICU for their survival. These newborns may have higher rates of disabilities (such as cerebral palsy, chronic lung disease, feeding difficulties, visual and hearing impairment, or intellectual disability) and even death.

Prior to discharge from the hospital or NICU, babies receive the hepatitis B vaccine to prevent chronic liver disease later in life. Depending on how long a baby is in the NICU prior to discharge, they may also receive other immunizations. Your nurse and physician will explain them to you and answer any questions you may have.

Premature babies are given extra medical attention and assistance immediately after delivery. Depending on how premature your baby is, your pediatrician or obstetrician may call in a neonatologist (a pediatrician who specializes in the care of premature or very ill babies) to help determine what, if any, special treatment is needed. Here are some of the most common conditions that occur in premature infants:

- Respiratory distress syndrome is a breathing disorder related to the baby's immature lungs. It occurs because the lungs often lack surfactant, which is a liquid substance that lines their tiny air sacs and allows the lungs to remain expanded at the end of each breath. Artificial surfactants can be used to treat some babies born prematurely. A high-flow nasal cannula (HFNC), a continuous positive airway pressure (CPAP) machine, or a breathing machine (ventilator) may also be used to help them breathe better and maintain adequate oxygen levels in their blood. Sometimes extremely preterm babies may need long-term oxygen treatment and may go home on supportive oxygen therapy.
- Bronchopulmonary dysplasia, or chronic lung disease, is a term used to describe a condition in which babies require oxygen for several weeks or months. Premature

infants born at later gestation usually outgrow this condition as their lungs mature and grow. However, those infants who have moderate to severe disease may have long-term health problems of lung growth and development. Your baby's neonatologist and other care providers will explain these to you prior to your taking the baby home.

- Apnea is usually a temporary pause (of more than twenty seconds) in breathing, and is commonly seen in premature infants. It often is associated with a decline in the heart rate, called bradycardia, and desaturation, a decline in the amount of oxygen in the blood. Apnea, bradycardia, and desaturation are monitored on cardiorespiratory (heart rate and breathing) monitors and by pulse oximetry. Apnea is treated by giving caffeine or by giving oxygen via a tube (nasal cannula) or CPAP; if the apnea is severe, treatment may also require the use of a breathing machine. Rarely, apnea can result from infection or other causes, such as anemia, low blood sugar, or necrotizing enterocolitis (NEC; see *page 28*). Your baby's care providers will explain to you the cause, the treatment, and its significance. The good news is that most infants outgrow the condition by the time they leave the hospital.
- Retinopathy of prematurity (ROP) is an eye disease featuring underdeveloped retinas, causing blood vessels at the back of the eye (retina) to bleed. Most cases resolve without treatment, although serious cases may need treatment with laser surgery and/or by injections of medication. Long-term complications include near-sightedness and blindness. A pediatric ophthalmologist or retina specialist will examine your infant to diagnose ROP or other visual problems and, if needed, recommend treatment.
- Intraventricular hemorrhage (IVH) is bleeding inside or around the ventricles (the spaces in the brain containing the cerebrospinal fluid). Intraventricular hemorrhage is most common in premature babies, especially very-low-birth-weight babies—those weighing less than 3 pounds 5 ounces (1,500 g). Bleeding can occur because blood vessels in a premature baby's brain are very fragile and immature, and rupture easily. Most premature babies

who develop IVH will do so within the first week after birth. It is diagnosed by doing an ultrasound examination of the head. Mild hemorrhages (grades 1 and 2) are most common, and often occur with no further complications. Severe hemorrhages (grades 3 and 4) are the most serious and may result in long-term brain injury to the baby. Hydrocephalus (too much cerebrospinal fluid in the brain) may develop after severe IVH due to blockage in the flow of the cerebrospinal fluid within the brain and/or the spinal cord. If the ventricle size increases, causing pressure on the developing brain, a small reservoir is surgically placed to facilitate removal of spinal fluid into the space around the intestines. Often hydrocephalus resolves spontaneously. However, if the head size increases and the baby weighs more than 4 pounds 6.6 ounces (2 kg), a ventriculoperitoneal shunt may have to be placed. Your neonatologist and neurosurgeon will explain its pros and cons to you prior to surgery. There is no specific treatment for IVH, except to treat any other health problems that may worsen the condition. Although care of sick and premature babies has advanced greatly, it is not possible to prevent IVH from occurring in some babies.

- Babies born prematurely, particularly those who have IVH or hydrocephalus, are at risk for cerebral palsy (CP), which is a disorder of the brain's control of movement, strength, or posture. Babies can be screened for CP using specialized examinations, and you should discuss this with your baby's doctors. Identifying babies at risk for CP is important, as earlier physical therapy can lead to improved outcomes.
- Preterm babies are at risk for infection. The symptoms of infection are like symptoms that premature babies have just from being premature. These include apnea (stopping breathing), bradycardia (low heart rate), desaturation (low oxygen), the need for increased support with a ventilator, increasing oxygen requirement, belly distension, feeding intolerance, and low blood pressure. If these symptoms occur, the baby may have a sepsis workup (getting blood count, blood cultures, urine cultures, and sometimes spinal fluid cultures). The baby may also receive antibiotics. If cultures are

negative after forty-eight hours, suggesting that there is no infection, the antibiotics will be stopped. Otherwise, if any of the cultures are positive, antibiotics will be given for seven to twenty-one days, depending on the type of infection.

- Necrotizing enterocolitis (NEC) is the most common and serious intestinal disease among premature babies. It happens when intestinal tissue, often in the small intestines (rarely the large intestine), is injured or inflamed. This can lead to death of intestinal tissue and, in rare cases, a hole (perforation) in the intestinal wall. Most cases of necrotizing enterocolitis occur in babies born before thirty-two weeks gestation. Babies with NEC usually develop it within the first two to six weeks after birth. It is diagnosed with signs of feeding intolerance or belly distension and is confirmed by ultrasound or X-ray examination of the abdomen. Not all feeding intolerance or belly distension is associated with NEC. Treatment involves stopping feedings for five to ten days and giving appropriate antibiotics. A pediatric surgeon is usually consulted if air is detected in the infant's bowel wall, so that they can follow the baby's condition with the neonatologist and be ready to intervene if necrotic (dead) bowel or intestinal perforation is suspected. They will discuss with you when surgery may be needed. Breast milk feeding is the single most effective means to prevent NEC in preterm infants. Research is currently under way on the role infant-specific probiotics play in decreasing the risk of NEC.
- Jaundice happens when a chemical called bilirubin builds up in the baby's blood as a result of the natural breakdown of red blood cells. The skin may develop a yellowish color. Treatment involves placing the undressed baby under special lights (while their eyes are covered). (For additional information about jaundice, see *pages 42–43*.)
- Developmental delays and disabilities are common in all children (one in six) but can be more common in those born prematurely. "Developmental delay" is a term used to describe a delay in how a child plays, learns, speaks, acts, and moves. Because premature babies were not yet done developing in utero, it is not expected that

they would show the same developmental skills at the same age as a full-term newborn. So, pediatricians often use a premature baby's corrected age (the age they would be if they were born on/after their due date) to determine if the child is showing any developmental delays. When a premature baby is in the NICU, the team may refer a child at risk for developmental delays for developmental services such as feeding therapy, speech therapy, or physical therapy. These early intervention services may start while the baby is still in the NICU or be provided later by your state's early intervention system, which is designed to support babies and toddlers in learning skills that typically developing children experience in the first three years.

- You can expect your pediatrician to ask about your child's development at each well-child visit, as they do with all children, and your child will have several developmental screenings done in the first few years. Parents and caregivers should always share any concerns that they have about their child's development with their pediatrician.
- Other conditions sometimes seen in preterm babies include anemia of prematurity (a low red blood cell count) and heart murmurs. (For additional information on heart murmurs, see *pages 611–13*.)

NATAL TEETH

Occasionally, a baby may be born with one or more teeth that have already erupted. The incidence of natal and/or neonatal teeth is far more frequent than previously supposed. Review of 359 recorded cases suggests an incidence of at least 1 in 3,000 births. About 70 percent of the natal and/or neonatal teeth are firmly fixed, but a small number can become loose.

How Your Newborn Behaves

Lying in your arms or in the crib beside you, your newborn makes a tight little bundle. Just as they did in the womb, your baby will keep their arms and legs close to their body and fists tightly clenched, although you should be able to gently straighten them. Your baby's feet will naturally curve inward. It may take several weeks for your baby's body to unfold from this preferred fetal position.

You'll have to wait even longer to hear the cooing or babbling we think of as "baby talk." However, from the beginning babies are noisy. Besides their crying when something is wrong, you'll hear a wide variety of grunts, squeaks, sighs, sneezes, and hiccups. Many of these sounds, just like your baby's sudden movements, are reactions to disturbances in the environment; a shrill sound or strong odor may be all it takes to prompt a startle or a cry.

These reactions, as well as more subtle ones, are signs of how your baby's senses are functioning. After months in the womb, your baby will quickly recognize the voice of the mother and often any other caregiver or partner who was around the baby during the pregnancy. If you play soothing music, your baby may become quiet or even move gently in time with it.

By using smell and taste, your newborn can distinguish breast milk from other liquids. You may notice your baby start to root when you hold them because you smell of breast milk.

Your baby's vision will be best within an 8- to 12-inch (20.3–30.5 cm) range, which means your baby can see your face as you hold and feed them. When you are farther away, you may notice a cross-eyed appearance. Don't worry about this in the first couple of months. Between 2 and 3 months of age, the eye muscles will mature, the vision will improve, and both eyes will remain focused on the same thing more of the time. If this does not happen, bring it to the attention of your baby's pediatrician.

Able to distinguish light from dark at birth and see bright colors, your infant will not yet see the full range of colors. While young infants who are shown a pattern of black and white or sharply contrasting colors may study them with interest, they are not likely to respond at all to a picture with closely related colors.

Perhaps the newborn's most important sense is touch. After months in the womb, your baby is now exposed to all sorts of new sensations—some harsh, some comforting. While your baby may cringe at a sudden gust of cold air, they'll love the feel of skin-to-skin contact with their parents/caregivers, a soft blanket, and the warmth of your embracing arms. Holding your baby gives them as much pleasure as it does you. It provides a sense of security and comfort, and it tells them they are loved. Research shows that close emotional bonding promotes growth and development for your baby.

Signs to Watch for in the First Days

During your baby's initial hospitalization, both you and your newborn will receive frequent checks from nursing staff and your doctors as well as daily exams. That said, if you notice any of the following, have someone come assess your baby:

- A blue appearance to the face or trunk. Blue or purple hands and feet are normal, but if you see the face turn blue, that could indicate a problem with the baby's heart or lungs.
- Breathing more than once every second or pulling of the skin between or below the ribs. Babies will often breathe fast then slow then fast again, but if you notice sustained fast or hard breathing, let your nurse know. Some babies breathe fine at birth but develop problems in the hours afterward.
- Rhythmic abnormal movements of one or more extremities. Newborns will quiver and shake, startling with even minor noises or changes in their environment, and this is all normal. But if you notice a sustained, rhythmic movement of the arms or legs, this could indicate a seizure.

Going Home

Most hospitals discharge you and your baby within forty-eight hours if you delivered vaginally. If you undergo a Cesarean section, you may go home at forty-eight hours, or if you have complications, you may stay at the facility for three or more days. If your baby is born in an alternative birthing center, you may go home within twenty-four hours. Nevertheless, just because a full-term, healthy infant could be discharged in less than forty-eight hours doesn't mean it should necessarily occur. The American Academy of Pediatrics believes that the health and well-being of the mother and the child are paramount. Since every baby is different, the decision to discharge a newborn should be made on a case-by-case basis.

If you are adopting, you may want to stay in the hospital and take care of the baby for the first couple of days after birth. If possible, plan ahead of time with the birth parent and the hospital to establish where you and the newborn will be and whether the birth parent will be involved in care during that time.

If a newborn does leave the hospital early, they should still receive all the appropriate newborn tests and measures, such as a hearing screen, newborn metabolic tests, vitamin K administration, antibiotic eye ointment, heart screening, and hepatitis B vaccine, and be seen by the pediatrician twenty-four to forty-eight hours after discharge. If latch or breastfeeding sessions are not going well, ask to see the lactation specialist or pediatrician and plan for follow-up after discharge for breastfeeding support. Call the doctor sooner if a newborn appears listless or is feverish, is vomiting, or has difficulty feeding, or if their skin develops a yellow color (jaundice).

Before you bring your baby home, your car should be equipped with at least the bare essentials. Make sure you have a federally approved car safety seat appropriate for your baby's size, and that it's correctly installed, rear-facing in the backseat of your vehicle. It is extremely important to follow the car safety seat manufacturer's instructions on installation and proper use. If possible, get your car safety seat installation checked by a certified child passenger safety technician to ensure you've gotten it right. (For more information on the choice and proper use of car safety seats, see *pages 321–30.*)

At home you'll need a safe place (crib, bassinet, or portable crib) for the baby to sleep, plenty of diapers, and enough clothing and blankets to keep your baby warm and protected.

Where We Stand

The timing of newborn hospital discharge should be a mutual decision between the parents and the physician caring for the infant. The American Academy of

Pediatrics believes that the health and well-being of the parent and baby should take precedence over financial considerations. Academy policy has established minimum criteria for discharge before forty-eight hours after birth. These include term delivery, feeding well, appropriate growth, and normal physical examination. It often takes forty-eight hours for all of these criteria to be met. The Academy supports state and federal legislation based on AAP guidelines as long as physicians, in consultation with parents, have the final authority in determining when to discharge the patient.

Parenting

Becoming a Parent

You may find your first few days with your baby to be a mixture of delight, pain, utter exhaustion, and—especially if this is your first child—some apprehension about your capabilities. Bringing home a baby you are fostering or adopting brings many of the very same feelings. Take comfort: You are not alone.

You may be so excited about your new arrival that you don't even notice how tired and sore you are. Despite the fatigue, it still may be difficult to fall asleep. If you deliver in a hospital and your baby is healthy, your baby will usually sleep in a hospital-supplied bassinet in your room. You should maximize your time enjoying skin-to-skin care with your baby, but be careful not to fall asleep with your baby on your chest, in bed, or on a chair or sofa.

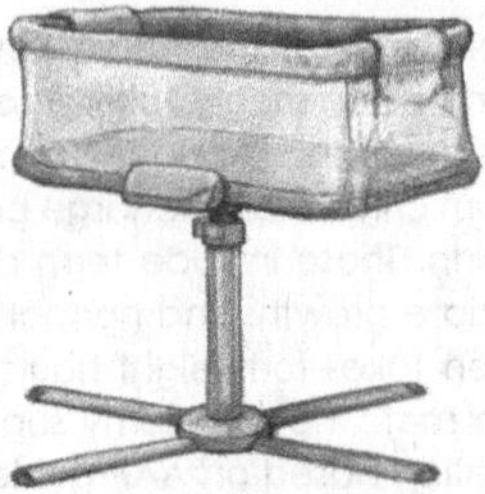

When you or your partner is tired or going to sleep, put your baby back in the bassinet on their back. Swaddling or using a sleep wrap may encourage sleeping apart from you. Take advantage of the time in the hospital to rest, learn from the trained professionals, and let your body recover. Once you are home, try to rest when you can. Being a new parent is an anxiety-provoking transition, so give yourself plenty of grace, as it will take a while to get used to routine baby care and for things to fall into place. Remember, you can rely on trusted friends, family members, and your pediatrician for help and advice. Although it is tempting to search online for answers, this may only end up adding more confusion. (For more information about postpartum blues and depression, see the description on *pages 35–36*.)

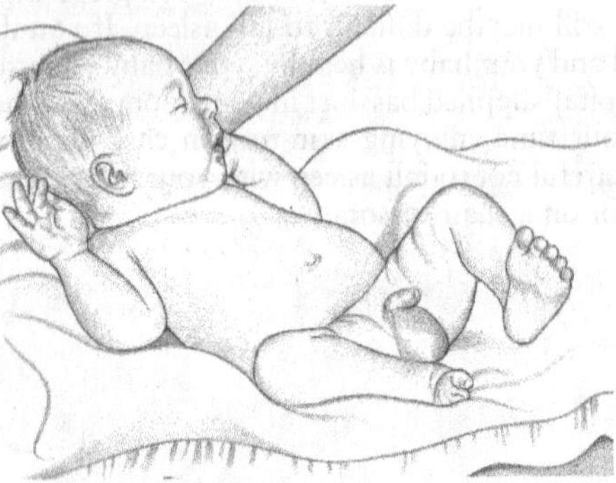

You have just given birth to a wonderful new being, but also to a new awesome responsibility.

If this is not your first child, there may be some questions on your mind, such as:

- *Will this new baby come between you and an older child?*

  This needn't happen, especially if you make a point of including your older child(ren) in your new routine. Toddlers are usually quite happy to help with giving the baby a bath or retrieving a clean diaper, and older children often take pride in checking for hazards (e.g., stray toys) and making sure all visitors wash their hands before touching the new baby. As you become more comfortable with your daily routine, be sure to include special times with your older child. Announcing this special time big and loud will make it more noticeable and memorable.

- *Will you be able to give the same intensity of love to the new child?*

  In fact, each child is special and will draw out different responses and feelings from you. Even the birth order may influence the way you relate to each other. It is often helpful to think that "new" isn't "better" or "worse," but usually just . . . different. This concept is important for both you and your child(ren) to remember. Providing your child with a sibling is a gift. Learning how to share, comfort, and compromise are all life skills learned first within a family context.

On a practical note, the prospect of taking care of multiple children may worry you. This only makes sense, but given time and patience, every family member will settle into new roles.

Most parents find that at some point the newness, fatigue, and seemingly unanswerable questions push them to tears. You won't be the first new parent to cry—or the last. The hormonal changes experienced by adolescents are minor compared to the hormonal shifts associated with pregnancy and the postpartum period.

The emotional changes can sometimes lead parents to experience sadness, fear, irritability, anxiety, or even anger toward their baby—feelings doctors call postpartum blues or baby blues. About three out of four new mothers experience this a few days after birth. For some these feelings will only last a few days, for others longer.

Some new mothers, however, have such severe sadness, emptiness, apathy, and even despair that doctors categorize this as postpartum depression. They also may experience even more extreme feelings of inadequacy and may begin to withdraw from family and friends. This may develop a few weeks after birth and affects about one out of three new mothers. The symptoms can last many months (or even more than a year), worsen with time, and become so intense that these mothers may feel helpless and incapable of caring for their baby and other children; they may even worry about harming themselves or their baby. Even the parent who didn't give birth themselves can suffer from postpartum depression; they, too, should be alert to the signs and seek help early on.

Discuss your feelings with your partner, your extended family, and close friends. Allow them to relieve you of being the primary caregiver, and try to reduce your stress and anxiety by embracing self-care. Sleep, exercise, meditate, connect with friends; take time to do whatever it is that renews your sense of well-being and energy. If this doesn't help and these feelings are severe and haven't subsided in about two weeks, talk to your obstetrician, primary care provider, or pediatrician, or seek help from a mental health professional; counseling and/or antidepressant medications may be recommended (many medications are safe, but check in with your pediatrician if you're using breast milk). Many pediatricians now screen for postpartum depression with a questionnaire at each well-child visit in the first six months.

Partner's Feelings

Even if you didn't carry and birth your baby, you may have made adjustments physically and emotionally as the due date approached and preparations for the baby became all-important. You may have been present and played an important supportive role during the delivery. Even if you felt that you didn't do as much as your partner, this is your baby, too.

When the baby finally arrived, you may have been relieved as well as excited and awed. If you witnessed your baby's birth, feelings of commitment and love that you had worried might never happen may have surfaced after all. You may also have experienced a greater admiration and love for the mother than ever before. At the same time, contemplating the responsibility of caring for this baby for the next twenty years or longer may feel more than a little unnerving.

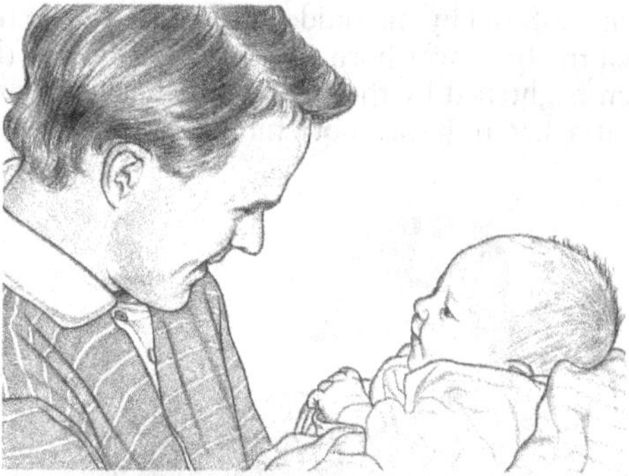

Become as involved as possible in caring for and playing with your new baby. You'll get just as emotionally attached to them as your partner will.

Depending on the hospital and your own schedule, you may have been able to room in with the mother and/or your baby until it was time to go home. This may help you feel less like a bystander and more like a key participant, allowing you to get to know your baby right from the start. It also allows you to share an intense emotional experience with your partner.

If conflicting emotions persist, how should you deal with them? The best approach is to become actively involved in parenting. Once the entire family is home, you can—and should—hold and comfort the baby, provide encouragement to your partner, and help them to rest whenever possible. During those times, you will gain confidence with diapering and even feedings. Doing these jobs helps you to bond with your child, and they are wonderful opportunities for the entire family to get to know, love, and welcome this new member home.

Siblings' Feelings

Older children may greet a new baby with open arms, closed minds, or a mixture of both. Their reaction will depend largely on their age and developmental level. For instance, there's little you can do to prepare a toddler for the changes that will come with a new sibling. To begin with, other children may have been confused by the sudden disappearance of their parents when the baby was born. Visiting the hospital, they may have been frightened by the sight of the birth parent in bed, perhaps attached to intravenous tubing.

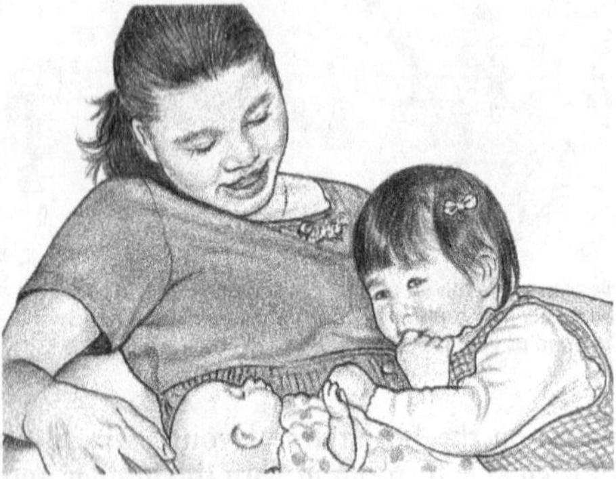

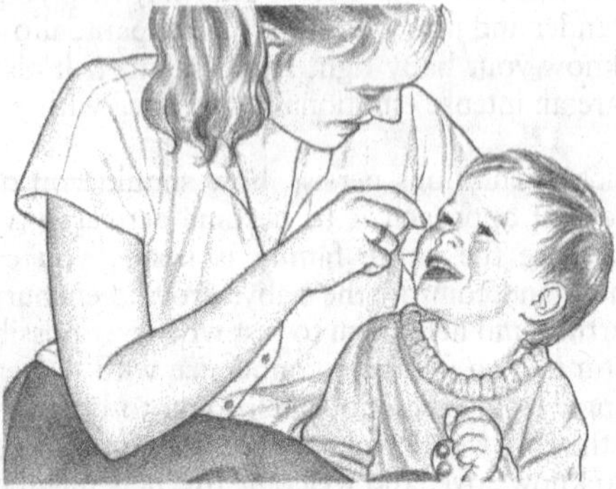

Make sure you reserve some special time each day just for you and your older child.

Siblings may also be jealous that their parents are holding someone else instead of them, and they may misbehave or begin acting younger (insisting on wearing diapers or suddenly having accidents several months after being toilet trained). These are normal responses to stress and change, and the best way to respond is simply to give extra love and reassurance rather than to punish them. Also, try very hard to catch them "being good" so they get attention for appropriate behaviors. Praise them for "acting like the big sibling," letting them know that they, too, have an important new role to play. Tell them that there's plenty of room in your heart to love both them and the new baby. Over time, their attachment to the baby will build. You'll want to supervise them with the baby at all times so that they can learn how to behave safely around their new sibling.

If your older child is a preschooler, they will probably better understand what's happening. If you prepared your older child as you waited for your baby, you may have helped ease their confusion, if not their jealousy. Saying things like "The baby is in my tummy" or "The baby will sleep in your old crib" often helps them be able to understand the basic facts of the situation and may make them very curious about this mysterious person.

If school-age, your child still needs to adapt to a new role. At the same time, they were probably fascinated by the process of pregnancy and childbirth and eager to meet the new baby. Once the infant arrives, they may become very proud and protective. Let them help take care of the little one at times, but don't forget they still need time and attention themselves.

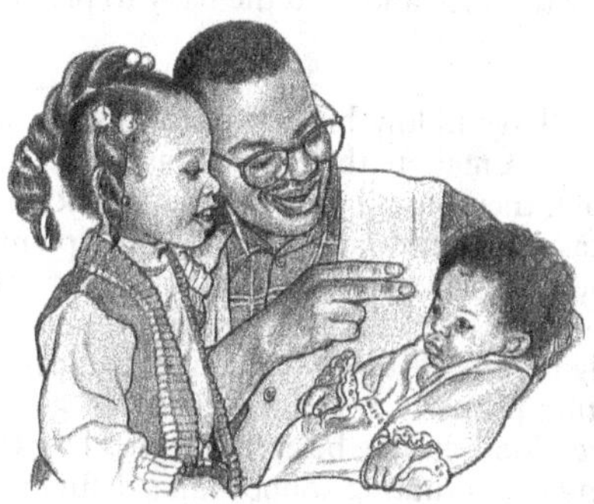

Let the older sibling know frequently that there's enough room and love in your heart for both children.

Health Watch

Some physical conditions are common during the first couple of weeks after birth. If you notice any of the following in your baby, contact your pediatrician.

Abdominal Distension. Most babies' bellies normally stick out, especially after a large feeding. Between feedings, however, they should feel soft. If your child's abdomen feels swollen and hard, and if the baby has not had a bowel movement for more than one or two days or is vomiting, call your pediatrician. Most likely the problem is due to gas or difficulty passing a stool, but it also could signal a more serious intestinal problem.

Birth Injuries. Babies can be injured during birth, especially if labor is long or difficult, or when babies are very large. While newborns recover quickly from some of these injuries, others persist. Occasionally a broken collarbone occurs, which will heal quickly. After a few weeks, a small lump may form at the fracture site, but don't be alarmed; this is a sign that new bone is forming to mend the injury, and it will soon be as good as new.

Muscle weakness is another common birth injury during labor, caused by pressure or stretching of the nerves attached to the muscles. These muscles, usually weakened on one side of the face or in one shoulder or arm, generally return to normal after several weeks. In the meantime, ask your pediatrician to show you how to nurse and hold the baby to promote healing.

Blue Baby. Babies may have mildly blue or purple hands and feet, which is usually normal. If their hands and feet turn slightly blue from cold, they should return to pink as soon as they are warm. Occasionally the face, tongue, and lips may turn a little blue when the newborn is crying hard, but once the baby is calm, the color should quickly return to normal. However, persistently blue skin coloring is a sign the heart or lungs are not operating properly and the baby is not getting enough oxygen in the blood. It may be accompanied by rapid and labored breathing or a grunting sound. Immediate medical attention is essential.

Bowel Movements. After birth, the staff will watch for your baby's first urination and bowel movement to make sure there are no problems with these important tasks. The initial bowel movement may be delayed twenty-four hours or more. The first bowel movement or two will be black or dark green and very slimy. It is meconium, a substance that fills the infant's intestines before the baby is born. If your baby does not pass meconium in the first forty-eight hours, further evaluation is required to make sure that no problems exist in the lower bowel. On occasion, newborns have a little blood in their bowel movements. If it occurs during the first few days, it usually means the infant has a little crack in the anus from stooling. This is generally harmless, but even so, let your pediatrician know about any signs of blood so that they can confirm the reason, since there are other causes that require further evaluation and treatment.

Coughing. If the baby drinks very fast, they may cough and sputter, but this type of coughing should stop as soon as the feeding routine becomes familiar. This may also be related to the speed at which the milk comes down if you are breastfeeding, especially with the initial let-down. If your baby coughs persistently or routinely gags during feedings, or excessively spits up, consult the pediatrician. These symptoms could indicate an underlying problem in the lungs or digestive tract.

Excessive Crying. All newborns cry, often for no apparent reason. If you've made sure that your baby is fed, burped, warm, and dressed in a clean diaper, the best tactic is probably to hold your baby and talk or sing to them until the crying stops. You cannot spoil a baby this age by providing too much attention. If this doesn't work, wrap your baby snugly in a blanket or try some of the approaches listed on *pages 102–4*. If you are worried about the degree of crying, call your pediatrician. Crying that doesn't stop can be stressful to any parent. If you find yourself starting to feel excessively frustrated, hand your infant to another caregiver or put your baby down in a crib or safe space and take a moment to calm down.

Forceps Marks. When forceps are used during delivery, they can leave red marks or even superficial scrapes on a newborn's face and head. These generally disappear within a few days.

Sometimes a firm, flat lump develops in one of these areas because of minor damage to the tissue under the skin, but this, too, will usually go away within two months.

Jaundice. Many normal, healthy newborns have a yellowish tinge to their skin, which is known as jaundice. It is caused by a buildup of bilirubin in the child's blood because the immature liver cannot clear it well. Mild jaundice is harmless. However, if the bilirubin level continues to rise and is not treated, it can lead to brain injury. Jaundice tends to be more common in breastfed newborns, most often in those not nursing well; breastfeeding mothers should nurse a minimum of eight times a day, but every two hours is more common, so ten to twelve times per day. Keeping the baby on task by feeding them in their diaper only and rubbing their back can help, especially when they are sleepy in the early days.

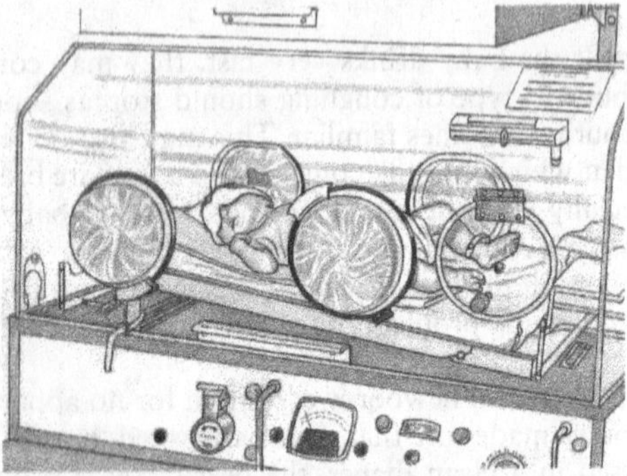

Phototherapy—or light treatment—can be delivered through different light sources, such as special lights or on a specialized blanket with the baby's eyes covered for protection.

Jaundice first appears on the face, then the chest and abdomen, and finally the arms and legs in some instances. The whites of the eyes may also be yellow. Hospitals now routinely screen newborns for jaundice twenty-four hours after birth using a painless handheld light meter. If the pediatrician suspects jaundice may be present—based on skin color as well as the baby's age and other factors—the doctor may order a skin or blood test to definitively diagnose the condition. If jaundice develops before the baby is 1 day old, a blood bilirubin test is always needed to help with the accurate diagnosis. If you notice a sudden increase in jaundice, your baby not feeding well, or a decrease in the number of wet diapers when your baby is at home, contact your pediatrician. At 3 to 5 days old, newborns should be checked by a doctor or nurse, since this is the time bilirubin levels are highest; for that reason, infants discharged before they are 3 days old should be seen by a pediatrician within two days of discharge. Some newborns need to be seen even sooner, including:

- Those with a high bilirubin level before leaving the hospital
- Those born early (more than two weeks before the due date)
- Those who are not feeding well
- Those with considerable bruising and bleeding under the scalp, associated with labor and delivery
- Those who have a biological parent or biological sibling who had high bilirubin levels and underwent treatment for it

An elevated bilirubin level can be treated with phototherapy, or light treatment. At either the hospital or home, an undressed infant is placed under special lights or on a specialized light blanket with eyes covered for protection. This kind of treatment can prevent the harmful effects of jaundice. In breastfed babies, jaundice may last for more than two to three weeks; in formula-fed babies, most cases go away by two weeks of age.

Lethargy and Sleepiness. Every newborn spends most of the time sleeping. As long as your baby wakes every few hours, eats well, seems content, and is alert part of the day, it's perfectly normal for them to sleep the rest of the time. But if your newborn is rarely alert, does not wake up for feedings, or seems too tired or uninterested to eat, you should consult your pediatrician. This lethargy—especially if it's a sudden change in your baby's usual pattern—may be a symptom of a serious illness.

Respiratory Distress. It may take your baby a few hours after birth to form a normal breathing pattern, but then you should notice no further difficulties. If your baby seems to be breathing in an unusual manner, it is most often due to blocked nasal passages. Using saline nasal drops, followed by suctioning the mucus from the nose with a bulb syringe (for its use, see *page 470*) or other device, may fix the problem; these are available over the counter.

However, if your newborn shows any of the following warning signs, notify your pediatrician immediately:

- Fast breathing (more than sixty breaths in one minute), although keep in mind that babies normally breathe more rapidly than adults
- Retractions (sucking in the muscles between the ribs with each breath, so the ribs stick out)
- Flaring of the nose
- Grunting while breathing
- Persistent blue lips or other areas of skin

Umbilical Cord. You'll need to keep the stump of the umbilical cord clean and dry as it shrivels and eventually falls off. There is no need to use alcohol on the cord; just keep it clean. Also, keep the diaper folded below the cord to prevent urine from soaking it. You may notice a few drops of blood on the diaper around the time the stump falls off; this is normal. But if the cord actively bleeds, call your baby's doctor immediately. If the stump becomes infected, it will require medical treatment. Although cord infections are uncommon, you should contact your doctor if you notice any of the following:

- Foul-smelling yellowish discharge from the cord
- Red skin around the base of the cord
- Crying when you touch the cord or the skin next to it

The umbilical cord stump should dry and fall off by the time your baby is 3 weeks old. If it persists beyond that time, a doctor's visit is needed.

Umbilical Granuloma. Sometimes instead of completely drying, the cord will form a granuloma, or a small reddened or brownish mass of scar tissue that stays on the belly button after the umbilical cord has fallen off. This granuloma may drain a light yellowish fluid. This condition will usually go away in about a week, but if not, your pediatrician may need to help dry or chemically cauterize the granulomatous tissue.

Umbilical Hernia. If your baby's umbilical cord area seems to push outward with crying, your baby may have an umbilical hernia—a small hole in the muscular part of the abdominal wall that allows the tissue to bulge out when there is increased abdominal pressure (i.e., crying). This is not a serious condition, and it usually heals by itself in the first twelve to eighteen months. In the unlikely event it doesn't heal by 3 to 5 years of age, the hole may need surgery. Don't put tape or a coin on the navel. It will not help the hernia, and it may cause a skin rash.

CHAPTER 3

FEEDING YOUR BABY

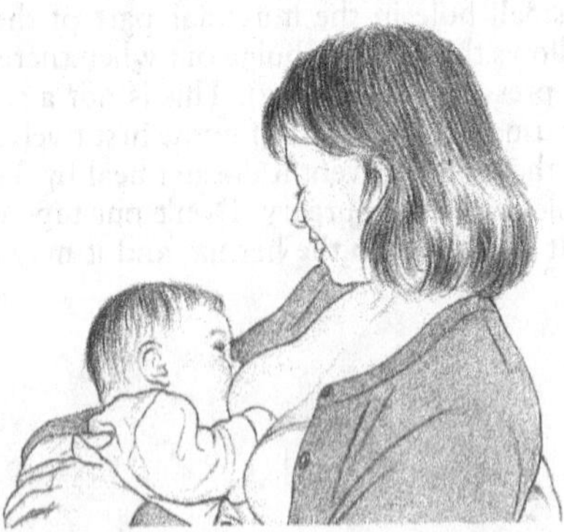

Your baby's nutritional needs during the rapid-growth period of infancy are greater than at any other time in their life. They will approximately triple their birth weight during their first year.

Feeding your infant provides more than just good nutrition. It also allows you to hold your newborn close, cuddle them, and make eye contact. These are relaxing and enjoyable moments for you both, bringing you closer together.

Before your baby arrives, you should consider how you are going to feed them. Major medical groups worldwide agree that, if possible, breastfeeding is best for the baby and the breastfeeding parent. That said, breastfeeding certainly can be difficult and might not be possible for some. This chapter will provide the basic information on infant feeding so that you can feel comfortable with your feeding decision.

It is important to note that not all parents who feed their babies with their own milk use the term "breastfeeding"; some transgender or non-binary parents may instead use the term "chestfeeding" to describe this process. Most scientific research on feeding breast milk has focused on breastfeeding. Because of this, we will use "breastfeeding" to describe feeding an infant milk from a mother. This chapter is written to address a breastfeeding mother, but the information may be helpful to partners or other supportive people in that parent's life. The AAP supports continued research and advocacy for all parents who wish to provide optimal nutrition for their infants.

Because of its nutritional composition and health-promoting properties, breast milk (also referred to as human milk) is the ideal food for human infants. Studies have shown that babies who are breastfed are at a reduced risk of acquiring upper respiratory infections and ear infections, wheezing in early childhood, and gastrointestinal infections that cause vomiting and diarrhea. Breastfeeding has been associated with reduced risk of sudden infant death syndrome (SIDS), which is a subcategory of sudden unexpected infant death (SUID), and childhood leukemia. Other studies have shown that breastfeeding may reduce the chance of overweight, obesity, and both type 1 and type 2 diabetes in childhood and later. Premature babies who receive breast milk may particularly benefit, with reduced risks of serious gut and blood infections. In addition, for those who breastfeed, studies show that breastfeeding helps a woman return to pre-pregnancy weight, helps prevent diabetes, and reduces the incidence of certain types of cancers later in life. As a result, most pediatricians recommend that new mothers breastfeed when possible.

Some women are uncertain about breastfeeding or cannot breastfeed for various reasons. If you have questions about breastfeeding, ask your prenatal care provider, your pediatrician, or a lactation consultant—someone knowledgeable with whom you can discuss your specific concerns, doubts, or fears. With support, most women are able to successfully breastfeed their babies. If you are unable to breastfeed, infant formula is an acceptable and nutritious alternative to breast milk. But you should thoughtfully weigh the many benefits of breastfeeding before making the choice to formula-feed. It's important to give it serious consideration before your baby arrives, since starting with formula and then switching to breast milk can be difficult if you wait too long. The production of milk (called lactation) is most successful if breastfeeding begins immediately after delivery.

Where We Stand

The American Academy of Pediatrics believes that breastfeeding is the optimal source of nutrition through the first year. We recommend exclusively breastfeeding for about the first six months, and then gradually adding solid foods while continuing breastfeeding for at least the first year. Thereafter, breastfeeding can continue for as long as both mother and baby desire it.

Breastfeeding should begin as soon as possible after birth, usually within the first hour. Newborns should nurse whenever they show signs of hunger—approximately eight to twelve times every twenty-four hours. The frequency of feedings and the amount of time for each feeding vary widely for each mother-baby pair. It is important to recognize signs that the baby is latching on to the breast and getting milk. The amount of milk a baby will get during each breastfeeding attempt is small during the first day (about 1 teaspoon) and increases on the second and third days. Before going home, it is important to identify the signs that your baby is getting milk during breastfeeding. (See Is Your Baby Eating Enough?, *page 68*.)

The American Academy of Pediatrics, the World Health Organization (WHO), and many other experts encourage breastfeeding for as long as possible, one to two years or longer, with a recommendation of six months of exclusive breastfeeding (see Where We Stand, *above*). Breast milk provides optimal nutrition and protection against infections. One survey found that 80 to 90 percent of pregnant women wanted to breastfeed. Of infants born in 2020, 84 percent were breastfed at birth and 57 percent were still being breastfed at 6 months of age (see the breastfeeding report card produced by the Centers for Disease Control and Prevention [CDC] at cdc.gov/breastfeeding-data/breastfeeding-report-card). Because most women want to breastfeed, and start out breastfeeding, national efforts have shifted to building a better support system for maintaining breastfeeding. That said, many workplaces and employers continue to lag in providing the support necessary for parents to successfully breastfeed.

Breastfeeding

Breast milk is the best possible food for any infant. Its major ingredients are water, sugar (lactose), easily digestible protein (whey and casein), and fat (digestible fatty acids). In addition, breast milk contains minerals and vitamins, as well as enzymes that aid the digestion and absorption. Formulas approximate these nutrients but don't provide all the enzymes, or the antibodies, growth-promoting factors, and many other valuable components that are involved in fighting infections.

There are many practical reasons to breastfeed your baby. The direct cost of breast milk is much less than the cost of buying formula retail—a slight increase in your caloric intake costs much less than what you would spend on formula. Breastfeeding uses about 500 calories a day to produce the milk. It's therefore especially important that mothers continue to eat a healthy, balanced diet while nursing, to avoid nutritional deficiencies. Breastfeeding also helps the uterus tighten and return to its normal size more quickly.

The psychological and emotional advantages of breastfeeding are just as compelling, for both mother and child. Nursing provides skin-to-skin contact, which is soothing for your baby and often pleasant for you. The same hormones that stimulate milk production and release also may promote feelings that enhance bonding. Almost all breastfeeding mothers find that the experience of breastfeeding makes them feel more attached and protective toward their babies and more confident about their own abilities to nurture and care for their children. The breastfeeding mother may feel an increased demand on her time. Studies, however, show that breastfeeding and formula-feeding take about the same amount of time. Bottle-feeding requires more time for shopping and for cleaning feeding utensils. Time spent with the baby is important for infant nurturing and development and can be pleasurable for the mother. Other family members can assist by covering household tasks, especially during the first few weeks when the mother needs extra rest and the baby demands frequent feeding.

THE HEALTH BENEFITS OF BREASTFEEDING

Research has shown that babies who are breastfed reap numerous benefits. Compared to those who are breastfed, babies who are formula-fed have higher rates of the following:

- Ear infections
- Eczema, food allergies, and asthma
- Gastrointestinal infections that cause vomiting and diarrhea
- Pneumonia and other respiratory diseases
- Obesity in adolescence and adulthood
- Type 1 and type 2 diabetes
- Childhood leukemia
- Sudden infant death syndrome (SIDS)
- Necrotizing enterocolitis (NEC), especially common in premature infants

Mothers who breastfeed longer than twelve months see improvements in maternal health, with decreasing rates of maternal type 2 diabetes, hypertension, breast cancer, and ovarian cancer.

Source: Adapted from American Academy of Pediatrics, ***New Mother's Guide to Breastfeeding***, ed. J. Y. Meek, 4th ed. (New York: Bantam Books, 2024).

Other family members can actively share in all aspects of baby care even though they do not directly feed them milk. Remain sensitive to the needs of fathers, partners, and siblings. A partner's non-nutritive cuddling with the baby plays an important role, as does comforting the mother and baby when needed. A partner can hold, burp, diaper, bathe, and walk with the baby. After breastfeeding is well established (about 3 to 4 weeks of age), the partner may feed expressed milk with a bottle.

CONSIDERING SPECIAL CIRCUMSTANCES

When parents are healthy, babies can thrive. It is very important that mothers prioritize their own health and take the medications their doctor recommends, such as medications for mental health diagnoses (including substance use disorders). Most medications, including many of those for depression or opioid use disorder, are safe for breastfeeding. If you're taking prescription or over-the-counter medications for any reason, let your pediatrician know before you start breastfeeding. The pediatrician can advise whether anything you are taking can pass through breast milk and cause problems. Some medicines can be switched to safer ones while breastfeeding. Also, be aware that just because something is labeled as a "dietary supplement" or "all natural" does not mean it can't cause harm to a baby when excreted in breast milk. (To get more information, you can visit LactMed, a database of drugs and dietary supplements that may affect breastfeeding: ncbi.nlm.nih.gov/books/NBK501922/. It includes information on the levels of such substances in breast milk and infant blood, and possible adverse effects in the nursing infant. It is also available as a free app for Android and iOS.) In rare situations, to protect the health of the mother, breastfeeding may not be recommended. You can still feed your baby in a loving, connected manner with infant formula; babies will know that their parent is giving them vital nutrition.

It's best for parents to discuss feeding issues openly to make sure everyone understands and supports the choices made before the baby arrives. Parents and care providers want a baby to receive the best possible nutrition from the start. If breastfeeding is well established (usually between 3 and 4 weeks of age) and the mother needs to be away from the baby for a period (e.g., because of the need to return to work or take some personal time), she can continue to provide milk by pumping and collecting breast milk for feeding from a bottle.

Some mothers may experience mild discomfort during early breastfeeding. But significant discomfort is not normal. If you experience pain, have difficulty getting the baby to latch on and feed well, or would like further support with nursing, seek help from an experienced health professional (pediatrician, nurse, or lactation specialist). All babies should be seen by a pediatrician, nurse, or lactation consultant within two to three days of hospital discharge to check on how both the parent and the newborn are adjusting to being home.

Seeking help from an expert early is a good way to prevent

and even overcome problems and maintain the skills and self-confidence necessary to continue breastfeeding. Occasionally some mothers have breastfeeding problems that lead to untimely weaning (before the mother had intended). Many women feel disappointed when breastfeeding does not work out as planned, but these situations are common, and formula provides a safe and nutritious alternative for growing infants. (Also see Bottle-Feeding, *page 80*.)

Getting Started: Preparing for Lactation

Your body starts preparing to breastfeed as soon as you become pregnant. The area surrounding the nipple—the areola—becomes darker. The breasts enlarge as milk-manufacturing cells multiply and the milk-carrying ducts develop. The increase in breast size is normal and a sign that your breasts are preparing to produce milk. Meanwhile, your body starts storing excess fat to provide the extra energy needed for pregnancy and lactation.

As early as the sixteenth week of pregnancy, the breasts are ready to produce milk as soon as the infant is born. Early milk, called colostrum, is a rich, slightly thick-appearing, orange-yellow substance produced for several days after delivery. Colostrum contains more protein, salt, antibodies, and other protective properties than later, "mature" breast milk, but it has less fat and fewer calories. Colostrum helps your baby establish their immune system. The colostrum gradually changes into transitional and then mature milk. The nutritional components of breast milk adjust to match the changing needs of your growing infant and will continue to do so for the duration of breastfeeding. This is a characteristic that infant formula cannot duplicate.

As your body naturally prepares for breastfeeding, there is little you need to do. Your nipples do not need to be "toughened up" to withstand your baby's sucking. Tactics such as stretching, pulling, rolling, or buffing the nipples may interfere with normal lactation by harming the tiny glands in the areola that secrete a milky fluid that lubricates the nipples in preparation for breastfeeding. In short, such efforts could make your nipples more likely to develop soreness and irritation.

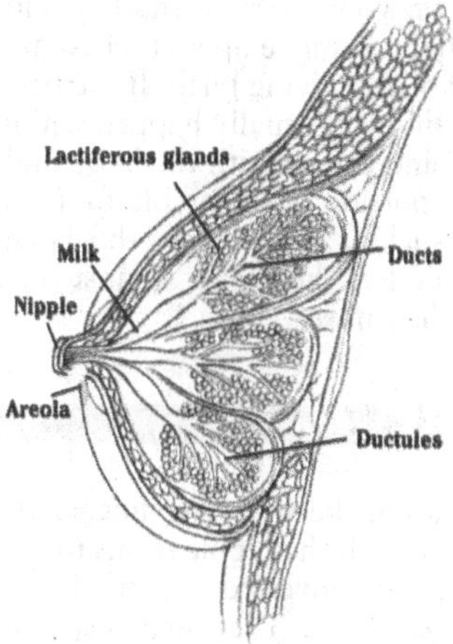

Milk is produced by the lactiferous glands. The milk then passes through the ductules into the ducts and out the nipple.

Normal bathing and gentle drying is the best way to care for your breasts during pregnancy. Although many women use lotions and ointments on their breasts, these are not necessary and may even clog skin pores. Salves, particularly those containing vitamins or hormones, are unnecessary and could cause problems for your baby if used while breastfeeding. On the other hand, some women find purified lanolin is helpful in soothing sore or irritated nipples. If lanolin makes nipple pain worse, it may be an indication of allergy to even the purified form of lanolin.

Some women start wearing nursing bras during pregnancy. They are more adjustable and roomier than normal bras and are more comfortable as the breast size increases. Nursing bras also have flaps that can be opened for breastfeeding or expressing milk. Pads may be inserted into the nursing bra to absorb leaking milk. Be aware that some mothers are allergic to some of these pads, so it is important to speak with your doctor if you develop a nipple rash or pain.

Letting Down and Latching On

By the time your baby is born, your breasts are already producing colostrum. As your baby nurses, your infant's actions let your body know when to start and stop the flow of milk. The placement of your baby on your chest in the first moments after birth allows your baby to move up your chest and latch on during the first minutes after giving birth. If the baby is not interrupted, the first feeding will usually happen within the first hour after birth. Latching begins with the baby finding and attaching onto a good portion of the areola (not just on the nipple) and starting to suckle. They will do this latching instinctively as soon as they feel the breast against their mouth and the nipple against their nose.

INVERTED NIPPLES AND BREASTFEEDING

Normally, when you press the areola between two fingers, the nipple protrudes and becomes erect. If the nipple seems to pull inward and disappear instead, it is "inverted" or "tied." Inverted nipples are a normal variation. They may begin to move out more as the pregnancy progresses. If you have questions about your nipples, discuss the issue with your prenatal professional or with a lactation specialist.

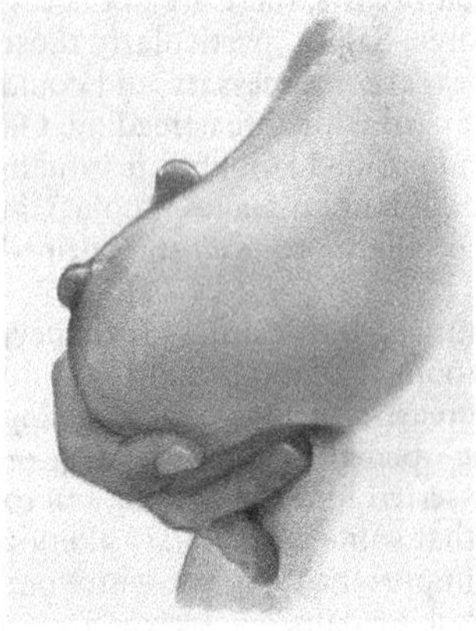

Normal nipple

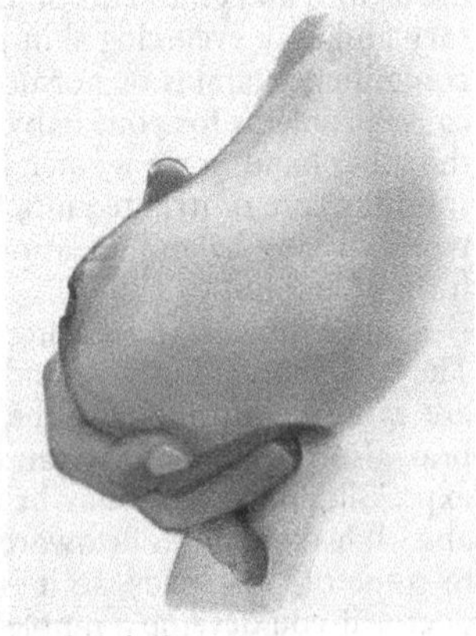

Inverted nipple

At times, inverted nipples are noticed only at delivery. In this case, the postpartum staff will assist you with early feedings. Working with a lactation consultant is often helpful. The consultant may recommend pumping briefly before nursing to help bring out the nipple, or temporarily using a nursing shield to help the baby latch on.

If you are having a vaginal delivery or a planned Cesarean, you will need to talk to your prenatal healthcare provider about skin-to-skin contact and breastfeeding immediately after birth. While on your chest, your baby will begin to move toward your breast and latch on to one of your breasts. If there are complications with delivery, or if your newborn needs immediate medical attention, you may have to wait a few hours. If the first feeding takes place within the first day or two, you should have no physical difficulty nursing. If nursing must be delayed beyond the first few hours after birth, the nursing staff will assist you with pumping or hand expression.

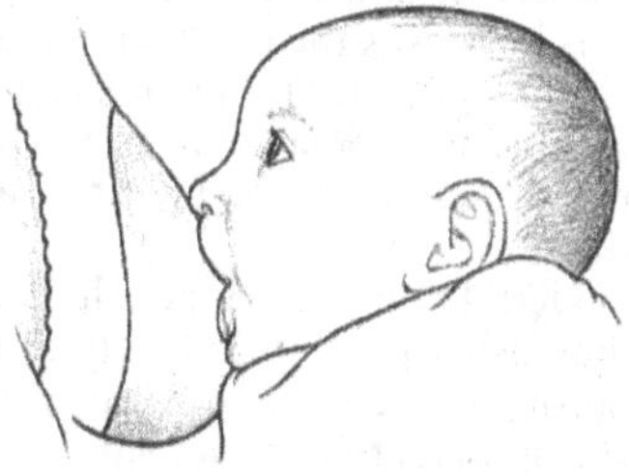

The baby has latched on to the breast correctly. The nose, lips, and chin are all close to the breast, allowing for effective breastfeeding.

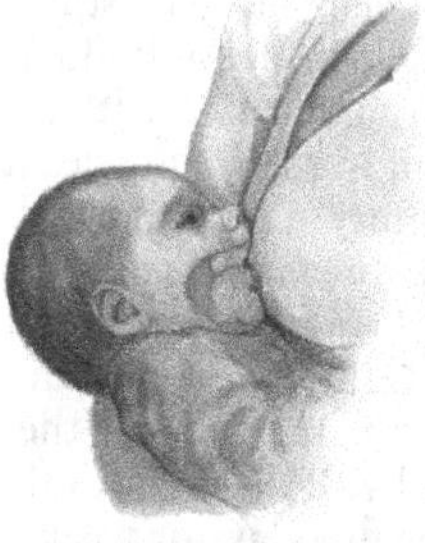

Most of the areola and nipple are in the baby's mouth.

When you begin breastfeeding, you may start by reclining and placing your baby on your chest between your breasts without a bra on. Just like in the delivery room, your baby will begin to move toward one of your breasts and latch on. You may also start by positioning your baby so that they squarely face the breast and then stroking their lower lip or cheek with the nipple or touching their chin to your breast. Doing this causes them to search for the nipple with the mouth (the rooting reflex). The infant opens their mouth widely and moves toward the breast. Using your hand to express a few drops of milk will also help your baby root and latch on to your breast, as the smell and taste will stimulate the latching reflex. The hospital staff or your birth attendant will show you how to hand-express your milk.

As your baby takes the breast into their mouth, their jaws should open wide and a good portion of the areola (not just the nipple) should be in their mouth. The baby's lips will pull back and look like fish lips on your skin, the gums encircling the areola. Their tongue will form a trough around the nipple and, in a wavelike motion, compress the milk reservoirs and empty the milk ducts. Putting your baby to the breast in the first hour after delivery will establish a good breastfeeding pattern at a time when infants are usually alert and vigorous. Later in the first day, your baby may be sleepy, but if they begin nursing in the first hour, they are more likely to successfully breastfeed.

When your baby suckles effectively at the breast, their movements will stimulate the breast and start milk flowing through the milk ducts. This is known as the let-down reflex; it is associated with the release of a pituitary hormone, oxytocin. In turn, the release of the hormone prolactin from the pituitary gland and the removal of milk from the breast cause the breasts to make more milk.

Oxytocin causes many wonderful things to happen. It gives a feeling of euphoria and diminishes pain immediately after birth. It enhances the feeling of love between you and your baby. It also causes the uterine muscles to contract, and so in the first days or weeks you may feel afterpains, or cramping of the uterus, each time you nurse. Although the pain may be annoying, the cramping helps the uterus return to its normal size and condition and reduces postpartum blood loss. These cramps are a good indicator that your baby is feeding effectively. Use some deep-breathing techniques or mild pain medications to ease the discomfort.

Once lactation has begun, it usually takes only a brief period of sucking before the milk lets down (begins to flow). Just hearing your baby cry may be enough to trigger milk flow. Signs of let-down vary from woman to woman and change with the volume of milk the baby demands. Some women feel a subtle tingling, while others experience a pressure that feels as if their breasts are overfull—sensations that are quickly relieved as the milk starts to flow. Some women never feel these sensations even though the infant is getting plenty of milk. The way the milk flows also varies widely. It may spray, gush, trickle, or flow. Some women have leakage with let-down or between feedings, and others don't; either case is normal. Flow or leakage also may be quite different in each breast—even gushing on one side and trickling on the other. There are slight differences in the ducts on either side, and this is no cause for concern as long as the baby is getting adequate milk.

When you nurse in the days right after birth, you might find it comfortable to lie on your side, with the baby facing you, opposite the breast. If you'd rather sit, use pillows to support your arms and cradle the baby slightly below breast level, making sure their entire body, not just their head, is facing your body.

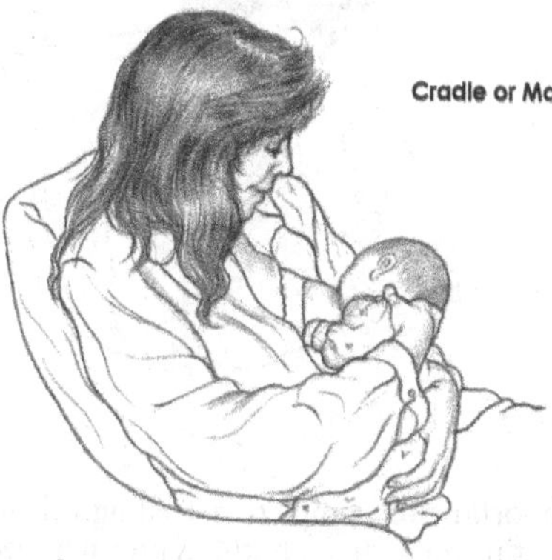

Cradle or Madonna hold

Following delivery, the most comfortable position may be a side hold, also called a football hold, in which you sit and the baby lies at your side facing you. Curl your arm underneath your baby and support their head at your breast. This position keeps the baby's weight off your abdomen, but the infant must squarely face the breast for the proper grasp.

If you stroke your newborn's lip with the nipple, they'll instinctively open wide, latch on, and begin to suck. Infants have been practicing this for some time in utero by sucking their hand, fingers, and possibly even their feet. (Some babies actually are born with blisters on their fingers from this sucking in the womb.) It takes little encouragement to get them to nurse, but you may need to help them properly grasp the areola. You can hold the breast with your thumb above the areola and your fingers and palm underneath it. Some gentle compression may be helpful to form a surface for latch-on. Then, when the baby opens their mouth very wide, pull them onto the breast. It is important to keep the nipple level or pointed slightly up, and to keep your fingers clear of the areola so that the baby can grasp it. Be sure your fingers are no closer than 2 inches from the base of the nipple. Let your baby nurse on one side as long as they wish, then put them on the other side if they are still interested in feeding.

Football or clutch hold

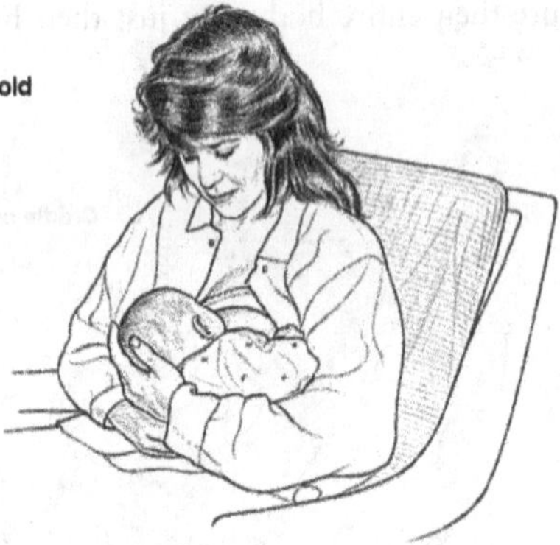

It is more important to complete a feeding on one breast than to have brief feedings from both. With each feeding, the earlier milk is more carbohydrate-packed, and as your baby consumes more, the hindmilk (later milk) becomes fattier and calorie-rich. Let-down, uterine cramping, swallowing sounds, and return to sound sleep by the baby are all signs of successful breastfeeding. In the beginning, it may take a couple of minutes for let-down to occur. Within a week or so, let-down will take place more rapidly and your milk supply will increase dramatically.

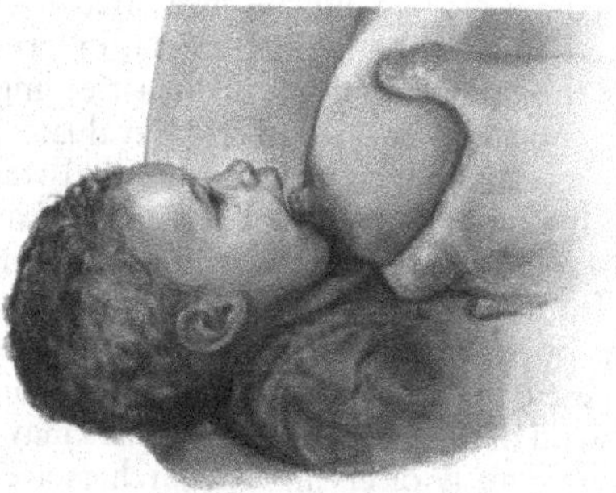

If you stroke your newborn's cheek or lip with your finger or with the nipple, they'll instinctively turn, latch on, and begin to suck. You may need to help them properly grasp the areola.

If you are not sure a let-down is happening, just watch your baby. Following a let-down, your infant should be swallowing after every few sucks. After five or ten minutes, they may switch to a more relaxed non-nutritive sucking that provides emotional comfort along with small amounts of creamier, fat-rich hindmilk. Other signs of let-down vary from woman to woman: uterine cramps the first days after delivery, let-down sensations, milk leakage from the opposite breast, the breast feeling full before and soft after feeding, or milk in or around the baby's mouth after feeding. The more relaxed and confident you feel, the quicker your milk will let down.

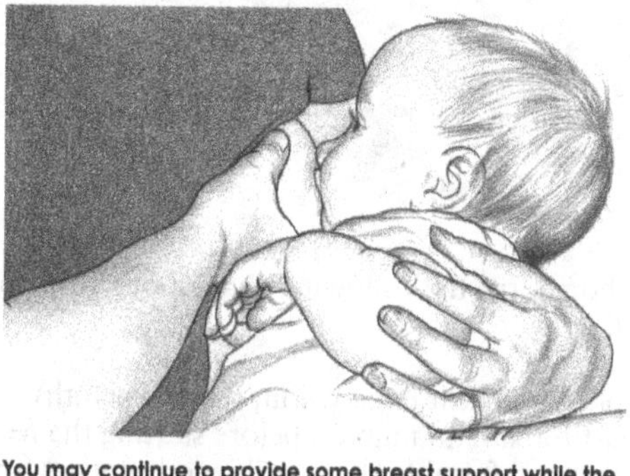

You may continue to provide some breast support while the baby is feeding, especially if your breasts are large.

The first feedings may be difficult. Breastfeeding should not cause sustained pain in the nipple, areola, or breast. If pain remains after the initial moments of breastfeeding, ask your doctor, nurse, or lactation specialist to evaluate the breastfeeding and suggest changes. Ask the hospital staff for help; they are usually very experienced at assisting nursing mothers and babies. In some cases, an infant will have trouble latching on. Suckling from the breast is different from sucking the nipple on a bottle or pacifier, and some infants are sensitive to the difference. These babies may simply lick, nibble, or chew with their jaws instead of using the tongue. Others may show frustration by pulling away or crying. Researchers are still uncertain if artificial nipples are the cause of breastfeeding problems or are just a response to a breastfeeding problem that already existed. Experts recommend that you avoid bottles and pacifiers for the first several weeks until you feel that breastfeeding is well established. During that time, if the baby seems to need more sucking, offer the breast again, or help them find their own hand or fingers to soothe themselves. If your baby has trouble latching on after you leave the hospital, you should call your baby's doctor for help or for a referral if needed.

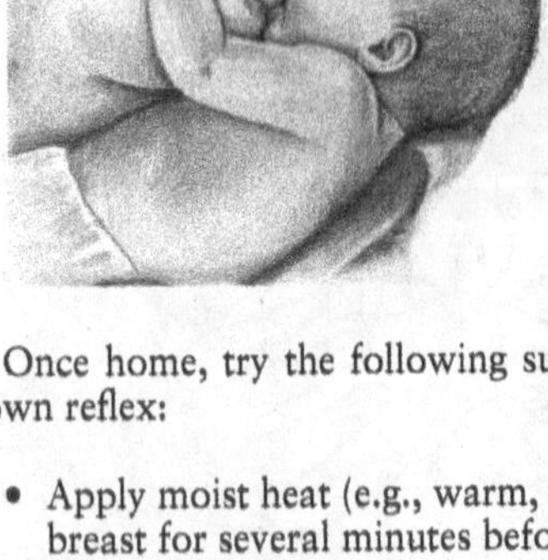

You can slide your finger into the corner of your baby's mouth if you need to interrupt the feeding before the baby is finished.

Once home, try the following suggestions to help the let-down reflex:

- Apply moist heat (e.g., warm, wet washcloths) to the breast for several minutes before starting the feeding.
- Sit in a comfortable chair, with good support for your back and arms. (Many nursing mothers recommend

rocking chairs or gliders, while others do best in a straight-back chair using propping pillows.) At night, when it is common for the baby to fall asleep during breastfeeding, it is best to breastfeed in bed instead of a sofa or chair, then return the baby to a separate sleep surface once the feeding is complete.

- Make sure the baby is positioned so that they squarely face the breast and are well latched on, as described earlier.
- Use some relaxation techniques, such as deep breathing or visual imagery.
- Listen to soothing music. Sip a nutritious drink, or drink water and have a nutritious snack during feedings.
- If your household is very busy, find a quiet corner or room where you won't be disturbed during feedings.
- Do not smoke, and avoid secondhand smoke. Do not use marijuana or illegal drugs (cocaine, heroin, ecstasy, etc.), as all contain substances that can interfere with let-down, affect the content of breast milk, and be harmful to mother and baby. Check with your obstetrician or pediatrician about any prescription or non-prescription drugs, as well as any herbal supplements, you may be taking. If you do drink alcohol, limit your consumption to one serving a day, ideally two hours or more prior to nursing.

If you still are not letting down after trying these suggestions, contact your pediatrician for additional help. If you continue to have difficulties, ask to be referred to a lactation expert.

Having a newborn can be a wonderful time for new parents to work with their doctors to address substance use, especially when breastfeeding. Reducing or eliminating tobacco and nicotine use is better for breast milk and better for the baby's and mother's health. Cannabis contains substances that pass into breast milk and can have effects on a newborn's developing brain, and it's better to eliminate use when breastfeeding. Other substances such as cocaine, ecstasy, and methamphetamine can be dangerous for babies and mothers, and should not be used, especially if breastfeeding. Opioids also pass into human milk and can affect the baby. Parents should work closely with their doctor regarding the use of opioids for pain and treatment for opioid use disorder to make a plan for safe breastfeeding. Alcohol can pass into breast milk. If breastfeeding, alcohol should be limited to one serving a day and at least two hours prior to nursing.

Mothers should talk with their doctors about all medications, including over-the-counter medicines and herbal supplements, and strategies to address substance use. A new baby can open opportunities for positive change for the whole family.

When Your Milk Supply Increases

For the first days after delivery, your breasts will be soft. But as the blood supply increases, your hormones change, and milk-producing cells start to function more efficiently, your breasts will become firmer. By the second to fifth day following delivery, your breasts should be producing transitional milk (milk that follows colostrum) and may feel very full. At the end of the baby's first week, you will see creamy white breast milk. After ten to fourteen days, the milk at the beginning of a feeding may look like skim milk, and as the feeding continues, the amount of fat in the milk will increase and the milk will look creamier. This is normal. Nursing your baby frequently and massaging your breasts prior to and during feeding may help minimize the feeling of fullness.

Engorgement occurs when the breasts become overfilled with milk and excess body fluids. This can be very uncomfortable and at times painful. The best solution is to nurse your baby whenever they are hungry, feeding at both breasts about eight to twelve times per day or before your breasts get swollen, firm, or painful. Sometimes the breasts are so engorged the baby has trouble latching on. If that happens, apply moist heat to soften the breasts, and if necessary, manually express some milk or use a mechanical breast pump before you start to nurse. Doing this may help the baby to get a better grasp and nurse more efficiently. (See *pages 69–73* regarding milk expression.) You also can try several techniques to ease the pain of engorgement, such as:

- Take a warm shower or use a warm washcloth. These techniques, when used just before breastfeeding or expressing milk, will encourage milk flow.

- Warmth may not help cases of severe engorgement, especially if no milk is flowing. In this case, you may want to use cool compresses in between or just after feeding.
- Express milk or pump just enough milk for comfort's sake.
- Try feeding your baby in more than one position. Begin by sitting up, then feed lying down. This changes the segments of the breast that are drained most at each feeding.
- Gently massage your breasts from under the arm and down the nipple. This will help reduce soreness and ease milk flow.
- The use of ibuprofen has been shown to be safe and effective for the treatment of engorgement. Take the dosage recommended by your doctor. Do not take any other medications without your doctor's approval.

Engorgement lasts only a few days, while lactation is getting established. However, your breasts can still get firm or overfilled anytime feedings are skipped and the breast is not emptied. The volume of milk produced increases dramatically over the first week. Your baby may take as little as 1 teaspoon (5 ml) at each feeding the first couple of days, and up to 1 ounce (30 ml) at each feeding by the fourth or fifth day. By the end of the week—depending on the size and appetite of the baby and length of feedings—you may be producing 2 to 6 ounces (60–180 ml) at each feeding. By the end of the first month, your infant should be consuming an average of 24 ounces (720 ml) of milk each day. (See *pages 73–74* for information on how to tell if your baby is getting enough.)

IS YOUR BABY NURSING CORRECTLY? A BREASTFEEDING CHECKLIST

Signs of Correct Nursing

- Your baby's mouth is open wide with lips turned out like the mouth of a fish.
- Your baby's chin is resting against the breast, with their nose close to the breast.

- Your baby has taken as much of the areola as possible into their mouth.
- Your baby is suckling rhythmically and deeply, in short bursts separated by pauses.
- You can hear swallowing regularly after the first couple of days as the baby feeds.
- Your nipple is comfortable after the first few suckles.

Signs of Incorrect Nursing

- Your baby's head is not in line with their body.
- Your baby is sucking on the nipple only, instead of on the areola with the nipple far back in their mouth.
- Your baby is sucking in a light, quick, fluttery manner rather than taking deep, regular suckles.
- Their cheeks are puckered inward, or you hear clicking noises.
- You don't hear your baby swallow regularly after your milk production has increased.
- You experience pain throughout the feed or have signs of nipple damage (such as cracking, bleeding, pinching, or blanching).

Source: American Academy of Pediatrics, ***New Mother's Guide to Breastfeeding***, ed. J. Y. Meek, 4th ed. (New York: Bantam Books, 2024).

WHAT ABOUT VITAMINS FOR BREASTFED BABIES?

Your breast milk provides your baby with all the vitamins they need, except for vitamin D. Even though breast milk (also known as human milk) provides small amounts of vitamin D, it is not enough to prevent rickets (softening of the bones). The current American Academy of Pediatrics recommendation is that all infants and children should have a minimum intake of 400 IU (10 mcg) of vitamin D per day beginning soon after birth, with 600 IU (15 mcg) per day in children over age 1. Prepared formula has vitamin D added to it. If your baby is drinking only formula and takes about 28 ounces (840 ml) per day, they will get the same amount of vitamin D as a supplement of 400 IU (10 mcg) per day. If you are breastfeeding and supplementing with formula, your baby will still require a vitamin D supplement. Some maternal vitamin D can make it into the breast milk. A mother needs to take 6,400 IU (160 mcg) of vitamin D per day for the baby to receive 400 IU (10 mcg).

Your baby also may need vitamin or iron supplements if born prematurely or if they have certain other medical problems. Discuss the need for supplements of vitamins or minerals with your doctor.

If you are a vegan (that is, you eat a diet that excludes all foods of animal origin), talk about your nutritional needs with your pediatrician. A vegan diet lacks not only vitamin D but also vitamin B12. A deficiency in B12 can lead to anemia and nervous system abnormalities.

(For more information about vitamin D and supplements, see Where We Stand, *pages 91–92*.)

BREASTFEEDING TWINS

Twins present a unique challenge to the nursing mother. At first it may be easier to feed them one at a time, but after lactation is established, often it's more convenient and time-saving to feed them simultaneously. Feeding them together can also increase your milk supply. You can do this using the football hold to position one at each side, or cradle them both in front of you with their bodies crossing each other.

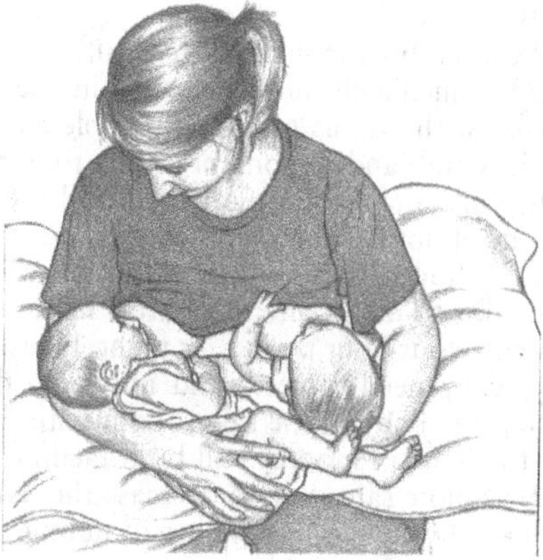

(For more information about raising multiples, seek out support groups like La Leche League or consider books such as ***Raising Twins: Parenting Multiples from Pregnancy Through the School Years***, 3rd edition, by Shelly Vaziri Flais, MD, FAAP, published by the American Academy of Pediatrics, 2019.)

How Often and How Long?

Breastfed newborns vary greatly in their feeding behaviors. They generally eat more frequently than formula-fed infants, eight to twelve (or more) times per twenty-four hours. As they get older, with enlarged stomach capacity and the mother's increased milk production, some can go longer between feedings. Others continue to prefer frequent, smaller feeds.

The best feeding schedule for a breastfed baby is the one they design on their own, called responsive feeding. Your baby lets you know they're hungry by waking and looking alert, putting hands toward their mouth, making sucking motions, whimpering, flexing arms and hands, becoming more active, and nuzzling against your breast (they can smell its location even through your clothing). It is best to nurse your baby before they start crying, a late sign of hunger. Whenever possible, use these signals rather than the clock to decide when to nurse. This way, you'll ensure they're hungry. In the process, your baby will stimulate the breast more efficiently to produce milk.

As stated earlier, breastfeeding is generally most successful when started immediately after delivery (in the first hour). Keep the baby with you as much as possible (rooming with them in the hospital) and respond promptly to hunger cues (a practice called demand feeding). A baby may have one or two 4-hour periods of not feeding, but then will feed frequently in the intervening hours. It is best to tally the feeds over the course of the day to make sure there are a minimum of eight feeds per twenty-four-hour period. At night, breastfeeding babies will typically need to feed, and not sleep through the night; keeping the baby in the same room with you at night for at least the first six months will both facilitate cue-based feeding and promote safe sleep to decrease the risk of sudden infant death syndrome. Long stretches of uninterrupted sleep are not typical for a breastfeeding baby until they are about 4 months old and generally weigh over 12 pounds (5.4 kg).

Allow your baby to nurse on the first breast as long as desired. When they stop for a prolonged period or withdraw from the breast, burp them. If they seem sleepy after the first breast, you may want to wake them up by changing their diaper or playing with them a little before switching to the second side. Since your infant suckles more efficiently on the first breast they use, you should alternate which breast you offer first from feeding to feeding. You might consider placing a safety pin or other marker on your clothing on the side last nursed as a reminder. Or you can start on the breast that feels fuller.

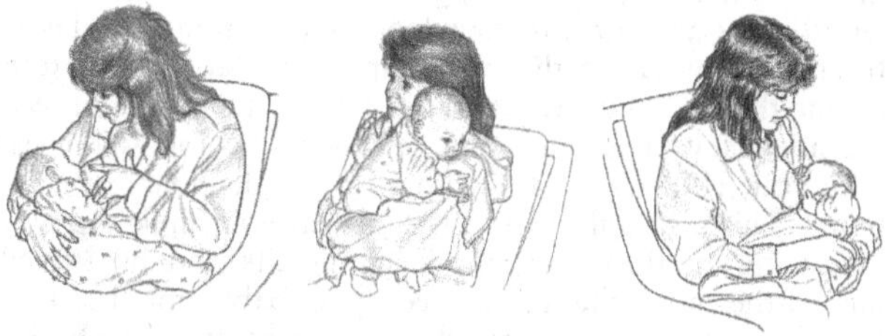

Your baby will generally feed for about ten to fifteen minutes on the first breast. Then your baby can be burped and offered the other breast.

Initially your newborn will probably nurse every couple of hours, regardless of whether it's day or night. By 6 to 8 weeks of age, many newborns have one sleep period of four to five hours. Establish nighttime sleep patterns by keeping the room dark, warm, and quiet. Don't use a bright light for nighttime feedings. If their diaper is soiled or wet, change it quickly and without fanfare before feeding and put them right back to sleep afterward. By 4 months, many—but not all—babies are sleeping six hours or more at night without awakening. However, some breastfed babies may continue to awaken more frequently for night feedings. (See Helping Your Baby Sleep, *page 105*.)

You'll also find that your infant may require long feedings at certain times and be satisfied quickly at others. They'll let you know when they're finished by letting go or drifting off to sleep between spurts of non-nutritive sucking. A few babies want to nurse around the clock. If your baby falls into this category, check with your pediatrician's office. You may be referred to a lactation specialist. There are several reasons infants behave this way, and the sooner the situation is evaluated, the easier it is to address the cause.

IS YOUR BABY EATING ENOUGH?

In the first week after birth, doctors will check your newborn to ensure that weight loss is not excessive (more than 10 percent of the birth weight), there is no excessive jaundice, and your baby is producing at least a few wet diapers and stools per day. Starting two days after birth, wet diapers and stooling are reliable signs of feeding. There should be four to eight wet diapers and three to four loose, seedy stools per day by the third day. Given that wet diapers and stooling patterns during the first two days can be unreliable indicators of feeding adequacy, it is important to schedule a follow-up visit with your pediatrician for within forty-eight hours of going home. This visit will help to ensure that your milk supply is increasing and that your baby is getting milk from breastfeeding. By the end of the second week, your baby should be back to birth weight or have gained some weight. If you've breastfed other children, lactation will probably be established more quickly this time, so the new baby may lose little weight and return to birth weight within days.

During the first month, after your milk supply increases, an adequate diet should produce six or more wet diapers a day and generally three or four (or more) bowel movements (often one little one after each feeding). Later, they may have less frequent bowel movements, and there may even be a day or more between them. If bowel movements are soft and your baby is otherwise thriving, this is typical. Another clue about intake is whether you can hear your baby swallow, usually after several sucks. Appearing satisfied for a couple of hours after a feeding is also a sign. On the other hand, a baby who is not getting enough to eat over several days may become very sleepy and seem "easy" to care for. In the early weeks, a baby who is excessively sleepy or feeds less frequently than eight times in a twenty-four-hour period should be seen by the pediatrician to make sure they are gaining weight as expected.

Once your milk supply is established, your baby should

gain between ½ and 1 ounce (14–28 g) a day during the first three months. Between three and six months, weight gain will taper off to about ½ ounce (14 g) a day, and after six months, weight gains each day will be even less. Your pediatrician will weigh the baby at every visit. If you have concerns between visits, call to schedule an appointment; don't depend on a home scale, as they are not very reliable for young infants.

When You Need to Give Expressed Milk

If circumstances keep you away from your baby, you will need to express breast milk, manually or mechanically, to stimulate continued milk production. The hospital staff will work with you to express your milk in a way that enables transitioning back to the breast, including using feeding techniques that avoid bottles and nipples. These techniques may include syringe or cup feeding, paced bottle-feeding, or feeding through a supplemental nursing system. Always check with your pediatrician or other expert before you stop giving your breast milk to your baby or begin supplementing with formula.

Once the milk supply is established, usually three or four weeks after delivery, you may decide to use a bottle for expressed milk so that you can be away during some feedings. Expressing breast milk in advance and storing it allows your baby to receive the benefits of your milk by bottle. In addition, using expressed breast milk will maintain your body's full milk production. An occasional bottle at this stage probably won't interfere with your baby's nursing habits, but it may lead to the problem of engorgement if the milk isn't expressed in a timely manner. Milk you express while you're away from your baby should be stored so that you can replace the breast milk used by other caregivers while you are away. Wearing nursing pads will help you manage leakage. (Some women wear nursing pads constantly during the first month or two to avoid milk stains.) It is important to either breastfeed or express your milk regularly throughout the day to avoid engorgement and potential problems from milk stasis, which may lead to decreased milk production or clogged ducts.

Milk Expression and Storage

Milk can be expressed most commonly with a double electric breast pump, covered by most insurances. Other options are a hand pump, a manual pump, or an electric pump. In any case, you must have the let-down reflex for the milk to flow. Manual or hand expression is easier to learn visually, rather than just reading about it, and can be quick and effective once learned, though it requires practice. Many hospitals teach mothers hand expression before leaving the hospital. Using breast pumps may seem easier than learning hand expression, but the quality of pumps varies widely. Luckily, there are many quality pumps available at various price points. A poor-quality breast pump will not remove milk effectively, resulting in engorgement or a gradually lower milk supply over time. Poor-quality breast pumps also may irritate the nipples or be painful.

Hand Expression and Handheld Pumps

If you choose to hand-express, wash your hands and use a clean container to collect the milk. Place your thumb above the areola and your fingers underneath. Gently but firmly roll the thumb and fingers toward each other while compressing the breast tissue and pushing toward the chest wall. Do not slide your fingers toward your nipple, as this can cause soreness. Transfer the milk to a clean bottle, rigid plastic container, or specially made plastic bag for storage in the freezer (see *pages 72–73*). If your baby is hospitalized, the hospital may give you specific and detailed information about milk collection and storage, and may lend you a double electric breast pump.

Another category of breast pump is the handheld pump with its own suction, which many moms use while feeding on one side to collect milk from the other side, or just to gently suction out and collect milk in lieu of actually "pumping." Note that it works best for breastfeeding women who already have an established milk supply, as it may not have enough suction to increase or establish supply.

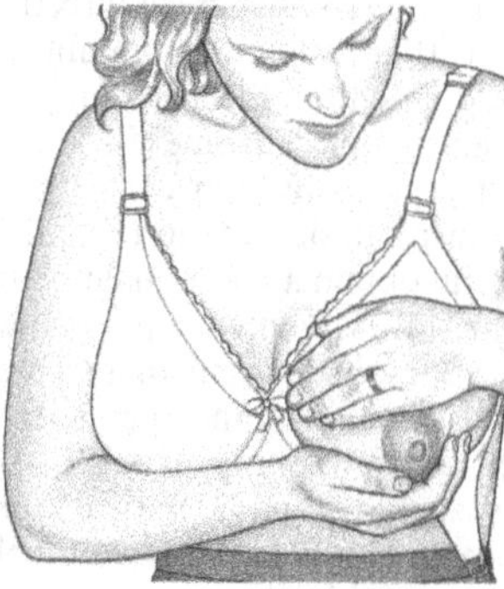

Expressing milk is easier if you stimulate the breast first by massaging it gently.

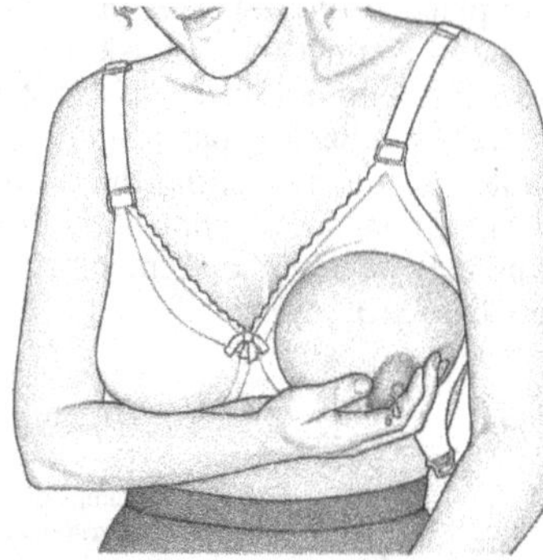

To use hand expression, hold the breast with the thumb and index finger at the edge of the areola on opposite sides of the breast, then press toward the chest wall with a rhythmic motion. Rotate the position of the fingers.

Electric Breast Pump

While manual breast pumps are available and may be easy to use while out and about, good-quality double electric breast pumps are optimal. Electric pumps can stimulate the breast more effectively than manual expression. These pumps have regulated pressures and are self-cycling for efficient milk removal. They are used primarily to induce or maintain lactation when a mother is unable to breastfeed directly for several days or more, such as with a hospitalized infant, or when the mother returns to work or school. Electric pumps are efficient but can be costly, ranging in price from $50 to $300 and up. If you need a pump temporarily, you can rent one from a medical supply store, hospital, or lactation rental agency.

In many states, you can obtain a good-quality pump through your insurance or your state's Women, Infants, and Children (WIC) program. Ask your obstetrician or pediatrician for a prescription and talk to your insurance provider to find out where to purchase a covered pump. The costs related to breastfeeding supplies, such as pumps, may also be a deductible item if you participate in a flexible spending plan.

When shopping for a double electric pump, make sure it creates a steady milking action with variable pressure, not simply suction. There are also bras and tops available to help hold both cones in place at once. Make sure that all parts of the pump that come in contact with the skin or milk can be removed for proper cleaning. Sterilization is not required for pumps and containers for a healthy baby; simply washing well with hot soapy water is fine, as is using the dishwasher. Talk to your pediatrician or lactation consultant for advice on which type of pump may be best. And remember to wash your hands immediately before pumping.

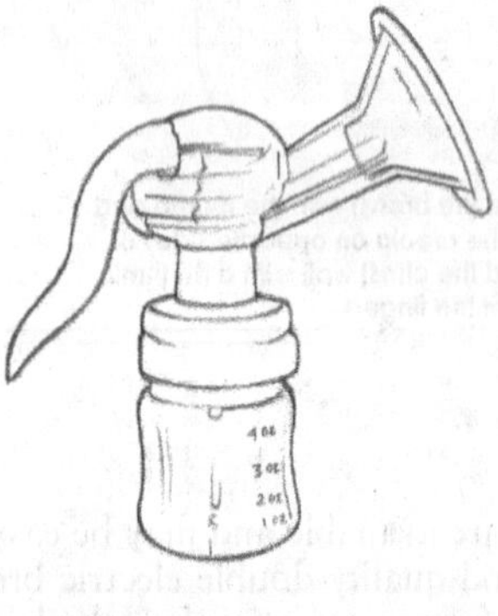

Hand pumps are available at most drugstores and baby stores.

Pumped milk should be stored in clean containers, preferably glass or rigid plastic, or special plastic bags. Baby bottle insert bags are not sufficiently strong or thick enough to protect the milk from contamination. Expressed breast milk can be stored safely at room temperature for three to five hours, in the refrigerator for up to three to five days, or in a freezer (0 degrees Fahrenheit [−20 degrees Celsius]) for up to nine months. Store frozen breast milk in the back of the freezer, where it's coldest. Write the date on each container, and use the oldest milk first. It's useful to freeze milk in the amount needed for a single feeding, about 3 to 4 ounces (90–120 ml). You also can freeze some 1- to 2-ounce portions (30–60 ml), which come in handy if the baby wants a little extra at any feeding.

When it's time to use stored milk, keep in mind that your baby is accustomed to breast milk at body temperature, so the milk may need to be heated to at least room temperature (68–72 degrees Fahrenheit [20–22 degrees Celsius]). Frozen milk may be thawed in the refrigerator, under warm running water, or in a container of warm water. Don't use the microwave to warm milk, as this leads to uneven heating and risk of scalding, and also damages the antibodies and other important components of breast milk needed for immunity and nutrient absorption. Once milk is thawed, its fat may separate, but this has no effect on quality. Swirl the container gently until the milk returns to a uniform consistency. Stored breast milk may have an altered smell or taste due to the breakdown of fat. This is not harmful to the baby. Thawed milk should be refrigerated and used within twenty-four hours. Never refreeze. If the infant does not finish all the thawed breast milk in the bottle, it should be consumed within one to two hours or discarded.

"IS MY NEWBORN GETTING ENOUGH MILK?"

Nearly all new mothers worry about whether their babies are properly nourished. Breastfeeding mothers cannot measure exactly how much milk their newborns take, but they can tell in other ways whether their babies are getting enough to eat. Your well-nourished newborn should:

- Lose no more than around 8–10 percent of their birth weight in the first few days after birth before starting to gain weight again.
- Have one or two bowel movements per day on days 1 and 2, with blackish, tarry stools, and at least two

stools that are beginning to appear greenish to yellow on days 3 and 4. By 5 to 7 days, their stools should be yellow and loose, with small curds, and should number at least three to four per day. When your milk production increases, your baby will often produce stool with each feeding for the first month after birth.

- Have six or more wet diapers per day, with nearly colorless or pale yellow urine, by 5 to 7 days.
- Seem satisfied and happy for an average of one to three hours between feedings.
- Nurse at least eight to twelve times every twenty-four hours.

Schedule your newborn's first checkup with the pediatrician or family physician for no more than forty-eight hours after hospital discharge. The weight check at that visit will help to determine the adequacy of feedings.

Source: Adapted from American Academy of Pediatrics, ***New Mother's Guide to Breastfeeding***, ed. J. Y. Meek, 4th ed. (New York: Bantam Books, 2024).

Not all breastfed babies react to the bottle the same way. Some accept it easily, regardless of when it is introduced and by whom. Others take an occasional bottle but may prefer a specific caregiver. It is possible that your baby will first accept a bottle if someone other than the mother offers it and if she is out of sight at the time. Once familiar with the bottle, your baby may take it from any caregiver. If your breastfed baby refuses a bottle, try a cup or sippy cup instead. Even premature newborns can cup-feed. Some breastfed babies go from breast to cup without ever using a bottle.

Possible Breastfeeding Concerns and Questions

For some, nursing goes well from the start and there are never problems. But breastfeeding can have its ups and downs, especially in the beginning. Fortunately, many common difficulties can be prevented with proper positioning and latch-on along with frequent feedings. Problems may resolve quickly if you seek advice right away. Don't hesitate to ask your pediatrician or office nurse for help with the following problems.

Sore and Cracked Nipples. Breastfeeding may produce initial mild soreness, especially with latch-on, in the first week or so. Breastfeeding should not cause sustained pain, discomfort, or open cracks. Proper latch-on is the most important factor in preventing sore and cracked nipples. If your nipples or other areas of the breast are painful, seek advice from your lactation expert.

During bathing, wash your breasts with mild soap, taking care to use only water on the nipple. Creams, lotions, and more vigorous rubbing are not necessary and may actually aggravate a problem. Also, try varying the baby's position at each feeding to help with nipple irritation.

You may use purified lanolin on cracked or dry nipples to protect them and allow them to heal. If this does not solve the problem, consult your doctor or lactation consultant for further advice; you might have a yeast or bacterial infection of the nipple, or may have a skin condition such as dermatitis that requires treatment.

Engorgement. As already mentioned, your breasts can become severely engorged if your baby doesn't nurse often or efficiently during the first few days after your milk comes in. While some engorgement is to be expected when lactation starts, extreme engorgement causes swelling of the milk ducts and of blood vessels across the entire chest area. The best treatment is to breastfeed frequently; express milk between feedings, either manually or with a pump; and offer both breasts at every feeding. If the baby feeds from only one side, it may help to manually express milk from the other side. Since warmth encourages milk flow, standing in a warm shower as you manually express may help. You also may get relief with warm compresses during nursing and cool compresses between nursing. If engorgement persists, it may lead to a decrease in milk production. This happens because breasts have a mechanism to turn off milk production when milk is not removed from the breast. To avoid problems with breast milk supply, it is important to relieve engorgement as soon as it is recognized.

Mastitis. Mastitis is an infection of the breast tissue caused by bacteria. Mastitis causes flu-like symptoms of fever, chills, headache, nausea, dizziness, and lack of energy. These general symptoms occur along with localized symptoms of redness, tenderness, swelling, heat, and pain in and around the breast. If you experience any of these symptoms, call your doctor at once. The infection is treated with milk removal (by feeding or pumping), rest, fluids, antibiotics, and pain medicine if needed. Your doctor will prescribe an antibiotic that is safe during breastfeeding. Be sure to take all the antibiotics even if you feel better. Do not stop nursing; doing so will worsen the mastitis and cause increased pain. The milk itself is not infected. Your baby will not be harmed by nursing during mastitis, and neither mastitis nor the antibiotics will change milk composition.

Mastitis may be a sign your body's immune defenses are down. Bed rest, sleep, and decreased activity will help you recover your stamina. Rarely, you may find it's too painful to nurse on the infected breast; in that case, let the milk flow from the painful breast onto a clean towel or absorbent cloth, relieving the pressure as you nurse from the opposite side. Then your baby can finish feeding on the infected side with less discomfort for you. Some women with severe pain find it is more comfortable to pump the breast than to feed the baby directly, even if just for a few feedings. The pumped milk can be stored or fed to the baby immediately after.

A mother's return to work is a peak time for the development of mastitis. It is important to express milk regularly, approximately on the same schedule as the baby would feed, to try to prevent the infection.

SUPPLEMENTAL NURSER (INFANT FEEDING DEVICE)

The amount of milk your breasts produce depends on the amount of milk removed from them. If you miss too many feedings, your body will decrease milk production. This can occur even if you express milk during missed feedings, since pumps do not stimulate or empty the breasts nearly as efficiently as your baby's sucking.

If your milk supply is not meeting the needs of your baby, if you miss a number of feedings because of illness, or if your baby is unable to nurse for some reason, you may be able to reestablish your milk supply by nursing more frequently (every hour for twenty-four hours) or by using a supplemental nurser (also known as a supplementer tube, infant feeding device, or nursing trainer). Unlike a bottle, which trains the baby away from the breast, this device provides supplemental expressed milk or formula while the infant is at the breast.

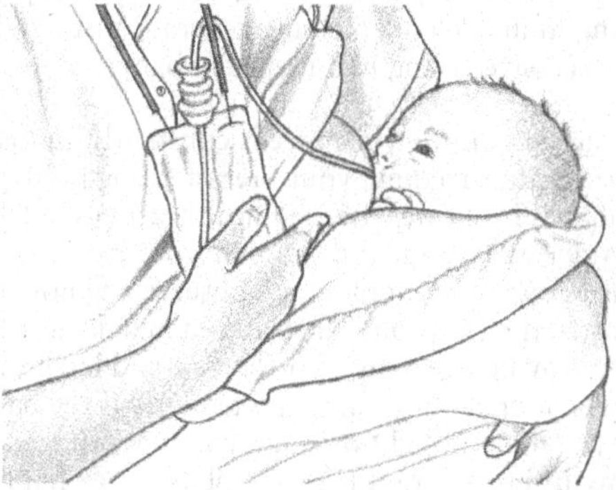

The supplemental nurser is also used to feed premature infants or to train babies with feeding problems. It even can help stimulate lactation in adoptive mothers, or in mothers who stopped breastfeeding for a prolonged period and wish to start again.

Hung from your neck, the container holding the formula or expressed milk has a thin flexible tube aligned along the breast with its tip adjacent to the nipple and placed in the corner of the baby's mouth as they suck. The suction draws the formula or breast milk from the container, so even if you aren't producing much milk, the baby will still get a full feeding. This reinforces the infant's desire to nurse at the breast. At the same time, the sucking stimulates your body to step up milk production.

Supplemental nursers are available from lactation specialists, medical supply stores, some pharmacies, or online. If possible, purchase the device from someone who can show you how to use and clean it. Most mothers and babies need a few days of practice to get comfortable with the device. Using a supplemental nurser requires commitment and dedication, as it may take weeks or months to rebuild the milk supply and the breastfeeding relationship.

Infant Fussiness. Sometimes babies, even breastfed babies, can be unusually fussy. Reasons for fussiness can range from normal personality variations to serious illness. Although most fussy babies do not have a serious medical problem, their constant crying can become extremely difficult for parents. The fussy baby wears on a parent's energy, time, and enjoyment of their young infant. Here are some general causes and suggestions for excessive crying in a breastfed baby:

- Hunger. If your newborn feeds constantly and is never satisfied after feeding, your breastfeeding needs to be evaluated by an experienced healthcare provider. Your provider will weigh and examine your baby, examine your breasts and nipples, and observe an entire breastfeeding session. The solution may be as simple as improving the baby's positioning and latch-on, or it may be more complicated, particularly if the baby has lost too much weight or is not gaining well.
- Growth spurt. A rapid growth phase often happens at 2 to 3 weeks of age, again around 6 weeks, and again at about 3 months. During these spurts, babies will want to nurse constantly. Many women think this is because the baby is not getting enough to eat (which is correct) and are tempted to give supplemental bottles. However, the baby is doing what is right. When you nurse constantly or every hour or so for several days, your breasts will make more milk. Remember, this is normal and only temporary; keep breastfeeding frequently, and do not give your baby other liquids. If this frequent feeding does not return to a more regular pattern after four to five days, or if you are tempted to start bottles, call your pediatrician's office for assistance. They should see the baby, check their weight, and evaluate the feeding process (or refer you to a lactation specialist if needed).
- Colic. Colic begins after 4 weeks of age. Colicky babies generally have at least one period each day when they appear to be in pain, crying hard, turning red, and drawing their legs up. They may act hungry, but then pull back and refuse the breast. Your baby's doctor can provide suggestions for managing colic. (For more on colic, see *pages 140–42*.)

- Oversupply or overactive let-down of breast milk. This could begin at any time in the first month. Your breasts will feel very full, and you may experience lots of leaking and spraying. Your baby will be gulping down milk very fast, sometimes pulling away to catch their breath or coughing or sputtering milk. As a result, the baby swallows lots of air and milk. Later, gas bubbles form, causing discomfort. Your pediatrician may guide you to a lactation consultant to assist with this problem. (Also see Engorgement, *page 75*.)
- Reflux (also called gastroesophageal reflux, or GER). Most newborns spit up after feeding. This is normal and requires no treatment. When spitting up results in problems such as fussiness, becomes more like vomiting (much larger amounts), or is associated with weight loss, your baby should be evaluated by your pediatrician. Physiological reflux is normal in all infants until 12 months of age and may be more prominent in preterm infants. Medication (antacid) is not required as long as your infant is gaining normal weight. (For more on reflux, see *pages 378–79*.)
- Allergies. Although infant crying is often blamed on food allergies, such allergies are much less common than some other reasons for fussiness. Allergies occur more often in babies from families where the mother, father, or siblings are affected by asthma, eczema, or other allergic diseases. Proteins in breast milk can be the source of allergy or irritation. The most common causes are dairy, eggs, peanuts, other nuts, soy, and wheat. It can be difficult to pinpoint the precise food, however, and symptoms can linger for more than a week after the food has been removed from the mother's diet. A milk protein allergy, also called food protein–induced allergic proctocolitis (FPIAP), can result in blood in the stool. If blood in the stool is the only symptom, then generally no treatment is necessary, but a pediatrician should evaluate the baby thoroughly to be sure. However, food allergies can be very serious, sometimes causing wheezing, hives, vomiting/diarrhea, and/or shock (collapse). Severe food allergies require the attention of your pediatrician.

- Other serious illnesses. Illnesses not related to feeding may cause babies to cry endlessly, unable to be comforted. If this occurs suddenly or seems unusually severe, call your pediatrician or seek emergency care immediately.

The Cancer Question. Most studies indicate that breastfeeding offers some protection against breast cancer, perhaps because nursing lowers the total number of menstrual cycles during a woman's lifetime (see cancer.org). If a woman has been diagnosed with cancer or has had a malignant tumor removed but is no longer on chemo or radiation therapy, breastfeeding should be safe (check with your physician). Breastfeeding is also safe after removal of a benign (noncancerous) breast lump or cyst.

Breastfeeding After Plastic Surgery on the Breasts. Plastic surgery to enlarge the breasts usually does not interfere with breastfeeding—provided the breasts were previously normal, the nipples were not moved, and no ducts were cut. Breastfeeding after breast reduction surgery is highly individual. Surgery to reduce breast size typically involves at least some disruption of breast tissue and often movement of the entire nipple and areola. Each mother-baby pair must be helped and followed individually. Your baby's weight should be checked more frequently, at least twice a week for the first few weeks, until the baby is gaining well. You can still breastfeed and supplement with formula if you aren't able to produce enough breast milk. This will provide your baby with some of the benefits of receiving breast milk. Make sure you discuss all concerns with your doctor. Your baby's pediatrician needs to be aware of previous breast surgery you've had so that your infant can be followed closely.

Bottle-Feeding

Even with tremendous effort and plenty of support, breastfeeding does not always go well for every mother-infant pair. In other cases, parents who recognize the benefits of breastfeeding may still prefer bottle-feeding. Some believe bottle-feeding provides more freedom and time for activities. Dad, grandparents, sitters, and even older siblings can feed an infant breast milk or formula in a bottle. This may give some mothers more flexibility. There are other reasons some feel more comfortable with bottle-feeding, such as knowing exactly how much food the baby is getting. Others prefer formula-feeding for reasons such as not needing to worry about the mother's diet or medications that might affect the milk.

Even so, it is impossible for formula manufacturers to reproduce the components that make breast milk from mothers so unique. Although formula does provide the basic nutrients for an infant, it lacks the antibodies, some of the specific components and sugars that feed good bacteria in a baby's gut, and many of the other components found in breast milk. Formula-feeding is also costly and may be inconvenient for some families. The formula must be bought and prepared or otherwise managed, and you'll need a reliable source of clean water for mixing the formula. This means trips to the kitchen in the middle of the night, as well as extra bottles, nipples, and other equipment.

If you have decided to bottle-feed your baby, you'll start by selecting a formula. Your pediatrician will help you pick one based on your baby's needs. Today there are several varieties and brands of commercial formulas from which to choose, all of which are equally safe and nutritious. The American Academy of Pediatrics does not recommend homemade baby formulas, since they can be deficient in vitamins and other important nutrients and may be contaminated with potentially harmful bacteria.

Why Infant Formula Instead of Cow's Milk?

Many parents ask why they can't feed their infant under 1 year of age cow's milk. The answer is simple: Infants cannot digest cow's milk as completely or easily as they do infant formula. Also, cow's milk contains high concentrations of protein and minerals, which can stress a newborn's immature kidneys and cause severe illness at times of heat stress, fever, or diarrhea. In addition, cow's milk lacks the proper amounts of iron, vitamin C, and other nutrients infants need. It may even cause iron-deficiency anemia, since cow's milk protein can irritate the lining of the stomach and intestine, leading to loss of blood in the stools. Cow's milk also does not contain the healthiest types of fat for growing babies. Your infant should not receive any cow's milk (or other non-human animal milk or milk substitute) for the first twelve months after birth.

Once over 1 year old, your child may consume whole cow's milk or reduced-fat (2 percent) milk, provided they have a balanced diet of solid foods (cereals, vegetables, fruits, and meats). Their intake should be limited to 2 cups (approximately 16 ounces [480 ml]) per day or less. More than 24 ounces a day (720 ml) has been associated with iron deficiency if toddlers aren't getting enough other healthy iron-rich foods. If your infant is not yet eating a broad range of nutrient-dense solid food, talk to your pediatrician about the best nutrition for them.

Most children over 1 year of age still need a higher fat content, which is why vitamin D–fortified whole milk is recommended. If your child has overweight or is at risk for having overweight, or if there is a family history of obesity, high blood pressure, or heart disease, your pediatrician may recommend 2 percent (reduced-fat) milk. Do not give your baby 1 percent (low-fat) or non-fat (skim) milk before their second birthday, as it does not contain enough fat for brain development. After 2 years of age, you should discuss your child's nutritional needs, including choice of milk products, with your pediatrician.

Dairy substitutes, such as milks made from nuts, rice, or soy, are increasingly popular in the grocery aisle; however, they usually do not provide appropriate nutrition for your baby. Typically, compared to cow's milk, they may contain less protein and fewer calories, although most do contain vitamin D. Check the labels to compare nutritional content when making a choice and always ask your pediatrician about the appropriateness of any milk substitution.

Choosing a Formula

To maintain safety standards, the US Food and Drug Administration (FDA) governs the nutrient content and safe manufacturing and distribution of all infant formulas sold in the United States. When shopping for infant formula, you'll find several basic types. Infant formulas with cow's milk, goat's milk, and soy protein isolate are all acceptable choices.

Cow's-milk-based formulas account for the majority of formula sold in the United States. Although cow's milk is the basis for many formulas, the milk has been heat-treated and fortified during the manufacturing process, making it safe for infants. The same is true for infant formula made from goat's milk. Both dairy milks are specifically treated during the process of making the infant formula in order to make the protein more digestible. More milk carbohydrate (lactose) is added to make the concentration more similar to that found in breast milk. Many US infant formulas use a skim or non-fat milk base and then add additional vegetable oils that support the infant's energy needs and also provide dietary essential fatty acids important for normal growth and development. The use of whole milk instead of skim milk is more common outside the United States and is growing in availability and acceptance in the US medical community. Whole-milk-based infant formula provides a natural nutrient base of fats with milk fat globule membrane (MFGM) and requires fewer vegetable oils to be added to meet nutrient requirements. However, all infant formulas contain vegetable oils to deliver the essential fatty acids needed to support normal growth and development.

All infant formulas have added iron. These iron-fortified formulas have dramatically reduced the rate of iron-deficiency anemia in infancy in recent decades. Some infants do not have enough natural reserves of iron, a mineral necessary for normal human growth and development. For that reason, the American Academy of Pediatrics currently recommends that iron-fortified infant formula be used for all infants who are not breastfed, or who are only partially breastfed, from birth to 1 year of age. Additional iron is available in many foods (including baby food), especially in meats, egg yolks, and iron-fortified cereals. Low-iron formulas are not recommended and should not be used. Some parents may worry about iron causing constipation, but the amount of iron in infant formula does not contribute to constipation. Most formulas also have docosahexaenoic acid (DHA) and arachidonic acid (ARA) added to them. These are fatty acids that are found in human milk and are important for the development of a baby's brain and eyes.

Some formulas contain probiotics, types of "friendly" bacteria thought to support gut health. Others may contain added prebiotics, such as oligosaccharides, in an attempt to mimic the natural breast milk oligosaccharides, which are substances that promote gut development and particularly support the intestinal lining. (For more information on probiotics, see *page 85*.)

Goat's-milk-based infant formulas are a newer type of formula in US markets. In recent years, a handful of goat's-milk-based infant formulas have been registered by the FDA and listed by the AAP as nutritionally complete. Goat's-milk-based formulas have a different dominant protein than most cow's-milk-based formulas. Because of this difference, FDA-registered goat's-milk-based infant formula can sometimes be a feeding option for babies who have difficulty digesting the proteins in cow's-milk-based formulas. However, raw goat's milk, like raw cow's milk, is not safe to feed a baby.

Soy infant formulas contain a soy protein isolate instead of dairy milk and include carbohydrates such as modified corn syrup instead of the lactose typically used in dairy-milk-based infant formula. Soy-protein-based infant formulas have typically been recommended when there is a concern about dairy milk protein sensitivity or intolerance or suspected allergic reaction to cow's milk, although around half of infants allergic to milk protein are also allergic to soy. Soy protein infant formulas are rarely used as a starter infant formula unless there is a history of intolerance with dairy-based feedings. Soy protein formulas may be recommended for infants with a rare genetic condition called galactosemia.

Another type of formula is called hydrolyzed formula, which contains varying levels of enzymatically digested protein that has been broken down into smaller pieces to support digestion. Elemental formulas or amino-acid-based formulas are also available for infants with allergies or other medical conditions and are well tolerated when needed. Ask your pediatrician to recommend a brand of hydrolyzed or elemental formula if one is needed for allergies or other medical conditions. These formulas do tend to be costlier than regular formulas.

With a milk protein allergy, also called food protein-induced allergic proctocolitis (FPIAP), which causes bloody stools in well infants, and possibly colic, failure to thrive, and diarrhea, the reaction is to the protein in the cow's-milk formula. Up to half the infants who have FPIAP are also sensitive to soy protein and thus must be given specialized formula (such as elemental or amino-acid-based), or breast milk while their mother eliminates milk and/or soy in her diet.

Some strict vegetarian and vegan parents choose to use soy formula because it contains no animal products. Remember that breastfeeding is the best option for vegetarian and vegan families. And while some parents believe a soy formula might prevent or ease the symptoms of colic or fussiness, there is no evidence to support this.

There are specialized formulas for infants with specific disorders or diseases, including for premature babies. If your pediatrician recommends a specialized formula, follow their guidance about feeding requirements (amounts, scheduling, special preparations), since these may be different from regular formulas.

PROBIOTICS

"Probiotic" (meaning "for life") is a word you may see when shopping for infant formula and supplements. Some formulas are fortified with probiotics, which are types of live bacteria.

Research is ongoing about the benefits of probiotics for health and which ones and in what doses they may be preferred. Before giving your baby a supplement or infant formula fortified with probiotics, discuss the issue with your pediatrician. (For more information about probiotics, see *page 360*.)

Feeding and Oral Health

As the number one chronic disease in US children, dental caries (cavities) should be a concern for all parents. Research has shown that diet and hygiene practices in the first 24 months after birth play a significant role in the risk of cavities as the child becomes older. While much more beneficial than cow's milk or formula, breast milk contains a sugar, lactose. Breastfeeding until up to 12 months of age decreases the risk of dental caries by half, most likely due to other immune-modulating effects and a protective microbiome, despite the lactose in breast milk.

It's not clear whether nighttime breastfeeding after 12 months causes dental caries, but the increased risk of dental caries with nighttime bottle-feeding has been more clearly established. To protect teeth from the natural sugars in breast milk and formula, the AAP recommends the nighttime routine of "brush, book, bed." This encourages nighttime toothbrushing and keeps kids from needing to feed in order to fall asleep. If it is not possible to brush before a nap or bedtime after feeds, the teeth should be wiped to minimize risk of caries. As children grow older and get more teeth, it is more important to protect teeth from the natural sugars in milk. Seeking counseling from a pediatric dentist to review individual dental caries risk factors by age 1 can help families make healthy choices for their situation.

Preparing, Sterilizing, and Storing Formula

Most infant formulas are available in ready-to-feed liquid forms and/or powders. Although ready-to-feed formulas are very convenient, they are also the most expensive. Formula from concentrate is prepared by adding water as the manufacturer directs. Unused concentrate may be covered and refrigerated for no more than forty-eight hours. Powder, usually the least expensive, comes either in premeasured packets or in a larger can. It's important to read the label and make sure you mix the right amounts of powder and water. Mix thoroughly to ensure that there are no clumps of undissolved powder. Always read the label instructions for mixing the formula properly. Please note that some international and specialty formulas, for example, may have different mixing instructions, so always use the scoop that comes with the container and follow the specific directions on the formula container you are using.

Powder is also light and portable. The powder will not spoil, even if it stays in the bottle several days before adding water. If you choose a formula requiring preparation, be sure to follow the manufacturer's directions exactly. Too much water and your baby won't get the calories and nutrients needed for proper growth; too little and the extra-concentrated formula could cause diarrhea or dehydration and will give your infant more calories than needed.

Use a safe water source to mix your infant formula. If you use well water or are concerned about the safety of your local tap water, or if your baby was born prematurely or has a weakened immune system, you can boil the water for approximately one minute, and then let it cool for approximately five minutes before adding it to the formula per the package directions. Make sure to let it return to room temperature before feeding. (If there is any concern, it may be a good idea to have your well water tested for bacteria or other contaminants.) You also can use bottled water.

Powdered infant formula is not commercially sterile and on rare occasions has been associated with a severe illness attributed to *Cronobacter* bacteria. However, the illness is very uncommon, and the World Health Organization has issued guidelines to improve the safety of powdered infant formula. The CDC and other US organizations recommend heating the water to at least 158 degrees Fahrenheit (70 degrees Celsius) before mixing with powder and allowing it to cool to a safe temperature to reduce the possibility of infection with this bacteria. These instructions may be found at cdc.gov/cronobacter/outbreaks/source-date/index.html.

Make sure all bottles, nipples, and other utensils used in preparation and feeding are clean. If your home has chlorinated water, a dishwasher or hot tap water with dishwashing detergent can be used. Rinse in hot tap water. If your home has non-chlorinated water, boil the utensils for five to ten minutes.

PREPARING FORMULA FROM POWDER

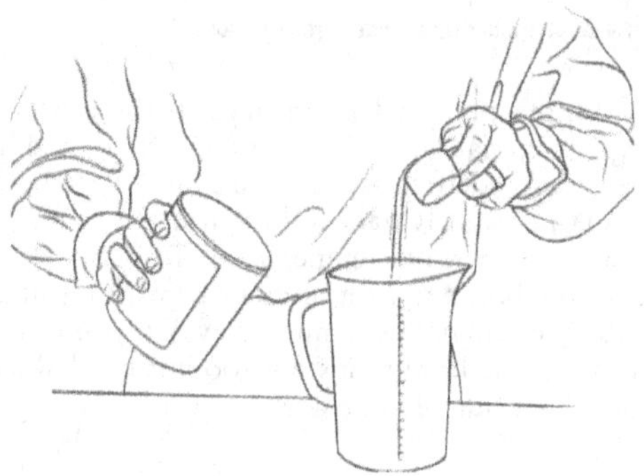

Wash your hands and then add powder.

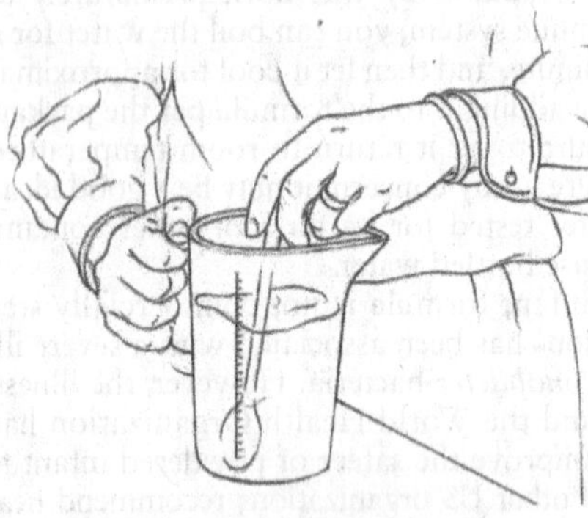

Measure water and stir to mix thoroughly.

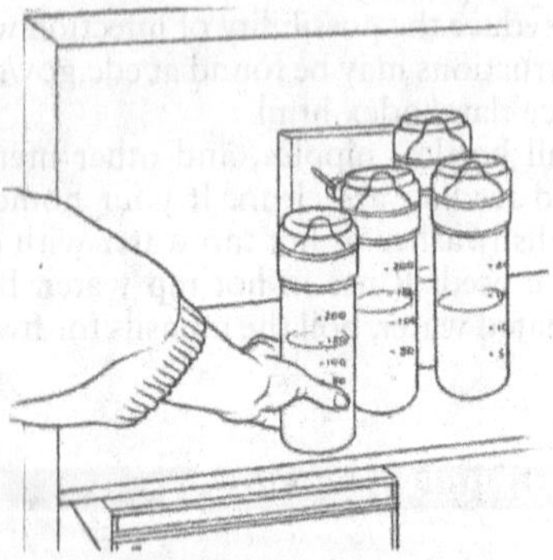

Fill clean bottles and place in refrigerator.

Store formula prepared in advance in the refrigerator to discourage bacterial growth. Unused refrigerated formula should be discarded after twenty-four hours. Refrigerated formula doesn't necessarily have to be warmed, but most infants prefer it at least at room temperature. To warm it, you can either leave the bottle out for an hour or warm it in a pan of hot water (again, do not use a microwave). If you warm it, test it in advance to make sure it's not too hot by shaking a few drops onto the inside of your wrist.

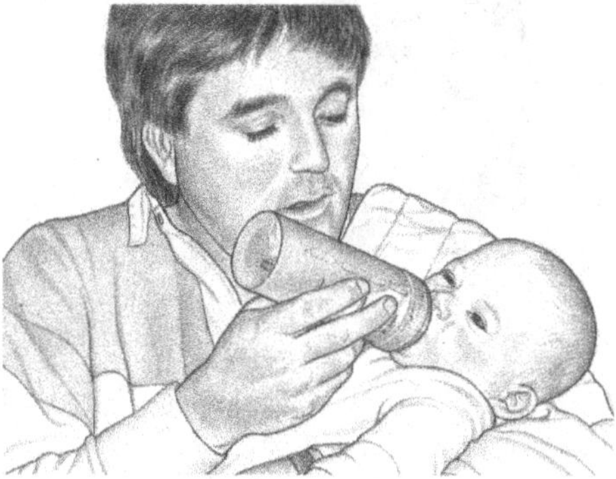

Bottles are usually made of glass, stainless steel, or BPA-free plastic. As your baby begins holding their own bottle, avoid using breakable glass bottles. Also, bottles designed to promote self-feeding are not recommended, as they may contribute to early childhood caries (ECC, formerly known as baby bottle tooth decay) by promoting constant feeding and overexposing the teeth to sugars. When milk or any other sugar-containing liquid sits in contact with tooth enamel over a prolonged period, bacterial overgrowth and acid production occur. ECC is most commonly seen in children 6 months and older who use a bottle or breastfeed to fall asleep or demand at-will feedings throughout the night. Also, self-feeding while lying on the back has been shown to contribute occasionally to ear infections. (See Middle Ear Infections, *page 471*.) Your baby should not have a bottle to suck on overnight. If you give your infant a bedtime feeding, take away the bottle and brush their teeth before they fall asleep to prevent ECC.

You may need to try several nipples before finding the one your baby prefers. There are standard silicone or rubber nipples, orthodontic ones, and special designs for premature infants and for babies with cleft palates. Whichever type is used, always check the size of the hole. If the hole is too small, your baby may suck so hard that they'll swallow too much air; if it's too big, the formula may flow so fast that they might choke. Ideally, formula should flow from an upended bottle at a rate of one drop per second and stop dripping after a few seconds.

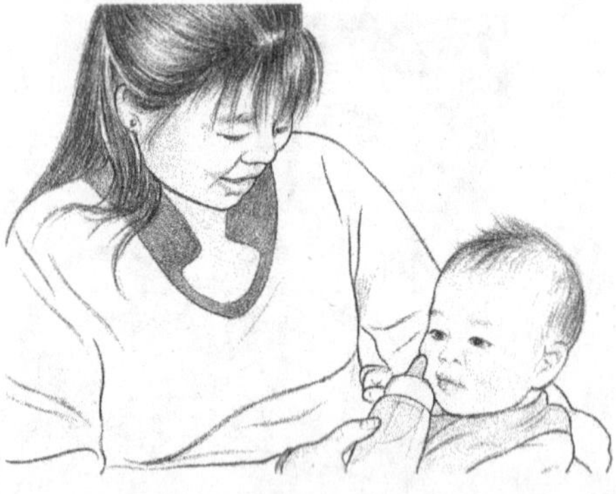

Feeding times should be relaxing, comforting, and enjoyable. They provide opportunities to show your love and to get to know each other. If you are calm and content, your infant will respond in kind. If you are nervous or uninterested, your baby may sense these negative feelings and a feeding problem can result.

You will probably be most comfortable in a chair with arms or with pillows that let you prop up your arms as you feed your infant. Cradle your baby in a semi-upright position and support their head. Don't feed your baby when they are lying down flat, as this will increase the risk of choking and may also cause formula to flow into the middle ear, leading to possible infection.

Hold the bottle so that formula fills the neck of the bottle and fills the nipple. This will prevent your baby from swallowing air as they suck. To get your baby to open their mouth and grasp the nipple, stimulate the rooting reflex by stroking the nipple against the lower lip or cheek. Once the nipple is in your baby's mouth, they will begin to suck and swallow naturally.

Amount and Schedule of Formula Feedings

Paced feedings are recommended to avoid overfeeding, a problem commonly seen with bottle-fed babies that can lead to reflux and obesity. In the first week after birth, babies should be eating no more than 1 to 2 ounces (30–60 ml) per feed. This volume increases gradually over the first month until babies take 3 to 4 ounces (90–120 ml) per feed, resulting in about 32 ounces (960 ml) per day. Formula-fed babies typically feed on a more regular schedule, such as every three to four hours. This happens because all of the nutrients in formula are always exactly the same. Breast milk components vary over the twenty-four-hour period and result in more irregular feeding patterns. Breastfed infants also take smaller, more frequent feedings than formula-fed infants. During the first few weeks, if your baby sleeps longer than four to five hours and starts missing feedings, wake them up and offer a bottle. By the end of the first month, your baby will be up to at least 3 to 4 ounces (120 ml) per feeding, with a fairly predictable schedule of feedings about every three to four hours. By 6 months, your baby will consume 6 to 8 ounces (180–240 ml) at each of four or five feedings in twenty-four hours.

On average, your baby should consume about 2½ ounces (75 ml) of formula a day for every pound (453 g) of body weight. But your baby probably will regulate their intake from day to day to meet their own specific needs, so let them tell you when they've had enough. If your baby becomes fidgety or easily distracted during a feeding, they're probably finished. If they drain the bottle and continue smacking their lips, they might still be hungry. There are high and low limits, however. If your baby consistently seems to want more or less, discuss this with your pediatrician. Your baby should usually drink no more than an average of about 32 ounces (960 ml) of formula in twenty-four hours, although this is not a strict maximum. Some babies have higher needs for sucking and may just want to suck on a pacifier after feeding.

Where We Stand

The American Academy of Pediatrics believes that healthy children receiving a normal, well-balanced diet do not need vitamin supplementation over and above the Recommended Dietary Allowances, which include 400 IU (10 mcg) of vitamin D a day for infants less than 1 year of age and 600 IU (15 mcg) a day for children over 1 year of age. Megadoses of vitamins—for example, large amounts of vitamin A, C, or D—can produce potentially dangerous symptoms, ranging from nausea to rashes to headaches and sometimes even more severe effects. Talk with your pediatrician before giving vitamin supplements to your child.

Initially it is best to offer formula-fed newborns a bottle on demand, or whenever they cry with hunger. As time passes, your baby will begin to develop a fairly regular timetable of their own. As you become familiar with their signals and needs, you'll be able to schedule feedings around your baby's routine.

Between 2 and 4 months of age (or when they weigh more than 12 pounds [5.4 kg]), most babies no longer need middle-of-the-night feedings. They're consuming more during the day, and their sleeping patterns have become more regular (although this varies considerably from baby to baby). Their stomach capacity has increased, too, which means they may go longer between daytime feedings—occasionally up to four or five hours. If your baby still seems to feed frequently or consume larger amounts, try distracting them with play or a pacifier. Sometimes patterns of obesity begin during infancy, so it is important not to overfeed your baby.

The most important thing to remember, whether you breastfeed or bottle-feed, is that your baby's feeding needs are unique. No book can tell you precisely how much or often they need to be fed or exactly how you should handle them during feedings. You will discover these things as you and your baby get to know each other.

TOO MUCH FEEDING

Some signs that your baby may be overfeeding:

- If bottle-fed, the baby is consuming more than 4 to 6 ounces (120 to 180 ml) per feeding.
- Your baby vomits most or all of the food after a complete feeding.
- Their stools are loose and very watery, and occur eight or more times a day. (Keep in mind that breastfed

babies normally tend to have much more frequent and looser stools.)

TOO LITTLE FEEDING

Some signs that your baby may be underfeeding:

- If breastfed, the baby falls asleep while feeding after a short time, and does not seem satisfied after the feeding.
- They wet fewer than four diapers per day; particularly if your baby has begun sleeping through the night, they may be feeding inadequately (since most babies feed at least once during the night), and may urinate less often and become mildly dehydrated.
- They have infrequent or very hard stools in the first month.
- They appear hungry, searching for something to suck shortly after feedings.
- Your baby becomes more yellow, instead of less, during the first week.
- They seem excessively sleepy or lethargic.

FEEDING ALLERGY OR DIGESTIVE DISTURBANCE

Signs of a feeding allergy or problem with digestion:

- Your baby vomits most or all food after a complete feeding or has copious watery diarrhea leading to dehydration.
- They produce loose and very watery stools eight or more times a day or have trouble gaining weight.
- They have blood in the stools.
- They have a severe skin rash.
- They have symptoms of anaphylaxis (combination of vomiting, hives, swelling, wheezing, or loss of consciousness) after feeding.

Supplementation for Breastfed and Bottle-Fed Infants

Water and Juice

Until your baby starts eating solid foods, they'll get all the water they need from breast milk or formula. In the first 6 months, additional water or juice is not needed for breastfed or bottle-fed infants. After 6 months, you may offer small amounts of water in a cup, but don't force it or worry if the baby rejects it. They may prefer to get the extra liquid from more frequent feedings. Juice is not recommended for babies in the first year. It is much healthier for infants to eat fruit and drink water instead of drinking juice.

Once your baby is eating solid foods, their need for liquid will increase. Getting your infant used to the taste of water is a healthy habit that will last a lifetime. When infants become used to drinking juice instead of water, they may want only sweet drinks as they get older, which has been associated with overweight and obesity.

Your baby may need extra fluids when ill, especially when a fever, vomiting, or diarrhea is present. The best fluid for a breastfed infant who is ill is breast milk. Ask your pediatrician what liquids are best and how much to give at these times.

Where We Stand

The American Academy of Pediatrics recommends fruit juice not be given to infants under 12 months of age, since it offers no nutritional benefit in this age group and may increase the risk of tooth decay while causing a preference for sweeter flavors instead of plain water. For children older than 12 months, fruit juice offers no nutritional benefits over whole fruit, but 4 ounces (120 ml) of juice per day given as part of a meal may be a reasonable option. Whole fruits also provide fiber and other nutrients. Children should not be given fruit juice at bedtime, nor as a treatment for dehydration or management of diarrhea.

Fluoride Supplements

Fluoride is a naturally occurring mineral that strengthens your child's enamel and prevents tooth decay. Babies under 6 months should not receive fluoride supplementation. After that time, breastfed and formula-fed infants need appropriate fluoride supplementation if local drinking water contains less than 0.3 parts per million (ppm) of fluoride. If you have well water, have the well tested to determine the amount of natural fluoride in the water. If your baby consumes bottled water or your home has a municipal water supply, check to see if the water is fluoridated. If your family prefers bottled water, you should consider purchasing water marketed for babies with fluoride added (sometimes called "nursery water"). It is available in the baby food aisle and can be used when mixing formula.

Your pediatrician or pediatric dentist can advise you on whether there is a need for fluoride drops, and can prescribe the appropriate dosage. Formula-fed infants receive some fluoride from their formula if the drinking water is fluoridated. The American Academy of Pediatrics recommends that you check with your pediatrician or pediatric dentist to find out if any additional fluoride supplements are necessary.

Remember, appropriate fluoride supplementation is based on each child's unique needs. A supplement should be considered by you and your doctor until all of a child's permanent teeth are present in the mouth.

Burping, Hiccups, and Spitting Up

Burping

Young babies naturally fuss and get cranky when they swallow air during feedings. Although this occurs in both breastfed and bottle-fed infants, it's seen more often with the bottle. When it happens, it may be helpful to stop the feeding rather than letting your infant fuss and feed at the same time. Continued fussing will cause your baby to swallow even more air, which only increases discomfort and may make them spit up.

One thing you can try is to burp the baby frequently, even if they show no discomfort. The pause and the change of position alone will slow gulping and reduce the amount of swallowed air. If your baby is bottle-feeding, burp them after every 2 to 3 ounces (60–90 ml). If nursing, burp them when they switch breasts. Some breastfed babies don't swallow very much air and therefore they may not need to burp.

Hiccups

Most babies hiccup from time to time. Usually this bothers parents more than the infant, but if hiccups occur during a feeding, change your baby's position, try to get them to burp, or help them relax. Wait until the hiccups are gone to resume feeding. If they don't disappear in five to ten minutes, try to resume feeding for a few minutes. Doing this usually stops them. If your baby gets hiccups often, try to feed your baby when they are calm and before they are extremely hungry. This will usually reduce the likelihood of hiccups occurring during the feeding.

Spitting Up

Spitting up is another common occurrence during infancy. Sometimes it means your baby has eaten more than their stomach can hold; sometimes they spit up while burping or drooling. Although it may be a bit messy, it's usually no cause for concern. It almost never involves choking, coughing, discomfort, or danger to your child, even if it occurs during sleep. Know that even if your baby has frequent spit-ups, the best position for sleep is on their back and with the mattress flat, not elevated.

HOW DO YOU BURP A BABY?

Here are a few tried-and-true techniques. After a little experimentation, you'll find which ones work best for your child.

- Hold the baby upright with their head on your shoulder to support their head and back while you gently pat their back with your other hand.

- Sit the baby on your lap, supporting their chest and head with one hand while patting their back with your other hand.
- Lay the baby on your lap with their back up. Support their head so that it is higher than their chest, and gently pat or rotate your hand on their back.

If your baby still hasn't burped after several minutes, continue feeding and don't worry; no baby burps every time. When they've finished, burp them again and keep them in an upright position for ten to fifteen minutes so they don't spit up.

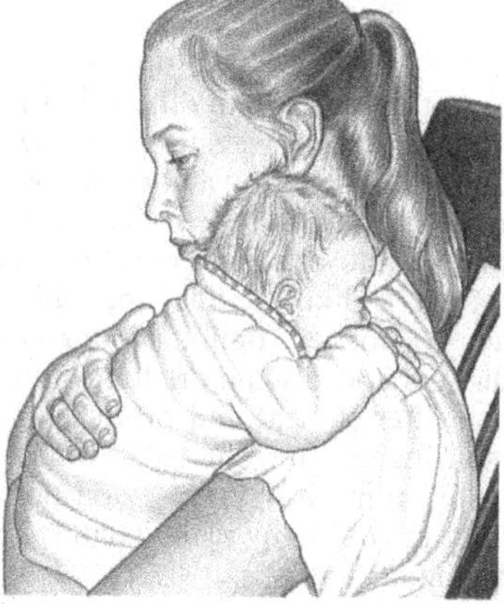

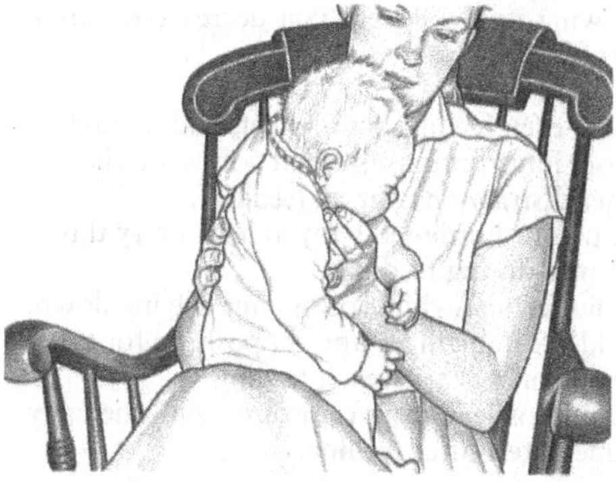

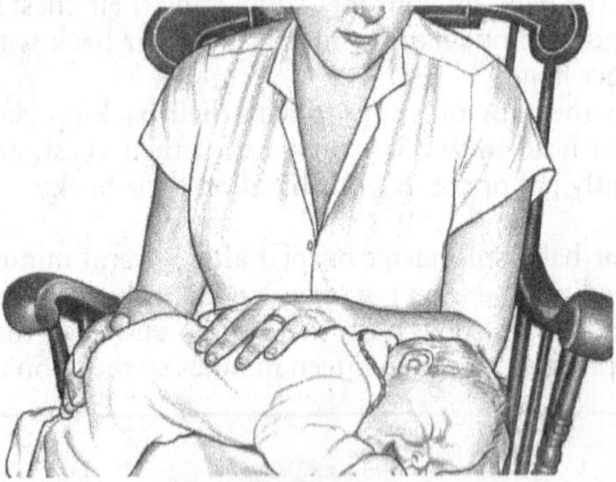

Some babies spit up more than others, but most are out of this phase by the time they are sitting. A few heavy spitters will continue until they start to walk or are weaned to a cup. Some may continue throughout their first year.

It is important to know the difference between spitting up and true vomiting. Unlike spitting up, which most babies don't even seem to notice, vomiting is forceful and usually causes great distress and discomfort for your child. It generally occurs soon after a meal and produces a much greater volume than spitting up. If your baby vomits on a regular basis (one or more times a day) or if you notice blood or a bright green color in your baby's vomit, consult your pediatrician. (See Vomiting, *page 377*.)

While it is practically impossible to prevent all spitting up, the following tips will help you decrease the frequency and amount of spit-up:

- Make each feeding calm, quiet, and leisurely.
- Avoid interruptions, sudden noises, bright lights, and other distractions during feedings.
- Burp your bottle-fed baby at least every three to five minutes during feedings.
- Avoid feeding while your infant is lying down.
- Hold the baby in an upright position for twenty to thirty minutes after each feeding.
- Do not jostle or play vigorously with the baby immediately after feeding.

- Try to feed your baby before they get frantically hungry.
- If bottle-feeding, make sure the hole in the nipple is neither too big (which lets the formula flow too fast) nor too small (which frustrates your baby and causes them to gulp air). If the hole is the proper size, a few drops should come out when you invert the bottle, and then stop.

BUILDING CONFIDENCE IN BREASTFEEDING

Breastfeeding is natural, sure, but it's also a skill that can take some time and assistance to master, for both you and your baby. There's plenty of help available, and you should take advantage of expert advice, counseling, classes, and group meetings. For example, you can:

- Talk to your obstetrician and pediatrician. They can provide not only medical information but also encouragement and support when you need it most.
- Talk to your prenatal instructors and attend a breastfeeding class; invite your partner to come with you.
- Watch online videos and talk to women who have breastfed or are breastfeeding successfully and ask their advice.
- Talk to members of La Leche League or other mother-to-mother support groups in your community. La Leche League is a worldwide organization dedicated to helping families learn about and enjoy the experience of breastfeeding. Information and support for parents is available at llli.org.
- See if there is a Baby Café in your area. Find out at babycafeusa.org.
- Read about breastfeeding. A recommended book is the American Academy of Pediatrics' ***New Mother's Guide to Breastfeeding***, ed. J. Y. Meek, 4th ed. (New York: Bantam Books, 2024).

(For more information on breastfeeding, visit HealthyChildren.org.)

Feeding your baby is one of the most important and, at times, confusing challenges you'll face as a parent. The recommendations in this section apply to infants in general. Please remember that your baby is unique and may have special needs. If you have questions that these pages have not answered to your satisfaction, ask your pediatrician to help you find the answers that apply specifically to you and your infant.

CHAPTER 4

BASIC INFANT CARE

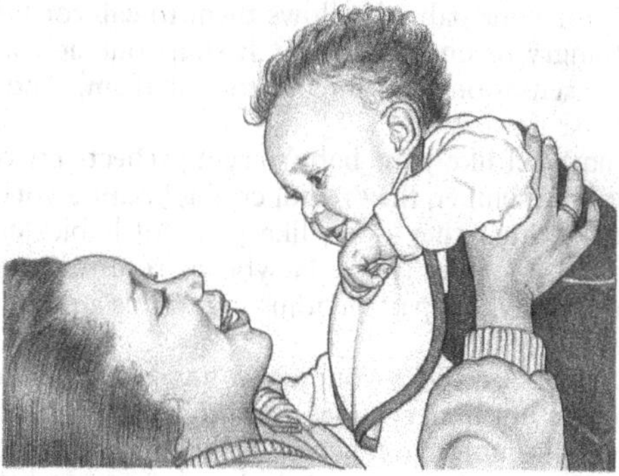

After all the anticipation and planning, the arrival of your new baby is a big transition. Routine tasks such as diapering and dressing them can fill you with anxiety—especially if you haven't spent much time around babies. But it doesn't take long to develop the confidence of an experienced parent, and you'll have help. While in the hospital, the nursery staff and your pediatrician will give you instructions and support. Family and friends can be helpful; don't be bashful about asking for assistance. Start to identify positive resources for you and your partner. Your baby will give you the most important information—how they like to be treated, talked to, held, and comforted. They'll bring out parental instincts that will guide you to many of the right responses, almost as soon as they're born.

The following sections address the most common questions and concerns during the first months after birth.

Day to Day

Responding to Your Baby's Cries

Crying is common for babies. Crying serves several useful purposes for your baby. It allows them to call for help when they're hungry or uncomfortable. It shuts out sights, sounds, and other sensations too intense to suit them. And it helps them release tension.

You may feel like your baby's crying reflects on your parenting, but remember, they're not crying because you're a bad parent or because they don't like you. All babies cry, often without any apparent cause. Newborns routinely cry one to four hours a day. It's part of adjusting to this strange new life outside the womb.

You may notice that your baby has fussy periods, even when they're not hungry, uncomfortable, or tired. At times it may seem like nothing can console them. Right after these spells, they may seem more alert than before, and then may sleep more deeply than usual. This kind of fussy crying seems to help babies get rid of excess energy to allow for a more contented state. As you get to know your infant's crying patterns, you may feel as if you can identify specific needs by the way they cry. Are they hungry? Angry? Distressed or in pain? Sleepy? Each baby will use their voice differently.

Sometimes different types of cries overlap. Newborns generally wake up hungry and crying for food. If you're not quick to respond, your baby's hunger cry may turn to a wail of rage. You'll hear the difference. As your baby matures, their cries will become stronger, louder, and more insistent. They'll also begin to vary more, as if to convey different needs and desires. The best way to handle crying is to respond promptly during their first few months. You cannot spoil a young baby with attention, and if you answer their calls for help, they'll cry less overall.

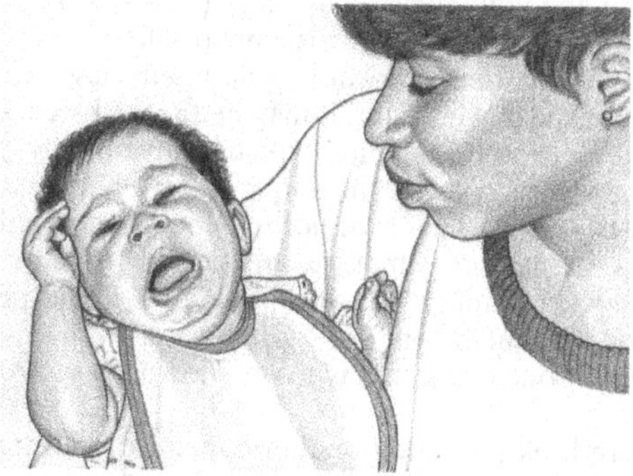

Respond promptly to your infant whenever they cry during their first few months. You cannot spoil a young baby by giving them attention.

When responding to your child's cries, try to meet their most pressing need first. If they're cold and hungry and their diaper is wet, warm them up, change their diaper, and then feed them. If there's a shrieking or panicked quality to the cry, consider if a piece of clothing or something else is making them uncomfortable. Perhaps a strand of hair is caught around a finger or toe. If they're warm, dry, and well fed but the crying won't stop, try the following consoling techniques. Find the ones that work best for your baby:

- Rocking, either in a rocking chair or in your arms as you sway from side to side
- Gently stroking their head or patting their back or chest
- Safe swaddling (wrapping them snugly in a receiving blanket)
- Singing or talking
- Playing soft music
- Walking them in your arms, a stroller, or a carriage
- Making rhythmic soft noise and vibration
- Burping them to relieve any trapped gas bubbles
- Giving them a warm bath (most babies like this, but not all)

Sometimes, if all else fails and your baby doesn't seem to be ill, the best approach is simply to leave the baby alone in a safe location such as a crib. Many babies cannot fall asleep without crying and will fall asleep quicker if left to cry. The crying shouldn't last long if the baby is truly tired.

If the crying does not stop, but intensifies and persists throughout the day or night, it may be caused by colic. Unfortunately, there is no definite explanation for why this happens. Most often, colic means simply that the baby is unusually sensitive to stimulation or cannot self-console or regulate their nervous system. As they mature, this inability to self-console—marked by constant crying—will improve. Some people try "gas drops" (simethicone) or "gripe water" (any number of ingredients), but research has never shown these products to work.

You can look into additional non-medication options such as reevaluating your diet, slow feeding, and ensuring appropriate burping. If bottle-feeding, try a slower-flow nipple and/or tipping the bottle to prevent milk flow for a few seconds intermittently to allow the baby to better organize their swallowing and breathing and realize when they are full. If your baby is inconsolable, they may be sick. Check their temperature (see Taking a Rectal Temperature, *page 127*). If you take it rectally and it is 100.4 degrees Fahrenheit (38 degrees Celsius) or higher, they could have an infection; contact your pediatrician.

The more relaxed you remain, the easier it will be to console your child. Even very young babies are sensitive to tension and react to it by crying. Hearing a wailing newborn can be agonizing, but letting your frustration turn to anger or panic will only intensify your infant's screams. If you start to feel you can't handle the situation, set the baby down in a crib and get help from a family member or friend. This will give you needed relief, and a new face can sometimes calm your baby. No matter how impatient or angry you feel, do not shake or hit the baby. Shaking an infant hard can cause blindness, brain damage, or even death. It's important to share this information on crying with anyone else who cares for your baby, including your spouse, partner, or babysitter.

No parent can console their baby every time they cry, so don't expect to be a miracle worker. Instead, take a realistic approach. Line up some help, get plenty of rest, and enjoy all those wondrous moments with your child.

Helping Your Baby Sleep

Initially your infant doesn't know day from night. Their stomach holds only enough to satisfy them for two to four hours, regardless of the time. There's no escaping the round-the-clock waking and feeding those first few months. But even at this age, you can begin to teach them that nighttime is for sleeping and daytime for play. Keep nighttime feedings as calm and quiet as possible. Don't turn up the lights or prolong diaper changes. Instead of playing, put them right back down after feeding and changing them. If they're napping longer than three or four hours, particularly in the late afternoon, wake them up and play with them. This will train them to save extra sleeping for nighttime. Also, begin to develop a routine before bedtime. Experiencing a strong sensation (like a sponge bath) followed by soothing time (like applying a bit of unscented, hypoallergenic moisturizing lotion and reading or singing) and then a final feeding followed by a short bedtime story can help signal to your baby that the longer nap is coming.

HOW YOUR BABY SLEEPS

Even before birth, your baby had periods of sleep and wakefulness. By the eighth month of pregnancy, their sleep periods had the same distinct phases we all experience:

1. Rapid eye movement (REM, "active") sleep, the times they do their active dreaming. Their eyes will move beneath their lids, almost as if they were watching a dream take place. They also may seem to startle, smile, twitch their face, and make jerking motions with their hands and feet. All are normal signs of REM sleep.
2. Non-REM (or quiet) sleep, which consists of four phases: drowsiness, light sleep, deep sleep, and very deep sleep. In newborns, however, non-REM sleep is undifferentiated, with well-defined stages appearing by 6 months of age. During the progression from drowsiness to deepest sleep, your baby becomes less and less active, and their breathing slows and becomes very quiet. In deepest sleep they are virtually motionless.

They may also make suckling movements. Very little, if any, dreaming occurs during non-REM sleep.

At first your newborn will probably sleep about sixteen hours a day, divided into three- to four-hour naps evenly spaced between feedings.

Each of these sleep periods will include relatively equal amounts of REM and non-REM sleep, organized in this order: drowsiness, REM sleep, light sleep, deep sleep, and very deep sleep.

After about 2 to 3 months, the order will change. As they grow older, they will cycle through all the non-REM phases before entering REM sleep. This pattern remains through adulthood. Young children achieve non-REM deep sleep fairly quickly upon sleep onset and it is difficult to wake them from it. With age, the amount of REM sleep decreases, and their sleep will generally become calmer.

Positioning for Sleep

The American Academy of Pediatrics recommends that healthy infants be placed on their backs for sleep, as this is the safest position for an infant to sleep. Placing your baby to sleep on their back decreases their chances of sudden unexpected infant death (SUID), which is responsible for more infant deaths in the United States than any other cause during the first year (beyond the newborn period).

In addition, recent findings suggest that certain regions of the brain may be underdeveloped in babies who die from SUID. When these sleeping babies encounter a situation challenging to their well-being, they may fail to wake up to remove themselves from danger. Babies who sleep on their stomachs sleep more deeply, and so it is harder for them to wake up; this is probably why stomach sleeping is so dangerous. Since it is impossible to identify which babies may not arouse normally, and because the relationship between SUID and sleep position is so strong, the Academy recommends that all infants be placed to sleep on their backs. Some doctors once thought that sleeping on the side might be a reasonable alternative to back positioning, but we now know that side sleeping is just as dangerous as stomach sleeping for babies. Babies placed to sleep on their sides can roll onto their stomachs, which increases the risk of SUID. Do not use a positioning device, like a wedge or blanket roll, to keep your baby on their back. These can lead to suffocation. It is enough just to put your baby on their back. All healthy babies, including those with gastroesophageal reflux, should sleep on their backs. Your pediatrician will tell you if your baby has one of the rare medical conditions that require them to sleep in a different position. Once the infant can roll both back to front and front to back, you may let them stay in the sleep position they choose.

It is also important to avoid placing your baby to sleep with or on soft surfaces such as pillows, quilts, comforters, bumper pads, or bean bags—even stuffed toys—in the infant sleep area, which may block their airway if they burrow their face into them. Also avoid having them sleep on an adult's chest because of the risk of the adult falling asleep while holding the baby. Waterbeds, sofas, and soft mattresses are also especially unsafe sleep environments for babies. Never put your baby to sleep in anything inclined or slanted: infant "bouncers," car safety seats (it's okay if a baby falls asleep in the car safety seat while riding in the car, but it is not safe for sleep outside of the car), strollers, swings, infant carriers, or slings. Especially under 4 months of age, infants cannot easily turn their heads if they're suffocating. A flat, firm (hard) crib mattress (in a safety-approved crib or bassinet) covered by a fitted sheet is the safest bedding. Do not pad the mattress with pillows or blankets to make it softer; this will make it more dangerous. Keep all soft toys and stuffed animals out of your child's crib throughout the first year. Keep the temperature in your baby's room comfortable. Use sleep clothing (such as a one-piece sleeper) with no other covering, instead of blankets. If you are worried that your baby will be cold, you can use layers of clothing, a wearable blanket sleeper, or a sleep sack as safe alternatives.

RECOMMENDATIONS FOR SAFE INFANT SLEEP

- Place your baby on their back to sleep for every sleep.
- Use a firm, flat, non-inclined sleep surface to reduce the risk of suffocation or wedging/entrapment.
- Feeding of breast milk is recommended because it is associated with a reduced risk of SUID/SIDS.
- It is recommended that infants sleep in the parents'

room, close to the parents' bed, but on a separate surface designed for infants, ideally for at least the first 6 months.

- Keep soft objects, such as pillows, pillow-like toys, quilts, comforters, mattress toppers, fur-like materials, and loose bedding, such as blankets and non-fitted sheets, away from the infant's sleep area to reduce the risk of SUID, suffocation, entrapment/wedging, and strangulation.
- Once breastfeeding is well established, offering a pacifier at nap time and bedtime is recommended to reduce the risk of SUID.
- Avoid smoke and nicotine exposure during pregnancy and after birth.
- Avoid alcohol, marijuana, opioids, and illicit drug use during pregnancy and after birth.
- Avoid overheating and head covering in infants during naps and bedtime.
- It is recommended that those pregnant obtain regular prenatal care.
- It is recommended that infants be immunized in accordance with guidelines from the American Academy of Pediatrics and the Centers for Disease Control and Prevention.
- Do not use home cardiorespiratory monitors as a strategy to reduce the risk of SUID.
- Supervised, awake tummy time is recommended to facilitate development and to minimize the risk of one side of the head becoming flat. Parents are encouraged to place the infant in tummy time while awake and supervised for short periods of time beginning soon after hospital discharge, increasing gradually to at least fifteen to thirty minutes total daily by 7 weeks of age.

Source: R. Y. Moon, R. F. Carlin, I. Hand, and the American Academy of Pediatrics Task Force on Sudden Infant Death Syndrome and Committee on Fetus and Newborn, "Sleep-Related Infant Deaths: Updated 2022 Recommendations for Reducing Infant Deaths in the Sleep Environment," *Pediatrics* 150, no. 1 (2022): e2022057990.

Many parents have felt the temptation to keep their babies in bed with them, especially when they are exhausted and the babies are fussy. Bed-sharing, however, raises the risk of infant death. Instead, place the baby's bassinet or crib in your room, where you can monitor them and comfort them as needed, always returning them to a safe sleep environment. Your baby is safest sleeping in your room on their own separate sleep surface close to your bed, ideally for the first 6 months.

Pacifiers may also help reduce the risk of SUID. However, if your baby doesn't want the pacifier or it falls out of their mouth, don't force it. If you are breastfeeding, wait until breastfeeding is well established, usually around 3 or 4 weeks of age, before using a pacifier. If you are formula-feeding or giving expressed breast milk, you can start the pacifier at any time. Pacifiers should not have strings, ties, or stuffed animals attached to them, since these can pose a strangulation risk.

Swaddling can help calm your baby, but it must be done safely. Swaddling should allow ample room for hip and knee movement to allow for proper leg development. Your baby has very sensitive hip joints that can be harmed by too much pressure or stress from abnormal hip positions or restricted motion, potentially causing lifelong problems like arthritis. Swaddling should be snug around the infant's chest, leaving enough space so that the caregiver's hand can fit between the blanket and the baby's chest. If the swaddle becomes loose, it can result in suffocation or strangulation. Always lay your swaddled infant on their back. When an infant exhibits signs of attempting to roll, it's time to stop swaddling, since a swaddled infant in the prone position is at high risk for SUID/SIDS and suffocation. Swaddles should not be weighted or have any weighting materials added to them.

Where We Stand

Based on an evaluation of current data on sudden unexpected infant death (SUID), the American Academy of Pediatrics recommends that healthy infants always be placed on their backs for sleep—whether for nap time or nighttime. Despite common beliefs, there is no evidence that choking is more frequent among infants lying on their backs (the supine position) when compared to other positions, nor is there evidence that sleeping on the back is harmful to healthy babies. Babies with gastroesophageal reflux (excessive spitting up) should still be placed on their backs.

Since 1992, when the American Academy of Pediatrics began recommending this sleep position, the annual SUID rate has declined more than 50 percent. However, there has also been an increase in accidental suffocation deaths. A safe sleep environment (baby on their back in a crib close to the parents' bed without any blankets or soft objects) is important to protect your baby from SUID or an accidental suffocation death.

While sleeping on the back is important, your baby should also spend time on their stomach when awake and being observed. This will help to develop your baby's shoulder muscles and head control and avoid flat spots on the back of their head. Be sure to spend part of their alert time every day playing with them in this position.

As their stomach grows, your baby will go longer between feedings. In fact, you'll be encouraged to know that while the average longest sleep period for infants from birth to 5 months is 5.7 hours, this increases to 8.3 hours by 6 to 24 months of age. Many infants can last for as long as 6 hours between feedings when they reach 12 or 13 pounds (5.44–5.89 kg). Larger babies may begin sleeping for longer periods at a time a little sooner. As encouraging as this sounds, don't expect the sleep struggle to end all at once. Most children swing back and forth, sleeping beautifully for a few weeks, even months, then returning abruptly to a late-night wake-up schedule. This may be due to growth spurts, when babies need more food; later, teething or developmental changes can cause increased awakenings.

From time to time, you will need to help your baby fall asleep or go back to sleep. Especially as a newborn, they will probably doze off most easily if given gentle continuous stimulation. Some infants are helped by rocking, walking, patting on the back, or using a pacifier. That said, if you always rock your baby to sleep, they may not learn to fall asleep on their own. Practice putting them to bed while they are sleepy but not fully asleep so that they can build this skill. For others, music can be very soothing if played quietly.

Diapers

Since disposable diapers were introduced about eighty years ago, they have been meeting the needs and expectations of most parents; however, diaper choice is a decision every new parent faces. Ideally, choose whether to use cloth or disposable diapers (or both) before the baby arrives, in order to stock up or make delivery arrangements. In planning, be aware that most newborns use about ten diapers a day.

HOW TO DIAPER YOUR BABY

Before you start, make sure you have all the necessary supplies within arm's reach. Never leave your baby alone on the changing table—not even for a second. Babies wiggle and squirm and can easily fall off a changing table. In addition, it won't be long before they can turn over, and if they do when your attention is diverted, a serious injury could result.

When changing a newborn, you will need:

- A clean diaper (possibly including fasteners if a cloth diaper is used)
- Unscented diaper wipes, or a small basin (or a mug or bowl) with lukewarm water and a washcloth; soft paper towels or cotton balls can also be used
- Diaper ointment or petroleum jelly

Do not use baby powder, since babies can breathe the dust from powder, potentially irritating the lungs.

This is how you proceed:

1. Remove the dirty diaper and use the unscented diaper wipes or the lukewarm water and the washcloth (or soft paper towel or cotton balls). Remember to wipe front to back on female infants.

2. Use the diaper ointment recommended by your pediatrician if needed. Make sure the diaper area is completely dry before applying it.

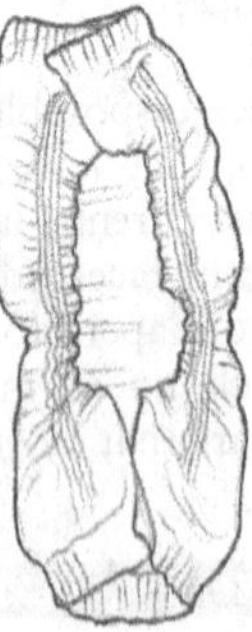

Disposable Diapers. Most disposable diapers consist of an inner liner designed to help keep wetness away from the skin, an absorbent core, and an outer waterproof covering. Some diapers now have a stripe that changes color to indicate wetness. Over the years, they have become thinner and lighter, while continuing to meet the needs for containment, comfort, ease of use, and skin care. When changing a soiled diaper, do not flush the diaper, as it can block plumbing. Wrap the diaper in its outer cover and discard in a waste receptacle. Afterward, always wash your hands.

Cloth Diapers. Like disposable diapers, reusable cloth diapers have improved over the years and are available in a variety of absorbencies and textures. If you want to use a diaper service, shop around; ideally, a diaper service should pick up dirty diapers and drop off clean ones twice a week. If you choose to wash diapers yourself, keep them separate from other clothes. After you dump stool into the toilet, consider rinsing the diaper with a diaper sprayer or pouring cold water over it into the toilet, then placing the damp diaper in a diaper pail until washing it in hot water and mild detergent. Some newer diaper types offer a disposable cloth liner with a reusable outer cover. Regardless, always remember to wash your hands afterward.

Diaper Choice. Diaper choice has been complicated in recent years by the debate on the environmental effects of diapers, mostly centered on disposable diapers and landfill space. Actually, a number of scientific studies have found that both cloth and disposable diapers have environmental effects, including raw material and energy usage, air and water pollution, and waste disposal. Disposable diapers add to municipal solid waste, while cloth diapers use more energy and water in laundering and contribute to air and water pollution. In the end, you must make your own decision about diaper type based on your concerns and needs or simply decide to use both.

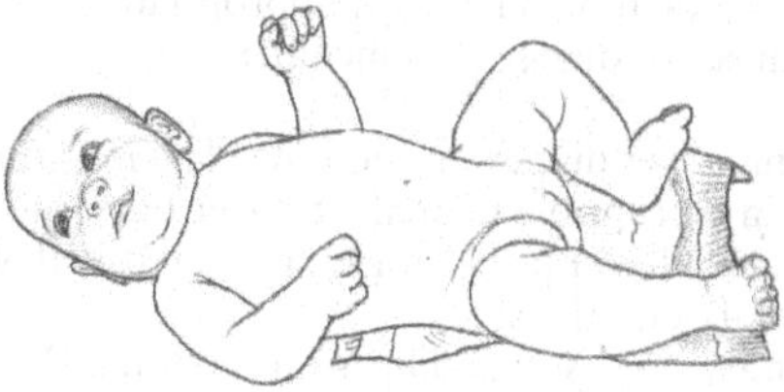

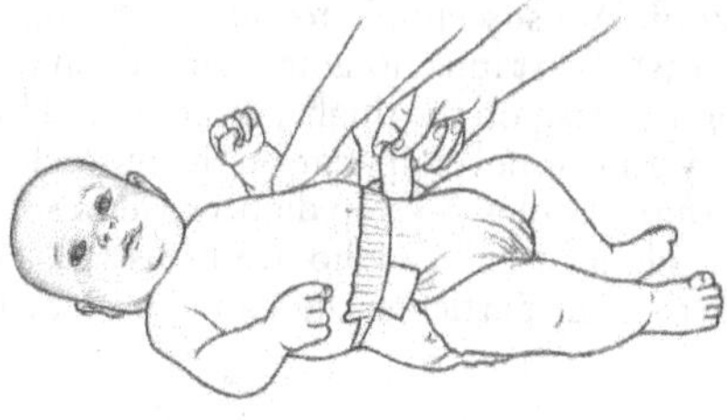

There are health aspects to consider as well. Excessively wet skin and contact with urine and stool can cause diaper rash. Because cloth diapers can't keep wetness away from your baby's skin as effectively as disposables, it's especially important to change cloth diapers quickly after they become wet or soiled. Some parents primarily use cloth diapers for their babies but use a disposable diaper at bedtime or on long outings to minimize contact with wetness when diapers can't be changed as often.

DIAPER RASH

"Diaper rash" describes a rash or irritation in the area covered by the diaper. The first sign of diaper rash is usually redness or small bumps on the lower abdomen, buttocks, genitals, and thigh folds—surfaces in direct contact with a wet or soiled diaper. This type of diaper rash is rarely serious and usually clears in three or four days with appropriate care. The most common causes of diaper rash include:

- Leaving a wet diaper on too long. The moisture makes the skin susceptible to chafing. Over time, the urine in the diaper decomposes, forming chemicals that can further irritate the skin.
- Leaving a stool-soiled diaper on too long. Digestive agents in the stool then attack the skin, making it more susceptible to a rash.

Regardless of how the rash begins, once the skin surface is damaged, it becomes even more vulnerable to irritation by urine and stool, and susceptible to subsequent infection with bacteria or yeast. Yeast infections are common in this area and often appear as a rash on the thighs, genitals, and lower abdomen, but they almost never appear on the buttocks.

Although most babies develop diaper rash at some point, it happens less often in babies who are breastfed. Diaper rash occurs more often at particular ages and under certain conditions:

- Among babies 8 to 10 months old
- If babies are not kept clean and dry
- When babies have diarrhea
- When a baby starts to eat solid food (probably due to changes in the digestive process caused by the new variety of foods)
- When a baby is taking antibiotics (because these drugs alter the germs in the gut and the acidity of the stool and encourage the growth of yeast organisms that can infect the skin)

To reduce your baby's risk of diaper rash, make these steps part of your diapering routine:

1. Change the diaper as soon as possible after a bowel movement. Cleanse the diaper area with a diaper wipe or soft cloth and water after each bowel movement.
2. Change wet diapers frequently to reduce skin exposure to moisture.
3. Expose the baby's bottom to air whenever feasible. When using diaper covers or disposable diapers with tight gathers around the abdomen and legs, make sure air can circulate inside the diaper.

If a diaper rash develops in spite of your efforts, begin using a diaper rash ointment as a barrier to prevent further irritation and to allow the skin to heal. The rash should improve noticeably within two to three days. If it doesn't improve or it gets worse (or if you see pimple-like pustules), consult your pediatrician.

Urination

Your baby will gradually increase the number of wet diapers in the first few days after birth. After the first week or two, your baby may urinate as often as every one to three hours or as infrequently as four to six times a day. If they're ill or feverish, or when the weather is extremely hot, their usual output of urine may drop by half and still be normal. Urination should never be painful. If you notice any signs of distress while your infant is urinating, notify your pediatrician. This could be a sign of infection or another problem in the urinary tract.

In a healthy child, urine is light to dark yellow in color. (The darker the color, the more concentrated the urine; the urine will be more concentrated when your baby is not drinking a lot of liquid.) In the first week after birth, you may see a pink or brick-red stain on the diaper, often mistaken for blood. In fact, this stain is usually a sign of highly concentrated urine, which has a pinkish color. As long as the baby is wetting at least four diapers a day, there is probably no cause for concern. If the pinkish staining persists, consult your pediatrician.

Newborn girls may have a small spot of blood in the diaper, also usually in the first week after birth; this blood is caused by the mother's hormones affecting the baby's uterus. After that time, however, the presence of actual blood in the urine or a bloody spot on the diaper is never normal, and your pediatrician should be notified. It may be due to nothing more than a diaper rash sore, but it also could be a more serious problem. If this bleeding is accompanied by other symptoms, such as abdominal pain, poor feeding, vomiting, fever, or bleeding in other areas, seek medical attention immediately.

Bowel Movements

For the first few days after birth, your baby's bowel movements will be a substance known as meconium. This thick black or dark green substance filled your baby's intestines before birth, and once the meconium has been passed, the stools turn yellow-green.

Stools vary in color and consistency due to the baby's immature digestive system. If your baby is breastfed, their stools should be yellow liquid mixed with some particles that remind many parents of little seeds. Until a baby starts to eat solid foods, the consistency of the stools may range from very soft to loose and runny. If babies are formula-fed, their stools will usually be tan or yellow in color. They will be firmer than a breastfed baby's but should be no firmer than soft clay. Green stools are not unusual, either, and they should not cause you alarm. If your formula-fed infant is having firm, dry, or formed stools, ensure you are mixing formula per the instructions, by adding the formula to the bottle first and then adding water.

Whether your baby is breast- or bottle-fed, hard or very dry stools may be a sign they are not getting enough fluid or are losing too much fluid due to illness, fever, or heat. Once solids are introduced, hard stools might indicate they're eating too many constipating foods, such as cereal, cow's milk, or cow's-milk-based formula, before their system can handle them. (Whole cow's milk is not recommended for babies under 12 months.) Underripe bananas can also be a common culprit of hard stools and constipation in babies and toddlers.

Here are some other important points to keep in mind about bowel movements:

- Occasional variations in color and consistency of the stools are normal. For example, if the digestive process slows down because of foods requiring more effort to digest (e.g., large amounts of cereal), the stools may become green, or if the baby is given supplemental iron, the stools may turn dark brown. If there is a minor irritation of the anus, streaks of blood may appear on the outside of the stools. However, if there are large amounts of blood or any blood in the stool of a newborn, or mucus or water in the stool, call your pediatrician immediately. These symptoms may warrant attention from your doctor.

- Because an infant's stools are normally soft and a little runny, it's not always easy to tell when a young baby has mild diarrhea. The telltale signs are a sudden increase in frequency (to more than one bowel movement per feeding) and unusually high liquid content in the stool. Diarrhea may be a sign of intestinal infection, or it may be caused by a change in the baby's diet.
- The main concern with diarrhea is the possibility of dehydration. If fever (a rectal temperature of 100.4 degrees Fahrenheit [38 degrees Celsius] or higher) is also present and your infant is less than 3 months old, call your pediatrician. If your baby is over 3 months and the fever lasts more than a day, check their urine output and rectal temperature, then report your findings to your doctor for consideration. Make sure your baby continues to feed frequently. As much as anything else, if they simply look sick, let your doctor know.

The frequency of bowel movements varies widely among babies. Many pass a stool soon after each feeding, a result of the gastrocolic reflex, which causes the digestive system to become active whenever the stomach is filled with food.

By 3 to 6 weeks of age, some breastfed babies have only one bowel movement a week and still are normal. Breast milk leaves very little solid waste to be eliminated from the child's digestive system. Thus, infrequent stools are not a sign of constipation and should not be considered a problem as long as the stools are soft and your infant is otherwise normal, gaining weight steadily, and nursing regularly. Babies with this breastfed stool variant usually have a large volume of stool if it has been a few days (so you should be prepared with lots of wipes to clean up).

If your baby is formula-fed, they should have at least one bowel movement a day. If they have fewer than this and appear to be straining, they may be constipated. Check with your pediatrician for advice on how to handle this problem. (See Constipation, *page 352*.)

Bathing

Your infant doesn't need much bathing if you wipe or wash the diaper area thoroughly during diaper changes. A short bath with a mild cleanser three times a week during their first year may be enough. More frequent bathing may dry out their skin, particularly if drying or irritating soaps are used or moisture is allowed to evaporate from the skin. Patting your baby dry and applying a fragrance-free, dye-free hypoallergenic moisturizer (ointment or cream is best) immediately after bathing can help prevent dry skin (see *page 122*).

In a warm room, lay the baby anywhere that's flat and comfortable for both of you—a changing table, bed, floor, or counter next to the sink will do. Pad hard surfaces with a blanket or fluffy towel. If the baby is on a surface above the floor, use a safety strap or keep one hand on them at all times to make sure they don't fall.

For sponge baths, have a basin of water, a damp, double-rinsed washcloth (with no soap residue), and a supply of mild baby cleanser within reach before you begin. Keep your baby wrapped in a towel and expose only the parts of their body you are washing. Use the dampened cloth with no soap to wash their face. Then use the soapy water to wash the remainder of their body, ending with the diaper area. Pay special attention to creases under the arms, behind the ears, and around the neck. Avoid cleaning the vagina/vulva with soap, as it can lead to irritation.

For uncircumcised boys, foreskin care during each bath time is important to prevent irritation and infection. In most newborns, the foreskin cannot be retracted due to natural adhesions to the head of the penis. Gentle retraction can be performed to allow cleaning of the foreskin and head where easily reached, but the foreskin should never be retracted forcefully, which can cause pain and scarring. It is very important to replace the foreskin after retraction. Each boy's foreskin can be completely retracted at variable times over childhood, but most can retract completely by puberty. Excellent educational videos are available from reputable sources online to improve comfort with foreskin care. For circumcised boys, the genital skin, including the head of the penis, can be cleaned with a regular cleanser and water. Once the circumcision is healed, some redundant or leftover foreskin may be present in circumcised boys, and it is safe to clean under this. The appearance of any redundant skin improves in most boys with natural growth.

Prior to the time when the umbilical cord dries and falls, you should avoid putting soap and water in the umbilical area, as it delays the cord's natural way of healing and may increase the risk of infection. It might be best to stick with sponge baths to avoid getting the stump wet. Do not clean the stump with alcohol or any other cleaning agents, as it might increase the risk of infection by killing the natural bacteria. Do not pull the stump. It is best to let the stump fall off on its own. If the skin around the stump becomes red or has any pus, this can be very dangerous and you need to seek urgent care with your pediatrician. Once the umbilical area is healed, you can try placing your baby directly in the water. Their first baths should be as gentle and brief as possible. They will probably protest; if they seem miserable, go back to sponge baths for a week or two, then try again. They will make it clear when they're ready.

Most parents find it easiest to bathe a newborn in a small bathtub, sink, or plastic tub lined with a clean towel. Fill the basin with 2 inches (5 cm) of water that feels warm—not hot—to the inside of your wrist or elbow. If you're filling the basin from the tap, turn the cold water on first (and off last) to avoid scalding yourself. The hottest temperature at the faucet should be no more than 120 degrees Fahrenheit (48.9 degrees Celsius) to avoid burns; in many cases you can adjust your water heater. Only place your baby in the basin once you have finished filling it and checked the final temperature.

Supplies should be at hand and the room warm before undressing the baby because babies lose body heat easily. You'll need the same supplies you used for sponge bathing, but also a cup for rinsing with clear water. When your baby has hair, you'll need baby shampoo, too.

BATHING YOUR BABY

Once you've undressed your baby, place them in the warm water immediately so that they don't get chilled. Bubble baths and other additives can be irritating; plain water is best. Use one hand to support their head and the other to guide your baby in, feet first. Speak encouragingly, and gently lower their body until they're in the tub. Most of their body and face should be well above the water level for safety, so you'll need to pour warm water over their body frequently to keep them warm.

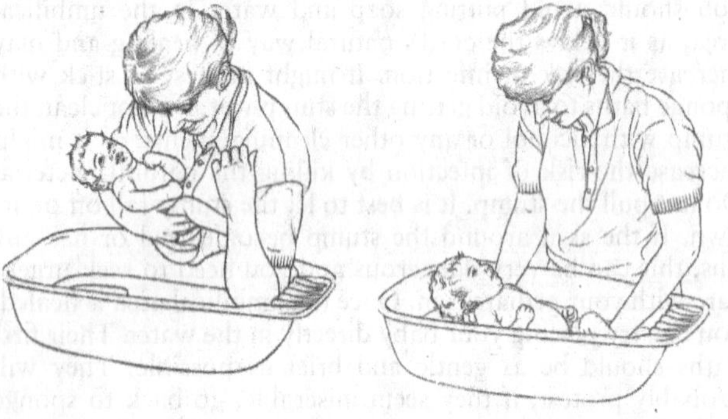

Use a soft cloth to wash their face and hair, cleansing once or twice a week. Massage their entire scalp gently, including over their fontanelles (soft spots). When you rinse the soap or baby shampoo from their head, cup your hand across their forehead so that the suds run toward the sides, not into their eyes. Should you get some cleanser in their eyes, simply take the wet washcloth and liberally wipe their closed eyes with plain, lukewarm water until the cleanser is gone, and they will open their eyes again. Wash the rest of their body from the top down.

If you've forgotten something or need to step away, you must take your baby with you, so keep a dry towel within reach. Never leave a baby alone in the bath, even for an instant.

If your baby enjoys their bath, give them extra time to splash and explore the water. The more fun your child has, the less they'll be afraid of the water. As they get older, bath time will lengthen until most of it is play. Bathing should be a relaxing and soothing experience, so don't rush unless they're unhappy.

Bath toys are not needed for very young babies. The stimulation of water and washing is exciting enough. Once a baby is old enough for the bathtub, however, toys become a fun addition. Containers, cups, age-appropriate toys, and even waterproof books make wonderful distractions as you cleanse your baby. Remember that bath toys can grow mold if they stay wet, so squeeze or shake out any water and give them a chance to dry between uses.

Baby towels with built-in hoods are the most effective way to keep your baby's head warm when the bath is over. Bathing a baby of any age is wet work, so be prepared to keep yourself dry.

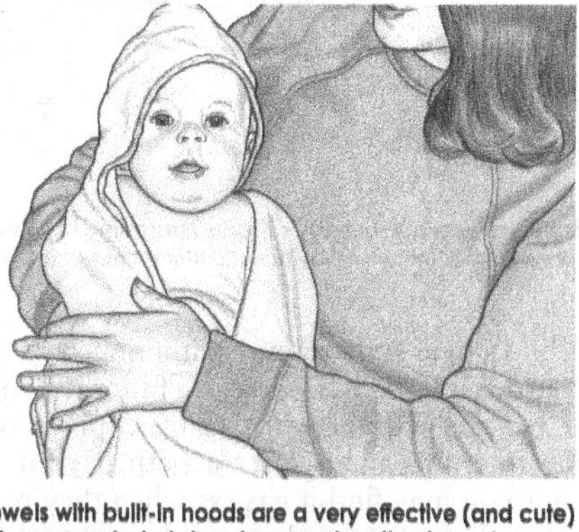

Baby towels with built-in hoods are a very effective (and cute) way to keep your baby's head warm when they're wet.

Many parents find that a bath is a relaxing way to prepare their baby for sleep if it works in their daily routines.

Skin and Nail Care

Your newborn's skin may be susceptible to irritation from chemicals found in new clothing and from soap residue on washed clothes. Double-rinse all baby clothes, bedding, blankets, and other washable items before exposing the child to them. It is common for a baby's skin to peel in the first few weeks, as their body is clearing away the extra skin cells from being in amniotic fluid.

Babies don't routinely need skin moisturizer during the first month after birth. If your baby's skin tends to be dry, or if you choose to give your baby a bath every day, it is helpful to apply an oil, lotion, cream, or ointment that contains no scents or coloring agents. If your baby has a persistent bumpy or dry rash, ask the pediatrician if your baby may have eczema (see *page 392*).

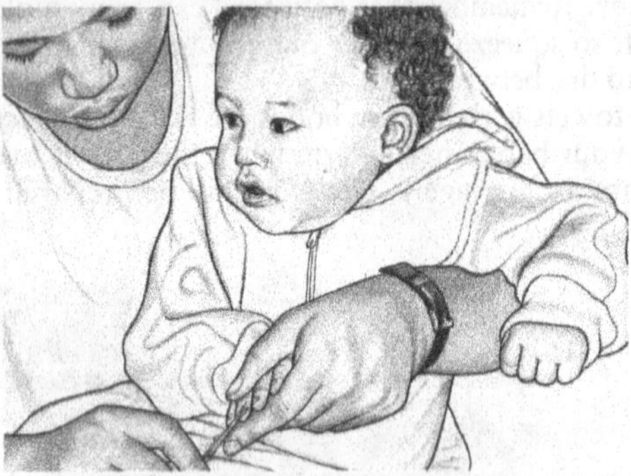

In the early weeks, your baby's fingers are so small and their nails grow so quickly that you may have to trim them twice a week.

Your child's nails only require trimming. You can use a soft emery board, baby nail clippers, or blunt-nosed toenail scissors, but be very careful when using clippers or scissors. A good time to trim nails is after a bath if your baby will lie quietly, but you may find it easiest when they're asleep. Keep their fingernails as short and smoothly trimmed as possible to help them avoid scratching themselves (or you). In the early weeks, their fingers are so small and their nails grow so quickly that you may have to trim them twice a week. Avoid the temptation to bite your child's nails as a way of trimming them, as this habit can lead to a skin infection.

By contrast, your baby's toenails grow much more slowly and are usually soft and pliable. They needn't be kept as short as fingernails, so they may only have to be trimmed once or twice a month. Because they are so soft, they sometimes look ingrown, but there's no cause for concern unless the skin alongside the nail gets red, inflamed, or hard, or you see an area of pus. As your baby gets older, their toenails will become harder and better defined.

DRESSING AND UNDRESSING YOUR BABY

Support your baby on your lap or changing table and stretch the garment's neckline to pull it over your baby's head. Use your fingers to keep it from catching on their face or ears.

Don't try to push your baby's arm through the sleeve. Instead, put your hand into the sleeve from the outside, grasp your baby's hand, and pull it through.

When undressing, take off the sleeves one at a time while you support your baby's back and head. Then stretch the neckline, lifting it free of your baby's chin and face as you gently slip it off.

Clothing

Unless the temperature is hot (over 75 degrees Fahrenheit [24 degrees Celsius]), your newborn will need several layers of clothing to keep warm. It's generally best to use an undershirt and diaper, covered by pajamas, and then wrap the baby in a receiving blanket. If your baby is premature, they may need still another layer of clothing until their weight increases and their body is better able to adjust to the temperature. A good rule of thumb is to dress the baby in one more layer of clothing than you are wearing.

SWADDLING

During the first few weeks, your baby may like to be wrapped in a receiving blanket. Not only does this keep them warm, but the slight pressure around the body seems to give some newborns a sense of security. To swaddle, spread the blanket out flat, with one corner folded over. Lay the baby face-up on the blanket, with their head at the folded corner.

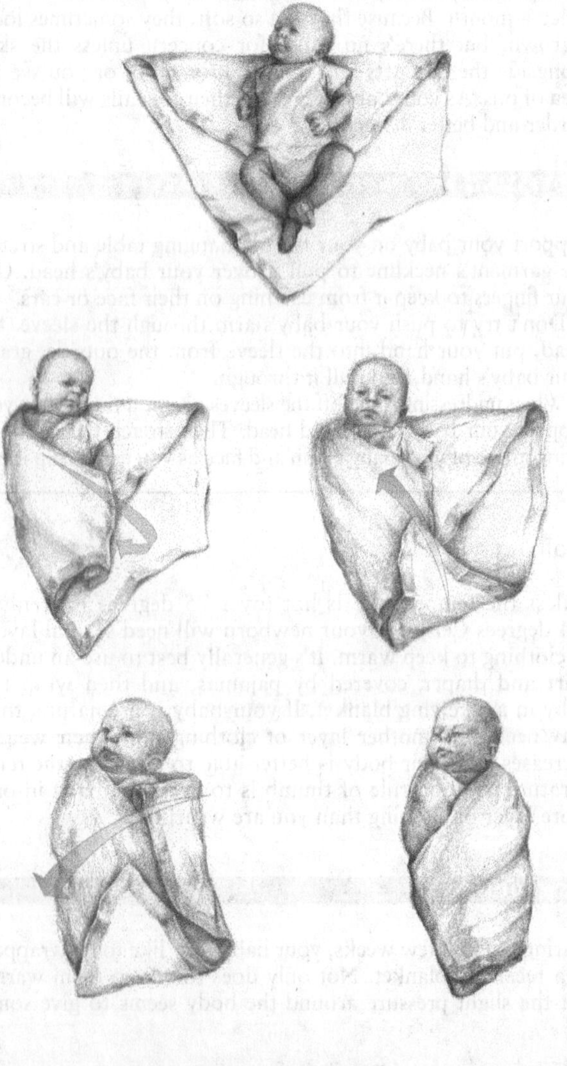

Wrap the left corner over their body and tuck it beneath them. Bring the bottom corner up over their feet, and then wrap the other corner around them, leaving only their head and neck exposed. As an option, you can keep their hands close to their chin, so that they can still self-soothe or display hunger cues. It is important that the hips and legs are allowed to move freely within the blanket. Tight swaddling of the hips could lead to dysplasia or even dislocation. Never place your swaddled baby in any position other than on their back. Stop swaddling as soon as your baby starts trying to roll over (even when they are not swaddled), usually around 2 to 3 months of age, because being on their stomach while swaddled can be dangerous. Babies born early may need to be swaddled for longer. (For more information on swaddling, visit HealthyChildren.org/swaddling.)

If you've never taken care of a newborn before, the first few clothing changes can be quite frustrating. Not only is it a struggle to get that tiny little arm through the sleeve, but your infant may shriek in protest through the whole process. They don't like the rush of air against their skin, nor do they enjoy being pushed and pulled through garments. It may be easier to hold them on your lap while changing the upper half of their body, then lay them on a bed or changing table while doing the lower half. When dressing them in one-piece pajamas, pull the pajamas over their legs before putting on the sleeves. Pull T-shirts over their head first, then guide one arm at a time through the sleeves. Use this opportunity to ask, "Where's the baby's hand?" As they get older this will turn into a game, with them pushing their arm through just to hear you say, "There's the baby's hand!"

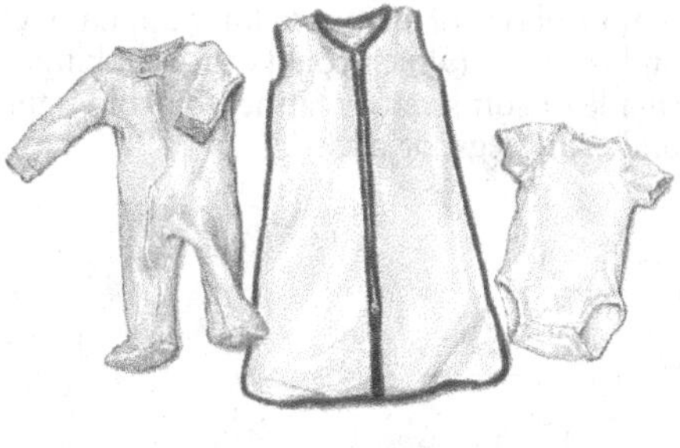

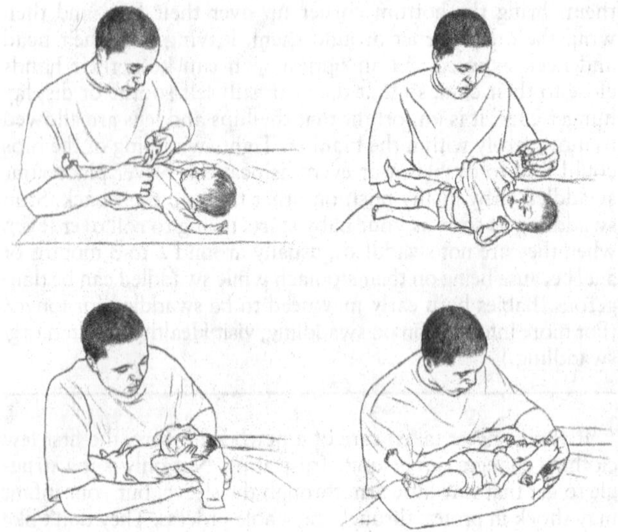

Certain clothing features can make dressing much easier. Look for garments that:

- Snap or zip all the way down the front, instead of the back
- Snap or zip down both legs to make diaper changes easier
- Have loose-fitting sleeves so that your hand fits inside to gently pull the baby's arm through
- Have no ribbons or strings to knot up, unravel, or wrap around the neck (which could cause choking)
- Are made of soft stretchy fabric (to avoid tight bindings around arms, legs, or neck)

Your Baby's Basic Healthcare

Taking a Rectal Temperature

Very few babies get through infancy without a fever, usually a sign of infection. A fever often indicates that the immune system is actively fighting viruses or bacteria, so—in this respect—it is a positive sign that the body is protecting itself. Because young babies give very few signs when ill, any child younger than 3 months with a fever needs an urgent evaluation by a physician to determine the cause; if it is due to a minor viral infection, it will usually resolve on its own, while a bacterial infection or more serious viral infection (e.g., herpes) will usually require immediate treatment with medications and frequently, in infants under 2 months of age, hospitalization.

An infant or toddler cannot hold a thermometer steady in their mouth for an oral temperature, and "fever strips" that are placed on the child's forehead are not accurate. While temporal artery thermometers (electronic devices that measure the skin temperature of the forehead) can be reliable, tympanic thermometers (devices that fit inside the ear canal) are unreliable in infants, especially under 6 months of age. An axillary (armpit) temperature can be a useful screen, but the best way to measure fever in an infant is rectally. Once you know how to take a rectal temperature, it is quite simple, but it's best to learn the steps in advance so that you're not nervous about them when your baby is actually sick. For a complete description of taking a rectal temperature properly, or other means of properly taking temperatures in infants and children, see *Chapter* 22, Fever.

Visiting the Pediatrician

You will probably see more of your pediatrician in your baby's first year than at any other time. The baby's first examination takes place immediately after birth. The schedules on *pages 692–93* list the minimum routine checkups from infancy through adolescence. Your pediatrician may want to see your baby more often.

Ideally, parents and/or regular caregivers should attend these early visits. These appointments give you and your pediatrician a chance to get to know each other and exchange questions and answers. Don't restrict yourself to medical questions; your pediatrician is also an expert on general childcare issues and a valuable resource if you're looking for childcare help, parent support groups, or other outside assistance. Many pediatricians offer information that covers common concerns, but it is a good idea to make a list of questions before each visit.

If only one parent or caregiver can attend, try to get a friend or a relative to join the parent who does. It's much easier to concentrate on your discussions with the doctor if you have a little help dressing and undressing the baby and gathering all of their things. While you're getting used to outings, an extra adult can help carry the diaper bag and hold doors.

The purpose of these early checkups is to make sure your baby is growing and developing properly and has no serious abnormalities. Specifically, the doctor will check the following areas.

Growth. You will undress your baby to be weighed on an infant scale. Their length may be measured on a flat table and their head size measured with a special tape. These measurements should be plotted in order to determine their growth curve from one visit to the next. (You can plot your baby's growth curve in the same way using the charts on *pages 699–702.*) This is the most reliable way to judge whether they're growing normally, and it will show you their position on the growth curve in relation to other children their age. If you are unsure about how your baby is growing, going into the office for additional weight checks may be reassuring.

Head. The soft spots (fontanelles, normal skin-covered openings in the skull) should be open and flat for the first few months. By 2 to 3 months of age, the spot in the back should be closed. The front soft spot should close between the ages of 18 and 24 months

Ears. The doctor will look inside both ear canals and at the eardrums with an otoscope. This detects any evidence of fluid or infection in the ear. You'll also be asked if the child responds normally to sounds. Formal hearing tests are done in the newborn nursery and later if a problem is suspected.

Eyes. The doctor will catch your baby's attention and track their eye movements. The doctor also may look inside the baby's eyes with a lighted instrument called an ophthalmoscope—repeating the internal eye examination first done in the hospital nursery. This is particularly helpful in detecting cataracts (clouding of the lens of the eye). (See Cataracts, *page 544*.)

Mouth. The mouth is checked for signs of infection and, later, for teething progress. The doctor may feel the roof of the mouth to look for a cleft palate, a condition where the bones or soft tissue does not close completely during development.

Heart and Lungs. The pediatrician will use a stethoscope on the front and back of your baby's chest to listen to the heart and lungs. This examination determines whether there are any abnormal heart rhythms, abnormal sounds, or breathing difficulties.

Abdomen. By placing their hand on the child's abdomen and gently pressing, the doctor is checking for enlarged organs or unusual masses or tenderness.

Genitalia. The genitalia are examined at each visit for any unusual lumps, tenderness, or signs of infection. In the first exam or two, the doctor pays special attention to a boy's circumcised penis to make sure it's healing properly. Pediatricians also check all boys to make certain both testes are down in the scrotum.

Hips and Legs. The pediatrician will check for problems with the hip joints. The movements your pediatrician will perform with your baby's legs are designed to detect dislocation or problems with the hip sockets. Doing this is important, as early detection can lead to proper referral and correction. Later, after the baby starts to walk, the doctor will watch them take a few steps to make sure the legs and feet are properly aligned and move normally.

Developmental Milestones. The pediatrician also asks about the baby's general development—how your baby plays, learns, speaks, acts, and moves. Among other things, they'll observe and discuss when your baby starts to smile, roll over, sit up, and walk, and how they use their hands and arms. During the exam, the pediatrician will test reflexes and general muscle tone. (See *Chapters 5 through 9* and the Appendix, *pages 692–95*, for details of developmental milestones.) If you have any concerns about your child's development, make sure to talk with your child's pediatrician. Families can monitor their child's development and share information with their child's doctor by knowing what milestones to expect at what age.

Immunizations

Your baby should receive most childhood immunizations before their second birthday. These will protect them against thirteen major diseases: hepatitis B, diphtheria, tetanus, pertussis (whooping cough), polio, *Haemophilus influenzae* type b (Hib) infection, pneumococcal infections, rotavirus, measles, mumps, rubella, chickenpox, and hepatitis A. In addition, after 6 months of age your baby will receive a yearly flu vaccine and possibly a COVID-19 vaccine. (See *Chapter 26*, Immunizations, for more information on each of these diseases, and see the Appendix, *pages 696–97*, for the immunization schedule recommended by the American Academy of Pediatrics.)

This chapter has dealt with basic infant care. However, your baby is a unique individual. Questions specific to them and them alone are best answered by your own pediatrician.

CHAPTER 5

YOUR BABY'S FIRST MONTH

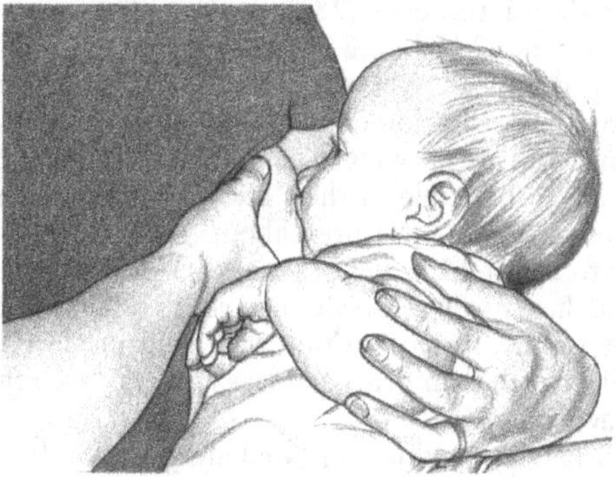

At first it may seem your newborn does nothing but eat, sleep, cry, and fill their diapers. By the end of the first month, they will be much more alert and responsive. Gradually their movements will be smoother and more coordinated—especially in getting their hand to their mouth. You'll realize your newborn will listen when you speak, watch you as you hold them, and occasionally move in response to you or to attract your attention. But before we explore their expanding capabilities, let's look at the physical changes during the first month.

Growth and Development

Physical Appearance and Growth

At birth, your newborn's weight included excess body fluid. This fluid was lost during the first few days. All newborns lose weight during the first seven days. Beginning on about the fifth day after birth, they should start gaining steadily, and by about 2 weeks of age they should have returned to their original birth weight. Almost all will have regained their birth weight by 3 weeks of age. You can plot your baby's growth on the charts in the Appendix, *pages 699–702*.

Most babies gain weight very rapidly, especially during growth spurts, which usually occur at 7 to 10 days and again between 3 and 6 weeks. The average newborn gains weight at a rate of almost an ounce (28 g) per day. They tend to grow between 1½ and 2 inches (3.8–5 cm) during this month.

Your pediatrician will pay attention to your newborn's head growth, a reflection of brain growth. The bones in your newborn's skull are growing faster during the first four months than at any other time in their life. The average newborn's head circumference measures about 13¾ inches (35 cm), growing to about 15 inches (38 cm) by 1 month.

During these first weeks, your newborn's body will straighten from the tightly curled position they held inside the uterus. They will stretch their arms and legs and may arch their back from time to time.

If your newborn's skull appeared misshapen at birth, it will soon resume its normal shape. Any scalp bruising or eyelid swelling that occurred during birth will be gone by the end of the first week or two. Any red spots in the eyes will disappear in about three weeks.

You may discover that the fine hair that covered your child's head at birth begins falling out. They may develop a temporary bald spot on the back of their head from sleeping on their back, even if the rest of their hair remains. This loss is not medically significant. The bare spots will be covered with new hair in a few months.

Another normal development is baby "acne"—pimples that break out on the face, usually during the third to fifth week. Doctors once thought this was due to maternal hormones stimulating glands in babies' skin, but they now think it may be a normal response to bacteria and yeast on the skin, and it has been renamed neonatal cephalic pustulosis. If your baby does have this pimply rash, washing the face gently once a day with a mild baby soap is sufficient. The rash usually resolves on its own in a few weeks. In severe cases, your pediatrician may prescribe a face cream. Drops of breast milk applied to the rash may also help.

Your newborn's skin may also look blotchy, ranging in color from pink to blue. Their hands and feet in particular may be colder and bluer than the rest of their body, the blood vessels being more sensitive to temperature changes and tending to shrink in response to cold. If you move their arms and legs, however, they will quickly turn pink again. Your baby's mouth, lips, and tongue should always appear pink or red.

Your baby's internal "thermostat," which causes them to sweat or shiver, won't be working properly for some time. Also, in these early weeks, they lack the insulating layer of fat that helps protect against sudden temperature shifts. It's important to dress your baby warmly in cool environments and lightly when it is hot (see *page 123*). Don't automatically bundle them up because they're a baby.

Between one and three weeks after birth, the stump from the umbilical cord should have dried and fallen off, leaving behind a clean, well-healed area. Occasionally a raw spot is left, and it may even ooze a little blood-tinged fluid. Just keep it dry and clean and it will heal by itself. If it is not completely healed and dry after three weeks, or if there is any oozing or redness that continues after it falls off, consult your pediatrician.

Checkups

After the newborn visit, your baby's next health maintenance exam will be at around 2 to 4 weeks of age. This visit is mainly to check growth and development and to help with any problems or adjustment hiccups you've encountered. There is an option to give the second dose of hepatitis B vaccine if a month has passed since the first dose, but otherwise there are no vaccines at this visit.

Reflexes

Much of your baby's activity in the first weeks is reflexive, meaning that it is involuntary or happens without the child intending it. If you put your finger in your newborn's mouth, they will reflexively suck your finger. Some reflexes remain for months, while others vanish in weeks.

In some cases, reflexes change into voluntary behavior. For example, your baby is born with a rooting reflex that prompts them to turn their head toward your hand if you stroke their cheek or mouth. This helps your baby find the nipple at feeding time. At first, babies will root from side to side, turning their head toward the nipple and then away in decreasing arcs. Soon, they will simply move their head into position and open their mouths widely to attach to the breast and suckle.

Sucking is another survival reflex present even before birth. If you had an ultrasound during pregnancy, you may have seen your baby sucking their thumb. After birth, when the baby attaches to your breast, they automatically begin to suck. This motion has two stages. First, your baby places their chin against your breast at the edge of the areola, or the dark circle that surrounds the nipple. Then, when your baby opens wide, point your nipple to meet the roof of your baby's mouth (or toward their nose and forehead). Your baby's nose will not touch your breast, and their chin will be buried in your breast. You should not feel any nipple pinching, rubbing, or pain. Your baby's attachment should feel comfortable to you, such that even if the baby feeds frequently, your nipples would not be sore. If you feel any discomfort, use your pinky finger to break the seal and reattach your baby until it feels comfortable to you and/or reach out for help from a doctor with special training in breastfeeding or a lactation consultant. When attached effectively, your baby squeezes the breast behind your nipple between the tongue and palate (called expression); this action forces the milk out. In the second phase, or milking action, the tongue moves from the areola to the nipple. This whole process is helped by the suction that secures the breast to the baby's mouth.

Coordinating these rhythmic sucking movements with breathing and swallowing is a relatively complicated task for a newborn. So even though this is a reflexive action, not all babies suck efficiently at first. If you do not hear swallows while your baby is attached to the breast, use gentle breast compression to help the milk flow; consider also using hand expression after the feeding to give your body more signals to produce milk, and feed the expressed milk to your baby. For bottle-fed babies, consider trying a different nipple size. With practice, however, your baby will become an expert at breastfeeding. Most babies, by the time they are two to three weeks past their due date, have breastfeeding going well, and in the meantime, you can help them get what they need and send signals to your body that they are here and for how much milk your baby needs.

Offer the breast every time your baby shows signs of hunger. Babies need to eat at least eight to twelve times in twenty-four hours. Rooting, sucking, and bringing their hand to their mouth are considered feeding cues in the first weeks after birth.

A dramatic reflex during these first few weeks is the Moro (or startle) reflex. If your newborn's head shifts position abruptly or falls backward, or if they get startled by something loud or abrupt, they will extend their arms and legs and neck, then rapidly bring their arms together. They may even cry loudly. The Moro reflex, which is present in varying degrees in different babies, peaks during the first month and then disappears after 2 months of age.

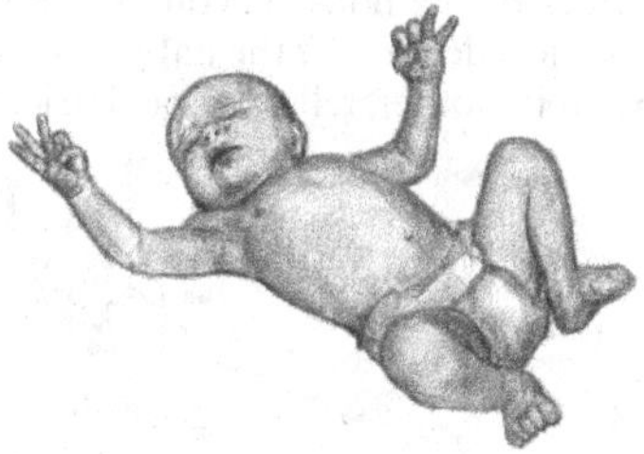

Moro reflex

A more interesting automatic response is the tonic neck reflex, or the fencing posture. You may notice that when your baby's head turns to one side, their corresponding arm will straighten, with the opposite arm bent, as if they're fencing. You may not see this response, however, since it is subtle, and if your baby is disturbed or crying, they may not perform it. It disappears at 5 to 7 months of age.

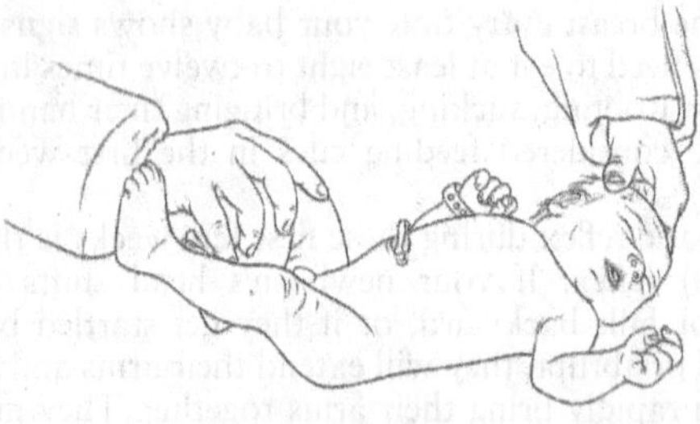

Tonic neck reflex

Both the Moro and tonic neck reflexes should be present equally on both sides of the body. If you note that the reflex seems different on one side, or that the baby moves one side of the body better than the other, tell your pediatrician.

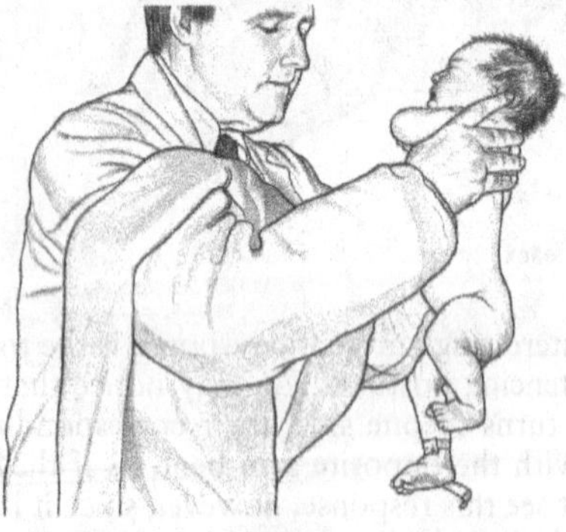

Walking/stepping reflex

EARLY BRAIN DEVELOPMENT

Research shows that during the first three years of a child's life the brain grows and develops significantly. Holding your baby skin-to-skin in the early weeks is especially important for these early brain connections. Patterns of thinking and responding are established. This means you have a special opportunity to help your baby develop appropriately and thrive socially, physically, and cognitively throughout their life. The first years last forever.

Studies have shown that children need certain elements in the early stages to grow and develop to their full potential:

- A child needs to feel special, loved, and valued.
- They need to feel safe.
- They need to feel confident about what to expect from their environment.
- They need guidance.
- They need a balanced experience of freedom and limits.
- They need to be exposed to a diverse environment filled with language, play, exploration, books, music, and toys.

While it may seem that a baby's brain activity would be relatively simple compared to an adult's, in fact a baby's brain is twice as active as an adult's. Seven hundred new connections, or synapses, form every second. During the first three years, a time neuroscientists have identified as especially important, the human brain has the greatest potential for learning. Not only is learning occurring rapidly, but basic ways of thinking, responding, and solving problems are being established. For example, notice how easy it is for a child to pick up words in a foreign language. How difficult is that same task for an adult?

This means that you and the environment you create will influence the way your baby deals with their emotions, the way they interact with people, the way they think, and the way they grow physically. By creating an appropriate environment, you are allowing normal brain development to take place. An appropriate environment is one that is child-centered and provides learning opportunities geared to your child's development, interests, and personality. Fortunately, components of a good environment include basic things that many parents naturally provide: proper nutrition; a warm, responsive, and loving family and other care providers; fun playtime; consistent positive reinforcement; engaging conversation; good books to read and to listen to; music to stimulate brain activities; and the freedom to explore and learn from their surroundings.

Review the following elements of children's health and how each one contributes to a child's brain development:

- Language. Direct face-to-face communication between parents (and other caregivers) and their baby supports language development, as does reading to them beginning in early infancy.
- Early identification of developmental concerns can help children receive services to support their development of typical early childhood skills. Due to the rapid development of the brain in early childhood, the earlier that delays are detected, the more effective interventions may be. Children with disabilities and other special healthcare needs also can greatly benefit from close monitoring of early brain development.
- Responsive feeding. Feeding based on your baby's cues as to when they are hungry and when they are full sets them up to eat only when they are hungry and not to overeat later in life.
- Positive parenting. Raising a child in a loving, supportive, and respectful environment enhances self-esteem and self-confidence, and has a great impact on the child's development. Your parental nurturing and your responsiveness to your infant will play a critical role in shaping your baby's future.
- Stimulating environment. Exploring and problem-solving in a variety of safe places promote learning.

More and more behavioral researchers are discovering how much environment plays a role in shaping a baby's life. This new science helps us understand exactly how significant our role is in a child's brain development.

To build a positive environment for your baby in your home and in your community, follow these suggestions:

- Those who are pregnant should find good prenatal care. Since brain development begins in the womb, good prenatal care can help ensure the healthy development of your child's brain. By starting prenatal care early, seeing a doctor regularly, and following their instructions—eating a balanced, healthy diet, taking prenatal vitamins, and avoiding recreational drugs, including alcohol, marijuana, and tobacco—those who are pregnant can contribute to their child's future health.

- Try to create a "village" around you. Since it's hard to raise a child on your own, seek support from your family, friends, and community. Talk to your pediatrician about parent support groups and activities.
- Interact with your child as much as possible. Talk with your child, read, listen to music, draw pictures, and play together. These kinds of activities allow you to spend time focused on your child's thoughts and interests, making your child feel special and important. You also can teach the language of communication that your child will use to form healthy relationships over a lifetime.
- Feed your baby when they show signs of hunger and do not overfeed them.
- Give your child plenty of love and attention. A warm and loving environment helps children feel safe, competent, and cared for, and it allows them to develop concern for others. Such attention cannot spoil a child.
- Provide consistent routines. Be sure you and other care providers are working with the same routines. Also, be sure your own guidelines are consistent while taking into account your child's growing competency. Consistency helps children feel confident about what to expect from their environment.

YOUR BABY'S STATES OF CONSCIOUSNESS

	Description	What Your Newborn Does
State 1	Deep sleep	Lies quietly without moving
State 2	Light sleep	Moves while sleeping; startles at noises
State 3	Drowsiness	Eyes start to close; may doze
State 4	Quiet alert	Eyes open wide; face is bright; body is quiet

State 5	Active alert	Face and body move actively
State 6	Crying	Cries, perhaps screams; body moves in very disorganized ways

Crying and Colic

From about 2 weeks on, infants cry. Some parents hesitate to pick up a crying baby, believing they'll spoil their child. But babies can't be spoiled, and their needs should be met as best as you can.

There are great variations in the crying patterns and temperaments of babies. Sometimes babies cry for no apparent reason, and it can be difficult to figure out what's behind the sobs. As the crying persists, parents can understandably become upset and stressed out.

Does your baby have a regular fussy period each day when it seems nothing will comfort them? This is quite common, particularly between 6 p.m. and midnight—just when you, too, are feeling tired from the day. These periods of crankiness may feel like torture, especially if you have other demanding children or work to do, but fortunately this phase usually improves within a few weeks or months. The length of this fussing usually peaks at about three hours a day by 6 weeks and then declines to one or two hours a day by 3 to 4 months. As long as the baby calms within a few hours and is relatively peaceful the rest of the day, there's no reason for alarm.

When you're feeling tense and anxious, have a family member or a friend look after the baby—and get out of the house. Even an hour or two away will help you maintain a positive attitude. If no other adult is available to help, it's okay to lay the baby on their back in the crib and leave the room for a few minutes. No matter how impatient or angry you become, a baby should never be shaken or hit. Shaking or slamming an infant can cause blindness, brain damage, or even death (see Abusive Head Trauma: Shaken Baby Syndrome, *page 142*). Let your personal doctor know if you are anxious or depressed or are having trouble dealing with your emotions, as they can recommend ways to help.

If the crying intensifies and persists, it may be caused by colic. About one-fifth of all babies develop colic, usually between the second and fourth weeks. It may occur even after changing your baby's diaper, feeding them, or soothing them by cuddling, rocking, or walking. Colicky children cry inconsolably, often screaming, extending or pulling up their legs, and passing gas. The crying spells can occur around the clock, although they often become worse in the early evening.

Unfortunately, colic has no definite explanation. Most often, colic means simply that the child is unusually sensitive to stimulation or cannot self-console or regulate their nervous system (also known as an immature nervous system). As they mature, this inability to self-console—marked by constant crying—will improve. Generally, colicky crying stops by 3 to 4 months, but it can last until 6 months. Colicky behavior also may signal a medical problem, such as a hernia or some type of illness. If you are worried about your baby's crying, consult your pediatrician.

Although you may simply have to wait it out, several things might be worth trying. First, of course, consult your pediatrician to make sure that the crying is not related to any serious medical condition that may require treatment. Then ask your doctor which of the following would be most helpful:

- If the fussiness seems directly related to feeds rather than time of day, consider talking with your pediatrician about dietary changes. If the baby is taking breast milk (inclusive of those bottle-feeding their infant breast milk), you can try to eliminate milk products, soy, eggs, and nuts from your own diet. This is a good thing to discuss first with your pediatrician, as a trial of elimination in your diet should be complete (checking all food products for the substance you are eliminating) and needs to be done for about two weeks before you can expect to see any changes. Be sure to eliminate only one thing at a time. If you're feeding formula to your baby, talk with your pediatrician about a protein hydrolysate formula. Less than 5 percent of colicky crying is due to food sensitivity, but in rare cases a change may help within a few days.
- Do not overfeed your baby, which could make them uncomfortable. If the baby is breastfed and you have a lot of milk, sometimes babies can get fussy because they are taking in too much milk. Your baby may be satisfied after eating on just one breast. You can offer the second

side if they are still hungry, and if not, then wait until they show signs of hunger and start on the other side for the next feeding. If you are bottle-feeding, consider trying different nipples to increase or decrease the flow rate based on your baby's hunger cues. You can also use paced feeding techniques to slow feeds and avoid overfeeding.

- Walk your baby in a baby carrier. The motion and body contact will help comfort and reassure your baby. Make sure you can always see your baby's face and that they are pink and comfortably breathing.
- Rock them, run the vacuum in the next room, or place them where they can hear the clothes dryer, a fan, or a white-noise machine. Steady, rhythmic motion and a calming sound may help them fall asleep. However, never place your child on top of the washer or dryer. Go for a ride in the car with your baby safely strapped in an approved car safety seat.
- Introduce a pacifier once breastfeeding is well established to help calm your baby and help them fall asleep. (See *pages 151, 317*.)
- Lay your baby tummy down across your knees and gently rub their back or give them a gentle massage. The pressure against their belly may help comfort them. If they fall asleep this way, you will want to place them in their crib on their back.
- Swaddle them in a large, thin, breathable cotton blanket so that they feel secure and warm. Make sure that their legs have kicking room, and that the blanket does not go above their shoulders, that their airway is clear, and that nothing is near their face.

ABUSIVE HEAD TRAUMA: SHAKEN BABY SYNDROME

Shaking a baby is a serious form of child abuse that occurs mostly with infants in the first year. The act of repeatedly shaking or slamming a baby—which may also include striking the baby's head—is often the result of a parent's or caregiver's frustration or anger in response to a baby's or toddler's constant crying or irritability. Shaking or striking a baby's head can cause serious physical and mental damage, even death.

Serious injuries associated with abusive head trauma may

include blindness or eye injuries, brain damage, damage to the spinal cord, and delay in normal development. Signs and symptoms may include irritability, lethargy (difficulty staying awake), tremors (shakiness), vomiting, seizures, difficulty breathing, and coma.

It is never okay to shake your baby. If you suspect that a care provider has shaken or hurt your baby—or if you or your spouse has done so in a moment of frustration—take your baby to the pediatrician or an emergency room immediately. Any brain damage that might have occurred will only get worse without treatment. Don't let embarrassment or fear keep you from getting treatment for your baby.

If you feel as if you might lose control when caring for your baby:

- Take a deep breath and count to ten.
- Put your baby in their crib or another safe place, leave the room, and let them cry alone for a few minutes.
- Call a friend or relative for emotional support.
- Give your pediatrician a call. Perhaps there's a medical reason your baby is crying.

The First Smile

A few of the most important developments during this month are your baby's first smiles and giggles. These start during sleep, for reasons not understood. While it's great fun to watch a newborn smile their way through a nap, the real joy comes near the end of this month when they begin to grin back at you intentionally during alert periods.

Those first loving smiles will help you tune in even more closely, and you'll soon discover you can predict a smile, a look, a sound, and, equally important, a pause from play. Gradually you and your child will recognize each other's patterns of responsiveness, so play becomes a kind of dance in which you take turns leading and following. By identifying and responding to your child's subtle signals, even at this young age, you are telling them that their thoughts and feelings are important and that they can affect the world around them. These messages are vital to their developing self-esteem and sense of fun.

Movement

For the first week or two, your baby's movements will be very jerky. Their chin may quiver and their hands may tremble. They'll startle easily when moved suddenly or from a loud sound, and the startling may lead to crying. If they appear overly sensitive to stimulation, they may be comforted if you hold them close or swaddle them snugly (see guidelines for safe swaddling on *pages 123–25*). There are even special blankets for swaddling small babies who are particularly difficult to console. (Babies should not be swaddled tightly when laid down to sleep, however, and they should never sleep in a weighted blanket.) By the end of the first month, as their nervous system matures and their muscle control improves, these shakes and quivers give way to smoother arm and leg movements that can look like they're riding a bicycle. Lay them on their stomach now and they will make crawling motions with their legs and may even push up on their arms.

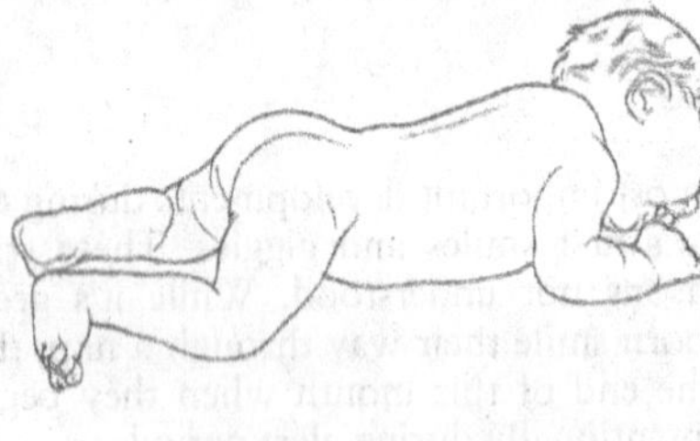

FIRST MOVEMENTS

- Makes jerky, quivering arm thrusts
- Brings hands within range of eyes and mouth
- Moves head from side to side while lying on stomach
- Head flops backward if unsupported
- Keeps hands in tight fists
- Strong reflex movements

Your baby's neck muscles also will develop rapidly, giving them more control over their head movements. Lying on their stomach, they may lift their head and turn it from side to side. However, they won't be able to hold their head up independently until about 3 months, so make sure you support it when holding them.

Your baby's hands, a source of endless fascination throughout much of this first year, will probably catch their eyes during these weeks. Their finger movements are limited, since their hands are likely clenched fists most of the time when they are awake. But they can flex their arms and bring their hands to their mouth or into their line of vision. While they can't control their hands precisely, they'll watch them closely as long as they're in view.

Vision

Your baby's vision will go through many changes this first month. They are born with better peripheral vision (the ability to see to the sides) than central vision, but they'll gradually be able to focus on a single point in the center of their visual field. They like to look at objects held about 8 to 12 inches (20.3–30.4 cm) in front of them, but by 1 month they'll focus briefly on things as far away as 3 feet (91 cm).

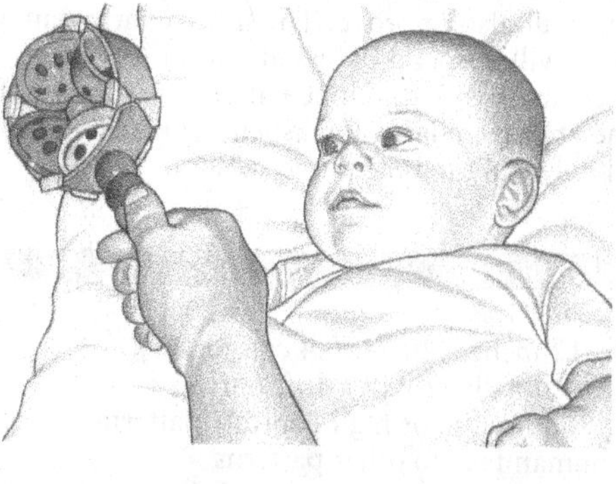

Your baby likes to look at objects held 8 to 12 inches (20.3–30.4 cm) in front of them.

At the same time, they'll learn to follow moving objects. Move your head slowly from side to side as they face you, or pass a patterned object up and down or side to side in front of them (making sure it's within their range of focus), and watch them follow your face or the object. At first, they may only be able to follow large objects moving slowly through a limited range, but soon they'll be following smaller, speedier movements.

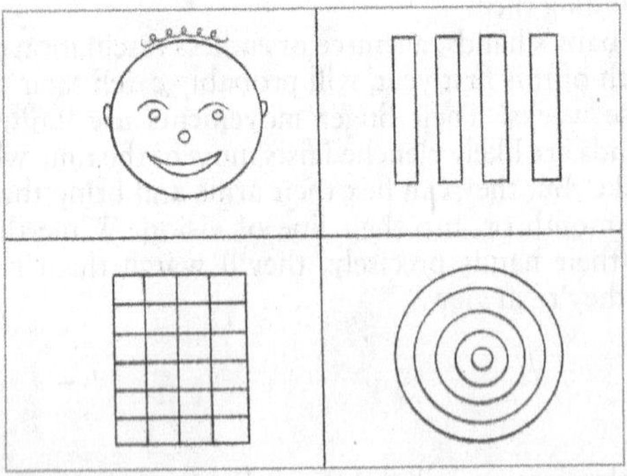

Babies are most attentive to black-and-white pictures or high-contrast patterns, such as stripes, bull's-eyes, checks, and very simple faces.

At birth your baby was very sensitive to bright light, and their pupils were smaller than those of an adult. At 2 weeks, their pupils will begin to enlarge and become more reactive to light. Some sensitive babies may cry when exposed to a very bright light. As their retinas develop, their ability to see and recognize patterns will also improve. The more contrast in a pattern, the more it will attract a baby's attention.

Color vision becomes more developed after 4 months, so if you show your newborn similar colors, such as green and turquoise, they probably can't tell the difference.

VISION AT 1 MONTH OLD

- Focuses 8 to 12 inches (20.3–30.4 cm) away
- Eyes may occasionally cross or drift outward
- Prefers black-and-white or high-contrast patterns
- Prefers the human face to other patterns

Hearing

Your baby should have had a hearing screen shortly after birth; in fact, the American Academy of Pediatrics recommends that newborn hearing screenings occur prior to discharge from the hospital, and parents should ask for the results. (See Hearing Loss [Hearing Impairment], *page 458*.)

Infants with normal hearing abilities will pay close attention to human voices during the first month, especially high-pitched ones speaking "baby talk." When you talk to them, they'll turn their head to search for you and listen closely. Watch carefully and you may even see them make subtle movements of their arms and legs in time with your speech.

Your infant also will be sensitive to noise levels. If you make a loud clicking sound in their ear or bring them into a noisy, crowded room, they may shut down, becoming as unresponsive as if they had heard nothing. Or they may be so sensitive that they startle, erupt into crying, and turn their entire body away from the noise. Substitute a soft rattle or quiet music, and they'll become alert and turn to locate the source of this interesting sound.

Not only does your baby hear well, but they'll remember some of the sounds. As some research supports, some mothers who repeatedly read a story aloud late in their pregnancy have found that their babies seem to recognize the story when it is read to them again after birth—the babies became quiet and looked more attentive. Try reading your favorite children's story aloud for several days in a row when your baby is alert and attentive. Then wait a day or two before reading it again. Do they seem to recognize it?

HEARING AT 1 MONTH OLD

- Hearing is fully mature
- Recognizes and reacts to loud sounds
- May look or turn toward familiar sounds and voices

Smell and Touch

As with patterns and sounds, babies are also particular about tastes and smells. They will breathe deeply to catch a whiff of your breast milk, vanilla, banana, or sugar, but will turn up their nose at the smell of alcohol or vinegar. By the end of their first week, if they're nursing, they'll turn toward their mother's breast but will ignore the breasts of other nursing mothers.

Babies are equally sensitive to touch and the way they're handled. They'll nestle into a soft piece of flannel but pull away from scratchy burlap. When they are stroked gently with a palm, they'll relax and become quiet. If picked up roughly, they'll probably take offense and start to cry. If rocked slowly, they'll become quiet and attentive. Holding, stroking, rocking, or cuddling will calm them when they're upset and make them more alert when they're drowsy. It also sends a clear message of a parent's love and affection. Long before they understand a word parents say, babies understand parental moods and feelings from their touch.

SMELL AND TOUCH AT 1 MONTH OLD

- Prefers sweet smells
- Avoids bitter or acidic smells
- Recognizes the scent of their own mother's breast milk
- Prefers soft to coarse sensations
- Dislikes rough or abrupt handling

Temperament

Consider these two babies, both from the same family:

- The first baby is calm and quiet, happy to play by themselves. They watch everything around them but rarely demand attention themselves. Left on their own, they sleep for long periods and eat infrequently.
- The second baby is fussy and startles easily. They thrash their arms and legs, moving almost constantly whether awake or asleep. While most newborns sleep fourteen hours a day, this baby sleeps only ten, and wakens at

> the slightest nearby activity. They seem in a hurry to do everything at once and even eat in a rush, gulping their feedings and swallowing so much air that they need frequent burping.

Both these babies are normal and healthy. One is no "better" than the other, but because their personalities are so far apart, the two will be treated very differently from birth.

Your baby will demonstrate many unique personality traits from the earliest weeks after birth. Discovering these traits is one of the most exciting parts of having a baby. Are they active and intense, or slow-going? Are they timid when faced with a new situation, such as the first bath, or do they enjoy it? You'll find clues to their personality in everything they do, from falling asleep to crying. The more you pay attention and respond appropriately to their unique personality, the calmer and more predictable your life will be in the months to come.

While most of these early character traits are built into the newborn's hereditary makeup, their appearance may be delayed in babies born prematurely. Premature babies don't express their needs—such as hunger, fatigue, or discomfort—as clearly as other newborns. They may be extra sensitive to light, sound, and touch, and these stimuli may cause them to become fussy and look away. When this happens, it's up to the parent to stop and wait until the baby is alert and ready for more attention. Eventually most of these early reactions will fade away, and the baby's natural character traits will become more evident. Neonatal intensive care units are now using developmental care that promotes attachment, taking into account a newborn's states of alertness and responsiveness to hearing their mother's voice, and providing kangaroo care when the baby's condition is stable enough to do so safely.

TOYS APPROPRIATE FOR YOUR 1-MONTH-OLD

- Mobile with highly contrasting colors and patterns (do not attach to the sleeping surface)
- Music players with soft music
- Soft, brightly colored, and patterned toys that make gentle sounds (remember not to leave these in the crib during sleep times)

Low-birth-weight babies—those who weigh less than 5½ pounds (2.5 kg) at birth—even if full-term, may also be less responsive than other newborns. At first, they may be very sleepy and not seem very alert. After a few weeks, they seem to wake up, eating eagerly but still remaining restless and hypersensitive to stimulation between feedings. This sensitivity may last until they grow and mature further.

From the beginning, your baby's temperament will influence the way you treat them and feel about them. If you had specific ideas about child-rearing, reevaluate them now to see if they're in tune with your baby's character. The same goes for expert advice—from books, articles, and especially from well-meaning relatives and friends about the "right way" to raise a child. The truth is, there is no single way that works for every child. You must create your own guidelines based on your child's unique personality, your own beliefs, and the circumstances of your family life. The important thing is to remain responsive to your baby's individuality. Don't try to box them into some previously set mold or pattern. Your baby's uniqueness is their strength, and respecting that strength from the start will lay the best possible foundation for their self-esteem and for loving relationships with others.

Basic Care

Bowel Movements

In the first week, your baby should have at least one bowel movement per day. If this is not happening, your baby should be seen by their pediatrician for a weight check. In the first few days, the stools will appear black and very tarry. By day 5, the bowel movements will be a bright mustard-yellow color. While we often refer to normal newborn stool as being yellow, soft, and seedy, normal stool colors can also vary widely, from light tan to forest green. The only colors that should prompt concern are white, which can indicate liver or gallbladder disease, and red at any point or tarry black after one or two meconium stools have passed, which can be a sign of bleeding within the stomach or intestines.

If your baby is having bowel movements that are not turning yellow by day 5 or that are hard like marbles or rabbit pellets, they should be checked by their pediatrician. Around

1 month of age, your breastfeeding baby's bowel movements may space out to once every few days or once a week. This is normal as long as the stools come out soft. If your infant is otherwise feeding normally, there is a wide range of acceptable bowel patterns.

Carrying Your Baby

A newborn has almost no head control and needs to be carried in a way that protects their head from flopping from side to side or snapping from front to back. This is done by cradling the head when carrying the baby in a lying position and supporting the head and neck with your hand when carrying them upright.

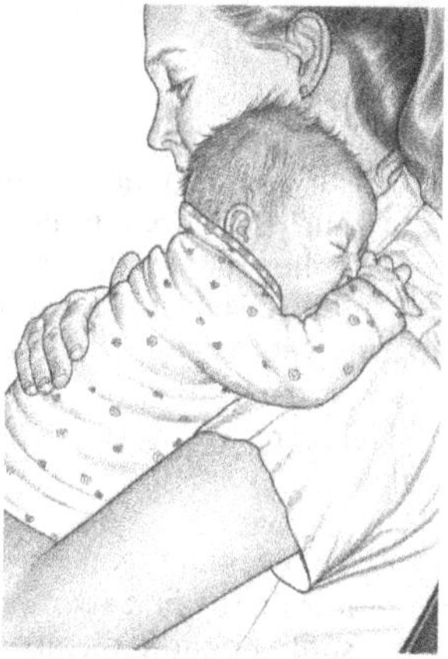

A very young infant who has not developed head control needs to be carried in a way that keeps their head from flopping from side to side or snapping from front to back.

Pacifiers

Once breastfeeding is well established, offering a pacifier when your baby is going to sleep may help reduce the risk of sudden unexpected infant death (SUID). However, if your baby doesn't want it or if it falls from their mouth, don't force it. Babies who suck their fingers or hands have an advantage, since hands are always available. Once older, your baby will have the hand coordination to find and replace the pacifier themselves.

Look for a pacifier model that is age-appropriate for your baby, has a soft nipple, is rounded in appearance (not flat on one side), and does not have any pieces that could break off and become a choking hazard (avoid models that break into two pieces). Clean pacifiers with warm, soapy water as needed.

Never fasten the pacifier with a cord, because of the risk of strangulation. Babies can choke or strangle on cords, strings, ribbons, and fasteners attached to pacifiers. Also, for safety reasons, it's never a good idea to make pacifiers out of bottle nipples. Babies have pulled the nipple out of such homemade pacifiers and choked on them. Follow the recommended age range on the packaging. Never attach objects, such as blankets, plush or stuffed toys, and other items that may present a suffocation or choking risk, to pacifiers.

Going Outside

Fresh air and a change of surroundings are good for both you and your baby, even in their first month, so take them out for walks when the weather is nice. Be sure to dress them properly for outings, since their internal temperature control isn't fully mature yet. As stated before, follow the one-light-layer-more-than-yourself rule.

Here are a few suggestions for those outings with your baby:

- Your infant's skin is extremely susceptible to sunburn during the first six months, so keep them out of direct sunlight and remember that water, snow, sand, and concrete can reflect enough sunlight to cause a sunburn. If you must take them out in the sun, dress them in lightweight and light-colored clothing, with a hat to shade their face. If you'll be staying in one place, make sure the spot is shady, and adjust their position as the sun moves. Sunscreen can be used on exposed areas if protective clothing, hats, and shade are not available. Apply it only on small areas such as the face and the backs of the hands as needed, testing ahead of time their sensitivity to it on a small patch on their back. Although sunscreen can be applied to all areas that the sun can reach, be careful to avoid the eyes.
- In hot-weather months, do not let baby equipment (such as car safety seats and strollers) sit in the sun for long periods. The plastic and metal parts can get hot enough to burn. Check the surface temperature of such equipment before allowing your baby to come in contact with it, and throw a blanket or towel over the car safety seat when the car is parked to keep it out of direct sunlight.

- In uncomfortably cold or rainy weather, keep your baby inside as much as possible. If you must go out, bundle them up and use a warm hat to cover their head and ears. You can shield their face with a blanket when you're outside, ensuring their mouth and nose are not covered, but make sure you can always see their face. If you need to drive, remember to remove thick coats and bulky clothes before strapping the baby into their car safety seat.
- To check whether they are clothed appropriately, feel their hands and feet and the skin on their chest. Their hands and feet should be slightly cooler than their body, but not cold. Their chest should feel warm. If their hands, feet, and chest feel cold, take them to a warm room, unwrap them, and hold them close so that the heat from your body warms them. Until their temperature is back to normal, these other methods are more effective to warm them before wrapping them in additional blankets or clothing.

Finding Help at Home

Many families need in-home help with a new baby. In two-parent households, if both are able to take off from work, this will help a lot. If not, one option is to ask a close relative or friend, or consider hiring a postpartum doula. Some families hire a professional baby nurse to help out. If you think you'll need the extra help, especially of a baby nurse, it is wise to make these arrangements in advance rather than waiting until after delivery.

Some communities have a visiting nurse or housekeeping service. Some neighborhoods and faith communities will arrange "meal trains." These services will not solve middle-of-the-night problems, but will provide an hour or two during the day to catch up on work or simply rest. It may be helpful to arrange these in advance if possible.

Be selective about the help you seek. Look for assistance from those who will really support you and your feeding and parenting decisions. Your goal is to reduce the stress level in your home, not add to it.

Before you start interviewing or asking friends or family for assistance, decide exactly what kind of help you need. Ask yourself the following questions:

- Do you want someone to help tend to the baby, or do the housework, or cook meals—or a little bit of everything?
- During what hours do you want help?
- Do you need someone who can drive (to pick up other children at school, shop for groceries, run errands, and the like)?

Once you know what you need, make sure the person you choose understands and agrees to meet those needs. Explain your expectations clearly, and if this is an employment situation, put those expectations in writing. This person should be someone you trust. If employing help, be certain a background check has been performed and the person has taken an approved CPR class (from the American Red Cross, for example) and has learned how to respond when a child is choking or not breathing. If the person will be driving, their driving record should be checked. Regardless of whether this is a relative, a friend, or an employee, ask this person to notify you if they become ill so that you can take steps to prevent the infection from being passed to your baby. (For example, that person should not come to work if ill. If they are only mildly ill, they might walk the dog or leave groceries on your front step rather than directly caring for your baby.)

Your Baby's First Sitter. Sometime in the first month or two, you may need to leave your baby for the first time. The more confidence you have in your babysitter, the easier this experience will be. Therefore, you may want your first sitter to be someone very close and trusted—a grandparent, close friend, or relative who's familiar with both you and the child.

After your first separation, you may want to look for a regular babysitter. Ask your friends, neighbors, and coworkers for recommendations, or see if your pediatrician or nurse practitioner can refer you to someone. Local childcare agencies or referral services are great resources. You might also contact the placement services at local colleges for a listing of child development or early education students who babysit. A number of online services can help you find a sitter and will even perform background checks and provide references, often for a small fee. It is absolutely essential you check references, inquiring about the sitter's responsibility, maturity, and ability to adhere to instructions and respect your parenting and feeding preferences—particularly for someone you've only recently met or don't know well.

Try to observe a candidate in person with your baby prior to hiring. You should be looking for someone who is affectionate, is capable, and supports your views about childcare. If you feel comfortable with the individual after talking, let them hold the baby so that you can see how they handle the infant. Ask if they've had experience caring for babies. Although experience, references, and good health are very important, the best way to judge a babysitter is by doing a trial run while you're home. It will give your baby and the babysitter a chance to get to know each other before they're alone, and it will give you an opportunity to make sure you feel comfortable with the sitter.

Whenever you leave your baby with a sitter, provide a list of all emergency phone numbers, including those where you or other family members can be reached; the sitter should know where you'll be and how to reach you at all times. Establish clear guidelines about what to do in an emergency and reinforce that the sitter should call the local emergency number; clearly post the home address on an emergency sheet to give to emergency responders. Show the sitter where all exits to your home are located, as well as smoke detectors and fire extinguishers. Make sure your sitter has taken an approved CPR class (from the American Red Cross, for example) and has learned how to respond when a baby is choking or not breathing. (See Cardiopulmonary Resuscitation (CPR) and Mouth-to-Mouth Resuscitation, *page 493*, and Choking, *pages 494, 703*.) Some local YMCAs or American Red Cross chapters can provide a list of babysitters who have taken CPR or babysitting safety courses. Give your sitter any other guidelines you feel are important (e.g., never open the door to strangers, including delivery people) and stress that the sitter can call you or a trusted neighbor if they are having difficulty with the baby and are getting frustrated. Let friends and neighbors know about your arrangement so they can help if there's an emergency, and ask them to tell you if they suspect any problems in your absence.

Traveling with Your Baby

Here are some tips for traveling with your baby:

- When traveling by car, make sure your baby is safely strapped into their car safety seat. (For more information, see Car Safety Seats, *page 321*.) The backseat is the safest place for children to ride. Rear-facing seats should never be placed in the front seat with a passenger-side airbag. At this age, a baby should always ride in the rear-facing position. The same car seat safety rules apply in rental cars, taxis, and any other vehicle your baby rides in. Give yourself extra time to properly install the car safety seat in such vehicles before you need to start traveling.
- If you can afford to, it is safest to use a car safety seat on planes, instead of holding the baby on your lap. This means your baby ideally would have their own ticket/seat on the plane. Besides protecting them from injuries in severe turbulence, riding in their familiar car safety seat may help keep your baby calm and quiet during the flight. It also ensures you will have a safe, appropriate car safety seat available at your destination. If you're not sure how to secure your baby safely on a plane, ask a flight attendant to help you.
- When breastfeeding, know that you are legally allowed to breastfeed your baby in the airport, in public places, and on the plane. Most airports now have private spaces to feed your baby and express your milk as needed.
- Always perform a safety inspection of any crib or play yard provided by a hotel for your baby to sleep in. (See Cribs, *page 300*.)

KEEPING SIBLINGS HAPPY

With all the excitement over the new baby's arrival, siblings will probably need some time to adjust. They may be upset over their parents' absence, especially if this was their first prolonged separation. Even after parents return home after the birth, siblings may have trouble understanding why their parents are tired and cannot play as much as they're used to. There are a number of ways you can help with the adjustment process by making special space for older siblings.

Here are some suggestions to help soothe your older children and make them feel more involved during the first month home with your new baby:

- If possible, have the siblings visit in the hospital.
- When the family comes home from the hospital, bring each sibling a special gift to celebrate, and have them help you "bring" the baby into the house and show the new baby their toys and room.
- Set aside a special time to spend alone with each sibling every day. Make sure that parents have time with each child, individually and together.
- While you're taking pictures of the new baby, take some of the older children—alone and with the baby.
- If both the new baby and the siblings want you at the same time, as long as you can hear the new baby's cries and you know they are safe, you can tend to the older child first and even say out loud to the baby, "I hear you, and I know you are hungry/want a diaper change, and I will be there as soon as I tend to your sibling."
- Ask the grandparents or other close relatives to take the older children on a special outing—to the zoo, a movie, or just dinner. This special attention may help them through moments when they feel abandoned.
- Have some small gifts for the older child and present them when friends come with gifts for the baby.
- Especially during the first month, when the baby needs to eat so often, older children can get jealous of the intimacy their parents have with the baby during feedings. One way to address this issue is to give a sibling a job to do, such as helping hold the bottle if you use one, picking out a burp cloth, or bringing you water.
- Reading stories that specifically deal with issues of jealousy encourages a toddler or preschooler to voice their feelings so that you can help them become more accepting. There are also a number of books about nursing a new baby geared to the older sibling that are fun for story time.

Health Watch

The following medical problems are of particular concern to parents during the first month. (For problems that occur generally throughout childhood, check the listings in Part 2.)

Breathing Difficulties. Normally, your baby should take twenty to forty breaths per minute. This pattern is most regular when they are asleep and healthy. When awake, occasionally they may breathe rapidly for a short period, then take a brief pause (less than ten seconds) before returning to normal breathing. This is called periodic breathing. A runny nose may interfere with breathing because your baby's nasal passages are narrow and fill easily. This condition can be eased by using a cool-mist humidifier and gently suctioning the nose with a bulb syringe (ordinarily given to you by the hospital; for its use, see *page 470*). Read and follow the cleaning instructions for humidifiers and bulb syringes carefully. Alternatively, you can use a breath-powered aspirator. Occasionally, mild salt-solution nose drops or a saline mist inhaler can help thin the mucus and clear the nasal passages. If your baby has a fever, their breathing may become faster, increasing by about two breaths per minute for each degree of temperature elevation. When the number of breaths exceeds sixty per minute, or if the baby's skin is pulling in between, over, or under their ribs (retractions), their nose is flaring, or they are coughing a lot, be sure to contact your pediatrician. A fever with a rectal temperature of 100.4 degrees Fahrenheit (38 degrees Celsius) or higher in a baby younger than 3 months old may be serious, and warrants urgent evaluation.

In the first month after birth, a baby with otherwise normal breathing at birth may develop stridor. Stridor is a high-pitched noise usually heard during inspiration (breathing in). Stridor results from rapid airflow across a narrowing, primarily at the level of the larynx (voice box) or trachea (windpipe). The most common cause is called laryngomalacia, which may worsen during feeds, while lying on the back, or during crying. Most babies with stridor from laryngomalacia are able to gain weight well and do not need any change in feeding pattern. Difficulty with feeding (coughing, choking, sputtering), inability to gain weight or maintain weight, or symptoms such as retractions, sleep difficulty, or changes in color warrant urgent evaluation by a pediatrician and/or a pediatric otolaryngologist.

Diarrhea. After feedings in the first month after birth, healthy and thriving breastfed babies may occasionally have frequent, watery, yellow, green, or orange-brown stools that some people mistake for diarrhea. The danger, especially at this young age, is fluid loss and becoming dehydrated. The first signs of dehydration are dry mouth and a significant decrease in the number of wet diapers. But don't wait for dehydration to occur. Call your pediatrician if the stools are very loose or occur more often than after each feeding (more than eight per day), or if you see any bright red blood in the stools.

Constipation. Constipation in babies presents as infrequent, very hard stools. Babies should be producing a stool at least once a day the first week after birth. If your baby is having fewer stools, skipping days, or having hard stools, it may be a sign that your baby isn't getting enough to eat or needs some extra fluid to push everything through. Call your pediatrician if your baby is stooling less often than usual, is having hard, pellet-like stools, or isn't feeding well.

Excessive Sleepiness. Since each baby requires a different amount of sleep, it's difficult to tell when a baby is excessively drowsy. If your infant starts sleeping much more than usual, it might indicate an infection, so notify your pediatrician. Another possible cause of sleepiness could be medication or herbal supplements taken by a breastfeeding mom. (Babies this age should not be taking any herbal supplements.)

Eye Infections/Tear Drainage Problems. Some babies are born with one or both tear drainage ducts partially or totally blocked, which may become noticeable when tear production increases starting at 2 to 4 weeks. If the ducts remain blocked, you may notice tearing and mucus because the tears are unable to drain into the nose and then flow back to the inner corners of the eyes. The ducts open up in most babies by 1 year of age without treatment. You may also help open them by gently massaging the area from the inner corner of the eye down the side of the nose. However, do this only at the direction of your pediatrician.

If the ducts remain blocked, the presence of mucus does not

necessarily mean your baby has an infection. This mucus may look like greenish yellow or white discharge at the inner corner of the eye, and the eyelashes may be stuck together when your baby wakes from sleeping. Because this discharge does not usually indicate an infection, it is often not treated with an antibiotic. (See Tear [or Lacrimal] Production Problems, *page 552*.) On the other hand, if an infection is suspected, it will usually be treated with antibiotic eye drops or ointment prescribed after examining the eyes. In many cases, only gentle cleansing with water is needed. When eyelashes are sticky, dip a cotton ball or soft washcloth in warm water and gently wipe the eyelid from the nose to the outer eyelid. Use a clean washcloth or cotton ball with each pass.

Although this type of discharge may recur several times, it will not damage the eye or affect the vision, and your baby will probably outgrow it. In rare cases, blocked tear ducts require surgical treatment, usually if they don't open by 9 to 12 months of age.

If the eye itself is bloodshot or pink with excessive discharge, your infant could have conjunctivitis (pinkeye), and you should notify your pediatrician (see Eye Infections, *page 545*).

Fever. Whenever your baby is unusually cranky or feels warm, take their temperature. (See Taking a Rectal Temperature, *page 127*.) If their rectal temperature reads 100.4 degrees Fahrenheit (38 degrees Celsius) or higher on two separate readings, and they're not overly bundled up, call your pediatrician at once. Fever can signal infection, and babies this age can become seriously ill quickly.

Floppiness. Newborn infants all seem somewhat floppy because their muscles are still developing, but if your baby feels exceptionally loose or floppy, it could be a sign of a more serious problem, such as an infection. Consult your pediatrician immediately.

Hearing. Pay attention to how your baby responds to sounds even if they passed their newborn hearing screening. Do they startle at loud or sudden noises? Do they become quiet or look toward you when you talk to them? If they do not respond normally to sounds around them, ask your pediatrician about formal hearing testing. (See Hearing Loss [Hearing Impairment], *page 458*.) Testing is recommended if your infant was extremely premature, if they were deprived of oxygen or had a severe infection at birth, or if your family has a history of hearing loss in early childhood. If there is any suspicion of hearing loss, your infant should be tested as early as possible, as a delay in diagnosis and treatment is likely to interfere with normal language development.

Jaundice. Jaundice is a normal yellowing of the skin that can appear shortly after birth and sometimes last for more than two to three weeks in breastfed babies. In formula-fed babies, most jaundice goes away within two weeks. If your baby is jaundiced for more than three weeks or the jaundice seems to be increasing at any time, see your pediatrician. (For additional information about jaundice, see *page 42*.)

Jitters. Many newborns have quivery chins and shaky hands, but if your baby's whole body seems to be shaking, it could be a sign of low blood sugar or calcium levels, or some type of seizure disorder. Notify your pediatrician so that they can determine the cause. If you can, try to take a video of the event, which can help your pediatrician determine how concerned to be.

Rashes and Infections. Common newborn rashes include the following:

- Cradle cap (seborrheic dermatitis) appears as scaly patches on the scalp. Washing the hair and brushing out the scales daily helps with control. It usually disappears on its own within the first few months but may need treatment with a special shampoo. (See Cradle Cap and Seborrheic Dermatitis, *page 653*.)
- Fingernail or toenail infections will appear as redness around the edge of the toenail or fingernail, which may seem to hurt when touched. These infections may respond to warm compresses, but for a baby at this age they should be taken seriously and be examined by a doctor, as they may require medication.
- Umbilical infections are rare, but if one occurs it often appears as redness around the umbilical stump. There's usually pus and often tenderness. Babies with these infections should be examined by your pediatrician. If

your baby is also running a fever, see your pediatrician right away, as they may need antibiotics or hospitalization. It is normal, however, to have a small amount of clear oozing, drops of blood, and a scab around the umbilical stump without any redness or fever. If this is the case, watch it for a few days; if it doesn't heal on its own, see your pediatrician.

- Diaper rash. See instructions for handling this problem on *pages 114–15*.

Thrush. White patches in the mouth may indicate that your baby has thrush, a common yeast infection. This condition is often treated with an oral antifungal medication prescribed by your pediatrician, but milder cases may resolve without treatment.

Vomiting. Although spitting up small amounts after feedings is very common, if your baby starts forcefully vomiting (shooting out several inches rather than dribbling from the mouth), contact your pediatrician at once to make sure they do not have an obstruction of the valve between the stomach and the small intestine (pyloric stenosis; see *page 378*). Any vomiting that persists for more than eight hours or two to three feedings, or is accompanied by diarrhea or fever or by fewer wet diapers, should be evaluated by your pediatrician.

Weight Gain. Your baby should be gaining weight rapidly (⅔ to 1 ounce [20–30 g] per day) after the first few days following birth. If they aren't, your pediatrician will want to make sure that they are getting adequate calories in their feedings and that they are absorbing them properly. Be prepared to answer these questions:

- How often does the baby eat?
- If breastfeeding, do you hear your baby swallowing? Do your breasts feel lighter after feeds? Does the baby seem satisfied?
- If bottle-feeding, what type of formula is used? How is it prepared? How much do they eat at a feeding?
- How many bowel movements does the baby have each day?
- What is the color and consistency of the stools?
- How often does the baby urinate?

If your baby is eating well and the contents of their diapers are normal in amount and consistency, there is probably no cause for alarm. Your baby may be getting off to a slow start, or their weight could have been inaccurately measured. Your pediatrician may want to schedule another office visit in two or three days to reevaluate the situation.

▪ YOUR BABY AT 1 MONTH OLD CHECKLIST ▪

Safety Check

Car Safety Seats

- Your baby should ride in a properly installed, federally approved car safety seat every time they ride in the car. If you are carrying your baby to the car in the car safety seat, make sure they are strapped in securely. Do not use the car seat as a place for the baby to nap in the house, because the angle of the car safety seat when removed from the car becomes an unsafe sleeping position. At this age, they should ride only in the backseat in the car safety seat in the rear-facing position. Never place a baby in the front seat of a car, as the passenger-side airbag can cause serious life-threatening injury. Car safety seats have an expiration date, so if you are using an older car safety seat, check to see if it is still within date. If your car was manufactured after 2002, you can use the Lower Anchors and Tethers for Children (LATCH) system or the vehicle seatbelt (not both) to attach the car safety seat (see *pages 326–28*).

Bathing

- A separate baby bathtub may be more convenient and easier to manage than bathing your baby in a regular bathtub.
- Fill it and test the water temperature before you put your baby in the tub. Never leave the faucet running while your baby is in the sink; instead, fill the sink first, test the temperature, and then put the baby in the water.

The water should feel just slightly warm to the touch. Always hold your baby under their arms while bathing them. If you are bathing your baby in the sink, seat them on a washcloth or bath mat to prevent slipping and hold them under their arms. Never leave your baby unsupervised in the water, even for just a brief amount of time. Never run the dishwasher while bathing your baby in the kitchen sink; otherwise, you risk scald burns from the dishwasher's hot water.

- Adjust the maximum temperature of your water heater to 120 degrees Fahrenheit (48.9 degrees Celsius) or lower so that hot water can't scald the child. Any modern water heater should indicate where this setting is, so check your manual or call your plumber if you're unsure.

Changing Surfaces

- Never leave your baby unattended on any surface (such as changing tables, chairs, tables, sofas, beds, and countertops) above the floor. Always keep a hand on your baby if they are on a raised surface. Even at this young age, babies can wiggle and move and push against things, and these movements can result in a fall. Place your baby in a safe place such as a crib or play yard when you cannot be with them.

Suffocation Prevention

- Keep the crib free of all objects. Make sure the mattress fits tightly, and use a fitted sheet only.
- Don't have your baby sleep in your own bed next to you. Keep them in their crib or bassinet next to your bed.
- Do not cover your baby in loose blankets or comforters that they could get tangled in or suffocate under. Instead, dress them in appropriate-weight sleepwear (like a wearable blanket or sleep sack).
- Always place your baby on their back for sleep. They should not sleep on a soft comforter, sheepskin, soft

mattress, cushion, or pillow. Place them to sleep only on their back on a firm surface.

- Never leave plastic bags or wrappings where your baby can wiggle or roll into them.

Fire and Burn Prevention

- Do not use a microwave oven to heat formula or breast milk, as it can leave hot spots in the fluid. Be sure to test the temperature of formula or heated breast milk on your wrist before feeding it to your baby.
- Do not carry your baby and hot liquids like coffee, tea, or soup at the same time. Also, do not hold or cradle your baby near hot liquids on the stove or tabletops. Even a small splash could scald your baby.
- Install smoke and carbon monoxide detectors in the proper places throughout your home, and check them regularly to be sure they are working.

Supervision

- Never leave your baby unattended in the bathtub, yard, or car. If you need to walk away from your baby inside the house, place your baby in a crib or play yard.
- Never leave your baby in the car unattended, even for a minute. Placing a teddy bear or an infant toy in the front seat or an item you need, like your wallet or purse, in the backseat next to your baby can help remind you.
- Never place an infant car carrier (with infant buckled in) near the edge of a table or counter. An infant in a carrier can easily fall to the ground.

Necklaces and Cords

- Don't let strings or cords (e.g., from a window shade) dangle in or anywhere near the crib or around your baby. Keep cribs away from windows and blind or curtain cords. The US Consumer Product Safety Commission recommends using cordless window coverings in homes where young children live or visit, but if that is not possible, tie cords high out of reach and keep the crib at least 3 feet away.

- Don't attach pacifiers, medallions, or other objects to the crib or to your baby with a cord.
- Don't place a string or necklace around the baby's neck (including amber teething necklaces, which have never been shown to reduce pain).
- Don't use clothing with drawstrings.

Head Support

- Do not jerk or shake the baby. Cradle and rock them gently.
- Always support the baby's head and neck when holding or moving their body.

CHAPTER 6

YOUR BABY AT 2 MONTHS

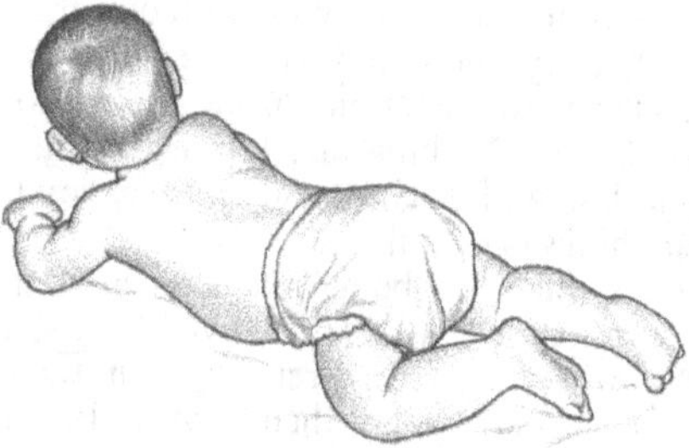

By the beginning of the second month, much of the awe, exhaustion, and uncertainty you may have felt has likely given way to more of a routine and self-confidence. You have hopefully settled into a fairly routine (if still demanding) schedule around your baby's feedings and naps. You've adjusted to having a new family member and are beginning to understand their general temperament. And you probably have already received the crowning reward that makes all the sacrifice worthwhile: their first true smile. This smile is just a glimmer of the delights in store over the next three months. Will the coming months continue to be frustrating and challenging? Of course. If you feel overwhelmed, activate your support network, and when you don't know where to turn, your child's pediatrician should be able to share some ideas.

You may also be returning to work and need to find infant-centered daycare. *Chapter 10* will help you select the proper type of childcare depending on your circumstances. Many new parents feel sad or anxious leaving their babies in others' care, but as you and the care team get to know each other, such feelings are likely to fade. Many childcare centers allow parents to visit during the day or to check on their children via remote video feeds; ask your center what policies they find work best for parents and staff.

Between 1 and 4 months, your baby will undergo a dramatic transformation from a totally dependent newborn to an active and responsive infant. They'll lose many of their newborn reflexes while acquiring control of their body. You'll find them inspecting their hands and watching their movements. They'll also become increasingly interested in their surroundings, especially people close to them. They'll often smile when they see or hear you. Sometime during their second or third month, they'll begin "talking" back in gentle but intentional coos and gurgles. With each new discovery, you'll see a new part of your child's personality.

Occasionally there will be moments when your baby's development seems to lag, usually followed by a spurt in progress. They may seem to be stretching out their nighttime feedings for several weeks, but then begin waking up again to feed more frequently. It's probably a sign they're about to take a major developmental leap forward. In a week or two (although this varies from child to child), they'll probably be sleeping longer at night again and maybe take fewer naps, although each nap may be longer. In addition, they'll have longer periods during the day where they will be considerably more alert and responsive to people and events. Many other types of developmental progress, including physical growth, may occur in spurts and pauses, with periods of setback or lag. As challenging as this may be, you'll soon learn to read the signals, anticipate these periods of change, and appreciate them.

Growth and Development

Physical Appearance and Growth

From months 1 through 4, your baby will continue growing at the same rate they did during their first few weeks. In general, babies gain between 1½ and 2 pounds (0.7–0.9 kg) and grow 1 to 1½ inches (2.5–4 cm) each month during this period. Their head size will increase in circumference by about ½ inch (1.25 cm) each month. These figures are only averages, so keep track of your child's development as it compares to the growth charts in the Appendix (*pages 699–702*).

At 2 months, the soft spots on your baby's head should still be open and flat, but by 3 months, the one at the back should be closed. Also, their head is more likely to be proportionately larger compared to their body, since it grows faster. This is normal; their body will soon catch up.

At 2 months, your baby will look round and chubby, but as they start using their arms and legs more actively, muscles will develop. Their bones will grow rapidly, and as their limbs loosen up, your baby will seem to stretch out, appearing taller and leaner.

Movement

Many of your baby's movements will still be reflexive at the beginning of this period. They may assume a "fencing" position every time their head turns (tonic neck reflex; see *page 135*) or extend their arms if they hear a loud noise or feel that they're falling (Moro reflex; see *page 135*). But, as mentioned, most of these common newborn reflexes will begin to fade by the second or third month. They may temporarily seem less active after the reflexes have diminished, but now their movements, however subtle, are intentional and will build steadily toward mature activity.

One of the most important developments of these early months will be your baby's increasing neck strength. Starting at birth, take a few opportunities every day to let them play with you on their tummy (tummy time). Before 2 months, they'll struggle to raise their head to look around. Even if they succeed for a second or two, they'll have a slightly different view of the world. These small exercises will strengthen the muscles at the back of their neck so that by around 4 months they'll be able to hold their head and chest up on their elbows. This is a major accomplishment, giving them freedom and control to look around at will. Giving them plenty of awake time off the back of their head will also help to prevent torticollis and plagiocephaly, or neck tightness and flattening of the back of their head.

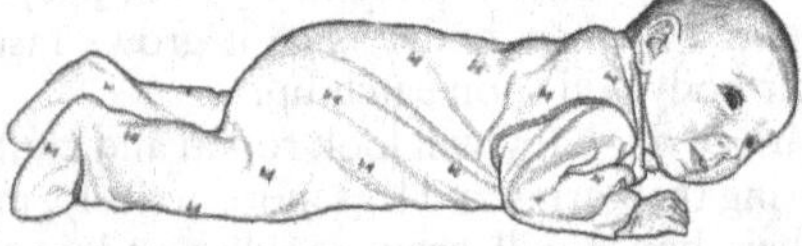

For you, it's also welcome because you no longer have to support their head as much when carrying them (although sudden movements or force will still require head support). If you use a front or back carrier, they'll now be able to hold their head up and look around as you walk.

A baby's control over the front neck and abdominal muscles develops more gradually, so it will take longer for your baby to raise their head lying on their back. At 1 month, if you gently pull your baby by the arms to a sitting position, their head will flop backward; by 4 months, however, they'll hold it steady in all directions.

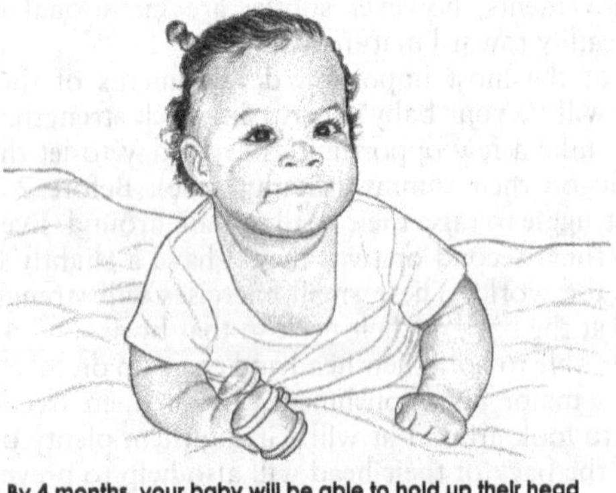

By 4 months, your baby will be able to hold up their head and chest as they support themselves on their elbows.

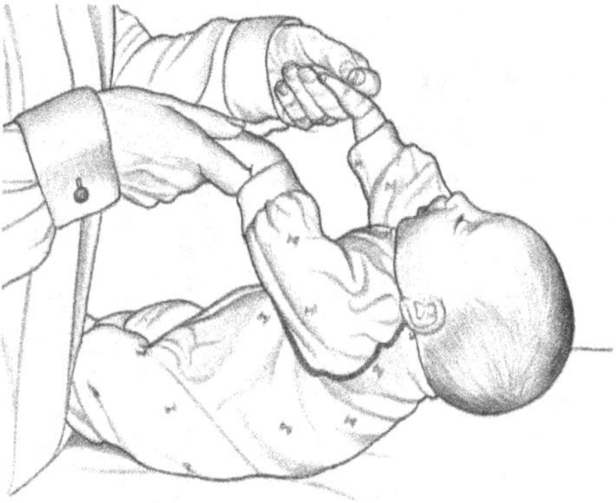

At 1 month, your baby's head will flop backward if you gently pull them to a sitting position (so always support your baby's head when picking them up).

Your child's legs also will become stronger and more active. During the second month, they'll start to straighten from their inward-curving newborn position. Although their kicks will remain mostly reflexive, they'll quickly gather force, and by the end of the third month they might even kick themselves over from front to back. (They probably won't roll from back to front until around 6 months old.) Since you cannot predict when they'll begin rolling over, you'll need to be especially careful whenever they're on the changing table or any other surface above floor level.

Another newborn reflex, the stepping reflex, allows them to take steps when they are held under their arms and their feet touch the floor. This reflex will disappear at about 2 months, and you may not see your baby step again until they're ready to walk.

MOVEMENT/PHYSICAL DEVELOPMENT MILESTONES FOR YOUR BABY AT 2 MONTHS

- Holds head up when on tummy
- Moves both arms and both legs
- Opens hands briefly

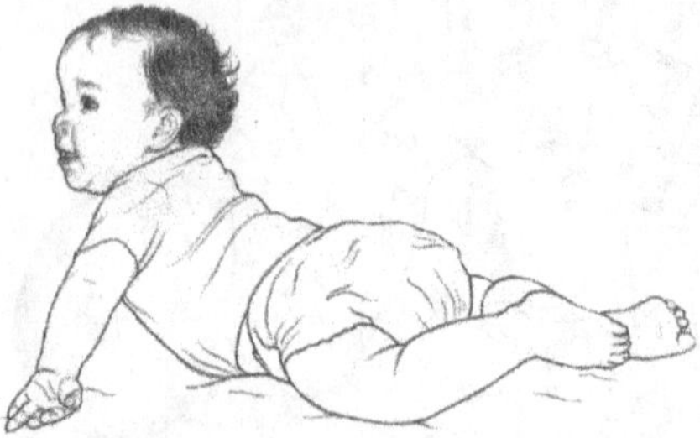

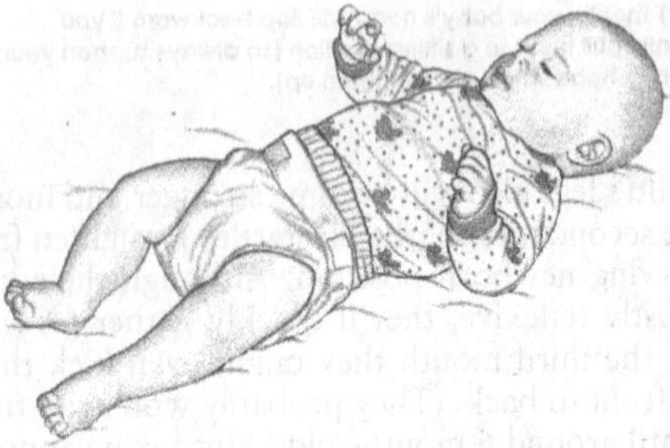

Many changes continue to occur within a month or two. Your baby's hands will relax and their arms will open outward. Over the next two months, they'll now bring objects to their mouth and drop them only after exploring them fully. (The more lightweight the toy, the better they can control it.) They'll never seem to tire of their hands themselves; just staring at their fingers will amuse them for stretches of time.

Vision

At 1 month, your baby still can't see clearly beyond 15 inches (38 cm) or so, but they'll closely study anything within this range, such as the crib corner or the mobile dangling above the crib. The human face is their favorite image, however. As you hold them, they are drawn automatically to your face, particularly your eyes. Often the mere sight of your eyes will make them smile. Gradually their visual span will broaden and they will take in your whole face. As this happens, they'll be more responsive to facial expressions involving your mouth, jaw, and cheeks.

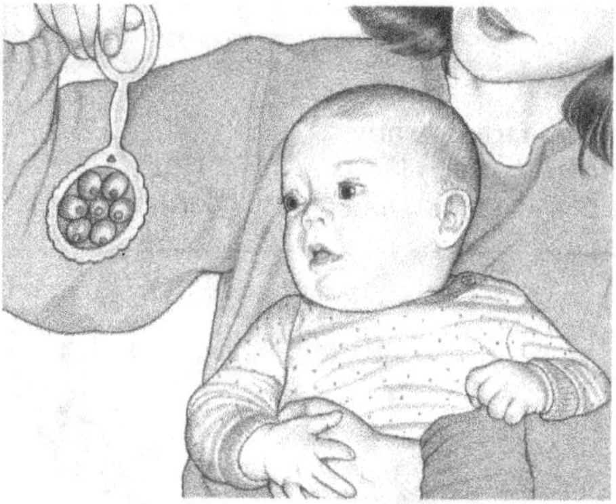

By 2 months your baby's eyes are more coordinated and can work together to move and focus at the same time.

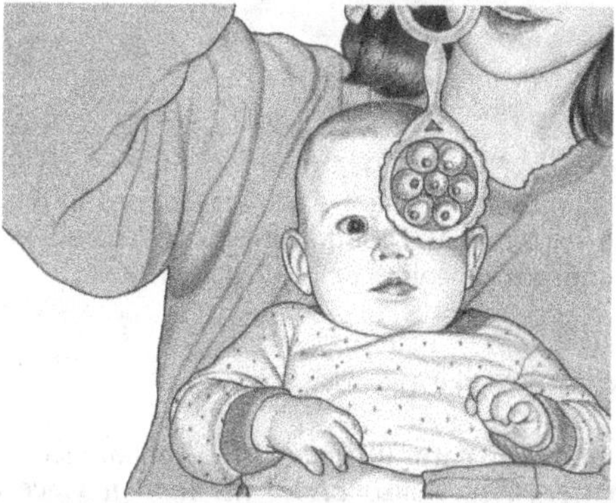

Soon they'll be able to track an object moving through an entire half-circle in front of them.

In their early weeks, your baby will have a hard time following an object moving in front of their face. If you wave an object quickly in front of them, they'll seem to stare through it. This will change dramatically by 2 months, when their eyes are better coordinated and can follow objects more smoothly, from their left to their right and back. This increased visual coordination and developing depth perception will help them look at objects as they move toward and away from them.

VISION DEVELOPMENTS FOR YOUR BABY AT 2 MONTHS

- Watches faces intently
- Follows moving objects
- Starts using hands and eyes in coordination

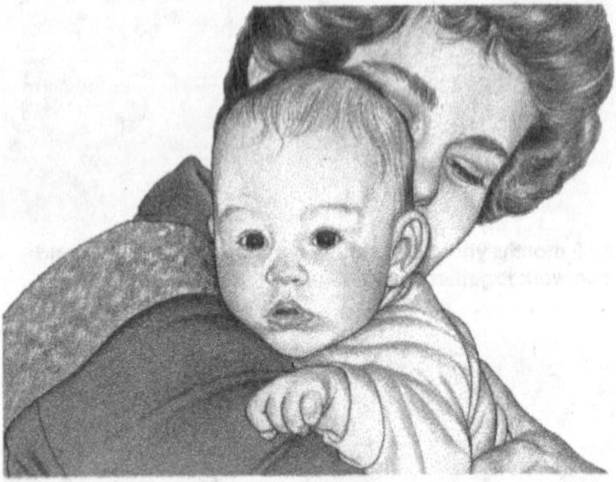

Your infant's color vision is also developing in the first few months after birth. At 1 month, they'll prefer bold patterns in sharply contrasting colors or black and white.

Hearing and Making Sounds

Just as your baby naturally prefers the human face over other visual patterns, they also prefer the human voice to other sounds. They will recognize and respond to those voices they hear most. They associate them with warmth, food, and comfort. Babies like high-pitched voices in general—a fact that most adults seem to understand intuitively and respond to accordingly, without even realizing it.

LANGUAGE/COMMUNICATION MILESTONES FOR YOUR BABY AT 2 MONTHS

- Makes sounds other than crying
- Reacts to loud noises

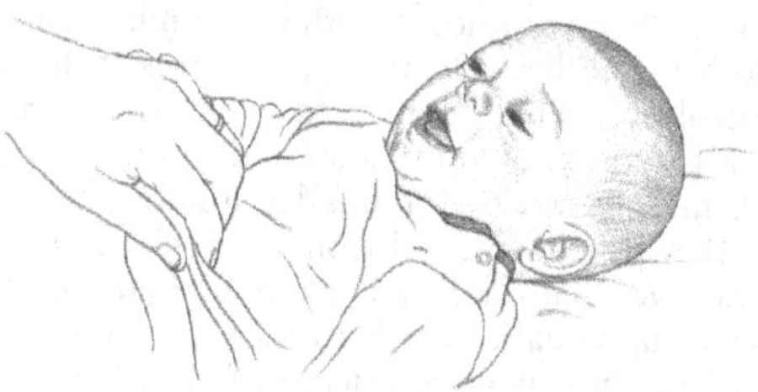

Listen to yourself the next time you talk to your baby. You'll probably notice that you raise your pitch, slow your speech, exaggerate syllables, and widen your eyes and mouth more than normal. This dramatic approach is guaranteed to capture almost any baby's attention—and usually makes them smile.

By listening to you and others, your baby will discover the importance of speech long before they understand or repeat specific words. By 1 month, they'll be able to identify you by voice, even if you're in another room. As you talk to them, they'll be reassured, comforted, and entertained. When they smile and gurgle at you, they'll see the delight on your face and realize talk goes both ways. These first conversations teach them many of the subtle rules of communication, such as turn-taking, vocal tone, imitation, pacing, and speed of verbal interaction.

Social/Emotional Development

By the second month, your baby will spend much of each day watching and listening to the people around them. Your baby learns that these people will entertain and soothe them, feed them, and make them comfortable. During their first month, they'll experiment with primitive grins and grimaces. Then, during the second month, these movements will turn to genuine signals of pleasure and friendliness.

If you've experienced their first true smile, then you know it's a major turning point for both of you; you'll do everything in your power to keep those smiles coming. For their part, your baby will suddenly discover that just by moving their lips they can have "conversations" with you. Smiling will also give them another way besides crying to express their needs and exert control over what happens to them. The more engaged they are with you and your smiles and the rest of the world around them, the more their brain development advances, and the more they'll be distracted from internal sensations (hunger, gas, fatigue) that once strongly influenced their behavior. Their increasing socialization is further proof that they enjoy and appreciate these new experiences. Expanding their world with these experiences is fun for both of you and important to their overall development.

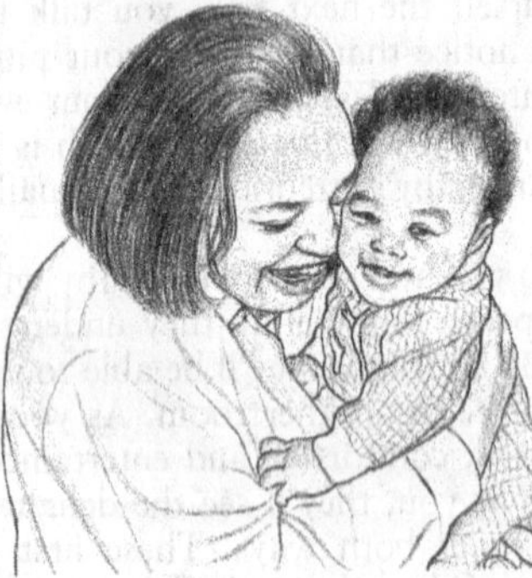

At first your baby may seem to smile past you without meeting your gaze, but don't let this disturb you. Looking away from you gives them some control and protects them from being overwhelmed. It's their way of taking in the total picture without being "caught" by your eyes. In this way, they can pay equal attention to your facial expressions, your voice, your body warmth, and the way you're holding them. As you get to know each other, they'll gradually hold your gaze for longer and longer periods, and you'll find ways to increase their tolerance—perhaps by holding them at certain distances, adjusting your voice level, or modifying your expressions.

SOCIAL/EMOTIONAL MILESTONES FOR YOUR BABY AT 2 MONTHS

- Calms down when spoken to or picked up
- Looks at your face
- Seems happy to see you when you walk up to them
- Smiles when you talk to or smile at them

Like adults, your infant may prefer certain people, often their primary caretakers. Grandparents or familiar sitters may receive a hesitant smile at first, followed by coos and body talk. By contrast, strangers may receive no more than a curious stare or fleeting smile. This selective behavior shows they're starting to sort out who's who in their life.

These early exchanges play an important part in their social and emotional development. By responding quickly and enthusiastically to their smiles and engaging them in these "conversations," you'll let them know they're important to you, can trust you, and have a certain amount of control in their life. By recognizing their cues when they're "talking," you'll also show you are interested in and value them. This contributes to their developing self-esteem.

As your baby grows, communication will vary with their needs and desires. On a day-to-day basis you'll find they have three general levels of need, each of which shows a different side of their personality:

1. When their needs are urgent—hunger or pain, for instance—they'll let you know, perhaps by screaming, whimpering, or using desperate body language. In time you'll learn to recognize these signals so quickly that you usually can satisfy those needs almost before your baby knows what they want.
2. When your baby is peacefully asleep, or alert and entertaining themselves, you've met all their needs for the moment. This is a welcome opportunity to rest or

take care of other business. Playing by themselves provides you with wonderful opportunities to observe—from a distance—how they are developing important new skills such as reaching, tracking objects, or manipulating their hands. These activities set the stage for self-soothing, which will help them settle down and ultimately sleep through the night. These are especially important skills to learn for more colicky or difficult-to-console babies.

3. Each day there will be periods when your baby's obvious needs are met but they're still fussy or fitful. They may whine, cry, have agitated movements, or exhibit spurts of aimless activity between moments of calm. They probably won't even know what they want, and any of several responses might help calm them. Playing, talking, singing, rocking, and walking may work. Simply repositioning them or letting them fuss it out may also be a successful strategy. This is okay as long as you have checked to make sure they don't need to be changed or fed, and that nothing else is bothering them. You might also find that while a particular response works momentarily, they'll soon become even fussier and demand more attention. This cycle may continue until you either let them cry a few minutes or distract them with something different—for example, taking the baby outside.

There may be times, however, when you feel frustrated, even angry, because your baby will not stop crying. People may not always talk about these feelings, but they are completely normal. The best thing to do here is to gently place them back in the crib and take a little break for yourself. It is most important you resist any temptation to shake or strike your baby in any way. Shaking or slamming your baby can cause serious harm and even death. "Shaken baby" situations are one form of child abuse that continues to be a problem around the world. If crying difficulties remain an issue, discuss this in detail with your pediatrician, who will give you other ideas for how to get through these episodes. Be sure you share these new techniques for quieting your infant with your childcare provider, who may feel similar frustrations with inconsolable crying.

Over time your baby's periods of acute need will decrease,

and they'll be able to entertain themselves for longer stretches. In part this is because you're learning to anticipate care for many of their problems. But also their nervous system will be maturing, and as a result, they'll be better at coping with everyday stresses. With greater bodily control, they'll amuse and console themselves and experience fewer frustrations. The periods when they seem most difficult to satisfy probably won't disappear for a few years, but as they become more active, it will be easier to distract them. Ultimately, they should learn to overcome these spells on their own.

During these early months, don't worry about spoiling your baby. Observe them closely and respond promptly when needed. You may not calm them every time, but it never hurts to show how much you care. At this age, they need frequent reassurance to feel secure about themselves and you. By helping them establish this sense of security now, you're laying a foundation for the confidence and trust that will allow them to gradually separate from you and become a strong, independent person.

Basic Care

Feeding

Your baby will continue exclusively nursing or bottle-feeding until 4 to 6 months of age. The best way to monitor whether your baby is getting enough is by monitoring their growth. Your doctor will measure their weight, length, and head circumference at each visit. Most breastfed babies will continue to feed on demand throughout the day and night. Pay attention to your baby's cues for hunger and fullness when deciding how much to feed; these are even more important than the amount of breast milk or formula your baby consumes.

Infants fed formula or expressed breast milk in a bottle will usually increase the amount of formula or breast milk from 2–4 ounces (60–120 ml) per feeding to 4–6 ounces (120–180 ml) per feeding by 4 months of age. When babies are solely breastfeeding, they will continue to feed eight to twelve times in each twenty-four-hour period. At times a breastfed infant may start demanding to eat more often, such as every ninety minutes to two hours. This is your baby's way of telling you that they are having a growth spurt and need more milk.

The more frequent feedings will send messages to your brain to make more hormones that produce breast milk, your milk supply will increase, and your baby will then return to feeding less frequently. It usually takes two to three days for the milk supply to increase. If your baby still seems persistently hungry after four to five days, call your pediatrician for a weight check appointment. If a breastfeeding infant is not gaining weight, your milk supply may have decreased. This can be associated with your return to work without adequate pumping, increased stress, longer sleeps for the baby, or a variety of other factors. Your pediatrician can help determine the cause of your decreased milk supply and suggest techniques to increase your milk supply and the baby's intake. This may include increasing the feeding frequency and using a breast pump between or after feedings to increase milk production as well as ensuring that you are getting enough nutrition and fluids in your diet. You may hear that adding cereal to the bottle will help your baby sleep through the night, but this is a myth, and it can lead to overweight and obesity.

Frequent or repeated coughing during feeds is not normal and should be brought to the attention of the pediatrician. Frequent pauses during feeds or facial color changes that require the child to pull off the breast or bottle to breathe may indicate that your baby is having a hard time breathing; these should be brought to the attention of your pediatrician.

Even without any additions to your baby's diet, you'll probably notice a change in their bowel movements. Their intestines can hold more and absorb a greater amount of nutrients, so their stools may be more solid than they were during the first month. The gastrocolic reflex (see *page 117*) is also diminishing, so they should no longer have bowel movements after each feeding. In fact, between 2 and 3 months, stool frequency in both breastfed and formula-fed babies may decrease dramatically; some breastfed babies have only one movement every three or four days, and a few perfectly healthy breastfed infants have one a week. As long as your baby is eating well and gaining weight, and their stools are not too hard or dry, there's no reason to be alarmed by this decrease in stool frequency. If you are worried about stool changes, call your pediatrician.

Some breastfed infants who are getting close to 4 months of age may begin to sleep more than five hours at a stretch during the night. These babies may feed more often during the day, and these fortunate mothers usually appreciate a longer stretch of sleep at night. At this stage, there is no need to wake a breastfed baby during the night to feed.

As mentioned earlier, some mothers will need to return to work between six weeks and six months after giving birth. This can be more stressful for the breastfeeding mother than for the baby. For mothers who will be returning to work, begin offering expressed breast milk in a bottle occasionally by the time your infant is 1 month of age. This will allow a mother to get used to breast milk expression and the baby to get used to sucking from a bottle. This also will allow a breastfed baby to feed if the mother is away for a period of time. A mother can get information from her baby's pediatrician, a lactation consultant, and in many cases her state's Women, Infants, and Children (WIC) program on choosing a breast pump and learning how to use it.

In the month before returning to work, many mothers will start expressing breast milk regularly once or twice a day between feedings and freezing the milk to get a supply of frozen breast milk for the daycare or caregiver. It is important for a mother returning to work to discuss her return and need to express milk during work hours with the appropriate work management before her actual return date.

Returning to work part-time rather than full-time can make it easier to express breast milk and continue breastfeeding. A new mother may want to ask her manager if she can return on reduced hours for the first one to two months of work. Mothers may notice a decrease in milk supply when they return to work, possibly from the stress of returning to work.

Mothers also will need to discuss with the baby's daycare program or caregiver that they will be supplying expressed breast milk. It is more than a full-time job to return to work and care for the household and yourself, so be prepared to ask for and accept help with jobs that can be done by others.

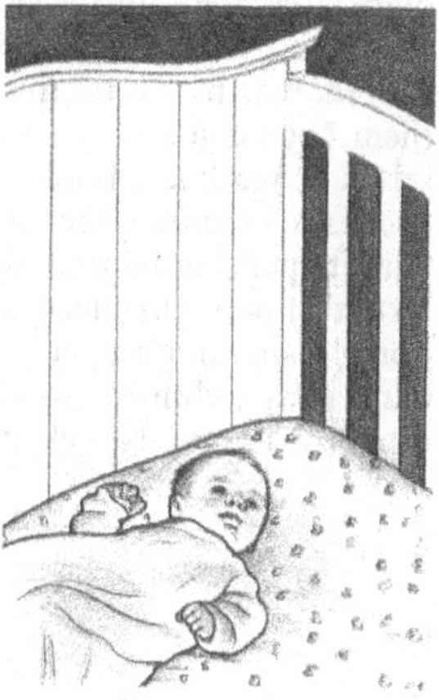

Your child should be placed on their back when going to sleep.

Sleeping

By 2 months, your baby will be more alert and social, and will spend more time awake during the day. Meanwhile, their stomach capacity will be growing, and they'll need fewer feedings; they may soon start spacing out their night feedings.

Remember, your baby should be placed to sleep on their back. (See *Chapter 30*, Your Child's Sleep, for more information.)

Siblings

By the second month, although you may be used to having a new baby, your older children still may be adjusting. Especially if the baby is your second child, your first may be saddened by not being the primary focus.

Sometimes older children might display frustration by talking back, doing something known to be forbidden, or literally shouting for attention. A child might also regress, suddenly wetting the bed or having daytime accidents even though they've been toilet trained for months. To a child there is no such thing as negative attention. They would rather get attention for inappropriate behavior than be ignored. This can quickly escalate into a vicious cycle of undesirable behavior associated with receiving more and more attention. One important way to reverse this frustrating cycle is to actively catch them "being good." Giving them praise for playing by themselves or reading a book makes those activities more likely to occur the next time they're looking for attention. Having each parent spend some time with them alone each day may help, too. You may also need to pick your battles. If your child is doing something to get your attention that is not harmful or dangerous (whining, for example), ignoring the behavior is often the best way to change it.

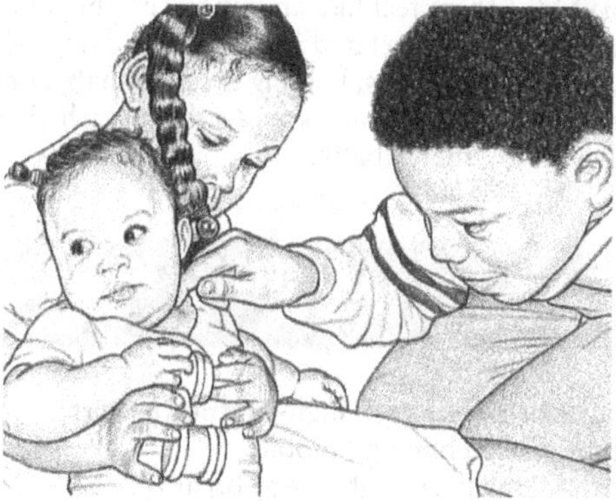

Invite older siblings to play with the baby.

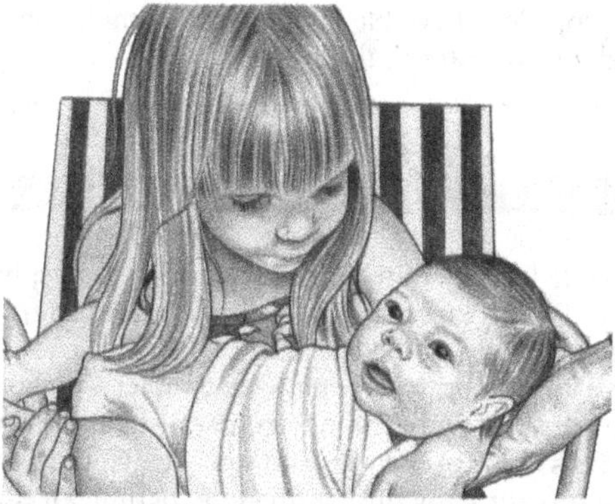

Set clear and consistent rules, such as never picking up the baby without permission.

However, you'll need to take more direct action if your older child takes out their frustration on the baby—interfering with feeds or even hitting the baby. Sit down and talk with them. Be prepared to hear things like "I wish that baby had never come here." Try to keep the older child's frustration and their other feelings in mind as you confront them. Reassure them you still love them very much, but explain firmly they must not hurt the baby. Make an extra effort to include them in all family activities, and encourage them to interact with the newborn. Make them feel like an important "big kid" by giving them specific baby-related jobs, such as carrying the diaper bag, putting away toys, helping dress the baby, or being in charge of making sure visitors and others wash their hands before they hold "their" baby.

TOYS AND ACTIVITIES APPROPRIATE FOR YOUR 2-MONTH-OLD

- Images or books with high-contrast patterns
- Bright, varied hanging mobile
- Rattles (sturdy enough not to break)
- Singing to your baby
- Playing soft music on low volume
- Appropriate chewable toys for oral stimulation between feedings to foster oral sensing

STIMULATING INFANT BRAIN GROWTH: AGE 2 MONTHS

- Provide healthy nutrition as your baby grows; have periodic checkups and timely immunizations from a regular source of medical care.
- Give consistent, warm, physical contact—hugging, skin-to-skin, body-to-body contact—to establish your infant's sense of security and well-being. Talk, read, and sing to your baby during dressing, bathing, feeding, playing, walking, and driving. Use simple, lively phrases and address your baby by name. Respond to their gestures, as well as to the faces and the sounds they make.
- Read to your baby every day, starting at birth. This time provides close physical contact, helps them learn your voice, and develops a wonderful lifelong habit.
- Be attentive to your baby's rhythms and moods. Learn to read their cues and respond to them when they are upset as well as when they are happy. Babies cannot be spoiled.

- Provide colorful objects of different shapes, sizes, and textures that they can play with. Show them children's picture books and family photographs.
- Your face is by far the most interesting visual object at this age. Play peekaboo with your baby.
- If you speak multiple languages, use them all at home.
- Avoid subjecting your baby to stressful or traumatic experiences, physical or psychological.
- Make sure other people who provide care and supervision for your baby understand the importance of forming a loving and comforting relationship with your child and also provide consistent care.

Health Watch

Newborns can get very sick very quickly, so if your infant is under 3 months and has a rectal temperature of 100.4 degrees Fahrenheit (38 degrees Celsius) or higher, call your pediatrician. The following medical problems are common between the ages of 2 and 4 months. If you are concerned your baby has any of these conditions while younger than 2 months, contact your pediatrician. Check Part 2 of this book for these and other illnesses and conditions that occur throughout childhood.

Diarrhea (see Diarrhea, *page 354*)

Ear Infections (see Middle Ear Infections, *page 471*)

Eye Infections (see Eye Infections, *page 545*)

Spitting Up (see Gastroesophageal Reflux [GER], *page 378*)

Rashes and Skin Conditions (see Eczema, *page 392*)

Respiratory Syncytial Virus (RSV) Infections (see Bronchiolitis, *page 408*)

Upper Respiratory Infections (URIs) (see Colds/Upper Respiratory Infections, *page 468*)

▪ YOUR BABY AT 2 MONTHS OLD CHECKLIST ▪

Immunization Update

Your baby should receive the hepatitis B vaccine soon after birth and before they are discharged from the hospital, and again at least four weeks after the first dose.

At 2 months, your baby should receive:

- Diphtheria, tetanus, pertussis (DTaP) vaccine
- Inactivated polio vaccine
- *Haemophilus influenzae* type b (Hib) vaccine
- Pneumococcal vaccine
- Rotavirus vaccine
- Hepatitis B vaccine (if not given at 1 month of age)

(For detailed information, see *Chapter 26*, Immunizations, and the Appendix, *pages 696–97*.)

Safety Check

Falls

- Never place the baby in an infant seat on a table, chair, or any other surface above floor level.
- Never leave your baby unattended on a bed, couch, changing table, or chair. (For more information about changing tables, see *page 302*.)
- On all kinds of gear, always buckle the safety straps.

Burns

- Never hold your baby while smoking, drinking a hot liquid, or cooking by a hot stove or oven.
- Never allow anyone to smoke around your baby.

Choking

- Routinely check all toys for small parts that could be pulled or broken off. Also look for sharp edges, which can pose a danger. Check and follow the age recommendations for toys.
- For this age group, do not attach a toy to the crib, since the baby could pull it down or become entangled in it.

CHAPTER 7

YOUR BABY AT 4 MONTHS

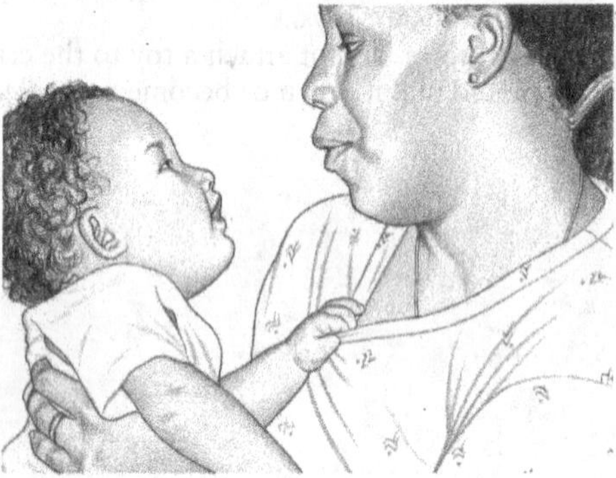

By your infant's 4-month birthday, you'll probably have more of a daily routine for their feeding, napping, bathing, and sleeping at night. This routine helps your baby feel secure while allowing you to budget time and activities. The schedule should be flexible, though. During a growth spurt, your baby will eat more frequently; if they're ill, they may have trouble sleeping. And sometimes you might want to have some spur-of-the-moment fun. Short strolls when the sun finally appears on a dreary day, an unexpected lunch visit from grandparents, or a family excursion to the zoo are all wonderful excuses to break the routine. Being open to life events and impulses will make life together more enjoyable and help your baby learn to adapt to the changes in their life ahead.

Many parents will be going back to work during this time, and this may cause added stress during the first year. As exciting as it is to have a new baby, you and your family are still adjusting, and it's natural to feel tired and worried. If those feelings become overwhelming, however, reach out for help.

For the time being, the most important changes are internal. At 4 months of age, babies will learn to coordinate their emerging perceptive abilities (vision, touch, and hearing) and their increasing motor abilities to develop skills like holding their head steady, making grasping motions, and bringing their hands to their mouth. The control evident in their budding motor skills will extend to every part of their life. Instead of reacting primarily by reflex, they'll now choose what they will and won't do. As a newborn, they sucked on almost anything placed in their mouth, but now they have definite favorites. Before, they merely looked at a strange new toy, but now they can use their arms to swing or bat at toys, and soon they will be able to mouth a toy, manipulate it, and explore its qualities. Infants who have experienced adversity, such as a stay in the NICU, prenatal substance exposure, or neglect, may still need more support with safe and nurturing routines.

Your baby will better communicate their emotions and desires now, and they'll voice them frequently. They'll cry not only when they're hungry or uncomfortable, but also when they want a different toy or a change in activity.

However, in these months before stranger anxiety, your child will probably go through a period of delightful showmanship, smiling and playing with everyone they meet. Their personality will be coming out in full bloom, and even people first meeting your baby will notice their many unique character traits. Take advantage of their sociability and acquaint them with people who will care for them in the future, such as babysitters, relatives, or childcare workers. This may help smooth the waters later when your baby hits the stranger-anxiety period.

Growth and Development

Physical Appearance and Growth

Your baby will grow rapidly over the next few months, but every baby is different. The best way to track growth is for your baby's doctor to measure their weight, length, and head circumference and compare them to charts from the World Health Organization. If you want to keep track as well, sample growth charts are provided in the Appendix (*pages 699–702*).

Movement

By 3 or 4 months, your baby will flex and straighten their legs at will. Lift them upright with their feet on the floor and they'll push down and straighten their legs so that they're virtually standing by themselves (except for the support you're providing). Then they'll try bending their knees and will discover they can bounce. Although parents are often concerned that this kind of bouncing may be harmful, it is perfectly healthy and safe.

Previously, your baby established the muscle control needed to move both their eyes and head so they could follow objects. They'll now begin to take on even greater challenges. They'll accomplish this as their back and neck muscles gradually strengthen and they develop better balance in their trunk, head, and neck. First they'll raise their head and hold it up while lying on their stomach. Encourage this by placing them on their stomach and extending their arms forward when they are awake; then get their attention with an attractive toy and coax them to hold their head up and look at you. This also is a good way to check their hearing and vision.

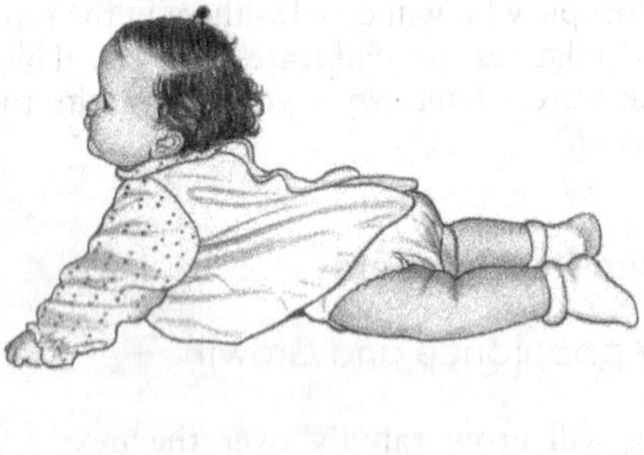

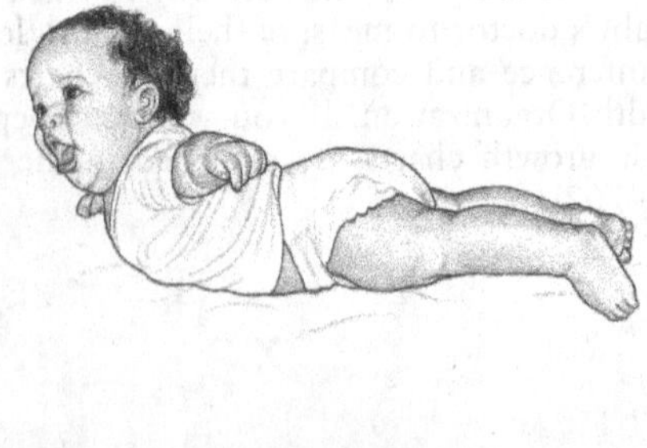

Once able to lift their head, your baby will start pushing up on their arms, first on their elbows and then with straight arms, arching their back to lift their chest. This strengthens their upper body, which will be essential to remaining steady and upright when they are learning to sit between 6 and 9 months of age. At the same time, they may rock on their stomach, kick their legs, and "swim" with their arms. These abilities, which usually appear at about 5 months, are necessary for rolling over and crawling. By the end of this period, they'll probably be able to roll over in both directions, although the time frame varies for different babies. Most children roll from stomach to back before the opposite direction, although doing it in reverse is perfectly normal.

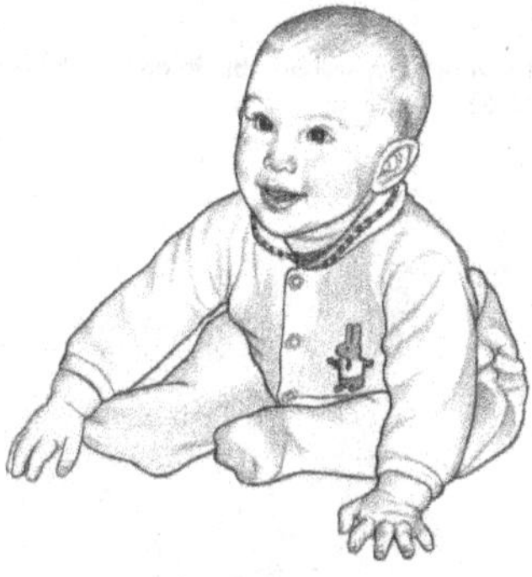

Once your baby can raise their chest, help them practice sitting up. Hold them up or support their back with pillows as they learn to balance themselves. By 6 months, they will learn to "tripod," leaning forward as they extend their arms to balance. Interesting toys in front of them will give them a focus as they gain their balance. It will be some time before they can maneuver themselves to sitting without your assistance. Helping your baby develop their balancing skills will help them learn to sit and discover all the wonderful things the world has to offer from this new vantage point.

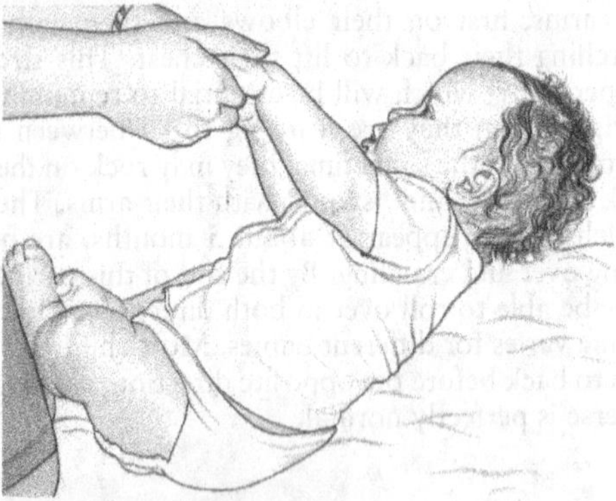

By 4 months, your baby will be able to hold their head steady in all directions.

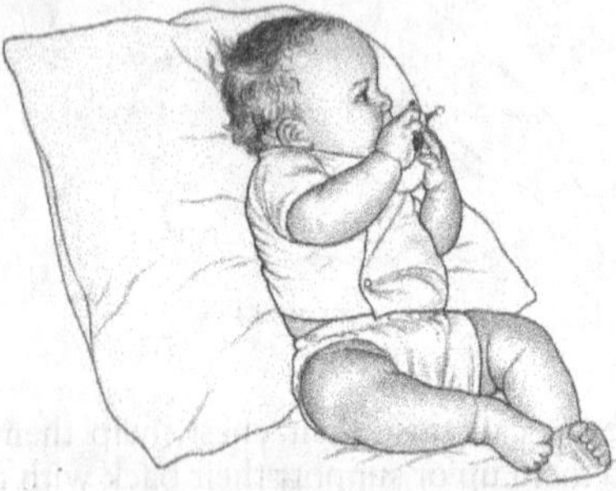

Your baby's hand and arm movements will also develop rapidly during these months. During the third month, their hands will be half open most of the time, and you'll notice them carefully opening and shutting them. In the beginning, their hands are tightly clenched fists with their thumb inside; if you uncoil the fingers, they'll grasp objects automatically, yet they won't be able to move them or bring them to their mouth. They'll gaze at their hands with interest when they are in view, but they probably won't be able to bring them to their face on their own.

By the fourth month, your baby can easily bring their hands

to their mouth and are able to use their arms to swing and bat at toys. By 6 months your baby will easily reach for, grab, and put things in their mouth. So, if you have not already done so, remove any objects from their environment that they could choke on or injure themselves with.

MOVEMENT/PHYSICAL DEVELOPMENT MILESTONES FOR YOUR BABY AT 4 MONTHS

- Holds head steady without support when you are holding them
- Holds a toy when you put it in their hand
- Uses their arms to swing at toys
- Brings hands to mouth
- Pushes up on elbows/forearms when on tummy

TOYS APPROPRIATE FOR YOUR BABY AT 4 MONTHS

- See-through rattles that show the pieces making noise
- Cloth books with colorful pictures
- Unbreakable plastic or Mylar mirror
- Soft balls, including some that make soft, pleasant sounds
- Textured toys that make sounds

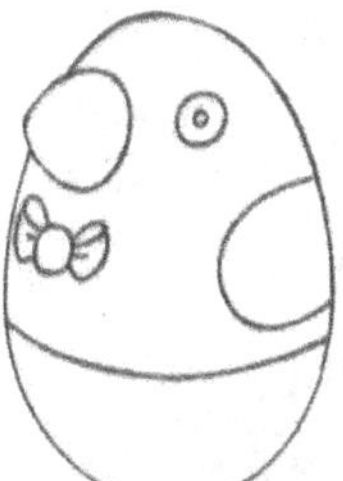
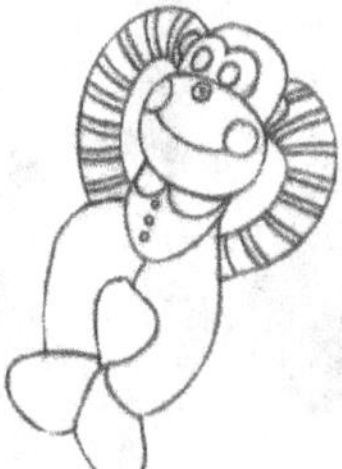
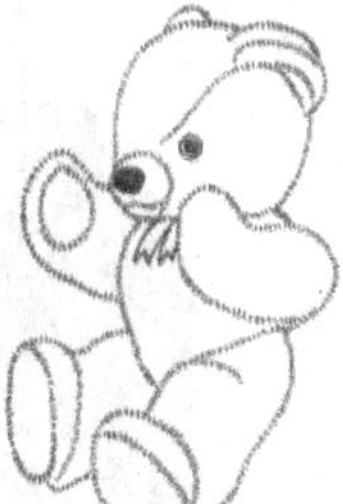

Vision

As your baby works on their motor skills, have you noticed how closely they watch everything they're doing? Their concentration reaching for a toy may remind you of a scientist engrossed in research. It's obvious their good vision is playing a key role in their early motor and cognitive development. Conveniently, their eyes become fully functional just when they need them most.

Although your baby could see at birth, their total visual ability has taken months to develop. Only now can they distinguish subtle shades of reds, blues, and yellows. Don't be surprised if you notice they prefer red or blue to other colors; these seem to be favorites among many infants this age. Most babies also like increasingly complex patterns and shapes as they get older—something to keep in mind when shopping for picture books or posters for your child's nursery.

By 4 months, they'll also have the arm and hand control needed to bat at objects as they move close to them; their aim won't be very good yet, but the practice will help them develop hand-eye coordination. If you think your baby's eyes may not be tracking together by 3 months of age, talk with your pediatrician.

Your baby's distance vision also is developing. You may notice them smiling at you halfway across the room or studying a toy several feet away. By 4 months, you'll catch them staring at the distant wall hanging or looking out the window. These are clues to normal development.

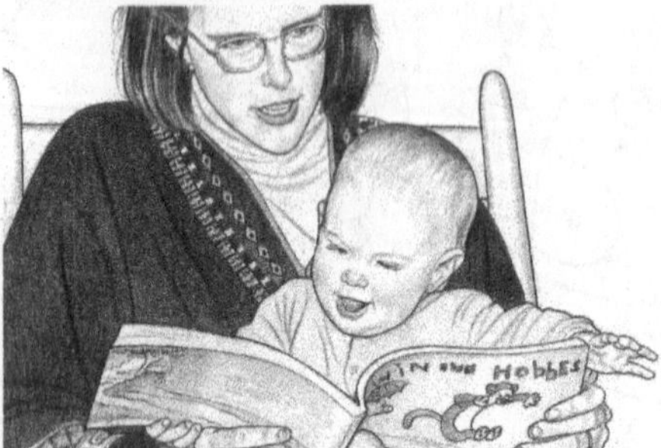

By 4 months, your baby will begin noticing not only the way you talk but also the individual sounds you make.

By 4 months, your baby's visual range has increased to several yards or more, and it will continue to expand. (See *Chapter 20*, Eyes, for more information on eye maturity.) At the same time, they'll follow faster and faster movements with their eyes. In the early months, if you rolled a ball across the room, they couldn't track it, but now they'll follow moving objects easily. As their hand-eye coordination improves, they'll be able to grab these objects around 6 months of age. Because of these improvements in vision, babies can be easily distracted while breastfeeding, so nursing in a quiet, darker space may be necessary during this phase.

A mobile over the crib or in front of an infant's bouncy seat is an ideal way to stimulate a young baby's vision. However, your baby may quickly get bored and search for other things. Also, some babies may already be sitting up and reaching and might pull down or tangle themselves in a mobile. Be sure to remove any mobiles when your baby is able to get up on their hands and knees or at 5 months old, whichever comes first. Hold your baby's visual interest by keeping them moving—around the home, down the block, to the store, or on special excursions. Help them find things they've never seen before and name each one out loud for them.

A mirror is another source of endless fascination for babies this age. The reflected image is constantly changing, and, even more important, it responds directly to your child's movements. This is a clue the person in the mirror is actually themselves. It may take a while to come to this realization, but it will probably register during this period.

Your child's visual awareness should clearly have increased by the age of 4 months. Watch how they respond when introduced to new shapes, colors, and objects. If they are not interested in looking at new things, or if one or both eyes turn in or out, inform your pediatrician.

VISION DEVELOPMENTS FOR YOUR BABY AT 4 MONTHS

Your baby may be most interested in circular patterns (bull's-eyes, spirals)—one of the reasons faces, full of circles and curves, are so appealing to them. By about 4 months, your baby will finally respond to the full range of colors and their many shades, and as their eyesight develops, your infant will naturally seek out more stimulating things to see.

Language Development

Your baby learns language in stages. From birth, they receive information about language by hearing people make sounds and watching them communicate. At first, they are most interested in the pitch and level of your voice. When you talk in a soothing way, they'll stop crying because they hear you want to comfort them. By contrast, if you shout out in anger, they will probably cry and show signs of being frightened because your voice is telling them something is wrong. By 4 months, they'll notice not only the way you talk, but also the individual sounds you make. Your baby will listen to the vowels and consonants and begin to notice how these combine into syllables, words, and sentences.

At about 2 months, your infant began cooing and repeating some vowel sounds (ah-ah-ah, ooh-ooh-ooh). By 4 months, imitate them cooing, while adding simple words and phrases to your "conversations." Your baby will not only be making noises to communicate with; they will turn their head toward you, smile, and act excited by moving their arms and legs to keep you engaged in having a "conversation" with them. Reading to your baby from birth is a wonderful and enjoyable way to help develop their language skills, even if they don't yet seem to understand the words.

By 4 months, your infant will babble routinely, often amusing themselves for long periods by producing strange new sounds (muh-muh, bah-bah). They'll also be more sensitive to your tone of voice and the emphasis you put on words or phrases. As you move through each day together, they'll learn from your voice when you're going to feed them, change their diaper, go for a walk, or place them in their crib. The way you talk teaches your baby about your mood and personality, and the way they respond shows you a lot about them. If you speak in an upbeat or comforting way, they may smile or coo. Yell or talk angrily, and they'll probably startle or cry.

Besides hearing sounds, your baby has also been producing them from the very beginning, first as cries and then as coos. At about 4 months, they'll start to babble, using many rhythms and characteristics of their native language. Although it may sound like gibberish, if you listen closely, you'll hear them raise and drop their voice as if they were making a statement or asking a question. Encourage them by talking to them throughout the day. When you recognize a syllable, repeat it back and then say some simple words that contain that sound. If their sound of the day is "bah," introduce "bottle," "box," "bonnet," "baa, baa, black sheep," and so on.

LANGUAGE/COMMUNICATION MILESTONES FOR YOUR BABY AT 4 MONTHS

- Makes sounds like "oooo," "aahh" (cooing)
- Makes sounds back when you talk to them
- Turns head toward the sound of your voice

Special equipment is used to check a very young baby's hearing. All newborns should be tested for hearing loss soon after birth, usually before they leave the hospital. In addition, your observations are the early warning system for whether further testing is needed. If you suspect a problem, you might ask your pediatrician for a referral to a children's hearing specialist.

Cognitive Development

Previously, you might have wondered if your baby really understood what was happening around them. This reaction is not surprising. After all, although you knew when they were comfortable or not, signs of actually thinking were likely few. But studies show from the minute they are born, your baby is learning about the world around them. Now, as their memory and attention span increase, you'll see evidence they're not only absorbing information but also applying it to their day-to-day activities.

During this period, they'll refine their concept of cause and effect. They'll probably stumble on this notion somewhere between 4 and 5 months. Perhaps while kicking their mattress, they'll notice the crib shaking. Or maybe they'll realize their rattle makes a noise when hit. Once they understand they can cause these interesting reactions, they'll continue to experiment.

COGNITIVE MILESTONES FOR YOUR BABY AT 4 MONTHS

- If hungry, opens mouth when they see breast or bottle
- Looks at their hands with interest

Social/Emotional Development

At age 4 months, your baby's social and emotional development will continue to blossom and bring you delightful moments of connection and interaction, and also moments of understandable frustration. Your baby will begin to show more interest in engaging with others, including family members and caregivers. You'll notice that they laugh in response to your facial expressions and sounds, sometimes even when you're not trying to be funny! They will also demonstrate increased awareness of their own emotions and those of others, which might be expressed through a wider range of facial expressions and vocalizations. As they learn to tell family members apart from strangers, they may also start to display stranger anxiety, becoming more cautious or wary of unfamiliar faces. Encouraging social interactions, responding to their emotional cues, and providing a secure and loving environment will help foster their social and emotional growth during these crucial months.

As your baby develops, your own habits will change as well. You and your baby will both benefit from establishing stable sleep routines, with a consistent bedtime and wake-up time. Now that your infant can express their desires more clearly, you may find yourself having to pause and take a breath when you can't respond immediately. Feeds may need to move to a quieter, less distracting place now that your baby is increasingly aware of and interested in the things going on all around them.

SOCIAL/EMOTIONAL MILESTONES FOR YOUR BABY AT 4 MONTHS

- Smiles on their own to get your attention
- Chuckles (not yet a full laugh) when you try to make them laugh
- Looks at you, moves, or makes sounds to get or keep your attention

---

By 4 months, your baby will be a master of "smile talk." Sometimes they'll start a "conversation" with a broad smile and gurgling to catch your attention. Other times they'll lie in wait, watching your face until you give the first smile before beaming back their enthusiastic response. Their whole body will participate. Their hands will open wide, one or both arms will lift, and their limbs will move in time with your speech. Their facial movements also may mirror yours, especially if you stick out your tongue!

Basic Care

Introducing Solid Foods: Allergy Prevention

Exclusive breastfeeding is recommended until around 6 months of age. However, some babies show signs of readiness to start solid foods around 4 to 6 months of age, such as the ability to hold their head up steadily. There is emerging guidance on food allergy prevention that indicates some benefit to introducing certain allergenic foods around 4 to 6 months of age.

Talk to your pediatrician at your 4-month checkup about when is the best time to introduce solid foods for your baby. For more information and guidance on introducing solid foods, see Introducing Solid Foods, *page 213*.

Babies are born with a tongue thrust reflex, and a young infant will push their tongue against anything inserted into their mouth, including food. Most babies lose this reflex at about 4 to 5 months, so when this reflex disappears, that's a good time to begin "practicing" with solid food. It may be that when they show interest in eating they can try some of the foods you are eating as well. Remember that while your baby is learning to eat solid food, the main source of nutrition remains breast milk or infant formula.

Research has shown that introducing peanut and egg products to infants between 4 and 6 months of age and keeping them in the diet consistently may prevent the development of allergies to those foods. (Never feed whole nuts before 3 years of age due to choking risk.) If your child has severe eczema or an allergy to any foods, talk to your doctor first before starting solid food. In addition, there is no evidence that waiting to introduce baby-safe (soft) allergy-causing foods, such as eggs, dairy, soy, peanuts, or fish, beyond 4 to 6 months of age prevents food allergy. This is why most allergists and pediatricians now recommend early introduction of allergy-causing foods to a baby's diet. So, feel free to introduce a variety of healthy foods in a form that your baby can tolerate around 4 to 6 months of age, when they show signs of readiness to begin eating solid food. You can find a guide to introducing peanut protein to your child's diet in the Appendix (*page 704*).

As your baby develops, their hunger and fullness (satiety) cues will become stronger. If your baby is looking around like they're hungry, offer to nurse. If they're trying to grab your fork, try offering a taste of soft food. If they turn away or keep their mouth closed, take a break on feeding. Now is a great time to teach your baby to pay attention to their own hunger and satiety, which can build healthy habits for life.

Dietary Supplements: Vitamin D

The American Academy of Pediatrics currently recommends that infants be fed breast milk exclusively for the first 4 to 6 months after birth. Exclusive breastfeeding means that the infant does not receive any additional foods (except vitamin D) or fluids unless medically recommended.

Most of the population in the United States has lower-than-recommended levels of vitamin D, probably due, in part, to spending more time inside. Vitamin D deficiency can produce diseases such as rickets (a severe form of vitamin D deficiency characterized by bone softening). Our bodies produce vitamin D after exposure to sunlight, but excessive sunlight exposure increases the risk of skin cancer later in life. Parents can take several steps to decrease the risk of sunburn and skin cancer. Infants and children can be dressed in protective hats and clothing when outdoors. If possible, family activities can be timed before and after the hours of peak sun exposure (10 a.m. to 4 p.m.). Seeking shade is important. Sunscreen can be applied, even to young infants, to areas not covered by clothing and hats. The American Academy of Pediatrics recommends that all infants receive a vitamin D supplement (unless they are consuming more than 28 ounces [840 ml] per day of commercial formula that has vitamin D added). Vitamin D supplements of 400 IU (10 mcg) per day are recommended for babies up until age 1 year, with 600 IU (15 mcg) per day for children over 1 year of age. For families that are breastfeeding, a maternal dose of 6,400 IU (160 mcg) per day will cross into the breast milk and meet the baby's vitamin D needs.

Sleeping

Between 4 and 6 months of age, your baby's brain is developing, and their stomach can hold more food. You'll notice that sleep periods are growing longer and more regular, sometimes even lasting all night. However, it is essential to recognize that every baby is unique, and there is a wide range of normal sleep behaviors during this period. Some babies may still require nighttime feedings, while others may start sleeping through the night. It's crucial to approach sleep with flexibility and adaptability, paying close attention to your baby's individual cues and needs.

A nurturing sleep environment will help promote healthy sleep habits. Start with a regular routine that may involve a bath, a book and/or song, and a safe sleep surface in a dark, quiet place. Some people find that quiet white noise is helpful. Some infants this age will still cry when you place them down for sleep, which is often a normal part of transitioning from a wakeful state to a sleeping state. If your baby does this, there are a variety of ways to help them learn to make this transition, including taking a little longer to respond every few nights or spending a little less time at the crib. If the crying seems excessive, talk to your pediatrician about what might be going on. It may be tempting to bring your baby into bed with you, but babies this age are highly vulnerable to sudden unexpected infant death (SUID), and maintaining a safe sleep environment remains critical.

Siblings

At about 3 or 4 months, your baby will become intrigued by other children. If they have brothers or sisters, you'll see your baby beaming as their siblings talk. This fascination with children will increase as they get older.

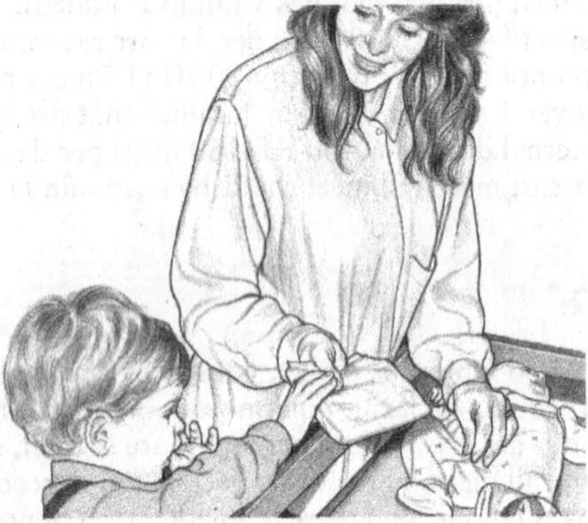

Health Watch

Don't be surprised if your baby catches their first cold or ear infection soon after their 4-month birthday. Now that they can actively reach for objects, they'll come into physical contact with many more things and people.

The first line of defense is to keep your baby away from anyone known to be sick. Be especially careful of highly contagious diseases such as influenza (the flu), RSV, COVID-19, chickenpox, and measles (see Mumps, *page 600*; Chickenpox [Varicella], *page 650*; Measles, *page 657*; and Rubella [German Measles], *page 667*). If someone in your play group has one of these diseases, keep your baby away from the group until you're sure no one else is infected. However, children and adults are contagious a day or so before they have symptoms, so it is impossible to prevent some exposures.

STIMULATING BRAIN GROWTH: AGE 4 MONTHS

- Respond positively to your baby. Act excited, smile, and talk to them when they make sounds. This teaches them to take turns "talking" back and forth in conversation.
- Provide safe opportunities for your baby to reach for toys, kick at toys, and explore what is around them. For example, put them on a blanket with safe toys.
- Allow your baby to put safe things in their mouth to explore them. This is how babies learn. For example, let them see, hear, and touch things that are not sharp, hot, or small enough to choke on.
- Talk, read, and sing to your baby. This will help them learn to speak and understand words later.
- Limit screen time (TV, phones, tablets, etc.) to video calling with loved ones. Screen time is not recommended for children younger than 2 years of age. Babies learn by talking, playing, and interacting with others.
- Give your baby safe toys to play with that are easy to hold, like rattles or cloth books with colorful pictures.
- Let your baby have time to move and interact with people and objects throughout the day. Try not to keep your baby in swings, strollers, or bouncy seats for too long.
- Set steady routines for sleeping and feeding.
- Lay your baby on their back and show them a bright-colored toy. Move the toy slowly from left to right and up and down to see if they watch how the toy moves.
- Sing and talk to your baby as you help them "exercise" (move their body) for a few minutes. Gently bend and move their arms and legs up and down.
- Play with your baby by holding them securely under their arms with their feet on your lap. Let them bounce up and down.
- Play games, such as peekaboo. You can cover your eyes with your hands and then uncover and say "peekaboo." Watch for your baby's smile or other signs they are enjoying the game.
- Pay close attention to how your baby reacts to different things. This will help you learn what they like and don't like and what makes them feel good.

- Copy your baby's sounds and see how long your baby "talks" back and forth with you.
- Call your baby by their name to help them learn it. They will start to recognize it around 9 months. For example, "Are you ticklish, Jordan?"
- Playing on the floor or play mat with your baby every day helps them to move, learn, and explore.
- Hold and talk to your baby; smile and be cheerful while you do.
- Have quiet play times when you read or sing to your baby.

▪ YOUR BABY AT 4 MONTHS OLD CHECKLIST ▪

Immunization Update

At 4 months, your baby should receive:

- Second DTaP vaccine
- Second polio vaccine
- Second Hib vaccine
- Second pneumococcal vaccine
- Second hepatitis B vaccine (may be given between 1 and 4 months)
- Second rotavirus vaccine (may be given as early as four weeks after the first dose)

Safety Check

Car Safety Seats

- Buckle your baby into an approved, properly installed rear-facing car safety seat before you start the car. The seat should be equipped with a five-point harness. If your car was manufactured after 2002, you can use either the seatbelt or the Lower Anchors and Tethers for Children (LATCH) system to secure all car safety seats (see *page 326*). The backseat is the safest place for all children to ride. Never place a rear-facing car safety seat in the front seat of a car with a passenger-side airbag.

Drowning

- Never leave a baby alone even for a moment in a bath or near a pool of water, no matter how shallow. Infants can drown in just a few inches of water. Baby bath seats or supporting rings are not a substitute for adult supervision. Practice touch supervision by staying within arm's reach anytime your baby is in or near water.

Falls

- Never leave the baby unattended on any place above floor level, such as on tabletops, on changing tables, or near stairs. If they do fall and seem to be acting abnormally in any way, call the pediatrician immediately.

Burns

- Never smoke or eat, drink, or carry anything hot while holding a baby.
- Keep all hot liquids, like coffee and tea, out of baby's reach.
- Prevent scalding by making sure the water coming out of the faucet is no more than 120 degrees Fahrenheit (48.9 degrees Celsius).

Choking

- Never give a baby any food or small object that could cause choking. All foods should be mashed, ground, or soft enough to swallow without chewing.
- Make sure they cannot get tangled up in cords such as electrical cords or those on window shades. Ideally, use cordless window coverings.

CHAPTER 8

YOUR BABY AT 6 MONTHS

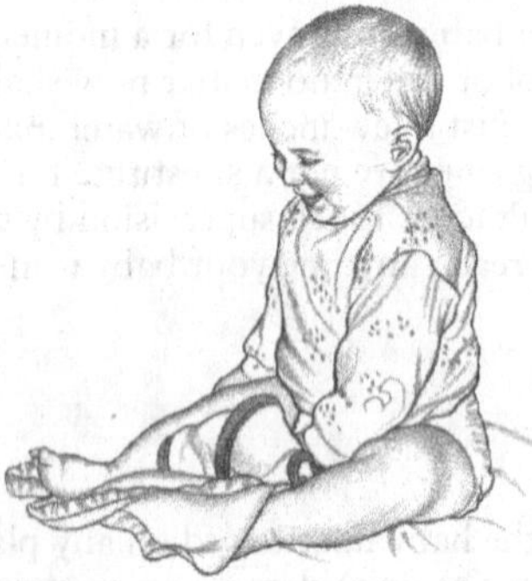

These are glorious months for you and your baby. As their personality emerges, their laughter, giggles, and joy at being with you and all they see are a wonder every day. Each day for them has new surprises and new accomplishments, and for you there is a growing sense of just how special the experience is.

You may find that your 5- or 6-month-old occasionally cries when you leave the room or when they're confronted by a stranger. They're developing a strong attachment to those who regularly care for them. They now associate you with their own well-being and can distinguish you from other people. Even if they don't cry out for you, they show this new awareness by curiously and carefully studying a stranger's face. By 8 or 9 months, they may openly object to strangers who come too close. This is a normal developmental stage known as stranger anxiety.

You and your baby are each unique, and your relationship is unique as well. What works for one baby may not work for another. You must discover what succeeds for you through trial and error. While your neighbor's child may fall asleep easily and sleep through the night, your baby may need some extra holding and cuddling. This can be frustrating and cause stress during the first year. While your first child might have needed a lot of hugging and comforting, your second might prefer more time alone. These individual differences don't indicate that your parenting is "right" or "wrong," only that each baby is unique.

Over time, you will get to know your child's individual traits, and you'll develop patterns of interaction designed especially for them. If you remain flexible and open to their special traits, they'll help steer your actions as a parent in the right direction. (Also see Social/Emotional Development, *page 211*.)

Growth and Development

Physical Appearance and Growth

Your child's specific weight and height are not as important as their growth rate. By now you should have established their position on the growth curve in the Appendix (*pages 699–702*). Continue to plot their measurements at regular intervals to make sure they maintain their growth rate. If you find they start following a different curve or are gaining weight or height unusually slowly, discuss it with your pediatrician.

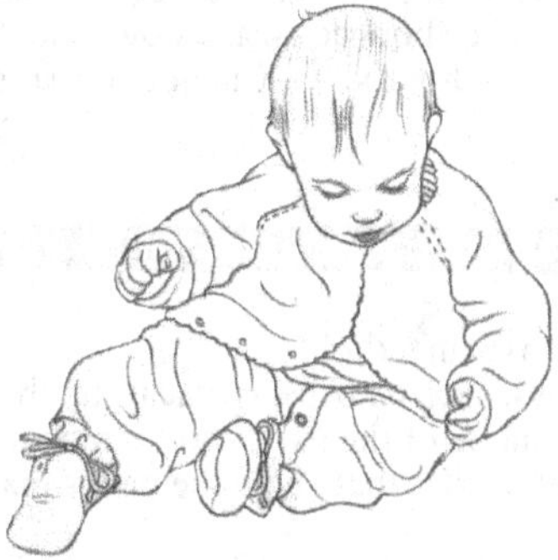

Movement

During their next four months, your baby will begin to use their fingers and thumbs in a mitten- or claw-like grip or raking motion, and they'll manage to pick up many things. They won't develop the pincer grasp with index finger and thumb until they're about 9 months old, but by 6 to 8 months, they'll learn to transfer objects from hand to hand, and turn and twist them.

MOVEMENT/PHYSICAL DEVELOPMENT MILESTONES FOR YOUR BABY AT 6 MONTHS

- Rolls from tummy to back
- Pushes up with straight arms when on tummy
- Leans on hands to support themselves when sitting

As their physical coordination improves, your baby will discover new parts of their body. Lying on their back, they can now grab their feet and toes and bring them to their mouth. While being diapered, they may reach down to touch their genitals. When sitting up, they may slap their knee or thigh. Through these explorations, they'll discover many new and interesting sensations. They'll start to understand the function of body parts. When you place their feet on the floor, they may curl their toes and stroke the surface, use their feet and legs to practice "walking," or bounce up and down. Watch out! These are all preparations for the next major milestones: crawling and standing.

TOYS APPROPRIATE FOR YOUR 6-MONTH-OLD

- Toys that have fingerholds
- Musical toys, such as bells, maracas, tambourines (make sure none of the parts can become loose)
- See-through rattles that show the pieces making the noise
- Books with bright pictures for you to show them
- Baby books with board, cloth, or vinyl pages

Vision

Just a couple of months ago, your baby's distance vision was about 20/100, which means they could see objects clearly at a distance of about 20 feet that adults with normal vision can see clearly at 100 feet. Now, however, their visual acuity has improved to about 20/40, which is close to what an adult with very mild nearsightedness can see. You may notice they start to respond to people and objects all the way across a room, or even farther!

Your infant also now has better color vision. Six-month-old infants are better able to discriminate between colors in the blue-green part of the spectrum compared to 4-month-olds, who have difficulty distinguishing between shades of blue and green.

Finally, at 6 months old, babies have developed better depth perception and the ability to perceive motion. This means they can track moving objects more accurately and reach for objects with greater precision. You'll notice your baby reaching out with increasing accuracy with both hands to grasp anything that catches their attention.

By this age, your baby's eyes should always be pointed in the same direction. The visual pathways in the brain that carry signals from one eye to the other have matured to the point that even if one is closed, it still knows what the other is seeing. If you notice your baby going "cross-eyed" or one or both eyes drifting to the side at this age, be sure to tell their pediatrician.

VISION DEVELOPMENTS FOR YOUR BABY AT 6 MONTHS

- Develops full-color vision
- Distance vision matures
- Ability to track moving objects improves

Language Development

Participation in your child's language development becomes even more important after 6 or 7 months, when they begin actively imitating the sounds of speech. Up till then, they might repeat one sound for a whole day or several days at a stretch before trying another. Now they'll become much more responsive to the sounds they hear you make, and they'll try to follow. Introduce them to simple syllables and words: "baby," "cat," "dog," "go," "hot," "cold," and "walk," as well as "mama" and "dada." Although it may be up to a year or more before you can interpret their babbling, your baby can understand many words well before their first birthday.

If they don't babble or imitate sounds by their seventh month, it could mean a hearing or speech development problem. A baby with partial hearing loss can still be startled by loud noises or will turn their head in that direction, and they may even respond to your voice. However, they will have difficulty imitating speech. If your baby does not babble or produce a variety of sounds by about 6 months, alert your pediatrician. If they had frequent ear infections, they might have fluid trapped in the middle ear space, which could interfere with hearing. A particularly important group of infants who need audiology follow-up at this age are those who were in the neonatal intensive care unit for any period of time. Usually they have a screening hearing test at birth and are recommended to have a behavioral hearing test by 6 months of age. You can discuss this with your primary care pediatrician, since often there is an audiologist that your doctor works with closely.

LANGUAGE/COMMUNICATION MILESTONES FOR YOUR BABY AT 6 MONTHS

- Takes turns making sounds with you
- Blows "raspberries" (sticks tongue out and blows)
- Makes squealing noises

Cognitive Development

Your baby will quickly discover that some things, such as bells and keys, make interesting sounds when moved or shaken. Before long, they'll begin dropping things intentionally to see you pick them up and to start a chain of responses from their audience, including funny faces, groans, and laughter. This is a way for them to learn about cause and effect, and their ability to influence their environment.

It's important to give your child what they need for these experiments and encourage them to test their "theories." Make sure everything you give them is unbreakable, lightweight, and large enough that they can't swallow it. If they lose interest in the usual toys, plastic or wooden spoons, unbreakable cups, jar or bowl lids, and boxes are endlessly entertaining and inexpensive.

Another major discovery your baby makes toward the end of this period is that objects continue to exist when out of their sight—a principle called object permanence. During their first few months, they probably thought the world consisted only of things they could see. When you hid a toy under a cloth, they thought it was gone for good, and so they wouldn't bother looking for it. But sometime after 4 months they began to realize the world is more permanent. You're the same person who greets them every morning. The block you hid under the can did not vanish after all. Playing hiding games like peekaboo and observing the people and things around them, your baby will continue to learn about object permanence for many months to come.

COGNITIVE MILESTONES FOR YOUR BABY AT 6 MONTHS

- Puts things in their mouth to explore them
- Reaches to grab a toy they want
- Closes lips to show they don't want more food

Social/Emotional Development

The subtle aspects of your baby's personality are determined largely by their temperament. Are they rambunctious or gentle? Easygoing or easily upset? Headstrong or compliant? To a large extent, these are inborn character traits. Just like their sizes and shapes, infants' temperaments differ as well and include their activity levels, persistence, and adaptability to the world around them. These traits will become increasingly apparent during these months. You won't necessarily find all of their personal characteristics enjoyable all the time—especially not when your determined 6-month-old screams in frustration as they lunge for the family cat. But in the long run, adapting to their natural personality is best. That personality is real, and it directly affects you and the rest of the family, so it's important to understand your child as completely as possible.

Your child's behavioral style will affect how you parent and sometimes even your feelings toward yourself. An agreeable, even-tempered child, for example, is more likely to make you feel competent as a parent than one who is constantly irritable. As you've probably discovered already, some infants of this age are "easy," calm, and predictable, while others are more difficult. Strong-willed and high-strung babies require an extra dose of patience and gentle guidance. They often don't adapt to changing surroundings easily and will become increasingly upset if pushed to perform before they're ready. You'll fare better and reduce stress by recognizing and accommodating their temperament rather than resisting and trying to change it.

Talking and cuddling sometimes will do wonders to calm the nerves of an irritable child. Distracting them can refocus their energy. If they scream because you won't retrieve the toy they dropped for the tenth time, move your baby to the floor so that they can reach it themselves.

The shy or sensitive child also requires special attention, particularly if you have more boisterous children who overshadow them. When a baby is quiet and undemanding, it's easy to assume they're content. If they don't laugh or smile a lot, you may not play with them as much. But this baby often needs personal contact even more than others. They may be overwhelmed easily and need you to show them how to be assertive and become involved. Give them plenty of time to warm up to any situation, and make sure other people approach them slowly. Let them sit on the sidelines before you attempt to involve them directly. Once they feel secure, gradually they'll become more responsive to the people around them.

Also let your pediatrician know if you have concerns about your baby's emotional development. Your pediatrician can help, but such concerns can often be difficult to detect in a routine office visit. That's why it's important to call the doctor's attention to your concerns and describe your day-to-day observations. Write them down so that you don't forget. And take comfort in the fact that with time and patience, some of the personality traits you wish you could change will evolve. In the meantime, enjoy them as they are.

SOCIAL/EMOTIONAL MILESTONES FOR YOUR BABY AT 6 MONTHS

- Knows familiar people
- Likes to look at themselves in a mirror
- Laughs

Basic Care

Introducing Solid Foods

At 4 to 6 months, depending on when your infant is ready, you can begin adding solid foods. Mothers who breastfeed do not need to avoid certain foods, unless instructed by your pediatrician due to an infant's allergy or intolerance. Breast milk offers many benefits, including possible protection against allergies. Talk with your pediatrician at the 4-month checkup about the timing of the introduction of solid foods, particularly if there is a strong history of food allergies in immediate family members or if your baby has severe eczema.

Once you begin, start solid foods at whichever time of day feedings work best for you and your baby. However, as they get older, they will want to eat with other family members, as family mealtimes provide significant benefits to the entire family, including improved nutrition habits, stronger family relationships, and—particularly helpful for a developing infant—exposure to lots of language, which stimulates brain development. To minimize the chances of choking, your baby should sit upright when you introduce solids. If they cry or turn away when you try, don't force the issue. It's more important you both enjoy mealtimes than for them to start foods by a specific date. Go back to exclusively nursing or bottle-feeding for a week or two, then try introducing solid food again. Just as you did with nursing or formula-feeding, follow your baby's cues to know when they are hungry and full rather than focusing on the specific amount they eat at each meal.

Options for experimenting with solid foods include using a spoon or a parent's fingers, or allowing your baby to explore the soft, pureed food with their hands. Putting solid foods in a bottle or infant feeder with a nipple is not recommended, as this can drastically increase food intake at each feeding, may be a risk for choking, and could lead to excessive weight gain. Besides, it's important for your baby to get used to the process of eating—sitting up, tasting new foods, resting between bites, and stopping when full. This early experience will lay the foundation for good eating habits throughout their life. There is no need to rub a new food on the skin before letting your baby eat it, as this is not an accurate test for allergy and can cause non-allergic skin irritation, which may raise undue concern.

Standard spoons may be too wide, but small spoons often work well; a rubber-coated baby spoon is also a good choice and can help avoid injury. Start with small amounts or tiny tastes, and talk your baby through the process ("Mmm, see how good this is?"). They probably won't know what to do the first time or two. They may look confused, wrinkle their nose, roll the food around in their mouth, or reject it entirely. This is an understandable reaction, considering how different their feedings have been.

One way to ease the transition is to give your infant small tastes of food, then finish off with their usual breast milk or formula. This will prevent them from being overly frustrated when they're very hungry, and it will link the satisfaction of nursing with this new experience of spoon-feeding. No matter what you do, the first few solid-food feedings are sure to wind up on their face and bib, so increase the size of their feedings very gradually, starting with just a teaspoonful or two, until they get the idea of swallowing solids.

What foods? Traditionally, single-grain cereals were introduced first. However, there is no medical evidence that introducing solid foods in any particular order has an advantage for your infant. Though many pediatricians recommend starting vegetables before fruits, there is no research indicating your infant will develop a dislike for or allergy to vegetables if they follow fruit. When you are breastfeeding, be sure to eat a variety of foods, including vegetables, as babies who are exposed to these tastes while nursing are less likely to reject them when they start eating solid foods.

While formula is fortified with iron, breastfed babies may not get enough iron from breast milk alone, so try to incorporate foods high in iron into your baby's diet, like beef, fish, dried beans (lentils, soybeans, black beans), dark green vegetables (spinach, chard), eggs, and tofu.

Many babies enjoy cereals. You may use premixed baby cereals or dry varieties mixed with breast milk or formula. Pediatricians now advise parents to choose iron-fortified whole-grain cereals rather than highly processed ones. There is no evidence that one whole-grain cereal is better than another, though some rice cereals particularly have been found to have higher levels of arsenic compared to other grains, so it is important to use a variety of grains rather than sticking with only rice cereal. Whichever you choose, make sure it is very soft or completely pureed until your baby is ready and able to safely manage and tolerate more texture.

Pediatricians recommend introducing new foods to your baby's diet, in any form your baby can handle, and watching for any signs of possible allergic reaction. Within two or three months of starting solid food, your baby's daily diet should include breast milk, iron-fortified whole-grain cereals, vegetables, meats (including fish), eggs, fruits, and nut butters (but never whole nuts) distributed among three meals. Remember that babies do not need the added sugars and salts that adults may have grown used to. Also know that if your baby rejects a given food the first ten times, they may come to love it on the eleventh try. Don't force it, but repeated exposure can be especially important when introducing some vegetables like broccoli and asparagus.

Once your baby sits independently, you can begin giving them finger foods to help them learn to feed themselves. Some parents skip pureed foods altogether in favor of very soft foods that babies can self-feed, a practice called baby-led weaning. Most infants can begin learning to self-feed without assistance around 6 to 8 months. Make sure anything you give is soft, is easy to swallow, and breaks down into small pieces they can't choke on. Well-cooked cut-up sweet potatoes, green beans, peas, shredded or diced chicken or other meat, small pieces of bread, and whole-grain crackers are good examples. Don't give any food that truly requires chewing, even if they already have teeth. After you are finished with the meal, it is a good idea to gently wipe your infant's teeth/gums with a wet cloth for proper oral care.

When feeding your baby solid foods, portion them into a small dish instead of directly feeding out of the container, jar, or pouch the food came in. This will prevent the food from becoming contaminated with bacteria from the baby's mouth. Discard the portion left in the dish rather than trying to save it.

While there is a huge variety of prepared baby foods available at the store, you don't have to rely on jars or packets to feed your baby, as making homemade baby food can be easy, inexpensive, and healthy. Everything you make should be soft and well-cooked. Cooked fresh vegetables and stewed fruits are easy to prepare. Although you can feed your baby mashed raw bananas, most other fruits should be cooked until soft. Immediately refrigerate any food not used, and then inspect carefully for signs of spoilage before giving it again. Never offer foods your baby might choke on, such as whole nuts, uncut grapes or cherry tomatoes, or raw carrots or celery.

Hold off on liquids other than breast milk (or formula if you are not breastfeeding) or small amounts of water in a sippy cup. The American Academy of Pediatrics recommends fruit juice not be given to infants, since it offers no nutritional benefit to babies in this age group, and giving fruit juice to infants and young children may get them used to sweet beverages, which can lead to excessive weight gain and tooth decay. In addition, cow's milk is not recommended until after 1 year of age because it doesn't have appropriate nutrition for young infants and can also cause intestinal bleeding and anemia.

If your infant seems thirsty between feedings, breastfeed them or give them formula, or, after 6 months, offer small sips of water. Getting a child used to plain water is a healthy habit for life. During hot months when your child loses fluid through sweat, offer water two or more times a day. If your water is fluoridated, this also will help prevent tooth decay. You can test your water with home kits to see if your water source is fluoridated. Most city water is fluoridated, and some well water naturally contains fluoride. Your pediatrician or dentist can guide you if additional fluoride is necessary. If you use well water, it is important to have the well water tested on a regular basis for contaminants such as bacteria and toxins. The CDC recommends testing wells used for drinking a minimum of every spring, or more often if there are certain contaminants; another option is the addition of a well filtration system.

By the time your baby is 6 or 7 months old, they'll probably sit well enough to use a high chair during mealtime. To ensure their comfort and safety, safety straps should be used, and the chair seat should be cleaned regularly. Also, look for a high chair with a detachable tray with a raised rim. (See *page 314* for safety recommendations.) The rim helps keep dishes and food in place during more rambunctious feeding sessions. The detachable tray can be cleaned easily, a feature you're bound to appreciate in the months to come. (There still may be days when the only solution is to put the entire chair in the shower for a complete wipe-down!) As your child's diet expands and they're feeding themselves more regularly, discuss their personal nutritional needs with your pediatrician. Poor eating habits established in infancy can lead to health problems later on.

Your pediatrician will help determine whether your baby is overfed, not eating enough, or eating too much of the wrong kinds of foods. By familiarizing yourself with the caloric and nutritional contents of what they eat, you can ensure they're eating a proper diet. Be aware of other food habits in your family. As your baby eats more and more table foods, they'll imitate the way you eat—the whole family should try to model a healthy, nutrient-rich diet to set a good example, and mealtimes should be a time for interaction and enjoyment, not struggles.

What if you're concerned your baby already has overweight? Even when infants are young, some parents are worried their babies are gaining too much weight. There has been a rise in childhood obesity and its potential complications (such as diabetes); thus it's wise to be sensitive to the problem, no matter your child's age. Some evidence indicates that bottle-fed infants gain weight more rapidly than breastfed babies, perhaps because some parents encourage their infant to finish a bottle. Always remember to let your baby's hunger cues drive how much they eat, rather than urging them to finish a set amount of food. Always check with your pediatrician regarding your child's growth curve, and never put your baby on a diet. Insufficient weight gain can be detrimental to your baby's brain development.

It is important to get your pediatrician's advice before making any dietary adjustments. During these months of rapid growth, your infant needs the proper balance of fat, carbohydrates, and protein for proper growth and development.

As soon as solid foods are started, your baby's stools will become more solid and variable in color. The stools will also have a much stronger odor. Peas and other green vegetables may turn the stool deep green; beets may turn it red. (Beets sometimes make urine red as well.) The baby's stools may contain undigested particles, especially hulls of peas or corn and the skins of tomatoes or other vegetables. This is normal. If the stools are extremely loose, watery, or full of mucus, however, it may indicate an irritated digestive tract. In this case, consult your pediatrician to determine if there is a digestive problem.

Sleeping

Most babies this age still need at least two naps a day, midmorning and midday. Some babies may nap a third time later in the afternoon. In general, it's best to let your baby sleep as long as they want, unless they have trouble falling asleep at their normal nightly bedtime. If this becomes a problem, wake them earlier from their afternoon nap.

Because your child is more alert and active now, they may have trouble winding down at the end of the day. A consistent bedtime routine will help. Experiment to see what works best, taking into consideration household activities and your baby's temperament. A warm bath, a massage, rocking, a story or lullaby, and a breast- or bottle-feeding will all help relax them and put them in a bedtime mood. Remember to begin these activities before your baby becomes overtired. Eventually they'll associate these activities with going to sleep, and that will help relax and soothe them.

Now that your baby is a little older, all the same rules of safe sleep apply (see Recommendations for Safe Infant Sleep, *page 107*), except that they are probably rolling over from back to front now on their own. Settle your baby in their crib while they're drowsy but still awake so that they learn to fall asleep on their own. Gently place them on their back, whisper your goodnight, and leave the room. If they cry, check on them and offer a few comforting words, then leave the room again. As the days pass, gradually give them less attention at night. If parents are consistent, most babies will cry less each night and will be more likely to learn self-soothing. (See *Chapter 30*, Your Child's Sleep, for more information.)

Teething and Dental Care

Teething usually starts during these months. The two front teeth (central incisors), either upper or lower, usually appear first, followed by the opposite front teeth. The first molars are next, followed by the canines, or eyeteeth.

There is great variability in the timing and pattern of teething. If your child doesn't show any teeth until later than this age period, or if they come in out of order, don't worry. The timing may be determined by heredity and doesn't mean anything is wrong.

Teething occasionally may cause mild irritability, crying, excessive drooling, and a desire to chew on something hard. More often, the gums around the new teeth will swell and be tender. To ease your baby's discomfort, try gently rubbing or massaging the gums with one of your fingers. Teething rings are helpful and should be made of firm rubber. (The teethers you freeze tend to get too hard and too cold and can cause more harm than good.) Never use teething gels to numb the gums; in rare cases, they can poison babies' blood cells and keep them from carrying oxygen. Homeopathic teething tablets also provide no benefit, and in some cases they have been made with potentially harmful toxins. Amber teething necklaces have not been shown to relieve pain, and they have caused cases of choking and strangulation; remember never to leave anything around your baby's neck. If your child seems particularly miserable or has a fever higher than 100.4 degrees Fahrenheit (38 degrees Celsius), it's probably not from teething, and you should consult your pediatrician, as your baby may be sick.

Your baby should see a dentist within 6 months after their first tooth erupts, but no later than 12 months of age, whichever comes first. Pediatric dentists are specially trained to see infants, and you can find a pediatric dentist for your baby at the American Academy of Pediatric Dentistry's website, aapd.org. But going to your family dentist for routine pediatric care is entirely adequate and may be covered by existing health insurance.

Brushing your baby's teeth at home is very important as

well. For cleaning when you first start seeing teeth, simply brush with a soft child's toothbrush and a smear of fluoridated toothpaste the size of a grain of rice. To prevent cavities, it's best not to let your baby fall asleep with a bottle or on the breast, either at nap time or at night. Doing this will keep milk from pooling around the teeth and creating a breeding ground for decay.

Swings and Play Yards

Many parents find that mechanical swings, especially with cradle attachments, can calm a crying baby when nothing else seems to work. If you use a device like this, check the weight limit and age recommendations on the device. Use only swings that stand firmly on the floor, not those that hang from door frames. Also, don't use a swing for more than half an hour twice a day; it may quiet your baby, but it is no substitute for attention. Secure your baby properly with the safety harness at all times. A swing is never a safe place for a baby to sleep, so if your baby looks sleepy, remove them right away and place them on their back in a crib or bassinet.

STIMULATING INFANT BRAIN GROWTH: AGE 6 MONTHS

Many connections are being made in your baby's brain during this time in their young life. Those connections are reflected in their behaviors, such as the strong attachments they have to you and others who take care of them, or their crying when you leave the room, when they are approached by a stranger, or when they want a particular toy. They are becoming more interested in the world and are better able to communicate their emotions and desires—all the while developing new skills such as grasping, rolling over, and sitting.

Without overstimulating your baby, try these activities to help strengthen the connections in their developing brain:

- Provide a stimulating, safe environment where your baby can begin to explore and roam freely.
- Give consistent, warm, physical contact—hugging, skin-to-skin, body-to-body contact—to establish your infant's sense of security and well-being.

- Be attentive to your baby's rhythms and moods. Respond to them when they are upset as well as when they are happy.
- Talk and sing during dressing, bathing, feeding, playing, walking, and driving. They may not yet understand the language, but as they hear it, their language skills will develop. Check with your pediatrician if your baby doesn't seem to hear sounds or imitate your words.
- Engage your child in face-to-face talk. Mimic their sounds to show interest.
- Read books to your baby every day. They'll love the sound of your voice, and before long they'll enjoy looking at the pictures and "reading" on their own.
- If you speak more than one language, use them all at home.
- Engage in rhythmic movement with your child, such as dancing together to music.
- Avoid subjecting your baby to stressful or traumatic experiences, physical or psychological.
- Introduce your baby to other children and parents; this is a very special period for infants. Be sensitive to cues indicating that they are ready to meet new people.
- Encourage your child to reach for toys. Give them baby blocks and soft toys that can stimulate their hand-eye coordination and their fine motor skills.
- Make sure other people who provide care and supervision for your baby understand the importance of forming a loving and comforting relationship with your child.
- Encourage your baby to begin to sleep for extended periods at night; if you need advice about this important step in your infant's development, ask your pediatrician.
- Spend time on the floor playing with your child every day.
- If your baby will be cared for by others, choose quality childcare that is affectionate, responsive, educational, and safe. Visit your childcare provider frequently and share your ideas about positive caregiving.

Once your baby starts to move about, you may need to use a play yard. Even before they crawl or walk, a play yard offers a protected place where they can lie or sit outdoors as well as in rooms where you have no crib or bassinet. (See Play Yards, *page 316*, for specific recommendations.) Be sure the play yard has not been recalled. Check the Consumer Product Safety Commission website (cpsc.gov) or saferproducts.gov for recalled products.

Siblings

If your baby has a big brother or sister, you may start to see signs of rivalry at this time, particularly if there is less than two years between the children. Earlier, the baby was more dependent, slept a lot, and didn't require your constant attention. But now that they are becoming more demanding, you'll need to ration your time and energy so that you have enough for the children individually and together.

Your older child may still be jealous at having to share your attention. Set aside special "big brother" or "big sister" chores that don't involve the baby. Doing this allows for some extra attention and gets housework done. Be sure to show the child how much you appreciate this help.

You also can help sibling relations by including the older child in activities with the baby. If the two of you sing a song or read a story, the baby will enjoy listening. The older child can also help care for the baby to some extent, assisting at bath or changing time. But unless the child is responsible and dependable enough, usually over age 12, don't leave your older child alone with the baby, even if they are trying to be helpful. Younger children can easily drop or injure an infant without realizing what they've done.

(For more information, see Siblings' Feelings on *page 38*. Many issues and guidelines described there also apply to children ages 4 through 7 months.)

Health Watch

No matter how you try to protect your baby, there will be times when they get sick. This is an inevitable part of growing up and will happen more frequently when they have more direct contact with other children. It's not always easy to tell when a baby is ill, but there are some signs. Do they look pale or have dark circles under their eyes? Are they acting less energetic or more irritable than usual? If they have an infectious disease, they'll probably have a fever (see *Chapter 22*, Fever), and they may lose weight due to loss of appetite, diarrhea, or vomiting. Some difficult-to-detect kidney or lung infections also can prevent weight gain in babies. At this age, weight loss could mean that the baby has a digestive problem, such as an allergy to wheat or milk protein (see Celiac Disease, *page 350*), or lacks the digestive enzymes needed to digest certain solid foods. If you suspect your child may be ill but you can't identify the exact problem, or if you have any concerns about what is happening, call your pediatrician and describe the symptoms.

YOUR CHILD AND ANTIBIOTICS

Antibiotics are among the most powerful and important medicines known. When used properly, they can save lives. When used improperly, antibiotics can harm your child. Understanding the rationale behind limiting antibiotic use is important.

Two main types of germs—viruses and bacteria—cause most infections. Viruses cause all colds and most coughs. There are no medicines effective against the common cold, and colds almost always clear up on their own with time. Antibiotics never cure common viral infections. Your baby recovers from these common viral infections when the illness has run its course. Antibiotics should not be used to treat viral infections.

Antibiotics are used to treat bacterial infections, but some bacteria have become resistant to certain antibiotics. If your child is infected with resistant bacteria, they might need a different antibiotic or even hospitalization, where more powerful medicines can be given intravenously. A few new strains of bacteria are already untreatable. To protect your child from antibiotic-resistant bacteria, use antibiotics only when your pediatrician has determined they might be effective, since repeated or improper use of antibiotics contributes to resistant bacteria and viruses.

When Are Antibiotics Needed? When Are They Not Needed?

These complicated questions are best answered by your pediatrician, and they depend on the specific diagnosis. If you think your child might need treatment, contact your pediatrician.

- Documented ear infection. Sometimes requires antibiotics.
- Sinus infections. These are very uncommon at this age, in large part because the sinuses are so small. Just because your child's mucus is yellow or green does not necessarily mean they have a bacterial infection. It is normal for mucus to get thick and change color during a viral cold.
- Bronchitis. Children rarely need antibiotics for bronchitis, since these infections are almost always caused by viruses.
- Colds. Colds are caused by viruses and sometimes can last for two weeks or more. Antibiotics have no effect on colds. Your pediatrician may have suggestions for comfort measures while the cold runs its course.
- Influenza. Once your baby reaches 6 months, they will be old enough for a seasonal flu shot. Until then, other family members—parents and older siblings—should receive theirs to protect the baby. There are antiviral medications for this infection, but not all are appropriate for newborns and infants, and they may not be as effective as prevention via immunization.

Viral infections sometimes may lead to bacterial infections. Keep your pediatrician informed if the illness gets worse or lasts a long time, so proper treatment can be given as needed.

If an antibiotic is prescribed, your child should take the antibiotic exactly as directed. Never save antibiotics for later use or let other family members use a prescription not intended for them.

The following illnesses and symptoms are the most common ones to occur at this age (all are described in Part 2 of this book):

Bronchiolitis (see *page 408*)
Colds/Upper Respiratory Infections (see *page 468*)
Conjunctivitis (pinkeye; see Eye Infections, *page 545*)
Croup (see *page 416*)
Diarrhea (see *page 354*)
Fever (see *page 572*)
Middle Ear Infections (see *page 471*)
Pneumonia (see *page 421*)
Sore Throat (Strep Throat, Tonsillitis) (see *page 480*)
Vomiting (see *page 377*)

▪ YOUR BABY AT 6 MONTHS OLD CHECKLIST ▪

Immunization Update

- First dose of influenza vaccine as soon as it's available in the fall; second dose given one month later
- Third DTaP vaccine
- Third polio vaccine (which can be given between 6 and 18 months)
- Third pneumococcal vaccine
- Third Hib vaccine (depending on vaccine type given for doses one and two)
- Third hepatitis B vaccine (can be given between 6 and 18 months)
- Third rotavirus vaccine (depending on vaccine type; one requires two doses and the other three)

Safety Check

See Safety Check in *Chapters 5* (*page 163*), *6* (*page 186*), and *7* (*page 204*).

CHAPTER 9

YOUR BABY AT 9 MONTHS

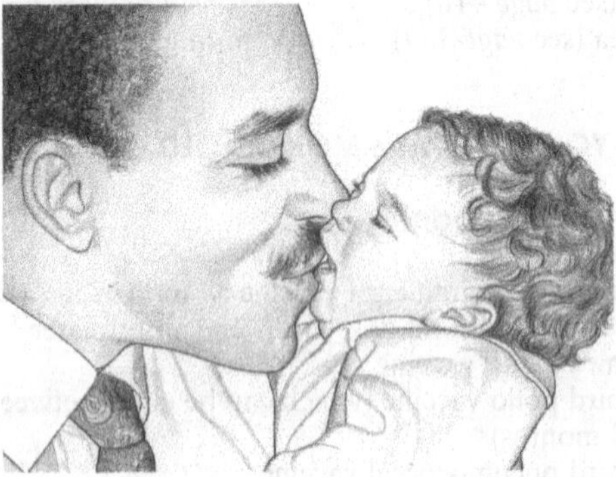

By 9 months, your baby is increasingly mobile, a development that will both thrill and challenge you. Being able to move gives your child a new sense of power and control—their first real taste of physical independence. And while this is exhilarating for them, the separation from you it causes is also frightening. So as they eagerly move out on their own to explore the farthest reaches of their domain, they may also wail if they wander out of your sight. Mobility does bring dangers that must be constantly monitored, which means there cannot be any unsupervised time.

For you, your baby's mobility may be a source of considerable concern as well as pride. Crawling and walking are signals they're developing on target, but these achievements also mean you'll have your hands full keeping them safe. If you haven't already fully childproofed your home, do it now. (See *Chapter 11*, Keeping Your Child Safe.) At their age, your baby has no concept of danger and a limited memory for warnings. The only way to protect them from the hundreds of hazards in your home is to secure cabinets and drawers, place dangerous and precious objects out of reach, and make perilous rooms such as bathrooms inaccessible unless they're supervised.

By childproofing your home, you'll also give your baby a

greater sense of freedom. After all, fewer areas will be off-limits, and thus you can let them make discoveries on their own. These personal accomplishments will promote their self-esteem; you might even think of ways of facilitating them. For example:

1. Fill a low kitchen cabinet or drawer with safe objects and let your baby discover it themselves.
2. Pad edges of a coffee table or sofa—or consider removing hard tables briefly and replacing them with soft-edged ottomans—and allow them to learn to pull up and cruise.
3. Equip your home with cushions of assorted shapes and sizes and let them experiment with the different ways they can move over and around them.

Knowing when to guide a child and when to let them act alone is part of the art of parenting. At this age, your child is extremely expressive and will give you cues on when to intervene. When they're acting frustrated rather than challenged, don't let them struggle. If they're crying because their ball is wedged under the sofa, or if they've pulled up to a standing position and can't get down, they need your help. At other times, however, it's important for them to solve problems. Don't let your impatience make you intervene more than necessary. You may be tempted to feed your 9-month-old because it's faster and less messy. However, that deprives them of a chance to learn how to feed themselves. The more opportunities you can give them to discover, test, and strengthen their new capabilities, the more confident and adventurous they'll be.

Growth and Development

Physical Appearance and Growth

Your baby will continue to grow rapidly during these months. The typical 8-month-old boy weighs between 17½ and 22 pounds (8–10 kg), with girls about ½ pound less. By the first birthday, the average child has usually tripled their birth weight and is 28 to 32 inches (71–81 cm) tall. Do not be alarmed if your child does not follow the typical growth curve in the middle, but follows their own curve. If they were born small, they may stay under the bottom line of the growth curve for the first few years. As long as they are following an upward curve, this is acceptable. Head growth between 8 and 12 months slows down from the first 6 months, a typical head circumference at 8 months being 17½ inches (44.5 cm) and at 1 year 18 inches (46 cm). Each baby grows at their own rate, however, so you should check your child's growth curves on the charts in the Appendix to make sure they're following the pattern already established.

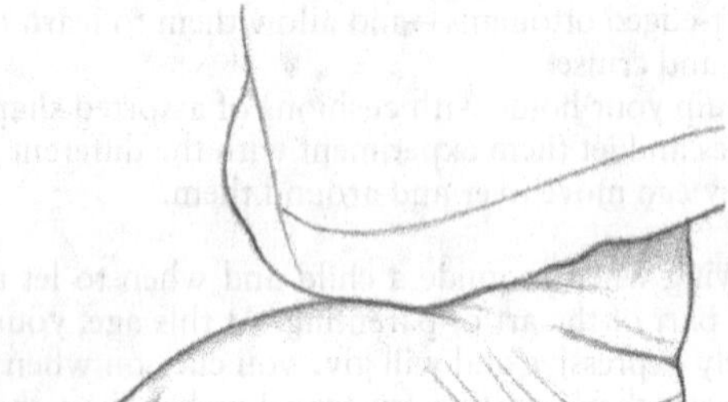

At this age, your child's feet will seem flat, the arch hidden by a pad of fat. In two to three years, this fat will disappear and their arches will emerge.

When your child first stands, you may be surprised by their posture. Their belly will protrude, their rear will stick out, and their back will sway forward. It may look unusual, but this stance is perfectly normal until they develop a confident sense of balance sometime in the second year.

When your child takes their first teetering steps, you may notice their feet turning outward. The ligaments of their hips are still loose, and their legs naturally rotate outward. During the first half of their second year, the ligaments will tighten and their feet should point straight.

Movement

At 8 months, your baby probably will be sitting without support. Although they may topple from time to time, they'll usually catch themselves with their arms. As the muscles in their trunk strengthen, they'll also start leaning over to reach objects. Eventually they'll figure out how to roll onto their stomach and get back up to a sitting position. If they are not sitting by themselves by 9 months, this is concerning and you should let your pediatrician know.

When lying on a flat surface, your baby is now in constant motion. When on their stomach, they'll arch their neck to look around, and when on their back, they'll grab their feet (or anything else nearby) and pull them to their mouth. They won't be content to stay on their back. They can turn over at will now and flip without a moment's notice. This can be dangerous during diaper changes, so you may want to retire their changing table, using instead the floor or bed, from which they're less likely to fall. Never leave them alone on a raised surface for even an instant at any time.

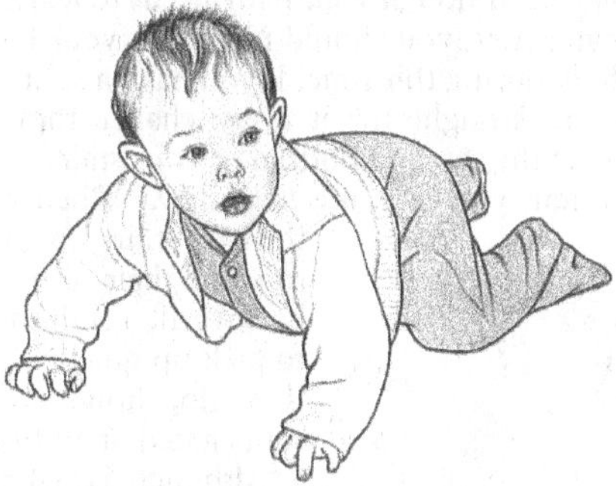

All this activity strengthens muscles for crawling, a skill usually mastered between 7 and 10 months. For a while they may rock on their hands and knees. Since their arms are stronger than their legs, they may even push themselves backward. But with time and practice they'll discover they can propel themselves forward across the room toward the target of their choice.

Some children never crawl. Instead, they use alternative methods, such as scooting on their bottoms or slithering on their stomachs. As long as your baby is coordinating both sides of their body and using each arm and leg equally, there's no cause for concern. The important thing is that they're able to explore their surroundings and strengthen their body in preparation for walking. If you feel your child is not moving normally, discuss your concern with the pediatrician.

How can you encourage your child to crawl? Try presenting them with intriguing objects just beyond their reach. As they become more agile, create miniature obstacle courses using pillows, boxes, and sofa cushions. Join in the game by hiding behind one of the obstacles and surprising them with a "peekaboo!" Don't ever leave your baby unsupervised, though. If they fall between pillows or under a box, they might not be able to get out. This is bound to frighten them, and they could even smother. Remember not to leave small objects on the floor, under the couch, or in any location where they can find them and put them into their mouth. Things like balloon fragments, small button batteries, and coins are especially dangerous.

Stairs are another ready-made—but potentially dangerous—obstacle course. Although your baby needs to learn how to go up and down stairs, you should not allow your baby to play on them alone during this time. If you have a staircase, they'll probably head straight for it every chance they get. Place sturdy gates at the top and bottom of your staircase. (To see a safe, horizontal-type gate, see *page 310*.) When you're with them on stairs, encourage them to work their way down them backward, a skill they're likely to pick up quickly. Even when they do, however, keep the stairs gated at all times.

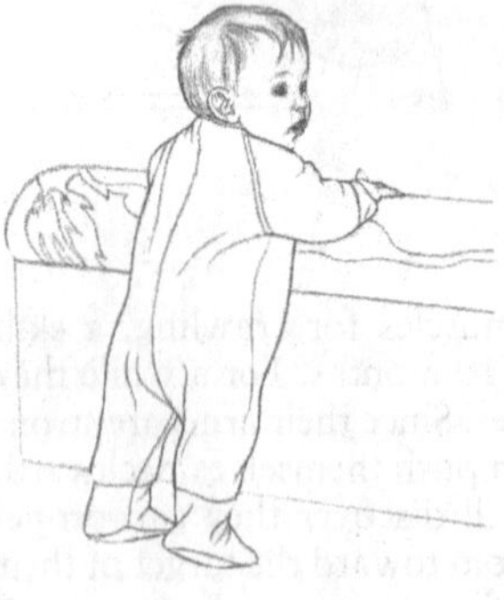

Although crawling changes dramatically how your baby sees and interacts with the world, don't expect them to be content for long. They'll see everyone else walking, and that's what they'll want to do. In preparation, they'll pull themselves to a standing position every chance they get—although when they first start, they may not know how to get down.

If they cry for help, physically show them how to bend their knees to lower themselves without falling. This may help and may save you many trips to their room when they're standing in their crib and crying because they don't know how to sit down. Once your baby feels secure standing, they'll try tentative steps while holding on for support. When your hands aren't available, they'll cruise alongside furniture. Just make sure whatever they use for support has no sharp edges and is properly weighted or attached to the floor.

As their balance improves, they may let go occasionally before seeking support again when they feel themselves totter. Their first steps will be shaky. They may take only one before dropping, either in surprise or in relief. Soon, however, they'll manage to keep themselves up and moving until you catch them several steps later. As miraculous as it may seem, most children advance from these first steps to confident walking within days.

Although both of you will feel excited over this dramatic development, you'll also be unnerved at times, especially when they stumble and fall. Even if you took pains to provide a safe environment, it's almost impossible to avoid bumps and bruises. Just be matter-of-fact about these mishaps. Offer a quick hug or a reassuring word and send them on their way again. They won't be unduly upset by these falls if you're not. Also, don't be alarmed if they choose to crawl at times after they have started walking; babies use whatever is easiest and fastest!

At this stage, or even earlier, some parents use a baby walker. Contrary to what the name suggests, these devices do not help children learn to walk. They actually eliminate the desire to walk. To make matters worse, they present a serious tipping hazard when the child bumps into an obstacle, like a small toy or a throw rug. Children in walkers are also more likely to fall down stairs and get into dangerous places otherwise beyond their reach. For these reasons, the American Academy of Pediatrics strongly urges parents not to use baby walkers.

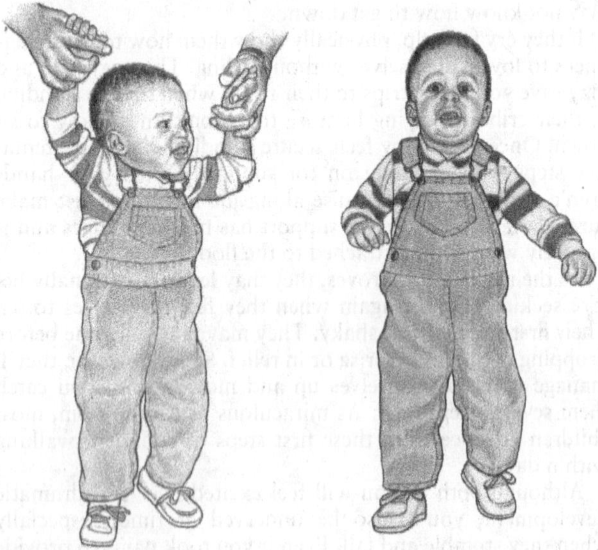

Soon your baby will manage to keep themselves up and moving until you catch them several steps later.

A stationary exercise saucer or activity center, with a rotating and bouncy seat but no wheels, is a better choice. You may also consider a sturdy wagon or kiddie push car. Be sure it has a bar to push and is weighted so that it won't tip when they pull themselves up on it.

As your child begins to walk outside, they'll need shoes. They should be closed-toe, comfortable, and flexible, with non-skid soles, and they should provide room to grow; sneakers are a great choice. Your child does not need wedges, inserts, high backs, reinforced heels, special arches, or other features designed to shape and support feet. These have no proven benefit for the average child and may actually make it harder to walk. Their feet will grow rapidly during these months, and their shoes will have to keep pace. Their first pair of shoes will probably last two to three months, but you should check the fit monthly during this formative period.

MOVEMENT/PHYSICAL DEVELOPMENT MILESTONES FOR YOUR BABY AT 9 MONTHS

- Gets to a sitting position by themselves
- Moves things from one hand to their other hand
- Uses fingers to "rake" food toward themselves
- Sits without support

Many babies' first steps are taken around their first birthday, although it's normal for children to start walking earlier or later. At first, your child will walk with feet wide apart to improve their shaky balance. During those initial days and weeks, they may get going too fast and fall when they try to stop. As they become more confident, they'll learn how to stop and change directions. Before long, they'll be able to squat, pick something up, and stand again. When they reach this level, they'll get enormous pleasure from push-pull toys—the noisier the better.

Hand and Finger Skills

Your baby's mastery of crawling, standing, and walking is bound to be their most dramatic accomplishment during these months, but don't overlook all the wonderful things they're learning to do with their hands. Their clumsy way of raking things toward them will lead to accurate grasping with their thumb and first or second finger. You'll find them practicing this pincer movement on any small object, from dust balls to cereal, and they may even try to snap their fingers if you show them how.

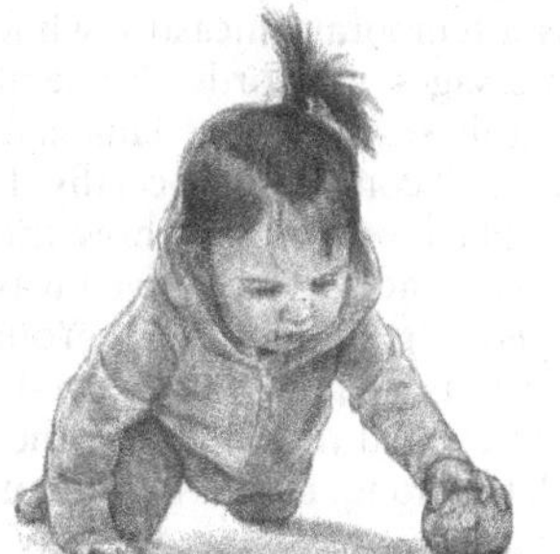

As your baby learns to open their fingers at will, they'll delight in dropping and throwing things. They'll fling small toys left on their high chair tray or in their play yard and then call loudly for someone to retrieve them so that they can do it again. If they throw hard objects like blocks, they might do some damage and increase the noise level in your household. Your life will be calmer if you redirect them toward softer objects, such as balls of various sizes, colors, and textures (include some with beads inside that make noise as they roll). One fun activity that allows you to observe your child's developing skills is rolling a large ball toward them. At first they'll slap it randomly, but eventually they'll learn to swat it so that it rolls back to you.

With improved coordination, your baby can now thoroughly investigate the objects they encounter. They'll pick them up, shake them, bang them, and pass them from hand to hand. They'll be particularly intrigued by toys with moving parts—those with wheels, levers, and hinges. Holes are fascinating to poke their fingers in and, when they're a little more skilled, drop things through.

Blocks are another favorite toy at this age. In fact, nothing motivates crawling better than a tower waiting to be toppled. Toward the end of this period, your child may even start building towers of their own.

Language Development

Toward the end of the first year, your baby will begin communicating what they want by pointing, crawling, or gesturing toward their target. They'll also imitate many gestures they see adults make as they talk. Non-verbal communication is a temporary measure while they learn how to phrase their messages in words. Remember that hearing problems can manifest as delayed language, so it is important to listen to others' concerns, especially if this is your first baby.

Have you noticed how the coos, gurgles, and screeches of earlier months have given way to recognizable syllables, "ba," "da," "ga," and "ma"? Your child may stumble into words such as "mama" and "bye-bye" accidentally, and when you get excited they'll realize they've said something meaningful. Before long, they'll use "mama" to attract your attention. At this age, they may also say "mama" just to practice. Ultimately, however, they'll use words when they want to communicate their meanings.

Even though you've been talking to your baby from birth, they now understand more language. Your conversations will take on new significance. Many babies can comprehend more words than you suspect, even before they can say them. Watch how they respond when you mention a favorite toy across the room. If they look toward it, they understand. To increase their understanding, keep talking to them as much as possible. Tell them what's happening around them, particularly as you bathe, change, and feed them. Make your language simple and specific: "I'm drying you with the big blue towel. It's so soft!" Label familiar toys and objects for them, and try to be consistent—that is, if you call the family pet a cat today, don't call it a kitty tomorrow.

Picture books can reinforce their budding understanding that everything has a name. Choose books with large board, cloth, or vinyl pages they can turn themselves. Also look for simple but colorful illustrations of things your child will recognize. Look at the pictures, point to things, and say the words for the objects in the book. The more words a child hears, the more they will learn. When you repeat the words as you look at the objects over and over, they will begin to understand that they are connected. At first, you can ask and answer questions like "What do you see? Do you see the ball?" Pause, and then say, "There is a ball. It is a blue ball."

BILINGUAL BABIES

If you speak a second language in your home, don't be concerned your child is going to become confused hearing two languages. More and more American families speak English and another language daily. Research and parental experience show that when children are exposed to two (or even more) languages at a very young age, particularly when they hear both consistently, they are able to learn both simultaneously. Yes, during the child's normal language development, they may be more proficient in one or the other, and at times they may mix words from the languages together. But with time, the two languages will become distinct and separate, and they should be able to communicate in both. (Some studies suggest that while they may be able to understand both languages, they will speak one of them better than the other for a time.)

Certainly, you should encourage your child to become bilingual. It's an asset, a skill that will benefit them the rest of their life. In general, the earlier both languages are introduced, the more proficient they'll be; by contrast, they may have a little more difficulty learning the second language if it is introduced during the preschool years after they've learned and spoken the first language exclusively.

Whether you're reading or talking to them, give them plenty of opportunities to join in. Ask questions and wait for a response. Let them take the lead. If they say "Gaagaagaa," repeat it back and see what they do. These exchanges may seem meaningless, but they tell your baby communication is two-way and they're a welcome participant. Paying attention to what they say also will help identify the words they understand and make it more likely you'll recognize their first spoken words.

These first words, incidentally, often aren't proper English. For your child, a "word" is any sound that consistently refers to the same person, object, or event. If they say "mog" every time they want milk, you should treat "mog" as a legitimate word by giving them milk when they say "mog." However, when you speak back to them, use "milk." Eventually they'll make the correction themselves.

Ages vary tremendously for when children begin to say recognizable words. Some can say two to three words by their first birthday. More likely, your baby's speech at 12 months will consist of gibberish with the tones and variations of speech. As long as they're experimenting with sounds that vary in intensity, pitch, and quality, they're getting ready to talk. The more you respond to them as if they were speaking, the more you'll stimulate their urge to communicate. Continuing to read to them daily will help tremendously. They will also enjoy simple songs. Make sure you turn off the television; having the television on in the background keeps parents from talking to their children and harms babies' language development. Limit your own screen time, as your baby needs your attention to learn.

LANGUAGE/COMMUNICATION MILESTONES FOR YOUR BABY AT 9 MONTHS

- Makes different sounds like "mamamama" and "babababa"
- Lifts arms to be picked up

Cognitive Development

An 8-month-old is curious about everything, but also has a short attention span and will move rapidly from one activity to the next. Two to three minutes is the most they'll spend with a single toy, and then they'll turn to something new. By 12 months, they may sit as long as fifteen minutes with a plaything, but they'll mostly be a body in motion. You shouldn't expect anything different.

Although toy stores are brimming with expensive playthings, the toys that fascinate children most at this age are ordinary household objects such as wooden spoons, egg cartons, and plastic containers of all shapes and sizes. Your baby will be especially interested in things that differ slightly from what they already know. If they're bored with the oatmeal box they've been playing with, renew their interest by putting a toy inside of it, or stacking two boxes on top of each other. These small changes will help them learn to detect small differences between the familiar and the unfamiliar. Also, when choosing playthings, remember that objects too much like what they've seen before will be quickly dismissed, while things too foreign may be confusing or frightening. Instead look for objects and toys that gradually expand their horizons. Pots and pans can be noisy but an inexpensive way of entertaining your child.

Often your baby won't need help discovering objects. As soon as they can crawl, they'll be off in search of new things to conquer. They'll rummage through drawers, empty wastebaskets, ransack cabinets, and conduct elaborate experiments on everything they find. (Make sure that any drawers or cabinets with potential hazards are secured with child safety locks.) They'll never tire of dropping, rolling, throwing, submerging, or waving objects to see how they behave. This may look like random play, but it's your child's way of learning how the world works. Like any good scientist, they're observing an object's properties, and from their observations they'll develop ideas about shapes (some things roll, others don't), textures (things can be scratchy, soft, or smooth), and sizes (some things fit inside others). They'll even begin to understand some things are edible and others aren't, although they'll still put everything into their mouth just to be sure. (Again, make sure there's nothing dangerous around that they can put in their mouth.)

Their observations during these months also help them understand that objects exist even when out of sight, a concept called object permanence. At 8 months, when you hide a toy under a scarf, they'll pick up the scarf in search of the toy—a response that wouldn't have occurred three months earlier. Additionally, if you hide the toy under the scarf and then remove it when they're not looking, they'll be puzzled. By 10 months, they'll be so certain the toy still exists they'll continue looking for it. To help your baby learn object permanence, play peekaboo with them. By switching between variations of this game, you'll maintain their interest almost indefinitely.

VARIATIONS OF PEEKABOO

The possible variations of peekaboo are almost endless. As your child becomes more mobile and alert, create games that let them take the lead. Here are some suggestions:

1. Drape a soft cloth over their head and ask, "Where's the baby?" Once they understand the game, they'll pull the cloth away and pop up grinning.
2. With baby on their back facing toward you, lift both their legs together—"Up, up, up"—until they conceal your face from them. Then open them wide: "Peekaboo!" As they get the idea, they'll move their legs themselves. (This is a great game at diaper-changing time.)
3. Hide behind a door or a piece of furniture, leaving a foot or arm in their view as a clue. They'll be delighted to come find you.
4. Take turns with your baby "hiding" your head under a

large towel and letting them pull the towel off, then putting it over their head and pulling it off.

As they approach their first birthday, your child becomes increasingly conscious that things have names and particular functions. You'll see their new awareness weave into their play as a very early form of fantasy. Instead of treating a toy telephone as an object to be chewed, poked, and banged, they'll put it to their ear just as they've seen you do. You can encourage important developmental activities like this by offering suggestive props—a hairbrush, toothbrush, cup, or spoon—and by being enthusiastic about your child's performances.

COGNITIVE MILESTONES FOR YOUR BABY AT 9 MONTHS

- Explores objects in many different ways (shaking, banging, throwing, dropping)
- Looks for objects when dropped out of sight (like a toy or spoon)
- Begins to imitate and use simple gestures (like lifting arms to be picked up, or shaking head no)
- Begins to use objects correctly (drinking from cup, brushing hair, dialing phone and putting it to their ear)

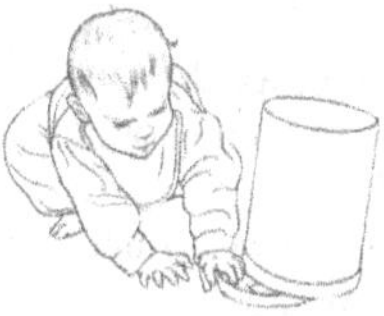

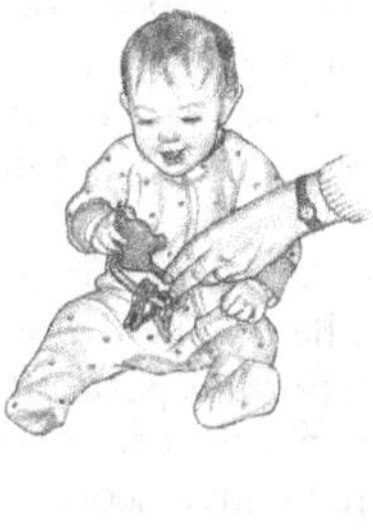

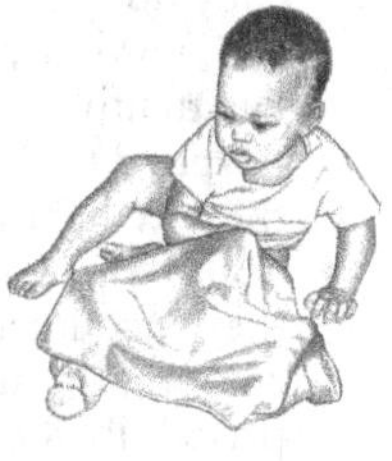

Brain Development

As you've read in this book, your child's early months are crucial to brain development. The environment they're exposed to and their experiences will have a powerful influence on their brain growth.

You have opportunities every day to nurture your child's brain. Just talking with them and encouraging them to say words they're learning will provide intellectual stimulation. You can give them a comfortable and safe environment to explore their world. You can provide them with simple toys to challenge their brain to develop. You can play games with them, sing songs, and continue reading to them every day to encourage their memory to stretch.

Following are day-to-day suggestions for interacting with your baby. They really can make a difference in your child's life, not only immediately but also as a foundation for brain growth for years to come.

STIMULATING INFANT BRAIN GROWTH: AGE 9 MONTHS

- Talk to your baby during dressing, bathing, feeding, playing, walking, and driving, using adult talk rather than baby talk. Check with your pediatrician if your baby does not seem to respond to sound or if syllables and words are not developing.
- Be attentive to your baby's rhythms and moods. Respond to them when they are upset as well as when they are happy.
- Your baby will be very tuned in to you and to others they encounter. Their ability to respond to your emotions is an important part of this developmental period. By 8 to 9 months of age, they can read your face for emotions, which underscores the need for you to temper strong negative expressions.
- Encourage your baby to play with blocks and soft toys. This helps them develop hand-eye coordination, fine motor skills, and a sense of competence.
- Provide a stimulating, safe environment where your baby can begin to explore and roam.

- Give consistent warm, physical contact—hugging, skin-to-skin, body-to-body contact—to establish your child's sense of security and well-being.
- Read to your baby every day.
- If you speak more than one language, use them all at home with your child.
- Try to be sure your baby is not exposed to events that could upset them or overwhelm them, or anything with content intended for older children or adults. This often means keeping the news or other TV shows off when your baby is in the room. You may forget these shows are on in the background, but the baby will notice scary sounds and pictures.
- Play games like peekaboo and pattycake to stimulate your baby's memory skills.
- Introduce your child to other children and adults.
- Provide toys that are age- and developmentally appropriate, safe, and inexpensive. Toys need not be costly—ordinary household objects are fine. It's much more important to give your child attention by talking, reading, and playing with them than to provide more toys.
- Sing songs that incorporate hand and body movements, repetitive words, etc.
- Teach your baby to wave bye-bye and to nod or shake their head for yes and no.
- Make sure other people who provide care and supervision for your baby understand the importance of forming a loving and comforting relationship with your baby.
- Understand that it's normal for your baby to be uncomfortable at times around people who are not their primary caregivers.
- Spend time on the floor playing with your child every day.
- Choose high-quality childcare that is affectionate, responsive, educational, and safe. Visit your childcare provider frequently and share your ideas about positive caregiving.

Social/Emotional Development

At times during these months, your child may seem like two separate babies. There's the one who's open, affectionate, and outgoing with you. Then there's another who's anxious, clingy, and easily frightened around unfamiliar people or objects. Some people may tell you your child is fearful or shy because you're "spoiling" them, but don't believe it. Your baby's diverse behavior patterns aren't caused by you or your parenting; they occur because your baby, for the first time, is able to tell the difference between familiar and unfamiliar situations. If anything, the predictable anxieties of this period are evidence of their healthy relationship with you.

Stranger anxiety is usually one of the first emotional milestones your baby will reach. You may think something is wrong when the same child who at 3 months interacted calmly with strangers is now beginning to tense up when they come too close. This is normal, and you need not worry. Even relatives and frequent babysitters once comfortable to them may prompt hiding or crying now, especially if they approach hastily.

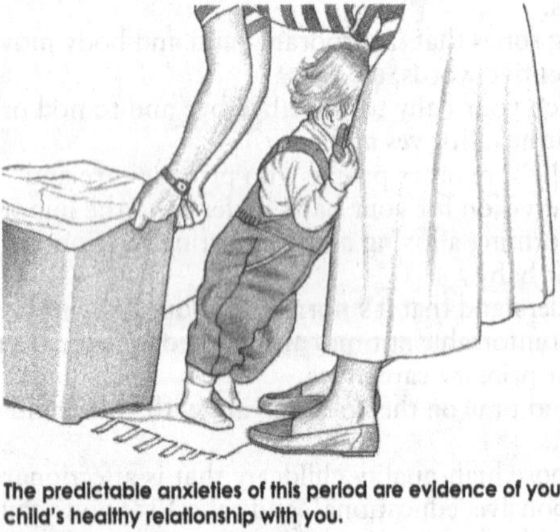

The predictable anxieties of this period are evidence of your child's healthy relationship with you.

SOCIAL/EMOTIONAL MILESTONES FOR YOUR BABY AT 9 MONTHS

- Is shy, clingy, or fearful around strangers
- Shows several facial expressions, like happy, sad, angry, and surprised
- Looks when you call their name
- Reacts when you leave (looks, reaches for you, or cries)
- Smiles or laughs when you play peekaboo

At about the same time, they'll become much more clingy about leaving you. This is the start of separation anxiety. Just as they're learning of each object's uniqueness and permanence, they'll also discover there's only one of you. When you're out of sight, they'll know you're somewhere not with them, and this may cause great distress. They'll have little sense of time and they won't know when—or if—you'll come back. Once they're older, their memories of you will comfort them when you're gone, and they can anticipate a reunion. For now, they're only aware of the present, so every time you leave their sight—even when you just go into the next room—they'll fuss and cry. When you leave them with someone else, they may scream as though their heart will break, although this crying will often resolve quickly once you're gone. At bedtime, they may refuse to leave you, and then wake up searching for you in the middle of the night.

Separation anxiety usually peaks between 10 and 18 months and then fades during the last half of the second year. In some ways this phase will be especially tender for both of you; in other ways it can be stressful. After all, their desire to be with you is a sign of their attachment to you—their first and greatest love. The intensity of their feeling as they hurtle into your arms is irresistible, especially when you realize that no one—including this same child, in the future—will ever again think you as perfect as they do at this age. On the other hand, you may feel suffocated by the constant clinging, but also guilty whenever you leave them crying. Fortunately, this emotional roller coaster will eventually subside, along with their separation anxiety. In the meantime, try to downplay your leave-taking as much as possible. Here are some suggestions:

- Your baby is more susceptible to separation anxiety when they're tired, hungry, or sick. If you know you're going to go out, schedule your departure to occur after they've napped or eaten. And try to stay with them as much as possible when they're sick.
- Don't make a fuss over your leaving. Instead, have the person caring for them create a distraction (a new toy, a visit to the mirror, a bath). Then say goodbye and leave quickly.
- Their tears will subside within minutes of your departure. Their outbursts are for your benefit, to persuade you to stay. With you out of sight, they'll soon turn their attention to the person they are with.
- Help them learn to cope with separation through short sessions at home. Separation will be easier when they initiate it. When they crawl to another room (one that's babyproofed), don't follow them right away; wait a couple of minutes in a place where you can see what they're doing. If they fuss, call to them instead of running to them. Gradually they'll learn that nothing terrible happens when you're gone and, just as important, that you always come back when you say you will.
- If you take your child to a sitter's home or a childcare center, don't just drop them off and leave. Spend a few extra minutes playing with them. When you do leave, reassure them you'll be back later.

ACQUAINTING YOUR BABY WITH A SITTER

Is your baby about to have a new babysitter for a few hours? Whenever possible, let your child interact with this new person while you're there. Ideally, have the sitter spend time with them on successive days before being left alone. If this isn't possible, allow an extra hour or two for this get-acquainted period before you leave. The same rules apply to daycare and anytime there will be a new caregiver.

During their first meeting, the sitter and your baby should get to know each other very gradually, using the following steps:

1. Hold the baby on your lap while you and the sitter talk. Watch for clues that your child is at ease before you have the sitter make eye contact with them. Wait until the baby is looking at them or playing contentedly by themselves.

2. Have the sitter talk to the baby while they stay on your lap. The sitter should not reach toward the child or try to touch them yet.
3. Once the baby seems comfortable with the conversation, put them on the floor with a favorite toy, across from the sitter. Invite the sitter to slowly come closer and play with the toy. As the baby warms up to them, you can move back gradually.
4. See what happens when you leave the room. If your baby doesn't notice you're missing, the introduction has gone well. Don't be discouraged, however, if they cry. That is normal and will improve with time.

You can use this leisurely introduction with anyone who hasn't seen the child recently, including relatives and friends. Adults often overwhelm babies this age by coming close and making funny noises or, worse yet, trying to take them from their mothers. Intervene when this occurs. Explain to these well-meaning people that your baby needs to warm up to strangers and that they're more likely to respond well if they go slowly.

If your child has a strong, healthy attachment to you, their separation anxiety will probably occur earlier than in other babies, and they'll pass through it more quickly. Instead of resenting their possessiveness during these months, maintain as much warmth and good humor as you can. Through your actions, you're showing how to express and return love. This is the emotional base they'll rely on in years to come.

From the beginning, you've considered your baby a unique person with specific traits and preferences. They, however, have had only a dim notion of themselves as a person separate from you. Now their sense of identity is coming into bloom. As they develop a growing sense of individuality, they'll also become increasingly conscious of you as a separate person.

One of the clearest signs of self-awareness is the way your baby watches themselves in the mirror. Up to about 8 months, they treated mirrors as fascinating objects. Perhaps they thought the reflection was another baby, or maybe a magical surface of lights and shadows. Now their responses will change, indicating they understand one of the images is theirs. Looking at a mirror, they may touch their nose or pull on a stray lock of hair. You can reinforce their sense of identity with mirror games. When you're looking in the mirror together, touch different body parts: "There is Olivia's nose. There is Mommy's nose." Move in and out of the mirror, playing peekaboo with the reflections. Make faces and verbally label the emotions conveyed.

As your child's self-concept becomes more secure, they'll have less trouble meeting strangers and separating from you. They'll also become more assertive. Before, you could count on them to be relatively compliant if they were comfortable. But now, more often than not, they'll want things a particular way. Don't be surprised if they reject certain foods or objects placed in front of them. And now that they're more mobile, you'll find yourself frequently saying no about things they shouldn't touch. However, even after they understand the word, they may still touch anyway. Just wait—this is only a forerunner of challenges to come.

TOYS APPROPRIATE FOR YOUR 9-MONTH-OLD

(Note: Look for toys labeled as appropriate/safe for < 1 year of age.)

- Stacking toys in different sizes, shapes, colors
- Cups, pails, and other unbreakable containers
- Unbreakable mirrors of various sizes
- Bath toys that float, squirt, or hold water
- Large building blocks
- "Busy boxes" that push, open, squeak, and move
- Squeeze toys
- Large dolls and puppets
- Cars, trucks, and other vehicle toys made of flexible plastic, with no sharp edges or removable parts
- Large balls
- Board books
- Music boxes, musical toys, and child-safe digital music players
- Push-pull toys
- Toy telephones

Remember that pets are not toys and supervision should be the rule at all times.

Your baby may also become afraid of objects or situations they used to take in stride. Fears of the dark, thunder, and loud household appliances are common. Later you can subdue these fears by talking about them, but for now, the only solution is to eliminate the source as much as possible: Use a nightlight, vacuum when they're not around, and so on. When you can't shield them from something frightening, try to anticipate their reaction and be close so that they can turn to you. Stay calm as you comfort them so that they understand you are not afraid. If you reassure them when they hear thunder or the roar of a jet overhead, their fear will gradually subside until all they have to do is look at you to feel safe.

TRANSITIONAL OBJECTS

You may still remember your favorite childhood blanket, doll, or teddy bear. Security objects such as these are part of the emotional support system every child needs in the early years.

Your child may not choose a blanket, of course, perhaps preferring a soft toy instead. Chances are your child will make their choice between months 8 and 12, and they'll keep it for years to come. When your child is tired, it will help them sleep. When they're separated from you, it will reassure them. When they're upset, it will comfort them. When they're in a strange place, it will help them feel at home.

These special comforts are called transitional objects. They help children make the emotional transition from dependence to independence. They work, in part, because they feel good: They're soft, cuddly, and nice to touch. They're also effective because of familiarity. This "lovey" has your child's scent on it, and it reminds them of the comfort and security of their room. It makes them feel everything is going to be okay.

Despite myths to the contrary, transitional objects are not a sign of weakness or insecurity, and there's no reason to keep your child from using one. In fact, a transitional object can be so helpful you may want to help them choose one and build it into their nighttime ritual.

You can also make things easier by having two identical security objects. Doing this allows you to wash one while the other is being used, thus sparing your baby (and yourself) a potential emotional crisis and a bedraggled lovey. If your baby chooses a large blanket for a security object, you can easily cut it into two. A baby has little sense of size and won't notice. If your child has chosen a toy instead, try to find a duplicate as soon as possible. If you don't start rotating them early, your child may refuse the second one because it feels too new and foreign.

Parents often worry that transitional objects promote thumb sucking, and in fact they sometimes do (but not always). But it's important to remember that thumb (or finger) sucking is a normal, natural way for an infant to comfort themselves. They'll gradually give up both the transitional object and the sucking as they mature and find other ways to cope with stress. Talk to your pediatrician if your child does not stop thumb sucking or finger sucking by 2 to 4 years of age. Thumb sucking longer than age 4 can impact how their adult teeth line up.

Basic Care

Feeding

At this age, your baby needs between 750 and 900 calories each day, of which about 400 to 500 should come from breast milk (or formula if breast milk is not available)—approximately 24 ounces (720 ml) a day. Babies receiving any amount of breast milk should also be supplemented with 400 IU (10 mcg) of vitamin D daily. Also, don't be surprised if their appetite is less robust now. Their rate of growth is slowing, and they have many new and interesting activities to distract them.

Starting around 6 to 9 months (once your baby can sit unsupported), your baby can be introduced to soft finger/table foods. Your baby can eat whatever your family is eating as long as it is soft. Great foods to offer include yogurt, oatmeal, banana, mashed potatoes, and roasted or steamed vegetables. Ground beef, shredded chicken, and eggs are excellent sources of protein, as are cottage cheese, yogurt, and avocado. Allow your baby to explore their foods with all five senses and use their fingers to feed themselves. It'll get messy, but that's okay.

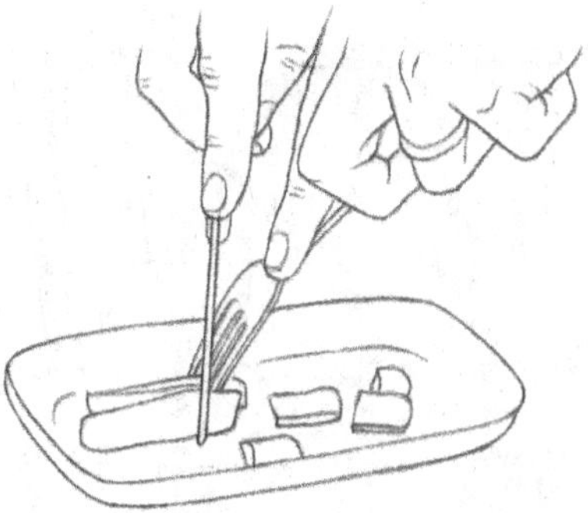

As your baby's hand use improves, give them a spoon and let them play with it at mealtimes. Once they've figured out how to hold it, dip it in their food and let them try to feed themselves. Don't expect much in the beginning. More food is bound to find the floor and high chair than their mouth. A plastic cloth under their chair will help minimize cleanup.

Be patient and resist the temptation to take the spoon away. They need the practice as well as the knowledge that you have confidence in their abilities. For a while you may want to alternate bites from their spoon and one that you hold. Once they can consistently find their mouth with a spoon (which might not be until after their first birthday), you may want to fill their spoon yourself to decrease the mess and waste but leave the actual feeding to them.

In the early weeks of self-feeding, things may go more smoothly when they're really hungry and more interested in eating than playing. Having your baby join the family at the table for mealtimes is a great way for them to observe how everyone else eats and encourages establishing an early habit of family mealtimes. You can also consider having your baby eat most of their meal first and then letting them occupy themselves with healthy finger foods at the table while the others eat.

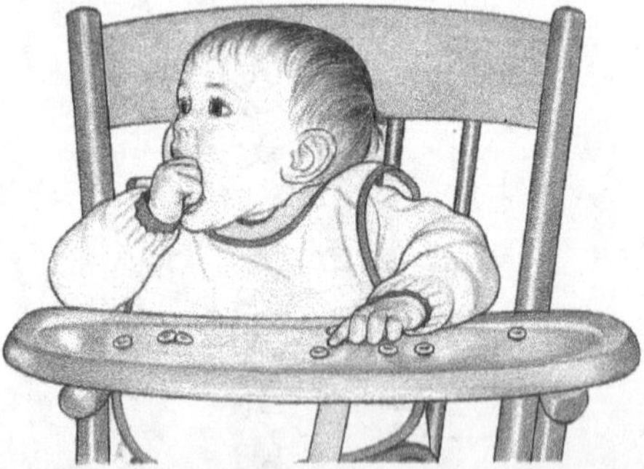

SAMPLE ONE-DAY MENU FOR YOUR 9-MONTH-OLD

(Please note that portion sizes may vary based on when your infant begins eating solids and how much breast milk or formula they are drinking.)

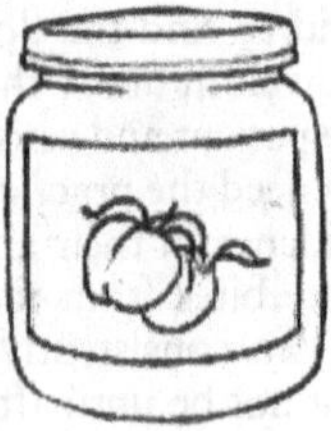

1 cup = 8 ounces = 240 ml
¾ cup = 6 ounces = 180 ml
½ cup = 4 ounces = 120 ml
¼ cup = 2 ounces = 60 ml

Breakfast
1–2 ounces cereal
½–1 ounce mashed or diced fruit
Breast milk or 2–4 ounces formula

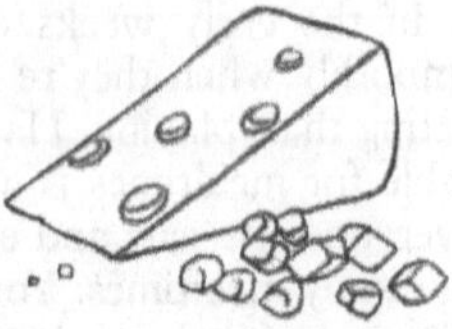

Snack
1–2 ounces cooked pureed or diced vegetables

Lunch
1–2 ounces yogurt or cottage cheese, or pureed or diced beans or meat

½–1 ounce cooked pureed or diced yellow or orange vegetables
Breast milk or 2–4 ounces formula

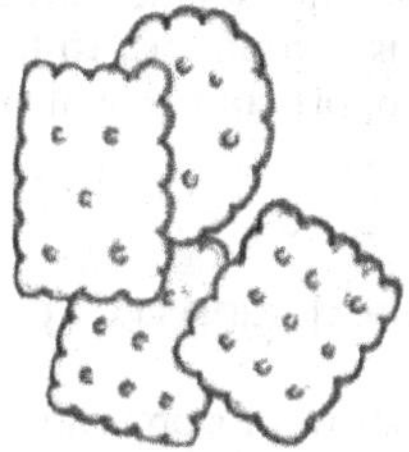

Snack

1 whole-grain cracker or teething biscuit
½–1 ounce fork-mashed or diced soft fruit

Dinner

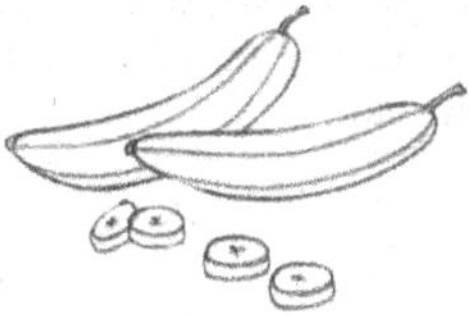

1–2 ounces diced poultry, meat, or tofu
½–1 ounce cooked green vegetables
1–2 ounces cooked soft whole-grain pasta, rice, or potato
½–1 ounce diced or mashed fruit
Breast milk or 2–4 ounces formula

Before Bedtime

Breast milk or 6 to 8 ounces formula, or water (if breast milk or formula, follow with water and brush teeth afterward)

Finger foods can include small pieces of steamed veggies, soft fruit such as bananas, well-cooked whole-grain pasta, small pieces of whole-wheat bread, chicken, scrambled eggs, or whole-grain cereals. Try offering a selection of flavors, shapes, colors, and textures, but always watch your baby for choking. (See Choking, *pages 494, 703*.) Also, because they're likely to swallow without chewing, never offer a baby chunks of peanut butter, large pieces of raw vegetables, whole nuts, whole grapes, popcorn, uncooked peas, celery, gum, hard candies, or other hard or round foods that could pose a risk for choking. Always observe your child eating. Choking can happen with hot dogs, grapes, chunks of cheese, or meat sticks (baby-food "hot dogs"), so these always should be cut lengthwise and then into smaller pieces before being fed to a child of this age. It is a good idea to have all family members take a basic life support course, which can be lifesaving during a choking episode.

Introducing a Cup

A straw or sippy cup can be introduced anytime after 6 months. Breastfed babies may transition to a cup more easily than to a bottle. To get started, use a trainer cup with two handles and a snap-on lid with a soft spout, an open cup, or a straw cup. Sippy and straw cups will minimize spillage as your child experiments with different ways to hold (and most likely throw) the cup.

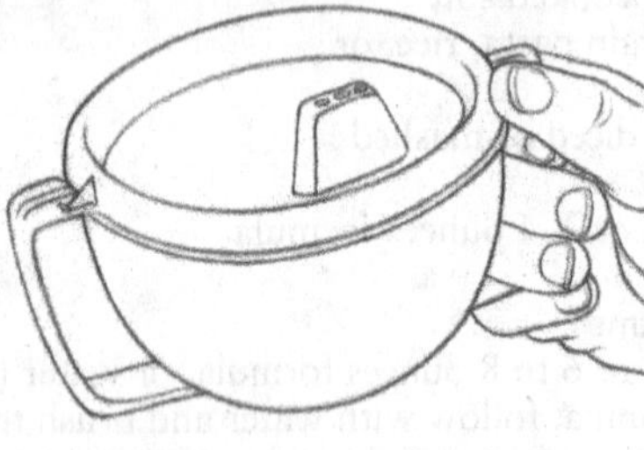

To start, fill the cup with a little water and offer it at one meal a day. Show your baby how to maneuver and tip it to their mouth so that they can drink. Don't become dismayed, however, if they treat it as a plaything for several weeks; most babies do. Just be patient until they're able to get most of the liquid down their throat or out of the straw without it dribbling down their chin or the cup flying around the room. Once they get the hang of the cup, put breast milk or formula in the cup to get them used to drinking milk from something other than a bottle.

There are advantages to drinking from a cup: namely, improved hand-to-mouth coordination, and preparation for the bottle-weaning process. Even under the best circumstances, the transition to using a cup may not take place overnight. Six months may pass before your baby takes all their liquid from a cup. Even so, you can start the process and proceed gradually, letting their interest and willingness guide you. You'll probably find it easiest to start with the midday feeding first. Once they have adjusted to this, try doing the same in the morning. The bedtime feeding probably will be the last, and for good reason: Your baby has become accustomed to this nighttime comfort, and it will take them time to give it up. If they're sleeping through the night and not waking up hungry, they don't physically need the extra nourishment from bedtime breast- or bottle-feeding. In this case, you might break the habit in stages, first by substituting water instead of milk for the bedtime bottle/feeding and then switching to a drink of water from a cup. Alternatively, just move the bedtime bottle/feeding earlier so that it's not associated with bedtime but instead is an evening snack.

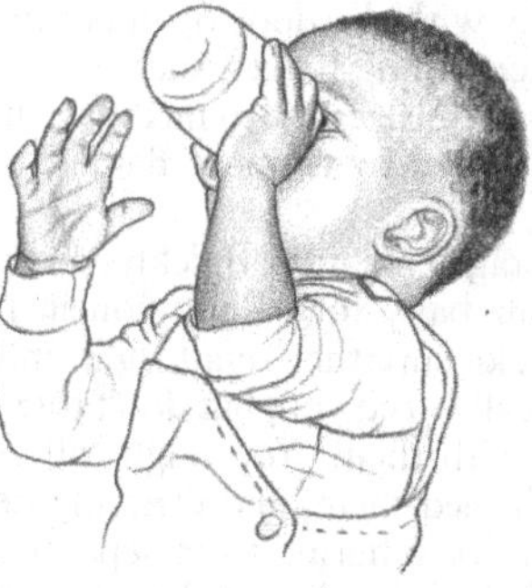

During this process, you may be tempted to put milk in their bottle to help them fall asleep, but it's not a good idea for several reasons. If they fall asleep while feeding, the milk will pool around their incoming teeth, and cause them to decay—a condition known as early childhood caries (formerly called baby bottle tooth decay). To make matters worse, drinking while lying flat on their back can contribute to their risk for middle ear infections.

Another disadvantage to prolonged bottle-feeding is that the bottle can become a security object, particularly if your baby keeps it beyond about age 1. To avoid this, don't let them carry or drink from a bottle while playing. Restrict the use to feedings when they're sitting down or being held. At all other times, give them a cup. If you never allow the bottle to go with them, they won't realize bringing it is even an option. Don't give in once this decision is made; be consistent or they may get confused and demand a bottle long after they have "officially" been weaned.

Sleeping

At 9 months, your baby probably still takes two naps, midmorning and midafternoon. They're also likely to sleep as much as ten to twelve hours at night without needing night feeding. However, as their separation anxiety intensifies in the next few months, they may start to resist going to bed, and they may wake up more often looking for you.

During this difficult period, you may need to experiment to find strategies that help your baby sleep. Some children go to sleep more easily with the door open (so they can hear you); others develop consoling habits, such as sucking their thumb or rocking. White noise can also be especially helpful, as long as the volume is quiet so as not to damage your baby's sensitive hearing.

To help this stage pass more quickly, don't do anything that will reward your baby for calling you in the middle of the night. Go to make sure they're all right and tell them you're nearby if they really need you, but don't turn on the light, rock them, or walk with them. You might offer them a drink of water, but don't feed them, and certainly don't take them to your bed. If they're suffering from separation anxiety, doing that will only make it harder for them to return to their crib.

When you do check on them, make them as comfortable as possible and confirm they aren't sick. Some problems, such as ear infections or croup, can come on suddenly at night. Once you're sure there's no sign of illness, check their diaper, changing it only if they've had a bowel movement or if their diaper is uncomfortably wet. Do the change as quickly as possible in dim light and then settle them back in their crib and on their back. Before leaving, whisper a few comforting words about how it's nighttime and time to sleep. If they still cry, wait a few minutes, then go back in and comfort them for a short time. This period can be extremely difficult for parents. After all, it's emotionally and physically exhausting to hear your child cry, and you'll probably respond with a combination of emotions. But remember, their behavior is not deliberate. Instead, they're reacting to natural anxieties and stresses. If you stay calm and follow a consistent pattern each night, they'll soon be putting themselves to sleep. Many parents will purchase a wireless baby monitor to watch and hear their baby from their own room. There are many different products available, so research them all before purchasing one. Doing so may make life much easier for both of you. (See *Chapter 30*, Your Child's Sleep, for more information.)

Teeth

By this age, your baby probably has at least one or two teeth, if not more. Don't worry if they don't; it's normal for babies as old as 12 months to still have no teeth. As soon as they do, however, it's time to start brushing with a soft toothbrush and a tiny bit of fluoride toothpaste, roughly the size of a grain of rice. They may or may not enjoy this experience. If they resist brushing, have them lie face-up on your or another person's lap while you make a game of gently cleaning each tooth. Brush their teeth at least once a day, front and back, ideally close to bedtime, since once you're done they should not eat or drink anything other than water. Sugar at night will undo all your hard work! You can also make their first dental appointment. Your child's first dentist visit should occur six months after the first tooth emerges or at 1 year of age, whichever comes first. The dentist may apply fluoride varnish to protect their new teeth. Your child's pediatrician may check the teeth and apply fluoride at well-child exams, but this does not substitute for a dental appointment.

Behavior

Discipline

Your baby's desire to explore is almost impossible to satisfy. As a result, they'll want to touch, taste, and manipulate everything they can get into. They're bound to find their way into places and situations that are off-limits or dangerous. Although their curiosity is vital to their overall development and shouldn't be discouraged unnecessarily, they can't be allowed to jeopardize their own safety or damage valuable objects. Whether they're investigating the burners on your stove or pulling up your flowers, you need to help them stop these activities.

Keep in mind that the way you handle these early incidents will lay the foundation for future discipline. Learning not to do something they very much want to do is a major first step toward self-control. The better they learn this lesson now, the less you'll have to intervene in years to come.

As we suggested earlier, distraction can usually deal effectively with undesirable behavior. Your baby's memory is still short, and you can shift their focus with minimal resistance. If they're headed for something they shouldn't do, you don't necessarily have to say no. Overusing "no" will blunt its effect. Instead, pick them up and direct them toward something they can play with. Look for a compromise that will keep them interested and active without squelching their curiosity. Never scream or yell at, shake, or hit your baby.

You should reserve your serious discipline for situations where your child's activities can expose them to real danger, like playing with electric cords. This is the time to say no firmly and remove them from the situation. Don't expect them to learn from one or two incidents. Because of their short memory, you'll have to repeat the scene over and over before they recognize and respond to your directions. Never depend on them to keep themselves away from danger, no matter how often you've corrected them. Find a spot where they can play safely—a zone where everything is safe and you don't have to say no.

To improve your discipline's effectiveness, consistency is critical. Make sure everyone taking care of your baby understands what the child is and isn't allowed to do. Keep rules to a minimum, preferably limited to potentially dangerous situations. Then make sure your baby hears "no" every time they stray into forbidden territory.

Immediacy is also important for good discipline. React as soon as you see your baby heading into trouble, not five minutes later. If you delay, they won't understand the reason you're reprimanding and the lesson will be lost. Likewise, don't be too quick to comfort after scolding. Yes, they may cry, sometimes as much in surprise as distress; but wait a minute or two before reassuring them. Otherwise, they won't know whether they really did something wrong.

It's important to not spank or strike your child in any way when disciplining. No matter the age or behavior, physical punishment is always an inappropriate response. Spanking only teaches a child to act aggressively when upset. Yes, it may relieve your own frustration temporarily, and for the moment you actually might believe it did some good. It may stop a particular behavior in the short term, but it is not an effective way of disciplining your child in the long term, and it certainly doesn't teach alternative ways to act. It may lead to physical injury, it undermines effective communication between you and your baby, and it weakens their own sense of security.

What's the alternative? The American Academy of Pediatrics recommends using time-outs and time-ins when your child is older, instead of spankings—putting a misbehaving child in a quiet place for a few minutes, away from other people, TV, electronics, or books. Parents of children with special healthcare needs may find it helpful to consult with a specialist to better understand their child's unique physical, emotional, and cognitive abilities. In some cases, consultation with a developmental-behavioral pediatrician may be helpful.

As you refine your own disciplinary skills, don't overlook the importance of responding positively to your baby's good behavior. This reaction is more important for their learning self-control. If they hesitate before reaching for the stove, notice their restraint and tell them how pleased you are. Give them a hug when they do something nice for others. As they grow, their good behavior will depend, in large part, on their desire to please you. If you make them aware now how much you appreciate the good things they do, they'll be less likely to misbehave to get your attention.

Some parents worry about spoiling a child this age by giving them too much attention, but you needn't be concerned. At 9 months, your baby still has a limited ability to be manipulative. You should assume that when they cry, it's not for effect but because they have real needs not being met.

These needs gradually become more complex, and as they do, you'll notice more variation in their cries—and in how you react to them. You'll come running to the shattering wail of something seriously wrong. By contrast, you may finish what you're doing before you answer the shrill "Come here, I want you" cry. You'll probably also recognize a whiny, muffled cry meaning roughly "I could fall asleep now if everyone would leave me alone." By responding appropriately to the hidden message behind your baby's cries, you'll let them know that their needs are important but that response comes only to deserving calls.

Incidentally, there probably will be times when you won't be able to figure out why your baby is crying. In these cases, they may not know themselves. The best response is comfort from you, combined with making sure they are safe and allowing whatever consoling techniques they choose. Try holding them while they cuddle their favorite stuffed animal or special blanket, or play a game or read a story with them. Both of you will feel better when they're cheered up. Remember, their need for attention and affection is just as real as their need for food and clean diapers.

Siblings

As your baby becomes more mobile, they'll be better able to play with siblings, and those brothers and sisters will usually be glad to cooperate. Older children, particularly 6- to 10-year-olds, often love to build towers for their baby sibling to destroy. Or they'll lend a finger to a baby learning to walk.

However, while mobility can turn your baby into a more active playmate for their brothers and sisters, it also will make them more likely to invade their siblings' private territory. This may violate an older child's budding sense of ownership and privacy, and it can present serious safety hazards for the baby, since older children's toys often contain small, easily swallowed pieces. You can ensure everyone is protected by giving older siblings a place where they can keep and play with their belongings without fear of a "baby invasion."

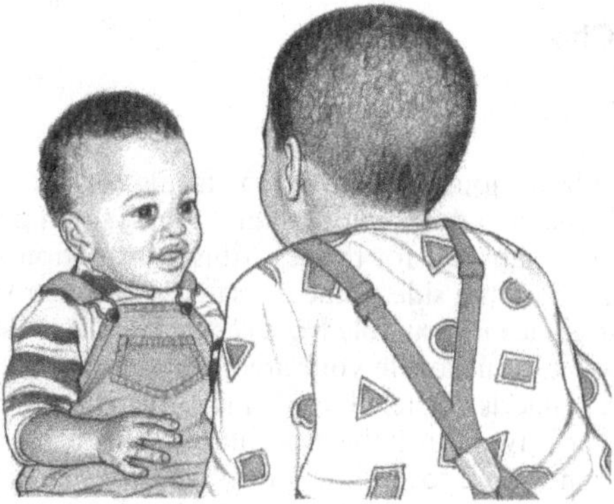

A baby this age can be a wonderful playmate to their siblings.

Also, now that the baby can reach and grab almost everything in sight, sharing is another issue. Children under 3 aren't capable of sharing without adult prodding and, in most cases, direct intervention. An adult should always be watching when children are playing together. As much as possible, try to sidestep the issue and encourage tandem play, each child with their own toys. When they do play together, suggest looking at books or listening to music, rolling a ball back and forth, playing hide-and-seek games, or other activities requiring limited cooperation. Remember that older siblings can become jealous, and they need attention, too.

▪ YOUR BABY AT 9 MONTHS OLD CHECKLIST ▪

Immunization Update

The third hepatitis B vaccine will be given between 6 and 18 months of age. In addition, a flu vaccine will be given if it is flu season. A COVID-19 vaccine may be recommended as needed; check with your pediatrician and the Centers for Disease Control and Prevention.

Safety Check

Car Safety Seats

- Children should remain in rear-facing car seats as long as possible, usually more than 2 years, so long as they are the right size for the seat (this information should be printed on the side of the car safety seat). Car safety seat advice is available from certified child passenger safety technicians in your area; you can find one at cert.safekids.org (click on "Find a Tech").
- Never leave your baby alone in the car when you're not in it, not even for a short time. Some cars have alarms that remind parents of this. You can also leave an item like a teddy bear in the front seat to remind you of the baby in the back, or you can put something you need (like your wallet, purse, or work ID) in the backseat to prompt you to check that it is empty.
- Buckle the baby into an approved, properly installed car safety seat before you start the car. It's important that properly installed seats are in all cars your baby will ride in, including those belonging to childcare providers, sitters, and grandparents. (There are other elements of car safety seats you need to be aware of, so for further information, see Car Safety Seats, *page 321*.)

Falls

- Use gates at the top and bottom of stairways, and in doorways to rooms not babyproofed.
- Do not allow an infant to climb on a kitchen chair, as the chair may tip over, resulting in head injury and possible leg or arm fractures.
- Do not use a baby walker. A stationary activity center is a much safer choice.

Furniture

- Ensure that any furniture or electronics your baby can reach are secured to the wall to prevent tipping. The manufacturer should provide a strap and an anchor to make this possible, or you can pick up a kit at the hardware store or order one online.

Burns

- Never smoke or carry hot liquids or foods near your baby or while holding your baby. When you must handle hot liquids or foods, put your baby in a safe place such as a crib, play yard, or high chair.
- Never leave containers of hot liquids or foods near the edges of tables or counters or on low surfaces, such as coffee tables.
- Do not allow your baby to crawl around hot stoves, floor heaters, or furnace vents.

Drowning

- Never leave your baby alone in a bath or around containers of water, including buckets, wading pools, swimming pools, sinks, or open toilets. Even a small amount of water can be a danger to a small child. Remove all water from containers immediately after use. If you have a swimming pool, install a four-sided fence at least 4 feet (1.2 m) high that completely separates the house from the pool.

Poisoning and Choking

- Never leave small objects on or near the floor where your crawling baby could find them. You should look at the floor from their level and crawl around to visualize what they see. Sometimes medications or other small items are dropped unknowingly.
- Have the Poison Help number nearby in case of an emergency (1-800-222-1222).
- Assess your windows and doors for peeling paint so that your child doesn't eat the paint chips and possibly get lead poisoning.

- Do not give your baby hard pieces of food, or any soft foods that could become lodged in their airway, such as chunks of hot dogs or uncut grapes.
- Store all medicines and household cleaning products high and out of the baby's reach. A lockbox can be used to securely store any substances that could be dangerous for your baby.
- Use safety latches on drawers and cabinets that contain potentially dangerous objects. It is best to store these items in high, out-of-reach, locked cabinets if possible.
- Make sure that your baby can't become entangled in electrical cords or window shade cords.
- Make sure that all places your child visits, such as their grandparents' house, follow these same guidelines.

CHAPTER 10

CHILDCARE

Who will care for your baby during the hours when you are away? Sooner or later you're bound to face this question. Whether you need someone to care for your child a few hours a week or nine hours a day, you'll want to feel confident about the person. But finding the right caregiver or team of caregivers for your baby can be a big challenge. When selecting childcare, your top priority should be the well-being of your child, overriding all other considerations. This chapter provides suggestions to make your search easier, and also contains guidelines for preventing, recognizing, and resolving problems once your choice is made.

To find good childcare, it is important to judge both the quality of the childcare program and the character and abilities of the caregivers involved with your child. Approximately six out of every ten families with children between 3 and 6 years of age use out-of-the-home center-based daycare. Parents may also choose to share care between themselves or have relatives or non-relatives provide care. Some children participate in different types of childcare at different times of the day or on different days of the week. If your child's caregiver is not a family member, chances are you will meet this person only a few times before entrusting your child to them. Even so, you will want to feel as confident about your choice as if they were a family member. While it is impossible to be absolutely sure under these circumstances, you can tell a great deal by observing caregivers at work for a day or two and by carefully checking references. Entrust your baby to someone only after you have watched them with your child and other children and you feel confident in their abilities and dedication.

What to Look for in a Care Provider

(For infants, see Your Baby's First Sitter, *page 154*.)

Children thrive when cared for in a safe, healthy environment by warm, affectionate, and supportive adults who help them learn, interact, and work out solutions while protecting them from making harmful choices. The following list describes several things to look for when observing someone who might take care of your child. More specific suggestions appear throughout this chapter, but remember they are general guidelines. They apply to all out-of-home and in-home care, including babysitters, nannies, and teachers during preschool and the early primary school years. Also, keep all this in mind as you play with your child or supervise groups of children.

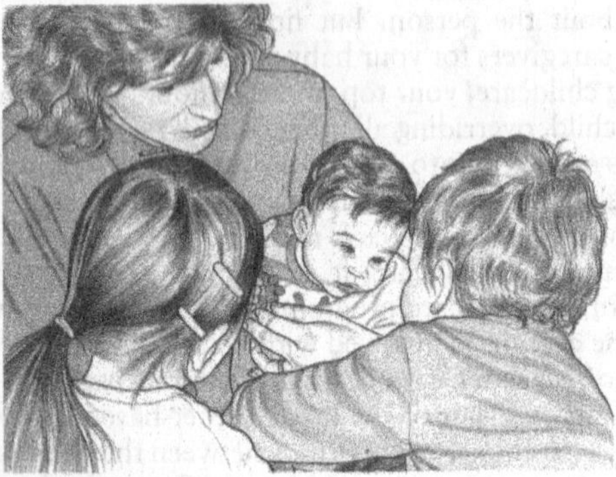

A good caregiver will:

- Listen carefully to children and observe their behavior
- Set reasonable limits for children and maintain them consistently
- Promote children's intellectual and physical growth and development through exposure to reading, singing, hands-on activities, and physical activity
- Tell children why certain things are not allowed and offer acceptable alternatives
- Deal with difficult situations as they arise, before they get out of control
- Anticipate trouble and intervene early to prevent it
- Live up to promises made to the children
- Join children at play without disrupting their activity
- Ease stressful transitions for children
- Encourage children to think of their own ideas before offering suggestions

- Reward children's efforts and relieve their "hurts" with an affectionate physical gesture, such as a hug or a pat
- Talk naturally and conversationally with the children about what they are doing
- Help children encourage each other by asking them to share their accomplishments
- Encourage children to complete projects, even if they take longer than originally planned
- Limit adult conversations in the children's presence
- Show respect for the children's ideas and decisions
- Avoid offering children choices when there are none
- Allow children to make mistakes and learn from them (as long as there is no danger involved in doing so)

Choices in Care

In addition to these general suggestions, you will want to identify your specific needs and desires. Before you meet and interview potential caregivers, questions you need answered should include:

- Where do I want my child to be during the day? At home? In someone else's home? In a childcare center? If out-of-home care, how far away? What other family members or friends will my child be near?
- What days and hours do I need or want childcare each week?
- How will I transport my child to and from the program? If the caregiver needs transportation during the day or evening, how will it be handled?
- What backup arrangements can I make? How will I handle days when my child is sick or when my child's caregiver is unavailable because of illness or personal business? What are the arrangements for holidays, summertime, and vacations?
- How much can I realistically afford?
- What size program do I want for my child? How much group interaction do I want for my child?
- How much structure and stimulation do I want for my child?
- What qualifications do I want the caregiver(s) to have?

- What type of discipline do I want used for my child?
- What other basic conditions would make me feel comfortable about leaving my child with someone else?

While a majority of young children in the United States are in some form of childcare, over a quarter of this care is provided by relatives, mostly grandparents. Not only are many grandparents caring for children for part of the day, but more and more are involved in taking children to and from other childcare arrangements.

If you have family members or friends whom you would like to care for your child and who live nearby, ask yourself if you are comfortable with their care and whether they would be willing to provide it (perhaps for a few hours a day or two to three days a week), either on a regular basis or as a backup if other arrangements fail. When possible, consider offering payment for these services to make the arrangement fairer and to create an additional incentive for the person to help you.

Other options include bringing someone into your home or taking your child to another person's home or a childcare center. Your financial resources, the age and needs of your child, and your own preferences about child-rearing will help you decide.

Remember that your child will grow and develop quickly, and that the correct choice today may not be the best choice tomorrow. Keep reevaluating your child's needs and the fit of your current childcare arrangement over time.

Here are suggestions to keep in mind when deciding among in-home care, family childcare, or a childcare center.

In-Home Care/Nanny

If you are returning to work while your child is an infant, one choice for childcare (often a more expensive one) is to have someone come into your home on a live-in or live-out basis. A person you hire to work in your home is not required to be licensed, so there are important considerations that should be part of your evaluation and the hiring process:

- Check references.
- Perform a background check, if possible.
- Ask for documented work experience (preferably for the previous five years).

- Ask about the person's approach to discipline, scheduling, feeding, comforting, and providing appropriate activities. Determine if that approach matches your style of child-rearing and is right for your child. Make sure the person you select shares your philosophy about how to react to excessive crying, how to respond when your child has an accident, or what to do when they don't want to take a nap or go to bed. (Sharing this kind of information is applicable no matter the type of care setting.)
- How will the caregiver report back about the child's day?

How Do I Find an In-Home Caregiver?

- Ask friends, work colleagues, and neighbors for recommendations.
- Scan or place ads online or in the paper (especially local publications for parents).
- Go through a service.
- Contact a childcare resource and referral agency in your community or an au pair service.

After Choosing an In-Home Caregiver

- Arrange a trial period of at least a week when you can be home to watch the caregiver work under your supervision.
- In the days and weeks ahead, carefully monitor the caregiver's performance.

Advantages of In-Home Care

1. Your child will stay in familiar surroundings and receive individualized care and attention.
2. They will not be exposed to the illnesses and negative behaviors of other children.
3. When your child is sick, you likely won't have to stay home from work or make additional arrangements to care for them.

4. Some caregivers do light housework and prepare family meals. If you want your caregiver to do household work in addition to childcare, make it clear from the start.

Disadvantages of In-Home Care

1. You may have difficulty finding someone willing to accept the wages, benefits, and confinement of working in your home; or you may find the costs of qualified in-home care prohibitive.
2. Since you will be considered an employer, you must meet minimum-wage, Social Security, and tax-reporting requirements.
3. The presence of a caregiver may infringe on your family's privacy, especially if they live in your home.
4. Because your caregiver will be alone with your child most of the time, you have no way of knowing exactly how they will perform their job.
5. Your caregiver may not always have backup help available for when they are sick, have a family crisis, or want time off. You will be responsible for securing a replacement.
6. Your caregiver will likely have less initial or ongoing training in child development and health and safety issues such as CPR, first aid, and medication administration. CPR and first aid are skills they have to learn. Consider signing them up for a class in these lifesaving skills, and offer to pay for it.
7. You may need to provide a car and car seat for your caregiver if you expect your child to be taken on outings.

Family Childcare

Many people provide informal care in their homes for small groups of children, often looking after their own children or grandchildren at the same time. Some even offer evening care or sick care. Family childcare is generally less expensive and more flexible than care offered by childcare centers. A small family childcare home typically has fewer than six children and one caregiver. Large family childcare homes may have up to twelve children and one caregiver and an assistant, though the exact numbers are dependent on the ages of the children and state and local regulations. (See the suggested child-to-staff ratios in the Appendix, *page 705*).

Family childcare may be licensed, registered, or unregulated. It is always best to seek out a licensed setting. (Licensing regulations vary from state to state and can be found at places like the website Child Care Technical Assistance Network, childcareta.acf.hhs.gov.)

In Choosing a Family Childcare Home

- Observe the caregiver's work.
- Look for signs of good-quality care, such as hygienic diaper changing and safety measures.
- Ask for references.
- Check certification and licensing compliance.
- Look over the home to ensure its safety.
- Find out how many children the provider has enrolled and during what hours. It also helps to know the ages of the other children and whether they have any special healthcare needs or behavioral challenges.
- Inquire about substitute arrangements when the caregiver is sick or cannot provide care.
- Request information on the caregiver's emergency situation plans.
- Ask the provider what training they have.
- Ask if the provider's program is accredited by the National Association for Family Child Care.
- Ask how the caregiver will report back about your child's day.
- Ask for the provider's approach to discipline, scheduling, feeding, comforting, and providing appropriate activities. Determine if that approach matches your style of child-rearing and is right for your child. Make sure the family care home you select shares your philosophy about how to react to excessive crying and squabbles between children, how to respond when your child has a bathroom accident or an injury, and what to do when they don't want to take a nap or go to bed.

How Do I Find a Family Childcare Provider?

- Ask friends for recommendations.
- Scan or place ads online and in local parenting-oriented publications.
- Contact a local resource and referral agency: Child Care Aware at 1-800-424-2246 or childcareaware.org. Or the National Association for Family Child Care, nafcc.org.

After Choosing a Family Childcare Provider

- Monitor your child's adjustment and carefully observe interactions between the caregiver and your child, and between your child and the other children.
- Keep the lines of communication open and address issues that arise.

Advantages of Family Childcare

1. In good family childcare settings, there is a favorable child-to-adult ratio. In general, the total number of children to adults should be no more than about three children for one adult, especially if some children are under 24 months. (See the Appendix, *page 705*, for additional information on optimal child-to-staff ratios.)
2. Your child will have the comforts of being in a home and can be involved in many of the same household activities they'd find at home.
3. When other children are present, your child will have social stimulation coming from having playmates.
4. Family childcare has the potential to be relatively flexible. Special arrangements can often be made to meet your child's individual interests and needs.
5. Your child may have more individualized attention and quiet time.
6. Your child may be exposed to fewer infectious diseases or less negative behavior from other children.

Disadvantages of Family Childcare

1. You cannot observe what happens to your child in your absence. While many providers carefully organize activities appropriate for children, there are instances where they may use the TV as a babysitter and even let children watch shows inappropriate for them.
2. Many family childcare providers work without supervision or advice from other adults.
3. The caregiver might share the care of your child with relatives, partners, or other people who might not give high-quality care.
4. Family childcare centers may have fewer protocols or trained staff for assisting with children and youth who have special healthcare needs. On the other hand, they may be able to provide more personalized care. During your selection process, if your child has special healthcare needs or if other children in the center have special healthcare needs, be sure to understand whether there are enough caregivers to address each child's needs.

Childcare Centers

Childcare centers may also be called daycare, child development centers, nursery schools, preschools, or other similar names. These facilities typically provide care for children in a non-residential building with classrooms for children of different age groups. Most centers are licensed, caring for children from birth to 6 years. Of the approximately 4 million children in childcare in the United States, about 2.7 million are in licensed facilities, meaning that about 25 percent are cared for in unlicensed and unregulated settings. Centers demonstrate a higher commitment to quality by participating in the accreditation process.

There are several types of childcare centers, most notably the following:

- Chain centers offer a wide variety of programs and appealing activities for children. Because they are chains and run under central management, some do not offer variation and room for individual creativity in their operations.

- Independent for-profit centers depend on enrollment fees to pay their overhead, typically earning a narrow profit for their owners. Because many of these programs are built around one or two dedicated people, they can be excellent—as long as those individuals remain actively involved in the daily operations.
- Non-profit centers are sometimes linked to religious institutions, community centers, universities, social service agencies, or independently incorporated facilities. Some have access to additional public funding, permitting discounted fees for lower-income families. Any income earned above expenses goes back into the program, directly benefiting the children.
- Head Start is a national child development program for children from birth to age 5, providing services to promote academic, social, and emotional development, as well as social, health, and nutrition services for income-eligible families.
- Centers for children and youth with special healthcare needs may be for-profit or non-profit chains or may have some public support. These centers are specially designed and staffed to meet the needs of children with developmental disabilities, chronic illnesses, or behavioral concerns.

How Do I Find a Childcare Center?

- The internet often lists childcare centers.
- Ask your pediatrician or other parents with children in childcare to recommend a center.
- Contact your community's health or welfare agency, or a local or national resource and referral organization, such as Child Care Aware at childcareaware.org or 1-800-424-2246.

Advantages of Childcare Centers

1. More information is generally available about them, since the majority of centers are regulated by licensing agencies.

2. Many centers have structured programs designed to meet children's developmental needs, functional abilities, and medical care needs.
3. Most centers have several caregivers, so you are not dependent on the availability of just one person.
4. Workers in these centers have higher educational requirements and tend to be better supervised than caregivers in other settings.
5. Some centers may allow you to arrange shorter hours or fewer days if you work part-time.
6. Many centers encourage parental involvement, so you can help make the center better. Co-op daycare centers rely on parents' involvement, and the daycare contract lists the days a parent must volunteer.

Disadvantages of Childcare Centers

1. Regulations for childcare centers vary widely based on the type of center.
2. Good programs in high demand may have waiting lists for admission.
3. Due to the number of children cared for in this type of program, your child may receive less personalized attention than in a smaller program.
4. Many childcare centers suffer from low pay and high staff turnover. Keeping staff skilled in the care of children with special healthcare needs can be challenging in these settings.

Selecting a Childcare Center

When considering childcare centers, you need to know the rules and practices that would affect your child. If the program is formal enough to have a printed or electronic handbook, this may answer many of your questions. Otherwise, ask the program director the following questions (some of which apply to in-home or family childcare as well):

1. What are the hiring requirements for staff members? (Regulations vary from state to state.) In many good programs, caregivers must have at least two years of college, pass minimum health requirements, and receive basic immunizations. Ideally, they will have some background in early child development and perhaps have children themselves. Directors generally have a college degree or many years of experience, qualifying them as experts in both child development and administration. Staff members should also have training in CPR and first aid.
2. What is the ratio of children to staff? Although some children need highly personalized attention and others do well with less, the general rule to follow is: The younger the child, the more adults are needed per group. Each child should have one primary caregiver responsible for that child's care, providing most of the child's feeding and diapering, and putting the child to sleep.
3. How many children are in each group? Generally, smaller groups offer children a better chance to interact with and learn from one another. While fewer children per adult is usually better, there is a desirable maximum ratio and group size for each age category. The designated ratios vary from state to state, and some good facilities do not reach the ideal child-to-staff ratios (see the Appendix, *page 705*).
4. Are there frequent staff changes? If so, this may suggest there are problems with the facility's operations. Ideally, most caregivers should have been with the program for several years, since consistency is desirable. Unfortunately, staff turnover in this profession is an issue for a variety of reasons, including low wages.
5. Are caregivers prohibited from smoking, even outside? This is important for your child's health.
6. Are caregivers required to have updated immunizations, including whooping cough (pertussis) and influenza vaccines?
7. What are the goals of the program? Some are organized and try to teach children new skills or attempt to change or mold their behavior and beliefs. Others are

relaxed, with an emphasis on helping children develop at their own pace. Still others fall somewhere in between. Decide what you want for your child, and make sure the program you choose meets your desires. Avoid programs offering no personalized attention or support for your child.

8. What are the admission procedures? Quality childcare programs require relevant background information on each child. Be prepared for specific questions about your child's individual needs, developmental level, and health status. You may also be asked about your child-rearing desires and about your other children.
9. Does the childcare provider have a valid license and recent health certificate, and does the provider enforce health and immunization requirements in the program? Standard immunizations and regular checkups should be required for all children and staff members.
10. How are illnesses handled? Parents should be notified if a staff member or child contracts a significant communicable disease (not just a cold, but illnesses such as chickenpox or hepatitis). The program should also have a clear policy regarding sick children. You should know when to keep your child home and how the center will respond if your child becomes ill during the day.
11. What are the costs? How much is it to start, and when are the payments due? What do the payments cover specifically? Do parents need to pay even when their child is absent for illness or vacations with the family?
12. What happens on a typical day? Ideally, there should be a mix of physical activity and quiet times. Some activities should be group-oriented, others individualized. Times for meals and snacks should be set. While a certain amount of structure is desirable, there also should be room for free play and special events.
13. How much parental involvement is expected? Some programs rely on parent participation, while others request very little. At the least, quality programs should welcome your opinions and allow you to visit during

the day. If the program maintains a closed-door policy for part or all of the day—typically for educational reasons—be sure you are comfortable with this practice.

14. What are the general procedures? A well-organized program should have clearly defined rules and regulations regarding:
    - Hours of operation
    - Transportation of children
    - Field trips
    - Meals and snacks, whether they are provided by parents or are prepared on-site
    - Administration of medication and first aid
    - Emergency evacuations
    - Notification of child's absence
    - Weather cancellations
    - Withdrawal of children from the program
    - Supplies or equipment parents must provide
    - Sleep arrangements, especially for infants
    - Special celebrations
    - How parents are to contact staff during the day or night
    - Exclusion of children while they are sick with certain illnesses
    - Security to ensure that everyone who enters the facility, including outdoor play areas, is screened by childcare personnel (strangers should not be able to enter any childcare area, indoors or out, nor should familiar adults who act oddly be allowed to stay)
    - How discipline or behavior challenges are addressed

Ask for their approach to discipline, scheduling, feeding, comforting, screen time, physical activity, outdoor time, and providing appropriate activities. Determine if their approach matches your style of child-rearing and is right for your child. Make sure the center you select shares your philosophy about how to react to excessive crying, how to respond when your child has an accident or an injury, and what to do when they don't want to take a nap or go to bed.

Once you've received this basic information, take a tour of the building and grounds during operating hours to see how the caregivers interact with the children. First impressions are especially important, since they'll influence all your future dealings with the program. If you sense warmth and a loving approach to the children, you'll probably feel comfortable placing your child there. Spanking or restraining a child too forcefully is not okay and should be reported.

Try to observe daily routines, paying attention to how the day is organized and what activities are planned. Watch how food is prepared and find out how often children are fed. Check how frequently children are taken to the toilet or diapered. While touring the childcare home or center, also check if the following basic health and safety standards are being met:

- The premises are clean and reasonably neat (without discouraging play).
- There is plenty of play equipment, and it is in good repair.
- The equipment is appropriate for the developmental skills of the children in the program.
- Children are closely supervised when crawling or climbing on playthings, roughhousing, or playing with blocks (which are sometimes thrown) and other potentially dangerous toys.
- Food is stored appropriately. If the childcare site is preparing the food and beverages, they are nutritious.
- Areas where food is handled are separate from toilets and diaper-changing areas.
- Diaper-changing areas are cleaned and sanitized before and after being used for each child.
- Handwashing sinks are available where needed and are used by the children and also staff members during the following:
  - Upon arrival
  - When moving from one childcare group to another
  - Before and after eating or touching breast milk, formula, food, and food preparation surfaces
  - Before and after giving medication
  - Before and after playing in water used by more than one person
  - After diapering
  - After using the toilet or helping children use the toilet
  - After handling any body fluid, such as nasal discharge, blood, vomit, drool, or sores
  - After playing in sandboxes
  - After handling garbage

- Potty chairs are avoided to decrease the risk of spreading diarrheal illnesses.
- Children are supervised by sight and sound at all times, even when napping.

While touring the childcare home or center, also check to see if basic health and safety standards are being met.

Once you are satisfied a particular program will provide your child with a safe, loving, healthy environment, let them test it out while you're present. Watch how the caregivers and your child interact, and make sure all of you are comfortable with the situation.

You can find a helpful childcare program checklist in the Appendix (*page 705*).

NAPPING IN CHILDCARE SETTINGS

Many parents know the importance of placing a baby to sleep on their back to minimize the risk of sudden unexpected infant death (SUID) or sudden infant death syndrome (SIDS). Obviously, this same precaution should be followed in childcare settings, where 20 percent of all SUID cases occur—a disproportionately high amount. Although the American Academy of Pediatrics stresses the importance of using the back-sleeping position to lower the incidence of SUID during childcare, not all states in the United States have licensing regulations to mandate that childcare facilities place infants on their backs to sleep.

If your baby will be napping at their childcare site, you must discuss this issue with the caregivers before making a final selection about a facility. Make sure the childcare setting you choose routinely follows this simple procedure. (For more information about SUID, see *pages 107–8*.) For older children, make sure that bedding is clean and hypoallergenic. (Additional information about crib safety is available on *pages 300–302*.)

Building a Relationship with Your Child's Care Providers

For your child's sake, develop a good relationship with the people who care for them in your absence. The better you get along with their caregiver, the more comfortable your child will feel as they interact with both of you. The better you communicate with the caregiver, the more continuity there will be in your child's care throughout the day.

Talk with the caregiver—even briefly—each time you drop your child off or return for your child. If something exciting or upsetting happened during the early morning, it might affect your child's behavior the rest of the day, so the caregiver should know about it. Share family stresses, both good and bad, like an expected birth or a family illness.

When you arrive for pickup, you should be told about any important events from the day, from a change in bowel movements or eating patterns to a new way of playing or their first steps. Also, if they've developed symptoms of illness, you and the caregiver should discuss the situation and agree on what to do if symptoms get worse.

A rivalry may develop between you and the caregiver for your child's affection and control of their behavior. When your child misbehaves, you may hear, "Funny, they never do that for me." Don't take this seriously, as children usually save their worst behavior for those they trust most.

If you treat caregivers as partners, they will feel you respect them and will probably be more enthusiastic about looking after your child. Here are some ways to build this sense of partnership on a daily basis:

- Show the caregiver something your child made at home, or talk about particularly funny or interesting things they've done. Explain that sharing this kind of information is important to you, and encourage two-way communication.
- Extend basic courtesy to your child's caregivers.
- Provide materials and suggestions for special projects the caregivers can do with your child and the group, or ask for ways you can help with planned activities.
- Help plan and carry out special activities with the caregiver.

- Make sure your child always knows you are leaving. Keep a positive tone, and be sure to say goodbye before you disappear, but leave without prolonging your departure. Don't just slip away.

Periodically, you and the caregiver should also have longer discussions to review your child's progress, discuss any problems, and plan for future changes. Schedule these extended conversations at a time when you won't be rushed, your child's caregiver isn't busy, and you are both in a place with no distractions. If possible, arrange for someone else to care for your child during the conversation. Allow enough time to discuss all of your child's achievements and concerns from both perspectives and agree on specific objectives and plans.

TIPS FOR TRANSITIONING TO CHILDCARE

Getting the day started can be a challenge. So here are some suggestions to make childcare drop-off a little easier for everyone.

Your Child's Developmental Stage	Your Response
0 to 7 months	
In early infancy, your baby primarily needs love, comforting, and good basic care to satisfy their physical needs.	Although this period may be a difficult time of separation for you, young infants generally will transition to a consistent childcare worker in almost any setting. Be patient during this initial settling-in period.

7 to 12 months	
Stranger anxiety normally occurs at this time. Suddenly your baby may be reluctant to stay with anyone outside their family. The unfamiliar setting of a childcare center also may upset them.	If starting childcare during this period, ease into it and know it may take a little longer to adjust. If your child is already in a program, take extra time each day before you say goodbye. Create a short goodbye ritual, perhaps letting them hold a favorite stuffed animal. Say goodbye and then quietly leave. Above all, be consistent from day to day.

Resolving Conflicts

Most parents are pleased with the childcare they've chosen. Nevertheless, whenever two or more people share responsibility for a child, conflicts sometimes arise. In many cases, you can resolve a disagreement about childcare simply by talking through the problem. You may find the conflict is nothing more than a misunderstanding of the situation. Other times, especially when several people are involved in the care of your child, you may need a more organized approach. The following step-by-step strategy can help:

1. Define the problem clearly. Understand who is involved, but avoid blaming anyone. If your child has been involved in a biting or hitting incident with another child, find out which caregivers were on hand at the time. Ask what they observed and focus your attention on realistic measures that can be taken to prevent the likelihood of further incidents. Maybe you can suggest an alternative way in which caregivers can respond if the incident recurs.
2. Listen to everyone's ideas to find other possible solutions.
3. Agree on a specific plan of action with clearly defined time limits and assignments to each of the caregivers—including you.

4. Consider everything that could go wrong with the plan and decide how these problems might be avoided or how they will be handled if they occur.
5. Put the plan into action.
6. Meet again at a specified time to decide whether the plan is working. If it's not, go through the process again to decide what changes need to be made.

The better you get along with the caregiver, the more comfortable your child will feel as they interact with both of you.

What to Do When Your Child Is Sick

If your child is like most, they will get their share of illnesses, whether they are in a childcare program or not. Most illnesses are colds or other respiratory infections, which tend to occur more often between early fall and late spring. At times your child may get infections one right after another and be sick for weeks. If both parents work full-time, this can be a problem and cause a great deal of stress, since often one will need to stay home with the ill child.

Even children who seem only mildly ill may be sent home from childcare programs; if the program's policies are based on sound principles, this may be for good reason. A sick child may be contagious and risks giving their illness to other children. Also, a sick child may need more individual care and attention than a provider can offer without interfering with the care of others.

States often have regulations requiring childcare programs to send sick children home. This makes sense, particularly when a child has a fever or symptoms like rashes that are weeping, vomiting two or more times in a twenty-four-hour period, or frequent diarrhea that is not contained in the diaper and/or more than two stools above normal, since those circumstances enable contagious diseases to spread. The ultimate goal is to provide your child with care and to limit the spread of contagious illnesses.

Ideally, you would stay home when your child is sick. However, there may be times when this option is particularly difficult or simply not possible. Be sure to talk to your employer ahead of time to see what arrangements might be available. You might suggest telecommuting, taking work home, or identifying co-workers who can fill in for you when this situation arises. Spouses, other family members, and trusted friends may be able to help as well.

If your job and your spouse's employer require full-time attendance, you will have to make other arrangements for a sick child. These are days when you might arrange alternative care, preferably where both the caregiver and the setting are familiar. If you rely on a relative or hire a sitter, make sure the caregiver understands the nature of the illness and how to manage it.

If your child requires medication, confirm your childcare provider's policies regarding giving medication to children, and always obtain written instructions from your pediatrician to give to your caregiver. Do not expect your caregiver to follow your instructions without a pediatrician's authorization. Also, both prescription and over-the-counter medications should have a pharmacy or drugstore label on them with the child's name, medication dosage, and expiration date. Giving medication to children is a significant responsibility and can be a challenge for caregivers. It should be requested only when necessary. Often medication dosages can be adjusted so that they are given in the morning, before childcare, and in the evening, after childcare. Address any questions to your pediatrician.

Your child's caregiver will need to know the reason for giving the medication, how it should be stored and administered (what doses, at what intervals, and for how long), and what side effects to look for and what to do if they occur. Again, this should all be put in writing. Do not disguise medicine as food or describe it as candy; instead, your child should know that it's medicine and why it's needed. Ask the caregiver to record the time each dose is given.

If your child is in a childcare center, be prepared to sign a consent form authorizing staff to administer medication. Also, expect your child's medications to come home each evening (regulations typically do not allow medicine to be kept at childcare facilities overnight).

A few communities have services specializing in care for mildly ill children. These include the following:

Home-Based Programs

- Family childcare homes equipped to care for both sick and well children. If a child becomes ill in such a program, they can continue attending in a segregated area, if necessary. Not all infections are contagious.
- Family childcare homes that care only for sick children. Some of these are associated with well-child care centers.
- Agencies or childcare centers that provide caregivers to work in your home.

Center-Based Programs

- Regular childcare centers that have trained staff members to care for sick children in the usual childcare setting, but apart from the main group.
- Centers offering a separate "get-well room" for sick children, staffed by a caregiver.
- Sick-child care centers set up specifically to care for ill children.

In sick-child programs, caregivers adjust the activity level to the child's ability to participate, and the children receive a lot of cuddling and personal attention. These programs should pay extra attention to hygiene for both caregivers and children. The premises and equipment, especially toys, should be cleaned thoroughly and often. Disposable toys may be necessary, depending on the nature of the illnesses. A pediatrician and public health consultant should be on call for every sick-child care facility.

Controlling Infectious Diseases

Whenever children gather, their risk of getting sick increases. Infants and toddlers are particularly affected, since they place their hands and toys in their mouths, making the spread of infections even easier.

While it's impossible for adults to keep toys and other objects in perfect sanitary condition, many precautions and practices can help control the spread of infection. Childcare programs should be extremely careful about maintaining good hygiene. Children and teachers should have easy access to sinks with soap. They should be reminded, and children assisted, to wash hands with soap and water after using the bathroom. Staff members also should wash at the times listed earlier in this chapter (*page 277*), and especially after changing diapers. Both the caregiver's and child's hands should be wiped after removing the soiled diaper, and then washed at the end of the diaper change routine. Handwashing or the use of alcohol-based hand sanitizers after blowing or wiping noses and before handling food or food surfaces can also significantly reduce infections.

If a center cares for infants, toddlers, and toilet-trained children, each group should have separate areas with accessible sinks for handwashing. The facility and all equipment should be cleaned at least daily. Changing tables should be cleaned after each diaper change, and toilets should be washed and disinfected regularly.

If an injury involving blood occurs, the caregiver should put on gloves and wash the wound, administer first aid, and apply a bandage. All blood-contaminated surfaces or clothing should be washed and disinfected. Also, since breast milk can transmit HIV and other viruses, be sure the childcare facility has procedures to prevent feeding one mother's breast milk to another mother's child. If such an incident occurs, the situation should be handled following the national standards described in "Caring for Our Children," published by the National Resource Center for Health and Safety in Child Care and Early Education (nrckids.org/CFOC). (Also see the description of HIV on *page 288*.)

As a parent, you can help control the spread of disease by keeping your child at home when they have a contagious illness with fever or one requiring medical attention. Also notify their caregiver as soon as anyone in your family is diagnosed as having a particular illness, and request that all parents be alerted if a child in the program has a serious or highly contagious illness. Many childcare centers exclude children with fever for twenty-four hours, although this measure has never been shown to reduce the spread of illness.

Immunizations can greatly reduce outbreaks of serious infectious diseases. Centers should require children to be immunized (at appropriate ages) against hepatitis B, rotavirus, diphtheria, tetanus, pertussis, polio, influenza, *Haemophilus influenzae* type b, pneumococcus, measles, mumps, rubella, hepatitis A, and chickenpox (also, the meningococcal vaccine is available for certain high-risk children). The immunity of your child's caregivers should be checked as well, and if there is any doubt, they should receive appropriate immunizations.

Teach your child proper hygiene and handwashing habits so that they are less likely to spread illnesses. Finally, educate yourself about common illnesses in childcare settings so that you know what to expect and how to respond if they occur. Such illnesses include the following.

Colds

Children in childcare typically have about seven to nine colds each year and are more likely to get these infections than infants cared for at home. Fortunately, the chances of contracting some of the most severe illnesses or complications associated with colds can be decreased by immunizing children. In childcare centers, toys, tables, doorknobs, and other surfaces touched by hands should be sanitized frequently.

Colds are spread by direct or close contact with the mouth or nose secretions of an infected individual, or by touching contaminated objects. In childcare settings, children can be taught to wash their hands frequently, and to sneeze into their upper arm rather than their hands. They should also be taught proper disposal of tissues and not to share cups or eating utensils. (For more information, see Influenza [Flu], *page 418*, and Colds/Upper Respiratory Infections, *page 468*.)

Cytomegalovirus (CMV) and Parvovirus Infection

Cytomegalovirus (CMV) and parvovirus usually cause no illness (or only mild illness) in children and adults. However, these viruses can be dangerous to pregnant women who are not immune to them and can sometimes also cause a serious infection in the unborn child. The infection is transmitted through direct contact with body fluids (tears, urine, saliva). Fortunately, most adult women are already immune to CMV and parvovirus, but if a woman is pregnant, has a child in daycare, or works in a childcare home or center, she has an increased risk of exposure and should discuss her risk with her obstetrician. Good hand hygiene is the most effective way to decrease transmission of CMV when caring for sick children. If necessary, her obstetrician can order a blood test to see if she has already had these diseases.

Diarrheal Diseases

The average child has one or two episodes of diarrhea a year. These illnesses can spread easily in childcare homes and centers. If your child has diarrhea, do not take them to childcare unless their stools have become manageable by normal diaper changes or by using the toilet. This will help avoid the chance of the infection being transmitted to others. If diarrhea is persistent with dehydration, or if stools have blood or mucus, the child should undergo medical evaluation; further lab tests may be required to identify the responsible bacteria, virus, or parasite for treatment and management before returning to childcare. (See Diarrhea, *page 354*.)

Eye and Skin Infections

Conjunctivitis (pinkeye), impetigo, scabies, and cold sores are common problems in young children. These infections of the skin and mucous membranes can spread by contact. Childcare staff should notify you if any child in the program contracts one of these illnesses. If so, watch for symptoms in your child and if symptoms appear, contact your pediatrician for early diagnosis and possible treatment. (See Herpes Simplex, *page 478*; Eye Infections, *page 545*; Impetigo, *page 656*; Ringworm (Tinea), *page 665*; Scabies, *page 669*.)

Head Lice

Head lice are small, tan-colored insects less than ⅛ inch long that live on blood they draw from the scalp. Although families and caregivers often become very upset about lice, the insects do not carry disease, though they do cause annoying symptoms such as itching. Lice are spread by direct contact with infested hair. By using medications that kill lice and nits, the infestation can be controlled. Children should not be excluded from childcare due to head lice.

Hepatitis A Virus

Because of the success of the hepatitis A vaccine, this infection in childcare settings is now rare, but it remains contagious. In infants and young children, most infections are asymptomatic or cause mild, non-specific symptoms. Older infected children may have only mild fever, nausea, vomiting, diarrhea, or jaundice (a yellowish skin color). However, adults who get this illness usually experience these symptoms to a much greater degree. (See Hepatitis, *page 368*.)

Hepatitis B Virus

Infants receive the hepatitis B vaccine series starting at birth. The virus can be acquired during birth from an infected mother or after birth by exposure to infected blood such as during a needle stick, but children also can contract the virus through frequent casual contact with household members. Transmission rarely occurs in a childcare setting, so there is no need to exclude a child with hepatitis B infection from group childcare. (Also see descriptions of hepatitis B, *page 369*, and hepatitis B vaccine, *page 626*.)

Human Immunodeficiency Virus (HIV)/AIDS

HIV (the virus that causes AIDS) can produce a serious chronic infection. Some children acquire HIV from their infected mothers before or during birth. HIV can also be transmitted from one child to another by exposure to blood; however, there have been no reports of HIV transmission in childcare. There is no need to exclude an HIV-infected child from childcare in the belief that this would protect others, since the risk of HIV transmission in this setting is extremely low when standard appropriate blood and body fluid precautions are used. If an injury involving blood occurs, see *page 285* for standard cleanup procedures.

Ringworm

Ringworm (or tinea) is not a worm but a mildly contagious fungal infection, causing red circular patches with raised edges. On the scalp, ringworm can lead to patchy areas of dandruff-like scaling. Ringworm is spread by direct contact with contaminated combs, brushes, towels, clothing, or bedding. The infection is easily cured with appropriate medication. Ringworm is a common condition and should not exclude a child from childcare settings. (See also Ringworm [Tinea], *page 665*.)

Preventing Injuries and Promoting Car Safety

Many injuries occurring at home or in childcare settings are predictable and preventable (see *pages 263–78* for sections on assessing and selecting childcare). Safety for children (and adults) in and around cars is a special concern. The center should have well-marked pickup and drop-off areas where children and adults are protected from street traffic, with "Children at Play" or similar signs placed in the pickup/drop-off areas as well as along nearby streets. The center should never allow a child in these areas, or in any area where cars come and go, unless they are being picked up or dropped off and are accompanied by an adult. Children should also never go behind vehicles that could back over them. Keep in mind that adults may need assistance dealing with more than one child in the car. Cars should not be left running and should always be driven slowly near childcare centers.

If your child shares a ride to and from childcare, be sure the drivers have good driving records and are using appropriate car safety seats for all infants and children. The driver must check to ensure that everyone is properly buckled in a car safety seat before pulling away, and that everyone has left the vehicle before locking up and leaving the car.

CAR POOL SAFETY

If you use a car pool, you are responsible for every child in the car in addition to your own child. This means making sure each child is properly restrained in a car safety seat appropriate for their size, installing each car safety seat correctly, not overloading the car, disciplining children who disobey safety rules, and checking that your insurance covers everyone on board. In addition, make sure you and other drivers observe the following precautions:

- Pick up and drop off children only in an area where they are protected from other cars. They should be dropped off on the same side of the street as the school to avoid having them cross the street in traffic areas.
- If possible, have each child's own parents or another responsible adult buckle them into the car safety seat and take them out when returning home.
- Turn all children over to the direct supervision of a parent or childcare staff.
- Close and lock all car doors, but only after checking that fingers and feet are inside.
- Open passenger windows only a few inches and lock all power window and door controls from the driver's seat if possible.
- Plan your routes to minimize travel time and avoid hazardous conditions.
- Have available emergency contact information (ideally in your phone) for each child.
- Ideally, equip each vehicle with a fire extinguisher and first-aid kit.
- Be sure no child is ever left in the car without a supervising adult.

If your childcare program includes swimming, appropriate safety precautions must be followed. Any pool, lake, creek, or pond used by children should first be checked by public health authorities. If the pool is at or near the childcare center, it should be entirely surrounded by at least a 4-foot-high (1.2 m), four-sided fence with a self-closing, self-latching gate that completely separates the center from the pool. For hygiene and safety reasons, portable wading pools should not be used.

Where We Stand

To ensure the safety of children while being transported to a childcare facility outside their home, the American Academy of Pediatrics strongly recommends all children travel in age-appropriate and properly secured child restraint systems in all motor vehicles.

The AAP has a long-standing position that new school buses should have safety restraints. Parents should work with school districts to encourage that new buses be equipped with lap/shoulder seatbelt restraints that can also accommodate car safety seats, booster seats, and harness systems. School districts should provide height- and weight-appropriate car safety seats and restraint systems for all children of preschool age; these systems include booster seats with a three-point belt.

When districts have policies on seatbelt use, children tend to be better behaved and less likely to distract the driver.

Caring for Babies with Special Healthcare Needs

If your baby has a developmental disability or chronic health condition, don't let that keep them from childcare. Quality childcare may be good for them. They are likely to benefit from the social contact, physical exercise, and variety of experiences of a group program.

The time your child spends in a childcare program will be good for you, too. Tending a child with special healthcare needs often places great demands on your time, energy, and emotions. The challenge is to find a program that encourages normal childhood activities and meets their special healthcare needs; fortunately, these are more available than in the past.

Safety Walk Checklist

Next time you walk through your child's childcare setting, use the following checklist to ensure the facility is safe, clean, and in good condition. If there is a problem with any item on the list, bring it to the attention of the director or caregiver and follow up later to ensure it has been corrected.

Indoors in All Programs

- Floors are smooth, are clean, and have a non-skid surface.
- Medicines, cleaning agents, and tools are locked up and out of children's sight and reach.
- First-aid kits are fully supplied and out of children's reach.
- Windowsills, walls, and ceilings are clean and in good repair, with no peeling paint or damaged plaster. (Windowsills are the highest-risk areas for lead poisoning.)
- Children are never left unattended.
- Bookcases, dressers, and other tall furniture are secured to the wall so that they cannot tip over if a child climbs on them. Televisions are mounted or strapped to the wall or secured to low, sturdy furniture that is designed to hold them.
- Electrical outlets are covered with childproof caps that are not a choking hazard.
- Electric lights are in good repair, with no frayed or dangling cords.
- Care is taken that batteries are not left around, particularly button batteries, which can be very damaging if swallowed.
- Heating pipes and radiators are out of reach or covered so that children cannot touch them.
- Ask if the hot-water heater is set at or below 120 degrees Fahrenheit (48.9 degrees Celsius) to lessen the risk of a scald burn.

- There are no poisonous plants or disease-bearing animals (e.g., turtles or iguanas).
- Trash containers are covered.
- Exits are clearly marked and easy to reach.
- Smoking is not allowed in the childcare facility.
- Windows at or above the second story have guards to prevent falls, and all drapery or window blind cords are secured out of children's reach. If possible, it is best to use cordless window coverings.
- Leaks are fixed promptly, and any mold is properly treated.

Outdoors in All Programs

- Grounds are free of litter, sharp objects, and animal droppings.
- Play equipment is smooth, well anchored, and free of rust, splinters, and sharp corners. All screws and bolts are capped or concealed.
- Outdoor playground equipment is mounted over impact-absorbent surfaces for a distance of at least 6 feet (1.8 m) on all sides of the equipment. Playground surfaces should be made of at least 12 inches (30 cm) of wood chips, mulch, sand, pea gravel, or other impact-absorbing material under and around areas where falls are more likely to occur (under monkey bars, slides).
- Swing seats are lightweight and flexible, and there are no open or S-shaped hooks.
- Slides have wide, flat, and stable steps with good treads; rounded rims along the sides to prevent falls; and a flat area at the end of the slide to help children slow down.
- Metal slides are shaded from the sun.
- Sandboxes are covered when not in use.
- Childproof barriers keep children out of hazardous areas.

Infant and Toddler Programs

- Toys do not contain lead or have any signs of chipping paint, rust, or small pieces that could break off. (A clue that suggests a toy might contain lead is that the toy feels unusually heavy or soft for its appearance.)
- High chairs have wide bases and safety straps.
- Toddlers are not allowed to walk around with bottles or take bottles to bed.
- Infant walkers are not used.
- Cribs, portable play yards, and beds meet safety standards and are free of pillows, blankets, bumpers, toys, and loose bedding.
- No recalled products or old products with broken or missing parts are used. Recalled products can be determined by checking the website of the Consumer Product Safety Commission: saferproducts.gov. Caregivers can subscribe to email alerts from the CPSC notifying them when any toy or other children's product is recalled.

Start your search with your pediatrician by asking about the best type of group programs for your child. Ask for referrals to suitable centers. Your pediatrician can draft an individualized care plan to address your child's special healthcare needs and help your childcare providers understand what is needed. Although only one appropriate site may be available in smaller communities, in many communities you will have several to choose from. The one you select should meet the same basic requirements outlined earlier, plus the following:

1. The program should include children with and without chronic health conditions and special healthcare needs, to the extent possible. Having relationships with typically developing playmates helps a child with a disability feel more relaxed and confident socially and helps build self-esteem. The arrangement also benefits the typically developing child and those with no special

healthcare needs by teaching them to look past surface differences and helping them develop sensitivity and respect.

If your child has a developmental disability or chronic health condition, they are likely to benefit from the social contact, physical exercise, and variety of experiences of a group childcare program.

2. The staff should be trained in the specific care your child requires. Some of the training needs can be specified in your child's care plan.
3. The program should have at least one physician consultant who is active in the development of policies and procedures affecting the type of special healthcare needs present. Your own pediatrician should also play an active role. Give permission for your childcare providers to discuss questions and issues with your pediatrician.
4. All children should be encouraged to be as independent as their abilities allow, within the bounds of safety. They should be restricted only in activities that might be dangerous or that have been prohibited by a doctor's order.
5. The program should be flexible enough to adapt to slight variations in the children's abilities. This may include altering equipment or facilities for physically challenged or visually or hearing-impaired children.
6. The program should offer special equipment and activities to meet the special healthcare needs of children, such as breathing treatments for children with asthma. The equipment should be in good repair, and the staff should be trained to operate it correctly.
7. The staff should be familiar with each child's medical and developmental status. The staff should recognize symptoms and determine when the child needs medical attention.
8. If the program includes off-site field trips or activities, the staff should be trained in safe transportation of children with special healthcare needs.
9. The staff should know how to reach each child's physician in an emergency and be qualified to administer any necessary emergency medications. Emergency planning should be specified in the child's care plan.

These are general recommendations. Because special health-care needs vary widely, it's impossible to advise more precisely how to determine the best program. If you're having trouble deciding among the programs your pediatrician suggested, go back and discuss your concerns with them. They will work with you to make the right choice.

Whatever your child's special healthcare needs, how they will be cared for in your absence is an important decision. The information here should help. However, you know your child better than anyone. Rely most heavily on your impressions when choosing a childcare arrangement.

CHAPTER 11

KEEPING YOUR CHILD SAFE

Everyday life is full of well-disguised dangers for children: sharp objects, shaky furniture, reachable hot-water faucets, pots on hot stoves, hot tubs, swimming pools, and busy streets. Adults navigate this minefield so well we no longer think of things like scissors and stoves as hazards. To protect your child from the dangers they'll encounter in and out of your home, you have to see the world as they do, and you must recognize they cannot yet distinguish hot from cold or sharp from dull.

Keeping your child physically safe is your most basic responsibility—a never-ending one. Unintentional injuries are a leading cause of death and disability in children over age 1, with drowning and car crashes accounting for a large number of injuries and deaths. Each year, children experience more than 6 million emergency department visits for unintentional injury, and almost 4,000 children and adolescents under the age of 15 die from injuries.

Many children are injured or killed by equipment designed specifically for them. In one recent twelve-month period, highchair-related injuries sent almost 8,000 children to the hospital. In 2017, toys caused almost 122,000 injuries serious enough to require an emergency department visit in children under 15.

These are worrisome numbers, but many injuries can be prevented. In the past, injuries were called "accidents" because they seemed unpredictable and unavoidable. Today we know injuries are not random but are often predictable and preventable. By understanding how a child grows and develops, and the risk of injury at each developmental stage, parents can take precautions to prevent many of these injuries.

Why Children Get Injured

Every childhood injury involves three elements: factors related to the child, the object that causes the injury, and the environment in which it occurs. To keep your child safe, you must be aware of all three.

Your baby's age greatly affects the kind of protection they need. The 3-month-old cooing in an infant seat requires different supervision from the walking 10-month-old or the toddler who's learned to climb. At each stage of your child's life, you must revisit the present hazards and consider how to eliminate them. As your child grows, you must repeatedly ask: How far and how quickly can they move? How high can they reach? What objects attract their attention? What can they do today that they couldn't yesterday? What about tomorrow versus today?

During the first 6 months, you can secure your baby's safety by never leaving them alone, even for a moment, in dangerous situations—for example, on a bed or a changing table where they might fall off. As they grow, they'll create dangers of their own—perhaps by creeping into places they shouldn't, or actively seeking out dangerous things to touch and taste.

For the baby on the move, you'll certainly tell them no whenever they approach something potentially hazardous, but they won't understand the significance of your message. Many parents find the ages between 6 and 18 months extremely frustrating, because the child doesn't seem to learn from reprimands. Even if you tell them twenty times a day to stay away from the toilet, they're still in the bathroom every time you turn your back. Your child is not being willfully disobedient; their memory isn't developed enough to recall your warnings when they're attracted by the forbidden object or activity. What looks like naughtiness is actually the testing and retesting of reality—the normal way a child this age learns.

Young children are extraordinary mimics and may try to take medicine as they've seen Mom do or play with a razor just as Dad does. Yes, your child may realize after the fact that the tugging of the cord is what pulled the lamp down on their head, but their ability to anticipate this is still months away.

Your child's temperament also may be a factor. Studies suggest that extremely active and unusually curious children have more injuries. At certain stages of development, your child is likely to be stubborn, easily frustrated, aggressive, or unable to concentrate—all characteristics that can be associated with injuries. When you notice your child having a bad day or going through a difficult phase, be especially alert with your supervision in terms of accident prevention.

Since you can't change your child's age and you have little influence over their basic temperament, most of your efforts to prevent injury should focus on objects and surroundings. By designing an environment where obvious hazards are removed, you can ensure the freedom your child needs to explore.

Some parents feel that childproofing their home is unnecessary because they intend to supervise their children closely. It's true that with constant vigilance, most injuries can be avoided. But even the most conscientious parents can't watch a child every moment. Most injuries occur not when parents are alert and at their best but when they're under stress. The following situations are often associated with injuries:

- Hunger and fatigue (e.g., the hour or so before dinner)
- Mother's pregnancy
- Illness or death in the family
- Changes with the child's regular caregiver or other change in routine
- Tension between parents or caregivers
- Sudden changes in the environment, such as moving to a new home or going on vacation

All families experience some of these stresses. Childproofing eliminates or reduces opportunities for injury, so even with a momentary distraction—the telephone or doorbell—your child is less likely to encounter harm-causing situations or objects.

The pages that follow include advice about how to minimize dangers in and out of the home. The intention is to alert you to hazards—particularly those that might seem harmless—so you can take the sensible precautions to keep your child safe and still allow them the freedom to grow up happy and healthy.

Safety Inside Your Home

Room to Room

Your lifestyle and your home's layout will determine which rooms should be childproofed. Examine every room where your child spends time (for most families, that means the entire house). It's tempting to exclude a formal dining or living room behind closed doors, but remember that the forbidden rooms are the ones your child will want most to explore. Any areas not childproofed require extra vigilance on your part, even if entrances are normally locked or blocked. At the very least, your child's room should be a place where everything is as safe as it can be.

Nursery

Cribs. Your baby is usually unattended in their crib, which should be a totally safe environment. Newborns are at risk for suffocation-related deaths and injuries, especially when there are soft materials in the crib or bassinet such as blankets, crib bumpers, pillows, or stuffed animals. In older infants and toddlers, falls are the most common injury associated with cribs, even though they can often be prevented. Children are most likely to fall when the mattress is raised too high for their height or not lowered properly as they grow.

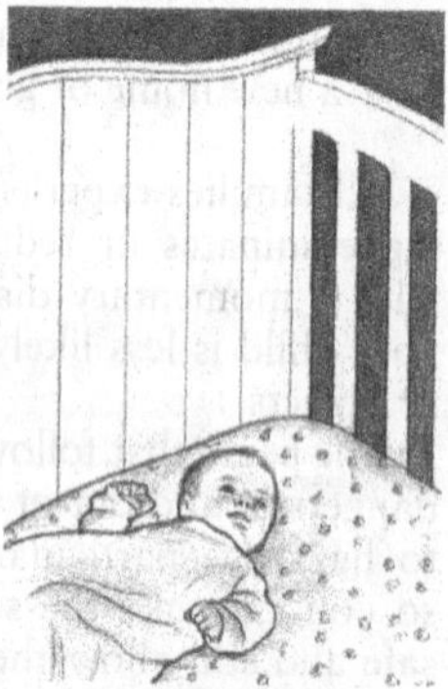

Your child should be placed on their back when going to sleep.

It is strongly recommended to use a crib manufactured after June 2011, when a stronger mandatory safety standard was implemented. If your crib has a side that lowers and raises, it is too old and should be replaced. Older cribs pose too high a risk of injury to infants.

No matter the age of your crib, inspect it carefully for the following features:

- Slats should be no more than 2⅜ inches (6 cm) apart so that a child's head cannot become trapped between them. Widely spaced slats can allow an infant's legs and body to fall through but will trap the infant's head, which can result in death.
- There should be no decorative cut-outs in the headboard or footboard, as your child's head or limbs could become trapped in them.
- If the crib has corner posts, they should be flush with the tops of the end panels, or else be very, very tall (such as posts on a canopy bed). For posts that stick up past the end panels, clothing and ribbons can catch on them and strangle an infant.
- All screws, bolts, nuts, plastic parts, and other hardware should be present and original equipment. Never substitute something from a hardware store for the original parts; obtain replacement parts from the manufacturer. They must be tightly fastened to prevent the crib from coming apart, as otherwise a child's activity could cause the crib to collapse, trapping and suffocating them.
- Before each assembly and weekly thereafter, inspect the crib for damage to hardware, loose joints, missing parts, or sharp edges. Do not use a crib if any parts are missing or broken.

Prevent other crib hazards with the following guidelines:

1. The mattress should be the same size as the crib, with no gaps to trap arms, body, or legs. If more than two fingers can be inserted between the mattress and sides or ends of the crib, the crib/mattress combination should not be used.
2. For a new mattress, remove and destroy all plastic wrapping that comes with it. It can suffocate a child.
3. Before your baby can sit up by themselves, lower the mattress to the level where they cannot fall out by leaning against the side or by pulling themselves over it. Set the mattress at its lowest position before your child learns to stand. Most falls occur when a baby tries to climb out. Move your child to another bed when they are 35 inches (89 cm) tall, or when the height of the

side rail is less than three-quarters their height (approximately nipple level).

4. Periodically check the crib to ensure that no rough edges, no sharp metal points, and no splinters or cracks in the wood have developed. If you notice tooth marks on the railing, cover the wood with a plastic strip (available at most children's furniture stores).
5. Do not use bumper pads in cribs. There is no evidence they prevent injuries, and there is risk of suffocation, strangulation, or entrapment. Infant deaths in cribs have been associated with bumper pads. In addition, toddlers can use a bumper guard to climb and fall out.
6. Pillows, quilts, comforters, sheepskins, stuffed animals, and other soft products should not be placed in a crib with an infant. Babies can suffocate on such items in the crib.
7. If you hang a mobile, be sure it is securely attached to the side rails. Hang it high and out of reach of the baby and remove it when they are able to get up on their hands and knees or reach 5 months, whichever comes first.
8. Crib gyms are not recommended, as infants and toddlers may injure themselves falling forward onto the gym or pulling it down on top of themselves.
9. To prevent the most serious of falls and to keep children from getting caught in window or drapery cords and strangling, don't place a crib—or any other child's bed—near a window. The Consumer Product Safety Commission recommends using cordless window coverings if possible.
10. Keep baby monitor cords at least 3 feet away from the crib and do not place any item with a cord near the crib or under the crib mattress.

Changing Tables. Changing tables make dressing and diapering easier, but falls from such a height can be serious. Don't trust vigilance alone to prevent falls; you should also consider the following recommendations:

1. Choose a sturdy, stable changing table with a 2-inch (5 cm) guardrail on four sides.
2. The top of the changing table pad should be concave, with the middle slightly lower than the sides.
3. Buckle the safety strap, but don't depend on it alone to keep your child secure. Always keep a hand on your

baby. Never leave a child unattended on a dressing table, even for a moment, even if they are strapped in.

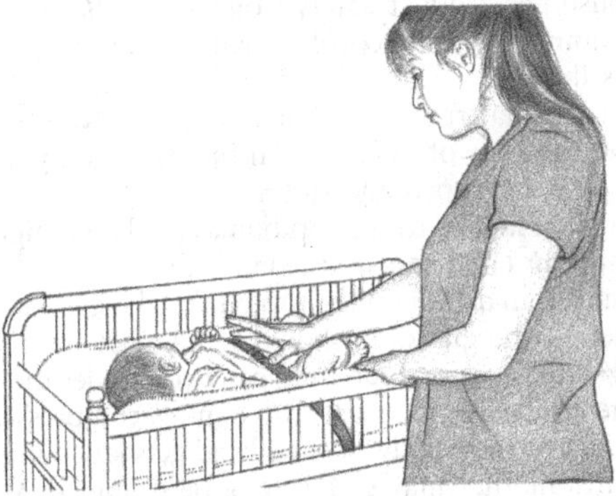

4. Keep diapering supplies within reach—but not your child's reach—so you don't have to leave your baby's side. Baby powder can get in your child's lungs and cause damage, so instead of powder use a diaper cream.
5. If you use disposable diapers, store them out of your child's reach and cover them with clothing when they wear them. Children can suffocate if they swallow torn-off pieces of the plastic liner.

Bunk Beds. Although some children love them, bunk beds pose several serious dangers. The child on the top bunk can fall out, and the child on the lower bunk can be injured if the top collapses. The bunk beds might be improperly constructed or assembled, resulting in dangerous structural flaws. Or a mattress that doesn't properly fit could entrap your child. If, despite these warnings, you choose to use bunk beds, take the following precautions:

1. Don't allow a child under 6 years to sleep in the top bunk. They won't have the coordination needed to climb safely or to keep from falling out.
2. Place the beds in a corner of the room so that there are walls on two sides. This provides extra support and blocks two sides from possible falls.
3. Don't place beds beside a window. This will help

prevent children from falling out of the window or being strangled by window or drapery cords. The Consumer Product Safety Commission (CPSC) recommends using cordless window coverings if possible.

4. The top mattress should fit snugly and not possibly slip over the edge of the frame. If there's a gap, your child might get trapped and suffocate.
5. Attach a ladder to the top bunk bed. Use a nightlight so that your child can see the ladder.
6. Install a guardrail on the top bunk. The gap between the side rail and guardrail should be no more than 3½ inches (8¾ cm). Be sure your child can't roll under the guardrail when the mattress on the top bunk is compressed by the weight of their body. If their head gets stuck under the guardrail, they may suffocate or be strangled. You may need a thicker mattress to prevent this.
7. Check the supports under the upper mattress. Wires or slats should run directly under the mattress and be fastened in place at both ends. A mattress supported only by the frame of the bed or unsecured slats could come crashing down.
8. If you separate bunks into two individual beds, remove all dowels or connectors.
9. To prevent falls and collapse of the bed, don't allow children to jump or roughhouse on either bunk.
10. Choose bunk beds with a label stating they comply with ASTM Standard F1427 to ensure they are designed and constructed to be as safe as possible.

Kitchen

The kitchen can be a very dangerous environment for young children. While your infant or toddler is with you in the kitchen, use a high chair or play yard. Your child should be within your sight, and if using a high chair they should be securely strapped in. Keep a toy box or drawer with safe play items in the kitchen to amuse them. Eliminate the most serious dangers by taking the following precautions:

1. Store strong cleaners, lye, furniture polish, dishwasher soap (especially detergent packets), and other dangerous

products in a high cabinet, locked and out of sight. Detergent packets pose a special risk for young children, who mistake them for candy; buy powdered or liquid detergent if at all possible. Lye is similarly dangerous and few households use it these days; it's better simply not to have it in the home. If you must store items under the sink, an automatically fastening child safety lock should be used (most hardware, baby supply, and department stores have them). Never transfer dangerous substances, recreational drugs, or illicit substances into containers that look as if they might hold food, as this may tempt a child to taste them.

2. In the kitchen, keep knives, forks, scissors, and other sharp instruments in a latched drawer separate from "safe" kitchen utensils. Store sharp cutting appliances such as food processors out of reach and/or in a locked cupboard.
3. Unplug appliances when not in use. Don't allow electrical cords to dangle where your child can reach and tug on them, possibly pulling a heavy appliance down on themselves.
4. Always turn pot handles toward the back of the stove so that your child can't reach up and grab them. Whenever you have to walk with hot liquid—coffee, soup—know where your child is so that you don't trip over them. Do not try to carry your child at the same time!
5. When shopping for an oven, choose one that's well insulated to protect your child from the heat if they touch the oven door. Never leave the oven door open.
6. If you have a stove, turn the dials firmly to the off position. If they're easy to remove, do so when you aren't cooking so that your child can't turn the stove on. If they cannot be removed easily, use child-resistant knob covers and block access to the stove as much as possible.
7. Keep matches and lighters out of reach and out of sight.
8. Don't warm baby bottles in a microwave oven. The liquid heats unevenly, and there may be pockets of milk hot enough to scald your baby. Also, overheated baby bottles have exploded when removed from the microwave.

9. If the microwave is within your child's reach, stay nearby when it is on and never permit your child to open the microwave or remove food or liquids that have finished heating.
10. Keep a fire extinguisher in your kitchen, and on every floor of your home, in a place you'll remember.
11. Do not use small refrigerator magnets your baby could choke on or swallow.

Laundry Room

Children love to help with laundry, but because this room contains several potential hazards, they should never be allowed into the laundry room without adult supervision. Here are some tips for laundry room safety:

1. Keep detergent, fabric softener, and other products in their original containers. Keep the containers closed tightly and store them in a high, locked cabinet.
2. Single-use detergent packets are highly concentrated and toxic. The packets can burst open if bitten or squeezed by a child, and the contents can shoot down the child's throat or into their eyes and cause breathing or stomach problems, coma, and even death. Detergent packets are often brightly colored and resemble candy or gummy treats. It is best to use traditional liquid or powder detergent products instead of concentrated packets until your child is at least 6 years old. If you do use detergent packets, the container must be sealed after each use and stored out of sight and reach in a locked cabinet.
3. Clean the dryer lint trap after each use to prevent fires.

Bathroom

The simplest way to avoid bathroom injuries is to make this room inaccessible unless your child is with an adult. This may mean installing a latch on the door at adult height or a top lock. Also, be sure any lock can be unlocked from the outside, in case your child locks themselves inside.

Prevent bathroom injuries with the following suggestions:

1. Children can drown in only a few inches of water. Never leave a young child alone in the bath, even for a moment. Practice touch supervision by staying within arm's reach of your child anytime they are in or near water, such as a bathtub or swimming pool. If you must leave the bathroom, wrap your child in a towel and take them with you. Bath seats and rings are strongly not recommended and will not prevent drowning if the infant is left unattended. Babies can slip out of the seat and be trapped underwater. Do not rely on a bath seat or ring to keep your baby safe, even for a moment. Never leave water in the bathtub when not in use.
2. Install no-slip strips on the bottom of the bathtub. Put a cushioned cover over the water faucet to prevent hurtful bumps on the head.
3. Get in the habit of closing the toilet lid, and use a toilet lid lock. A curious toddler playing in the water can lose their balance, fall in, and drown. A toddler's head is disproportionately heavy, and they may not be able to lift it out of the water.
4. To prevent scalding, the hottest temperature at the faucet should be no more than 120 degrees Fahrenheit (48.9 degrees Celsius). In many cases, you can adjust your water heater. If you're unsure how to set your water heater's temperature, check with the manufacturer. When your child is old enough to turn the faucets, teach them to start the cold water before the hot.
5. All medicine containers should have safety caps. However, remember these caps are child-resistant, not childproof. Store all medicines, recreational drugs, illicit substances, and cosmetics high and out of sight and reach in a locked cabinet. Don't keep toothpaste, soaps, shampoos, and other frequently used items in the same cabinet as medicines. Instead, store all medications, recreational drugs, or illicit substances in a hard-to-reach cabinet equipped with a safety latch or lock. Get rid of old or unused medications. Refer to the package insert or label for directions on safe ways to dispose of medications. If the label does not provide instructions on safe disposal, look for take-back programs in your community, often sponsored by your local hospital, law

enforcement, or waste management facility. For more information on safe medication use, storage, and disposal, visit HealthyChildren.org.

6. If you use electrical appliances in the bathroom, particularly hair dryers and razors, unplug and store them in a cabinet with a safety lock when not in use. All bathroom wall sockets should be GFCI outlets, which automatically shut off when in contact with water, to lessen the likelihood of electrical injury if an appliance falls into the sink or bathwater. It's even better to use appliances in another room where there is no water. Ask an electrician to check your bathroom electrical outlets and install GFCI safety outlets if needed.

Garage and Basement

Garages and basements are places where potentially lethal tools and chemicals are stored. Keep doors locked, with self-closing doors, and make both areas strictly off-limits. To minimize the risk when children do gain access to the garage and basement:

1. Keep paints, varnishes, thinners, pesticides, and fertilizers in a locked cabinet or locker. Always keep these substances in their original, labeled containers.
2. Store tools in a safe locked area out of reach. This includes sharp items like saw blades. Be sure power tools are unplugged and locked in a cabinet when not in use.
3. Do not allow your child to play near the garage or driveway where cars may be coming and going. Children have been killed when playing in the driveway when someone, often a family member, unintentionally backed over them. Most vehicles have large blind spots where a child cannot be seen even if the driver is watching the mirrors carefully. Even backup cameras are no match for small, fast-moving children.
4. If you have an automatic garage door opener, be sure your child is nowhere near the door before it's opened or closed. Keep the opener out of reach and sight. Make sure the automatic reversing mechanism is properly adjusted to avoid crushing a child as the door is closing.

5. Never leave a car running in the garage, as dangerous carbon monoxide gas can collect quickly in a partly enclosed space.
6. If, for some reason, you must store an unused refrigerator or freezer, remove the door so that a child cannot become trapped if they crawl inside.
7. Do not allow your child to ride on a riding lawnmower, as children can fall off and be injured by the blades. Do not mow while a child is playing on the lawn, since lawnmowers can send rocks and other dangerous projectiles flying at high speeds.

All Rooms

Certain safety rules and preventive actions apply to every room. The following safeguards against commonplace household dangers will protect not only your small child, but your entire family as well:

1. To prevent injuries from fire and carbon monoxide, install smoke and carbon monoxide detectors throughout your home, at least one on every level and inside and outside bedrooms. Check them monthly to be sure they are working. It is best to use smoke detectors with long-life batteries, but if these are not available, change the batteries annually on a date you will remember. Smoke and carbon monoxide detectors should be replaced after ten years of use; many states have passed laws requiring newly installed detectors to use ten-year batteries. If possible, install networked smoke detectors so that when one alarms they all alarm. Develop a fire escape plan and practice it so that you'll be prepared if an emergency does occur.
2. To prevent electrocution injuries, put non-choking-hazard safety plugs or covers in all unused electrical outlets so that your child can't stick their finger or a toy into the holes. If your child won't stay away from outlets, block access to them with furniture. Keep electrical cords out of reach and sight.
3. To prevent slipping, carpet your stairs where possible. Be sure the carpet is firmly tacked down at the edges. When your child is just learning to crawl and walk,

install safety gates at both the top and bottom of stairs. Avoid accordion-style gates, which can trap an arm or neck, and instead use gates firmly mounted to the home's wall studs.

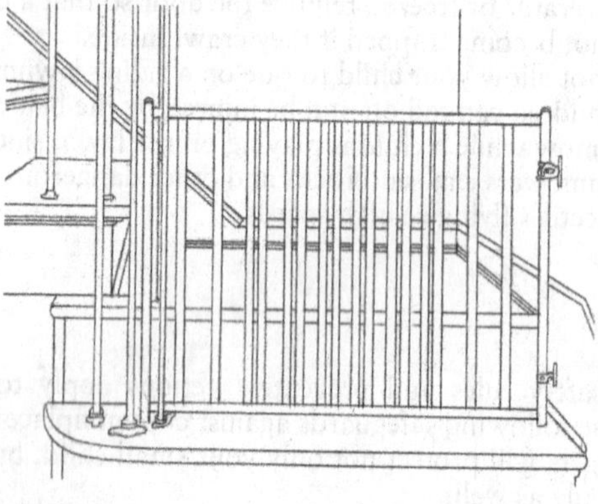

Safe, horizontal-type gate with slats 2⅜ inches (6 cm) apart

4. Certain houseplants may be harmful. The Poison Help line (1-800-222-1222) or the National Capital Poison Center (poison.org/articles/plant) has a list and descriptions of plants to avoid. You may want to forgo houseplants for a while or, at the very least, keep houseplants out of reach.
5. To prevent a choking injury, check floors constantly for small objects a child might swallow, such as coins, buttons, beads, pins, and screws. The best way to check is to get down at your child's level and see what's there. This is particularly important if someone in the household has a hobby involving small items, or if there are older children who have small items.
6. Button and coin batteries can cause life-threatening risks when swallowed. These batteries are found in many common household and personal electronic products, such as small remote controls, calculators, thermometers, digital scales, key fobs, musical greeting cards, cameras, garage door openers, flameless candles, watches, toys, flashing holiday jewelry or decorations, tracking devices, and hearing aids. If they are ingested, coin batteries can become stuck, and the battery can

cause serious damage to the esophagus in as little as two hours; severe injuries may result in death. If a button battery is placed inside the nose or ear canal, it can cause serious tissue injury and should be removed by a medical professional as quickly as possible. If you own any electronic devices that feature compartments that house a battery, be sure to check them often to ensure they are secure. It is important to always keep devices that are button- or coin-battery-controlled and any type of battery out of reach or locked away, especially for children ages 5 and under. If you know or suspect your child may have swallowed a battery, review the following steps:

- —Go immediately to the emergency department.
- —Do not induce vomiting.
- —Do not have your child eat or drink anything.
- —Call the 24/7 National Battery Ingestion Hotline (1-800-498-8666).

7. Children can suffer head injuries and cuts or injuries to their teeth when they fall while running. If you have hardwood floors, don't let your child run around in socks, which make slippery floors even more dangerous.
8. The Consumer Product Safety Commission recommends using cordless window coverings in all homes with children to prevent children from becoming strangled by cords. If your window products are not cordless, attach cords for window blinds and drapes to floor mounts that hold them taut, or wrap cords around wall brackets to keep them out of reach. Use safety stop devices on the cords. Cords with loops should be cut and equipped with safety tassels.
9. Pay attention to doors between rooms. Glass doors are particularly dangerous because a child may run into them. Fasten them open if possible. Swinging doors can knock a small child down, and folding doors can pinch little fingers. If you have either type of door, consider removing them until your child is old enough to understand how they work.
10. Sharp edges of furniture can injure a running or falling child. Check your home for furniture with hard edges and sharp corners that could injure your child (coffee tables are a particular hazard). If possible, remove dangerous furniture from traffic areas, particularly

when your child is learning to walk. You also can buy cushioned corner and edge protectors that can be applied to furniture.

11. To prevent crush injuries from furniture, test the stability of large pieces of furniture, such as floor lamps, bookshelves, and television stands. Put floor lamps behind other furniture, and anchor bookcases, dressers, and TV stands to the wall. Deaths and injuries occur when children climb onto, fall against, or pull themselves up on large pieces of furniture. Secure televisions to the wall or to a low, stable stand designed to hold them; children have died from being crushed by a falling television.
12. Keep computers out of reach so that your child cannot pull them over onto themselves. Cords should be out of sight and reach.
13. To prevent fall injuries from windows, open windows from the top if possible. If you must open them from the bottom, install operable window guards only an adult or older child can open. A screen is not strong enough to prevent a fall. Never put chairs, sofas, low tables, or anything else a child might climb on in front of a window. Doing so gives them access to the window and creates an opportunity for a serious fall.
14. To prevent suffocation injuries, never leave plastic bags lying around the house, and don't store children's clothes or toys in them, as children can suffocate inside them. Dry-cleaning bags are particularly dangerous. Knot them before you throw them away so that it's impossible for your child to crawl into them or pull them over their head. Even a small torn-off piece can become a potential choking hazard.
15. Think about the potential hazard of anything you put into the trash. Any trash container used for potentially dangerous items—spoiled food, discarded razor blades, batteries—should have a child-resistant cover or be kept out of reach.
16. To prevent burns, check your heat sources. Fireplaces, woodstoves, and kerosene heaters should be screened so that your child can't get near them. Gas fireplaces with glass doors get extremely hot, stay very hot long after the fireplace is turned off, and can cause severe burns

when touched. Check electric baseboard heaters, radiators, and even vents from hot-air furnaces to see how hot they get when the heat is on. They, too, may need to be screened.

17. If firearms are kept in the house, layers of barriers to prevent unauthorized access are essential to decrease the risk of intentional (e.g., suicide or homicide) or unintentional shootings. For safety, store the firearm unloaded, lock away the firearm, and store ammunition separately in a locked place. In other homes where your child spends time, it is also important to ask how firearms are stored. (Also see Where We Stand, *below.*)
18. Alcohol can be very toxic to a young child. Keep all alcoholic beverages in a locked cabinet and empty any unfinished drinks immediately.

Where We Stand

Firearms increase the risk of injury, both intentional and unintentional, in the home. Safety options include storing firearms away safely or removing them from the home and storing them in another location (e.g., shooting range, firearms store).

Baby Equipment

The Consumer Product Safety Commission takes an active role in setting safety standards to ensure the safety of equipment manufactured for children and infants. The Consumer Product Safety Improvement Act of 2008 started a process of strengthening safety standards for many durable juvenile products, so you must pay special attention to the safety of furniture made before then. The following guidelines will help you select the safest possible baby equipment, whether used or new, and utilize it properly.

High Chairs

Falls are the most serious danger associated with high chairs. To minimize the risk of your child falling:

1. Select a chair with a wide base, so it can't tip over.
2. If the chair folds, make sure the locking device is secure each time you set it up.
3. Strap your child in with the shoulder, waist, and crotch safety straps whenever they sit in the chair. Never allow them to stand in the high chair.
4. Don't place the high chair near a counter or table; your child may be able to push hard enough against these surfaces to tip the chair over. Never place the chair within reach of a hot or dangerous object.
5. Never leave a young child unattended in a high chair, and don't allow older children to climb or play on it, as this could cause it to tip over.
6. A high chair that hooks onto a table is not a substitute for a more solid one. But if you plan to use such a model when you eat out or travel, look for one that locks onto the table. Be sure the table is heavy enough to support your child's weight without tipping. Also, check to see whether their feet can touch a table support. If they can push against it, they may be able to dislodge the seat from the table.
7. Check that all caps or plugs on chair tubing are firmly attached and cannot be pulled off; these could be choking hazards.

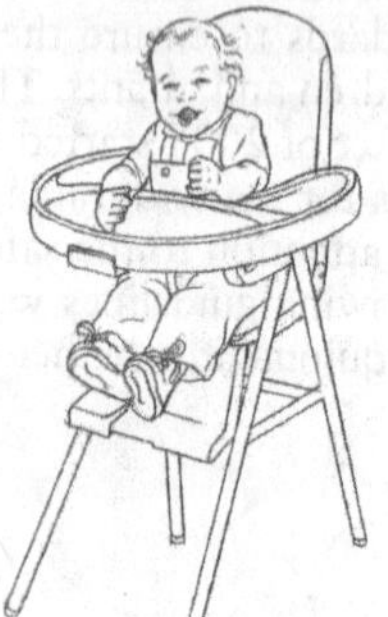

Infant Seats and Bouncers

Infant seats and bouncers should be labeled to meet CPSC safety standard F2167. Use care in selecting an infant seat. Check the weight guidelines provided by the manufacturer, and don't use the seat after your baby has outgrown it. Here are some other safety guidelines to follow:

1. Do not put the seat above floor level. The most serious injuries associated with infant seats occur when a baby falls from a high surface, such as a table, countertop, or chair. Even small infants can jiggle a seat or carrier off a surface and fall, suffering head trauma and other injuries. To keep an active, squirming baby from tipping the seat over, place it on a carpeted area near you and away from sharp-edged furniture. Infant seats also may tip over when placed on soft surfaces, such as beds or upholstered furniture; these are not safe places for infant seats.
2. Never leave a baby unattended in an infant seat.
3. Never use an infant seat as a substitute for a car safety seat. Infant seats are designed only for propping a baby up so that they can see, play, or be fed more easily.
4. Always buckle the safety strap and harness.
5. Choose a seat with an outside frame that allows the infant to sit deep inside. Be sure the base is wide, to prevent tipping over.
6. Look at the bottom of the infant seat to ensure that it's covered with a non-skid material.
7. Parents should remove the infant from the seat before moving the seat to avoid falling or other injuries to the baby.
8. Never place a baby in an infant seat or a car safety seat on the roof or back of a car, even for a moment.
9. Infants should never sleep in a sitting device. If your baby falls asleep in a car safety seat (while the car is not in motion) or bouncer, move them to a crib, bassinet, or portable play yard right away.

Play Yards

Most parents depend on play yards (sometimes called playpens) as a safe place to put a baby when parents aren't available to watch them every moment. Yet play yards, too, can be dangerous under certain circumstances. To prevent mishaps:

1. Choose a play yard with a label stating it meets ASTM F406, a safety standard that will ensure it is designed and built to prevent injuries. This standard is mandatory for all new play yards.
2. Do not add a supplemental mattress to the play yard. This is a suffocation hazard. Your baby will be comfortable using just the mattress that came with the play yard. If your baby sleeps in the play yard, follow safe sleep practices: Remove pillows, blankets, and stuffed toys, and put your baby on their back.
3. Never leave the side of a mesh play yard lowered. An infant who rolls into the pocket created by the slack mesh can become trapped and suffocate.
4. Do not tie toys to the sides or across the top of a play yard, as a baby or toddler can become entangled.
5. If your play yard has a raised changing table, always remove the changing table when your child is in the play yard so that they cannot become entrapped or strangled in the space between the changing table and the side rail.
6. When your child can pull themselves to a standing position, remove any boxes or large toys in the play yard they could use to climb out.
7. Teething children may gnaw on the top rails. Check them periodically for tears and holes in the fabric. If the tears are small, repair them with heavy-duty cloth tape; if more extensive, contact the manufacturer to find out how to repair.
8. Be sure a play yard's mesh is free of tears, holes, or loose threads and that the openings are less than ¼ inch (0.6 cm) across so your child cannot get caught in it. The mesh should be securely attached to the top rail and floor plate. If staples are used, they should not be missing, loose, or exposed. Slats on wooden play yards

should be no more than 2⅜ inches (6 cm) apart so that your child's head cannot become trapped between them.

9. Circular enclosures made from accordion-style fences are extremely dangerous. Children can get their heads caught in the diamond-shaped openings and the V-shaped border at the top of the gate. Never use such an enclosure, either indoors or out.

Walkers

The American Academy of Pediatrics does not recommend the use of mobile infant walkers. Children can fall down stairs, leading to head injuries. If the walker runs into a piece of furniture like a table or bookshelf, objects may fall off the furniture and injure the child. Walkers do not help a child learn to walk, and they can delay normal motor development. A stationary walker or activity center is a better choice. These do not have wheels, but seats that rotate and bounce. You may also consider a sturdy wagon or a kiddie push car. The toy should have a bar they can push, and it should be weighted so that it won't tip over when they pull themselves up on it.

Pacifiers

Pacifiers will not harm your baby. In fact, there is evidence that pacifiers may help reduce the risk of sudden infant death syndrome (SIDS) when your infant is being placed for sleep. However, for maximum safety, use the following tips when using a pacifier:

1. Do not use the top and nipple from a baby bottle as a pacifier, even if you tape them together. If the baby sucks hard, the nipple may pop out of the ring and choke them.
2. Purchase pacifiers that cannot possibly come apart. If you are in doubt, ask your pediatrician for a recommendation.
3. The shield between the nipple and the ring should be at least 1½ inches (3.8 cm) across so that the infant cannot take the entire pacifier into their mouth. Also, the shield

should be made of firm plastic or silicone with ventilation holes.

4. Never tie a pacifier to your child's crib or around your child's neck or hand. This is very dangerous and could cause serious injury or even death.
5. Pacifiers deteriorate over time. Inspect them periodically to see whether the material is discolored or torn. If so, replace them.
6. Follow the recommended age range on the pacifier, as older children can sometimes fit smaller newborn-size pacifiers in their mouths and choke.

Toy Boxes and Toy Chests

A toy box can be dangerous for two reasons: A child could become trapped inside, or a hinged lid could fall on your child's head or body while they are searching for a toy. If possible, store toys on open shelves your child can get to easily. If you must use a toy box:

1. Look for one with no top, a lightweight removable lid, or sliding doors or panels. However, little fingers can easily be injured under lids and between sliding doors and panels.
2. If you use a toy box with a hinged lid, be sure it has a lid support that holds the lid open at any angle. If your toy box didn't come with such a support, install one yourself—or remove the lid.
3. Look for a toy box with rounded or padded edges and corners, or add the padding yourself.
4. Children occasionally get trapped inside toy boxes. Your box should have ventilation holes or a gap between the lid and the box. Don't block the holes by pushing the box tight against a wall. The lid should not latch.

Toys

Most toy manufacturers want to produce safe toys, but they cannot always anticipate the way a child might use—or abuse—their products. In 2021, there were an estimated

206,000 toy-related injuries treated in US emergency rooms. Of these, 37 percent (76,220) involved children under age 5. If your child is injured by an unsafe product or you would like to report a product-related injury, visit saferproducts.gov. The Consumer Product Safety Commission keeps a record of complaints and initiates recalls of dangerous toys, clothing, jewelry, and other household products. Your report may protect not only your child, but others as well.

When selecting or using toys, always observe the following safety guidelines:

1. Match toys to your child's age and abilities. Follow the manufacturer's guidelines on the packaging.
2. Rattles—probably your child's first toy—should be at least 1⅝ inches (4 cm) across. An infant's mouth and throat are very flexible, and a smaller rattle could cause choking. Rattles should have no detachable parts.
3. Toys should be constructed of sturdy materials that won't break or shatter when a child throws or bangs them.
4. Check squeeze toys to ensure the squeaker can't become detached.
5. Before giving your child a stuffed animal or a doll, make sure the eyes and other parts are firmly attached; check them periodically. Remove all ribbons. If a doll comes packaged with accessories, don't allow your child to suck on a doll pacifier or any other accessory small enough to be swallowed.
6. Swallowing or inhaling small toy parts is a serious danger to young children. Inspect toys carefully for small parts that could fit in your child's mouth and throat. Look for toys labeled for children 3 and under, because they must have no small parts likely to be swallowed or inhaled.
7. Toys with small magnets are especially dangerous. If more than one magnet is swallowed, the magnets can attract each other in the child's body and cause intestinal blockages, perforations, and even death. Keep toys with small magnets away from children. High-powered magnets are extremely dangerous when more than one is swallowed; keep all high-powered magnets out of sight and reach of children.
8. Toys with small parts purchased for older children should be stored out of reach of younger ones. Impress

on your older child the importance of picking up all the pieces from such toys when they're finished playing. You should check that there are no items dangerous for your baby left out. Consider restricting the use of these toys to a small area or places inaccessible to the baby.

9. Don't let a child play with balloons; they may inhale a balloon if they try to blow it up. If a balloon pops, pick up and discard all the pieces. Mylar balloons are a safer choice than latex.
10. To prevent both burns and electrical shocks, don't give young children (under age 10) a toy that must be plugged into an electrical outlet. Instead, buy battery-operated toys. Be sure that the battery cover is securely fastened in an enclosure that requires a screwdriver or other tool to open, in order to prevent a loose battery from becoming a choking hazard. All newer battery-powered toys meet this guideline, but check older toys, and do not use them if the batteries can be accessed without a screwdriver. If a toy uses round button-cell batteries, cover old batteries with tape and discard them immediately in a secure trash can, and keep replacement batteries in their package in a high, locked cabinet out of sight and reach. Check toys' battery compartments periodically to ensure the screws have not loosened.
11. Ensure that teething children do not have access to electrical cords, which they might bite through, risking electrical burns.
12. Carefully inspect toys with mechanical parts for springs, gears, or hinges that could trap a child's fingers, hair, or clothing.
13. Register any applicable toys with the manufacturer in order to be informed of any recalls.
14. To prevent cuts, check toys to ensure they don't have sharp edges or pointed pieces. Avoid toys with parts made of glass or rigid plastic that could crack or shatter.
15. Don't allow your child to play with very noisy toys, including squeeze toys with unexpectedly loud squeakers. Noise levels at or above 100 decibels can damage hearing.
16. Projectile toys such as dart guns or slingshots are not suitable for children. They can easily cause eye injuries. Never give your child a toy that fires anything except water.

HOW TO REPORT UNSAFE PRODUCTS

If you become aware of an unsafe product used by children—or if your child suffers an injury related to a particular product—report it to the Consumer Product Safety Commission (CPSC) at saferproducts.gov. Your report is important for helping the CPSC identify hazardous products requiring further investigation or a potential recall.

Safety Outside the Home

Even if you create the perfect environment inside your home, your child will spend a lot of time outside, where surroundings are less controllable. Obviously, your personal supervision will remain the most valuable protection, but even a well-supervised child is exposed to many hazards. The following information will show how to eliminate many of these hazards and reduce the risk your child will be injured.

Car Safety Seats

Each year, an average of 3,460 children between the ages of 1 and 19 are killed in car crashes. Many deaths can be prevented if the children are properly restrained in a car safety seat when riding in a motor vehicle. Contrary to what some believe, a parent's lap is the most dangerous place for a child to ride. In a car crash or even a sudden stop or swerve, you wouldn't be able to hold on to your child, and your body would crush theirs as you were thrown against the dashboard and windshield. Not even the strongest adult can keep hold of a child while experiencing the massive forces of a crash. The single most important way to keep your child safe in the car is to buy, install, and use an approved car safety seat, appropriate for the age and size of your child, every time they ride in the car. Children should ride in the rear seat until they turn 13 years old in order to prevent brain or spine injuries from front seat airbags.

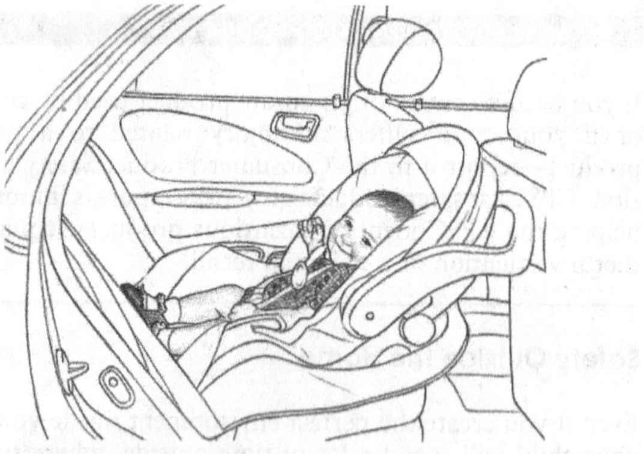

Rear-facing-only car safety seat

Car safety seats are required by law in all fifty states, the District of Columbia, and US territories. Unfortunately, studies consistently show that many parents do not use them properly. The most common mistakes include facing car safety seats in the wrong direction (facing forward too soon), not keeping your child in a car safety seat long enough, placing rear-facing seats in front of an airbag, failing to strap or fasten the child into the car safety seat, failing to securely fasten the child's car safety seat to the vehicle seat, not adequately tightening the straps, not using a booster seat for older children, and letting a child ride in the front seat. Remember that it is very important to use the car safety seat, even on short trips. Most fatal crashes occur within 5 miles (8 km) of home and at speeds of less than 25 miles (40 km) per hour. For all these reasons, children continue to be at risk. It's not enough to have a car safety seat—you must use it correctly, every time, in the backseat.

Choosing a Car Safety Seat

Here are guidelines for selecting a car safety seat:

1. The American Academy of Pediatrics annually publishes a list of car safety seats available, "Car Safety Seats: Product Listing," which can be found online at HealthyChildren.org/carseatlist.

2. No one seat is "safest" or "best." The "best" car safety seat is one that fits your child's size and weight and can be installed correctly in your car and used correctly on every trip.
3. Price does not always make a difference. Higher prices can mean added features that may or may not make the seat easier to use.
4. When you find a seat you like, try it out. Put your child in the seat and adjust the harnesses and buckles. Make sure it fits in your car and that the harnesses are easy to adjust when the seat is in your car. Some big-box stores will allow you to take a loaner seat out to your car to see how it fits.
5. If your baby is born preterm, they should be monitored in their car safety seat by hospital staff before leaving the hospital to ensure that the semi-reclined position does not cause low heart rate, low oxygen, or other breathing problems. If the pediatrician advises you that your baby needs to lie flat during travel, use a crash-tested car bed. If possible, an adult should ride in the backseat next to your baby to watch them closely.

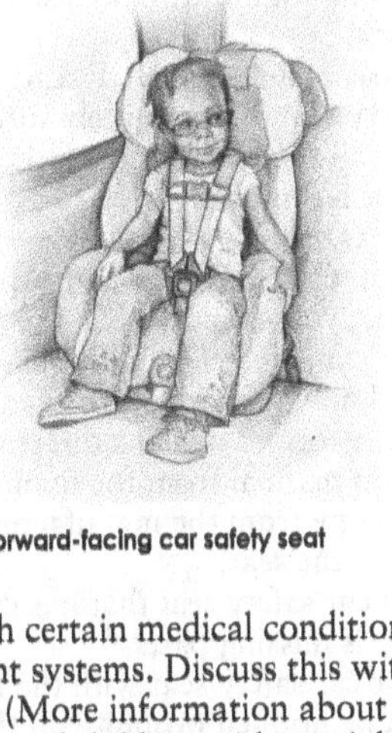

Forward-facing car safety seat

6. Children with certain medical conditions may need other restraint systems. Discuss this with your pediatrician. (More information about safe transportation of children with special healthcare needs is available from the Automotive Safety Program

by phone at 1-800-543-6227 or on their website at preventinjury.org.)

7. Do not use a car safety seat that is too old. The label has the date of manufacture. Many manufacturers recommend seats be used for only six years. Check the instruction manual for the expiration date; this may also be found on a label on the seat or stamped into the plastic shell. Over time, and with exposure to heat and cold, the car safety seat parts can become weakened. It is important not to use a car safety seat past the manufacturer's expiration date.
8. If a car safety seat was in a moderate or severe crash, it may have been weakened and should not be used, even if it looks fine. Seats that were in minor crashes may still be safe to use. A crash is considered minor if the vehicle can be driven away from the crash, the door closest to the car safety seat was not damaged, no one in the vehicle was injured, the airbags did not go off, and you can't see any damage to the car safety seat. Some manufacturers still recommend replacing a seat after even a minor crash. Check the instruction manual or call the car safety seat manufacturer if you have questions about your seat. Only use a seat if you know its full history.
9. It is best to use a new car safety seat. If you choose a used car safety seat, be absolutely sure it has never been in any crash, all the labels and instructions are present, and it has not been recalled.
10. Do not use a car safety seat missing a label with the date of manufacture and seat name or model number. Without these, you cannot check for recalls.
11. Do not use a car safety seat with missing instructions. You need to know how to use the car safety seat. Do not rely on the former owner's directions. Get a copy of the instruction manual from the manufacturer or download a copy from the manufacturer's website before you use the seat.
12. Do not use a car safety seat that has cracks in the frame of the seat or is missing parts.
13. Register your car safety seat with the manufacturer so that you can be notified promptly in the event of a recall. Newly purchased seats will have a registration card attached, or you can register the seat on the

manufacturer's website or by calling its customer service department.

14. You can find out if your car safety seat has been recalled by calling the manufacturer or the US Department of Transportation's Vehicle Safety Hotline at 1-888-327-4236 from 8 a.m. to 8 p.m. ET, Monday through Friday. This information is also available on the National Highway Traffic Safety Administration website: nhtsa.gov/recalls. If the seat has been recalled, follow instructions to fix it or get the necessary parts.

Types of Car Safety Seats

Infants/Toddlers

All infants and toddlers should ride in a rear-facing car safety seat as long as possible, or until they reach the highest weight or height allowed by the car safety seat manufacturer. They should be positioned in the backseat. This is the safest way to ride. Although your child may outgrow an infant-only rear-facing car seat at some point in the first two years of life, nearly all convertible car safety seats have rear-facing weight and height limits that allow most children to ride rear-facing well past the second birthday.

Installing a Car Safety Seat

1. Read your vehicle owner's manual for important information on how to install the car safety seat correctly in your vehicle.
2. To prevent head and spine injuries from the deployment of an airbag in the event of a crash, the safest place for all children to ride is in the backseat. Avoid driving more children than can be buckled safely in the backseat.
3. Never place a child in a rear-facing car safety seat in the front seat of a vehicle with a passenger airbag. All new cars have airbags. When used with seatbelts, airbags work very well to protect older children and adults. However, airbags are very dangerous when used with rear-facing car safety seats. If your car has a passenger

airbag, children in rear-facing seats must ride in the backseat. Even in a low-speed crash, the airbag can inflate, strike the car safety seat, and cause serious brain injury and death. Toddlers who ride in forward-facing car safety seats are also at risk from airbag injuries. Remember, all children younger than 13 are safest in the backseat.

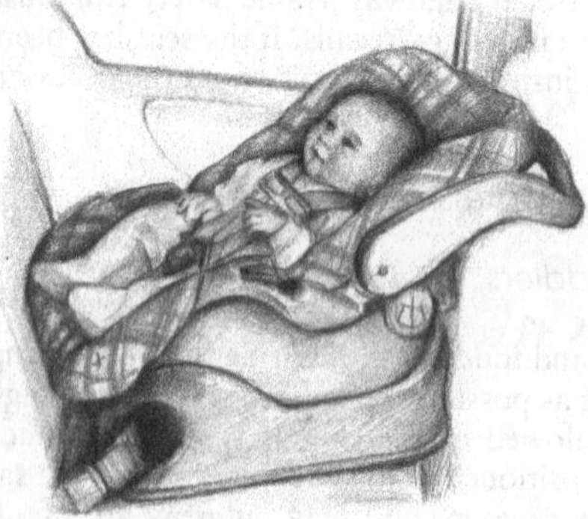

If you have a pickup truck without a backseat or with a backseat that is too small for a properly installed car safety seat, it may be possible in some cases to install a car safety seat in the front seat. Keep in mind, though, that a rear-facing car safety seat can never be installed in a seating position with an active front airbag. Do not rely on the vehicle sensor to disable the airbag; only use that seating position if the airbag can be deactivated with a key. Installing a car safety seat in a pickup truck, even in the backseat if there is one, can be more complicated than installing in other vehicles, so read the owner's manuals for both the pickup truck and the car safety seat and follow the instructions carefully.

4. Car safety seats can be installed using either the vehicle seatbelts or the LATCH (Lower Anchors and Tethers for Children) system. LATCH is a system of lower anchors located in the seat bight (where the vehicle cushions meet) and tether anchors located on the shelf behind the seat (in most sedans) or on the floor, ceiling, or back of the seat (in most minivans, SUVs, and hatchbacks). The systems are equally safe, but in some

cases, it may be easier to install a seat tightly using LATCH. You should use the seatbelt or LATCH, but not both, unless the car safety seat manual specifically allows using both at the same time.

5. Place the seat facing the correct direction for the size and age of your child. Route the seatbelt or LATCH strap through the correct path on the car safety seat (check your instructions to make sure) and pull it tight. Before each trip, check to make sure the car safety seat is installed tightly enough by pulling on the car safety seat where the seatbelt or LATCH strap passes through. It should not move more than an inch side to side or toward the front of the car.
6. If your infant's head flops forward, the seat may not be reclined enough. Recline the seat to the correct angle according to the manufacturer's instructions; there may be different recline settings for very young infants and for older babies. Your seat may have a recline indicator to help determine whether the angle is correct and a built-in adjuster for this purpose. If not, you may wedge firm padding, such as a rolled towel, under the seat's front base.
7. If the seatbelt buckle lies just at the point where the belt bends around the car safety seat, it may be impossible to make the belt tight enough. If you cannot get the belt tight, try another position in the car or consider using LATCH if it is available.
8. If you install a car safety seat using the vehicle seatbelt instead of LATCH, the seatbelt must be locked tightly in place. In many vehicles, you can lock the seatbelt by pulling the shoulder belt all the way out, then feeding it back into the retractor. In many cases, it may be easier to use (or the car safety seat manufacturer may advise using) a built-in lock-off that comes with the car safety seat to lock the seatbelt. Read your car owner's manual and car safety seat instructions to determine the best way to lock the seatbelt.
9. In rare situations, a lap-only belt may need a special, heavy-duty locking clip, available from the vehicle manufacturer. Check your car owner's manual for more information.
10. Before using LATCH, check the car safety seat and vehicle instructions for information, including the

weight limits for the lower anchors and attachments and which seating positions can be used for LATCH installation. Check the vehicle instruction manual to ensure you don't attach the tether to a cargo tie-down or other attachment point not designed as a tether anchor.

11. Tethers should always be used with forward-facing car safety seats. Most anchors are located on the rear window ledge, the back of the vehicle seat, or the floor or ceiling of the vehicle. Tethers give extra protection by keeping the car safety seat from being thrown forward in a crash. All new cars, minivans, and light trucks are required to have tether anchors for securing the tops of car safety seats. If your vehicle was manufactured before September 2000, it may be possible to have a tether anchor installed by a dealer, often at no cost.
12. For specific information about installing your car safety seat, consult a certified child passenger safety (CPS) technician. A list of certified CPS technicians is available by state or ZIP code at cert.safekids.org (click on "Find a Tech"). A list of inspection stations staffed by certified CPS technicians is also available online at nhtsa.gov/equipment/car-seats-and-booster-seats. In addition, the information can be accessed by telephone on the Department of Transportation's Vehicle Safety Hotline at 1-888-327-4236, from 8 a.m. to 8 p.m. ET, Monday through Friday.

Using the Car Safety Seat

1. A car safety seat protects your child only if they are buckled securely every time they ride—no exceptions, beginning with your baby's first ride home from the hospital. Help your child form a lifelong habit of buckling up by always using your seatbelt. If you have two cars, buy two seats or transfer the seat to the car in which your child will be traveling. Remember never to place a rear-facing car safety seat in the front seat if there is an airbag. The safest place for all children to ride is in the back.
2. Read and follow the car safety seat manufacturer's instructions, and always keep them with the car safety

seat. If you lose the instructions, call or write the manufacturer for a replacement. In many cases, you can download the instructions from the manufacturer's website.

3. Most children go through a stage when they protest whenever you put them in the car safety seat. Explain firmly that you cannot drive until everyone is buckled. Then back up your words with action.
4. Use the correct harness slots for the child. When riding rear-facing, the harness straps should be at or below your child's shoulder level. When riding forward-facing, they should be at or above the shoulders. Some seats do not have slots, but instead use a sliding mechanism to move the harness straps up and down. Read the instructions to see how and where to adjust the harness strap height.
5. The harness straps should be snug against your child's body. Dress your baby in clothes that allow the straps to go between their legs. Keep the straps snug so that they hold your child securely; if you can pinch a fold of webbing between your fingers, they are too loose. Be certain the straps lie flat and are not twisted.
6. If needed to keep your newborn from slouching, pad the sides of the seat and behind the crotch strap with rolled-up diapers or receiving blankets. Do not use add-on products behind the baby or between the baby and the harness straps; these can cause the straps to not restrain the baby properly in a crash. Some seats for newborns include an insert to improve the harness fit; these are okay to use, but never use any add-on products that did not come with your car safety seat or are not specifically allowed by the manufacturer's instructions.
7. In cold weather, dress your baby in thinner layers rather than thickly padded clothes, and tuck blankets around your baby after adjusting the harness straps snugly. Do not use bunting products that have a layer that goes underneath your baby.
8. In hot weather, drape a towel over the seat when the car is in the sun. Before putting your child in the seat, test the fabrics and metal buckle with your hand to ensure they aren't hot.

9. No matter how short your errand is, never leave an infant or child alone in a car. They can get overheated or too cold very quickly, even if the temperature outside seems mild, or they may become frightened and panicky when they realize they're alone. Children left alone in cars in hot weather can die from hyperthermia (overheating) in less than ten minutes. Any parent, no matter how loving and attentive, can accidentally forget a child in the car. Take steps to prevent this by incorporating visual reminders or check-ins into your routine:
    - Put something you need at your destination, like your purse or briefcase or a shoe, in the backseat, where you must open the back door to retrieve it.
    - Put a large stuffed toy in the car safety seat when your child is not in the car, and when your child rides with you, move the toy into the front seat where you will see it.
    - Ask your childcare provider to call if your child does not arrive when expected.
    - Be especially vigilant when the usual routine is changed; the risk of forgetting a child is higher during such disruptions.
    - Lock your car and set the parking brake when not in use so that children cannot get inside. Overheating deaths have occurred when children got into cars to play. If a child is missing, check the pool or other body of water first, and then check the car, including the trunk.
10. Always use your seatbelt. In addition to setting a good example, you'll reduce your own risk of injury or death in a crash by 60 percent.
11. Never let your infant sleep in a car safety seat outside of the car. It is fine to sleep in the car safety seat while riding in the car, but when you reach your destination, move your baby to a crib, bassinet, or portable play yard to finish napping.
12. Never place your infant in a car safety seat with unbuckled or partially buckled straps, as there is a risk of strangulation.

Airbag Safety

An airbag can save your life. However, airbags and young children do not mix. The following information will help keep you and your children safe. (This information is worth repeating.)

- The safest place for all infants to ride is in the backseat. When front seat airbags deploy, they can injure children's brains or spines.
- Never put a rear-facing car safety seat in the front seat of a car with an airbag. Your child can suffer a serious injury or death from the impact of the airbag against the back of the car safety seat. (See *page 326* of this chapter for information on pickup trucks and car safety seats.)
- Infants and toddlers should ride in a rear-facing car safety seat until they reach the height or weight limit set by the manufacturer. Nearly all convertible car safety seats have weight and height limits that allow most children to ride rear-facing well past the second birthday. Rear-facing is the safest way to ride. It is best to ride that way as long as possible.
- All children should be properly secured in car safety seats or booster seats correct for their age and size.
- Side airbags improve safety for adults in side impact crashes. When children ride next to side airbags, it is essential they be restrained in the proper position. Read your car safety seat manual for guidance on placing the seat next to a side airbag and refer to your vehicle owner's manual for recommendations that apply to your vehicle.

KEEPING YOUR CHILD HAPPY AND SAFE ON THE ROAD

As hard as you may try to enforce car safety seat and seatbelt use, your child may resist these constraints as they get older. Here are some tips to keep them occupied and content—and safe—while the car is in motion.

Birth to 9 Months

- Ensure your newborn's comfort by padding the sides of their car safety seat with receiving blankets if necessary to prevent slouching. Padding should only be added outside the harness straps, never under your baby or between your baby and the harness straps.
- If needed, place a small rolled-up cloth diaper or receiving blanket between the crotch strap and your baby to prevent their lower body from sliding too far forward.
- If your infant's head flops forward, double-check whether the seat has been reclined enough. Follow the manufacturer's instructions on how to achieve the proper recline angle.

9 to 24 Months

- Children this age love to climb and may want desperately to get out of the car safety seat. If this describes your child, remind yourself this is only a phase. As mentioned, insist in a calm but stern voice that they stay in their seat whenever the car is on the road. Let them know the car cannot move unless everyone is buckled in, then follow through if they try to escape their seat. Keep the harness straps snug and the harness clip at chest level to make it more difficult for them to escape.
- Entertain your toddler by talking or singing with them as you drive. However, never do this to the point where it distracts you from paying attention to driving.

Kids Around Cars

From a young age, teach children not to walk or play in the street or driveway. Young children are not safe around streets and should not play near them. While they have the skills to get to roads and streets, they do not have the ability to recognize that streets and cars are dangerous. Children move quickly and impulsively. They are curious. Yet they have difficulty seeing cars in their peripheral vision, localizing sounds, and understanding traffic and the meaning of signs and signals. They cannot judge speed and vehicle distance. Add in drivers who may be multitasking and not looking out for young children playing near the street, and a disaster could be in the making. If children are near streets, hands-on supervision is necessary for quick intervention if your child darts into the street to get a ball or to run after an older child.

To avoid injuries from vehicle back-overs, driveways, alleyways, and any adjacent unfenced front yards should not be used as play areas. Parents should remember the large blind spots behind cars (especially in bigger vehicles like SUVs and minivans) and the need to walk completely around the car before getting in and starting the engine. Never assume that having a backup camera is adequate to prevent backing over a fast-moving small child. Adults should make a point of knowing where the children are before putting a vehicle in reverse.

Where We Stand

All fifty states require children to ride in car safety seats. The American Academy of Pediatrics urges that all newborns discharged from hospitals be brought home in rear-facing car safety seats. The AAP has established car safety seat guidelines for low-birth-weight infants, which include having them ride in a rear-facing seat and supporting them with ample padding around the sides, outside the harness system. A convertible car safety seat is recommended as a child gets older.

Infants and young children must always ride in car safety seats—preferably in the backseat. Never use a rear-facing car safety seat in the front seat of a vehicle equipped with a passenger-side airbag. An infant or child should never ride in an adult's arms. Children age 12 and younger should ride in the rear seat.

Older children should use booster seats until the vehicle safety belt fits well, meaning the shoulder belt crosses the middle of the child's chest, the lap belt is low and snug across the thighs, the child can sit all the way back on the vehicle seat with knees bent at the edge, and the child is able to sit this way the entire ride. This position helps avoid injuries to the neck and internal organs from the seatbelt in case of a crash.

Baby Carriers: Backpacks, Front Packs, and Slings

Back and front carriers for infants are very popular. For your baby's—and your own—comfort and safety, follow these guidelines when purchasing and using baby carriers:

1. Infants born prematurely or with respiratory problems should not be placed in backpacks or other upright devices, as the positioning in these devices may make it harder for them to breathe.
2. Some sling carriers may curl your baby's body into a C-shape, which greatly increases the risk of breathing problems. If you use a sling, your baby's neck should be straight and their chin not pressed into their chest, and make sure you can always see their face.
3. In any type of carrier, check frequently to ensure that your baby's mouth and nose are not blocked by fabric or your body and that airflow is not restricted. The CPSC warns about the suffocation hazard to infants, particularly those younger than 4 months, carried in infant sling carriers. When infant slings are used for carrying, it is important to ensure that the infant's head is up and above the fabric, the face is visible, and the nose and mouth are clear of obstructions.
4. Take your baby with you when you shop for the carrier so that you can match it to their size. Make sure the carrier supports their back and the leg holes are small enough that they can't possibly slip through. Look for sturdy material.
5. If you buy a backpack, the frame should be padded so that your baby won't be hurt if they bump against it. A sunshade is also a good idea to shield your baby from the sun.
6. Check the pack periodically for rips and tears in the seams and fasteners.
7. When using a baby carrier, bend at the knees, not the waist, if you need to pick something up. Otherwise, the baby may tip out of the carrier, and you may hurt your back.
8. Babies over 5 months old may become restless in the carrier, so continue to use the restraining straps. Some children will brace their feet against the frame or

against your body, changing their weight distribution. You should be certain your child is seated properly before you walk.

9. Do not cook or handle hot foods or liquids while using a baby carrier, even if the baby is behind you on your back.

Strollers

Look for safety features and take the following precautions:

1. If you string toys across your stroller, fasten them securely so that they can't fall on the baby. Remove such toys as soon as the baby can sit or rise on all fours.
2. Strollers should have easy-to-operate brakes. Use the brake whenever stopped, and ensure your child can't reach the release lever. A brake that locks two wheels rather than just one provides an extra measure of safety.
3. Select a stroller with a wide base, to avoid tipping.
4. Children's fingers can become caught in the folding hinges of the stroller. Keep your child at a safe distance when opening and closing it. Securely lock open the stroller before putting your child in. Check that your baby's fingers cannot reach the stroller wheels.
5. Don't hang bags or other items from the handles of your stroller—they can make it tip backward. If the stroller has a basket for carrying things, be sure it is low and near the rear wheels.
6. The stroller should have a five-point harness (with straps over both shoulders and hips, and between the legs) that should be used whenever your child goes for a ride. For infants, use rolled-up baby blankets on either side of the seat if necessary to prevent slouching.

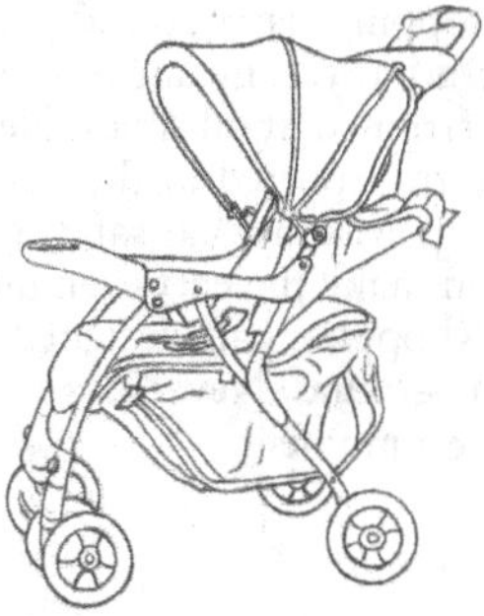

7. Never leave your child unattended in a stroller.

If they fall asleep in their stroller, make sure you can always see them.

8. If you purchase a side-by-side twin stroller, the footrest should extend all the way across both sitting areas. A child's foot can become trapped between separate footrests.
9. There are also strollers that allow an older child to sit or stand in the rear. Be mindful of weight guidelines, and be especially careful that the child in the back doesn't become overly active and tip the stroller.

Shopping Cart Safety

More than 20,000 children are treated in emergency departments for shopping-cart-related injuries each year. The most frequent kinds of injuries are contusions, abrasions, and lacerations, and most injuries are to the head or neck. Shopping-cart-related injuries can be serious enough to require hospitalization, often because of head injuries and serious fractures. Some deaths have even occurred.

Shopping carts are often unstable; it may take as little as 16 pounds (7.26 kg) of force on the handle to tip a cart. The design of shopping carts makes them tip over easily when a child is in the cart or in a car safety seat snapped onto the cart near the handle. The seats attached to the top of shopping carts or built into them won't prevent a child from falling out if they aren't properly restrained; these seats also won't prevent the cart from tipping over even if the child is restrained.

If possible, seek an alternative to placing your child in a shopping cart; consider using a stroller or baby carrier instead. If you must use a shopping cart, make sure your child is restrained at all times. Never allow them to stand in the cart, be transported in the basket, or ride on the outside. Do not snap an infant car safety seat onto the built-in cart seat, as this can make the cart even more unstable. If one is available, use a shopping cart designed to carry children in a seat lower to the ground. Never leave a child alone in a shopping cart, even for a moment.

Your Backyard

Your backyard can be a safe play area for your child if you eliminate potential hazards:

1. If you don't have a fenced yard, teach your child the boundaries where they should play. They may not always follow your guidelines, so watch them very closely. Always have a responsible person supervise outdoor play, as young children may wander off or get injured.
2. Check your yard for dangerous plants, and teach your child never to pick and eat anything from a plant, no matter how good it looks, without your permission. Plants are a leading cause of poisoning. If you are unsure about the plants in your yard, call the Poison Help line (1-800-222-1222) and request a list of poisonous plants common to your area. You can also see an extensive list of poisonous plants, with photos of each, at poison.org/articles/plant. If you have poisonous plants, either replace them or securely fence and lock that area of the yard.
3. If you use pesticides or herbicides in your yard, it's important to choose products labeled "safe for use around people and pets," as this means the product is registered with the EPA and poses no unreasonable risk to human health when used as directed. Always read and follow the instructions carefully on any products.
4. Don't use a power mower to cut the lawn when young children are around. Mowers may throw sticks or stones with enough force to injure children. Never allow your child on a riding mower even when you are driving. It is safest to keep young children indoors while the lawn is being mowed.
5. When you cook food outdoors, screen the grill so that your child cannot touch it, and explain that it is hot like the stove in the kitchen. Store propane grills so that your child cannot reach the knobs. Be sure charcoal is cold before dumping it.

Water Safety

Water is one of the most dangerous hazards your child will encounter. Young children can drown in only a few inches of water, even if they've had swimming instruction. All children should learn to swim, but parents should know swimming instruction and skills do not provide "drownproofing" for children of any age. Evidence now shows that children ages 1 to 4 may be less likely to drown if they have had formal swimming instruction with a focus on water survival. Even so, because the studies are small, and because they don't define what type of lessons work best, the American Academy of Pediatrics recommends swim lessons as a layer of protection against drowning that can begin for many children starting at age 1. A parent's decision to enroll young children in swim lessons should be based on the child's frequency of exposure to water, their emotional development, their physical abilities, and certain health concerns related to pool water infections and pool chemicals. The following can be helpful when considering swimming lessons:

1. You may be lulled into being less cautious because you think your child can swim, and children themselves may be emboldened to enter water without supervision.

Where We Stand

The American Academy of Pediatrics feels strongly that parents should never—even for a moment—leave children alone near open bodies of water (lakes, swimming pools), or near water in homes (bathtubs, spas). For backyard pools, rigid, motorized pool covers are not a substitute for four-sided fencing, since pool covers are unlikely to be used appropriately and consistently. Parents should learn CPR and keep a telephone and emergency equipment (e.g., life preservers) at poolside. Parents should stay within arm's length of young children whenever they are swimming and avoid distractions such as mobile phones.

2. Young children repeatedly immersed in water may swallow so much that they develop water intoxication. This can result in convulsions, shock, and even death.

Children under age 1 may participate in swimming programs with a parent as a fun, recreational activity, but because there is no evidence that programs intended to prevent drowning in infants less than 1 year are effective or safe, they should not be given this type of swim lessons.

When selecting a swimming program, choose a class that adheres to guidelines established by the national YMCA. Remember, even a child who knows how to swim needs to be watched constantly. Whenever your child is near water (e.g., swimming pools, ponds, oceans, lakes), follow these safety rules:

1. Be aware of small bodies of water your child might encounter, such as fishponds, ditches, fountains, rain barrels, watering cans—even a 5-gallon bucket used for car washing. Empty water containers when done using them. Children are drawn to water and need constant supervision to ensure they don't fall in. Remember that bacterial and chemical contamination can render any body of water unsafe, so check advisories before allowing your child to swim anywhere.
2. Children who are swimming—even in a shallow toddler's pool—always should be watched by an adult, preferably one who knows CPR. (See Cardiopulmonary Resuscitation (CPR) and Mouth-to-Mouth Resuscitation, *page 493*, and Choking, *page 494*.) The adult should provide touch supervision, remaining within arm's reach, whenever young children and those without swimming skills are in or around water. Empty and put away inflatable pools after each play session.
3. Enforce safety rules: No running near the pool and no pushing others underwater.
4. Don't allow your baby to use inflatable toys or mattresses to keep them afloat. These toys may deflate suddenly, or your child may slip off them into water that is too deep.
5. Be sure the deep and shallow ends of any pool are clearly marked. Never allow your child to dive into the shallow end.
6. If you have a home swimming pool, it should be completely surrounded with a four-sided fence that is at

least 4 feet (1.2 m) high and not attached to the house. It should have a self-closing, self-latching gate that opens away from the pool. Check the gate frequently to ensure that it is in good working order. Keep the gate closed and locked at all times. Be sure your child cannot manipulate the lock or climb the fence. No opening under the fence or between uprights should be more than 4 inches (10 cm) wide. Keep toys out of the pool area when not in use so that children are not tempted to get through the fence.

7. If your pool has a cover, remove it completely before swimming. Also, never allow your child to walk on the pool cover; water may have accumulated on it, making it as dangerous as the pool itself. Your child also could fall through and become trapped underneath. Do not use a pool cover in place of a four-sided fence because it is unlikely to be used appropriately and consistently.
8. Keep a safety ring with a rope beside the pool at all times. If possible, always have a phone at hand in the pool area, and keep emergency numbers in your contacts list.
9. Spas and hot tubs are dangerous for young children, who can easily drown or become overheated. Don't allow young children to use these facilities unless the temperature is turned down to 98 degrees Fahrenheit (36.6 degrees Celsius) and you are within arm's reach at all times. Even then, limit soaks to no more than fifteen minutes.
10. Your child should always wear a life jacket, or "boat coat," when swimming or riding in boats. A life jacket fits properly if you can't lift it off over your child's head after the child is fastened in. For the child under age 5, particularly the non-swimmer, it also should have a flotation collar to keep the head upright and the face out of the water.
11. Adults should not drink alcohol or use sedating medications when swimming or boating. It presents a danger for them as well as children they might be supervising. Adult supervisors should know CPR and how to swim.
12. Eliminate distractions while children are in the water. Talking on the phone, working on the computer, and other tasks need to wait until children are out of and

away from water. Consider assigning a "water watcher" whose sole responsibility is to keep close watch on children in or near the water, and rotate the responsibility frequently.

Safety Around Animals

Children are more likely than adults to be bitten by domesticated animals, including your family pet. This is particularly true when a new baby is brought home. At such times, the pet's response should be observed carefully, and it should not be left alone with the infant. After a two- or three-week get-acquainted period, the animal may become used to the baby. However, it is always wise to be cautious when the animal is around, regardless of how much your pet seems to enjoy the relationship.

If you are getting a companion pet for your child, wait until they are mature enough to handle and care for the animal—usually around age 5 or 6. Younger children have difficulty distinguishing an animal from a toy, so they may inadvertently provoke a bite through teasing or mistreatment. Remember that you have ultimate responsibility for your child's safety around any animal, so take the following precautions:

1. Look for a pet with a gentle disposition. An older animal is often a good choice, because a puppy or kitten may bite out of sheer friskiness. Avoid older pets raised in homes without children, however.
2. Treat your pet humanely so that it will enjoy human company. Don't tie a dog on a short rope or chain. Extreme confinement may make it anxious and aggressive.
3. Never leave a young child alone with an animal. Many bites occur during periods of playful roughhousing because the child doesn't realize the animal is overexcited.
4. Teach your child not to put their face close to an animal.
5. Don't allow your child to tease your pet by pulling its tail or taking away a toy or a bone. Make sure they don't disturb the animal when it's sleeping or eating.
6. Have all pets—both dogs and cats—immunized against rabies.

7. Obey local ordinances about licensing and leashing your pet. Be sure your pet is always under your control.
8. Find out which neighbors have dogs, so your child can meet animals they're likely to encounter. Teach your child how to greet a dog: After asking the owner for permission, the child should stand still while the dog sniffs them; then they can slowly extend their hand to pet the animal.
9. Wild animals can carry serious diseases that may be transmitted to humans. You (and family pets) need to avoid contact with rodents and other wild animals (raccoons, skunks, foxes) that can carry diseases ranging from hantavirus to plague, toxoplasmosis to rabies. To avoid wild animal bites, notify the health department or animal control whenever you see an animal that seems sick or injured, or one acting strangely. Don't try to catch the animal or pick it up. Teach your child to avoid all undomesticated animals.

In the Community and Neighborhood

Many parents worry about keeping their child safe in and around the neighborhood. Fortunately, child abductions are rare, although they understandably get plenty of media attention when they occur. Most abductions occur when children are taken by non-custodial parents, although a smaller number of abductions by strangers do take place each year.

Here are some suggestions to help keep your child safe:

- When shopping with your child, always keep an eye on them. They can move quickly in and out of sight—in an instant. You might encourage your child to hold on to your hand whenever you're out.
- When choosing a childcare center, ask about safety issues. Make sure a policy exists where your child is picked up only by a parent or another designated person.
- When hiring babysitters, always check references and/or ask for recommendations from friends and family members.

- For more information, contact the National Center for Missing & Exploited Children (1-800-843-5678; missingkids.com).

When planning ways to keep your child safe, remember they are constantly changing. Strategies that protect them from danger when they're 1 year old may no longer be adequate as they grow and become stronger, more curious, and more confident. Review your family's home and habits often to ensure your safeguards remain appropriate for your child's age, and balance supervision with opportunities for them to learn and play independently.

PART 2

The information and policies in this section, such as first-aid procedures for the choking child and cardiopulmonary resuscitation (CPR), are constantly changing. Ask your pediatrician or other qualified health professional for the latest information on these procedures.

It is rare for a child to become seriously ill with no warning. Based on your child's symptoms, you should always contact your pediatrician for advice. Timely treatment of symptoms can prevent an illness from getting worse or turning into an emergency. Although the focus of this publication is on the first year of life, some of the information in this section will also benefit your growing child beyond the first year.

CHAPTER 12

ABDOMINAL/ GASTROINTESTINAL TRACT

Children of all ages experience abdominal pain occasionally, but the causes of such pain in infants tend to be quite different from what they are in older children. Children of different age groups also react to pain differently. An older child may rub their abdomen and tell you they're having a "bellyache" or "tummyache," while a very young infant will show their distress by crying and pulling up their legs. Vomiting or excessive burping also may accompany crying in babies with abdominal pain.

Fortunately, most stomachaches disappear on their own and are not serious. However, if your child's complaints continue or worsen over a period of three to five hours, or if they have a fever, a severe sore throat, or an extreme and sustained change in appetite or energy level, you should notify your pediatrician immediately. These symptoms may indicate a more serious disorder.

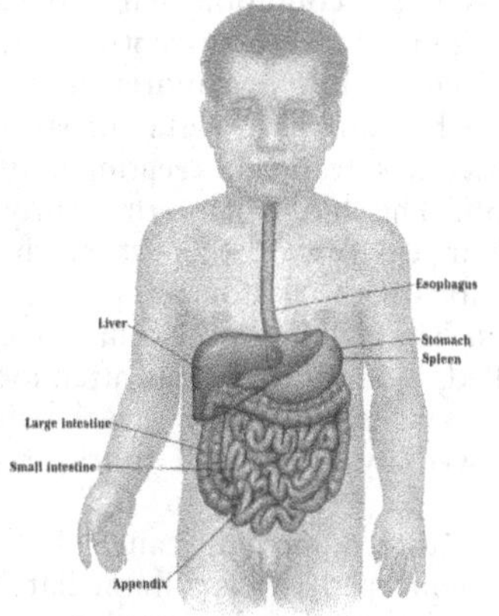

Abdomen/Gastrointestinal Tract

In this section, you'll find descriptions of problems that lead to abdominal pain in children, from colic to intestinal infections. You'll be referred to other sections of this chapter as well as other chapters in the book for more detailed descriptions of some of these disorders.

Abdominal Pain

Colic usually occurs in infants between the ages of 10 days and 3 months. It typically improves after three months, resolving by 1 year of age at the latest. While no one knows exactly what causes it, colic certainly looks like abdominal discomfort. The discomfort often is more severe in the late afternoon and early evening, and may be accompanied by inconsolable crying, pulling up of the legs, frequent passage of gas, and general irritability. You can try a variety of approaches to colic, which might include rocking your baby, walking with them in a baby carrier, swaddling them in a blanket, or giving them a pacifier. Some probiotic supplements have shown promise in easing colic symptoms, but so far, no medication or supplement has proven it can help colic symptoms. (For more information, see Crying and Colic, *page 140*.)

Intussusception is a rare condition that may cause abdominal pain in young infants. Intussusception is the most common abdominal emergency in children under age 2. This problem occurs when one part of the intestine slides inside another and becomes trapped, creating a blockage that causes severe pain. The child will intermittently and abruptly cry and pull their legs toward their stomach. This will be followed by periods without stomach pain and often without any distress. These children also may vomit and have dark, mucus-filled, bloody stools that often look like blackberry jelly. The pain is frequently severe, with periods of screaming followed by periods of quiet or even periods of lethargy.

It is important to recognize this cause of abdominal pain and to talk to your pediatrician immediately. They will want to see your child and perhaps order an ultrasound or an X-ray called an air contrast or barium enema. Sometimes doing this test not only enables the diagnosis but also unblocks the intestine. If the enema does not unblock the intestine, an emergency operation may be necessary to correct the problem.

Viral or bacterial infections of the intestine (gastroenteritis) are usually associated with diarrhea and/or vomiting. On-and-off abdominal pain is often also present. Most cases are viral, require only hydration and supportive care, and will resolve on their own within several days to a week; the pain itself generally lasts one or two days and then disappears. One exception is an infection caused by the *Giardia lamblia* parasite. This infestation may produce periodic recurrent pain not localized to any one part of the abdomen. The pain may persist for weeks or months and can lead to a marked loss of appetite and weight. Treatment with appropriate medication can cure this parasitic infection and the abdominal pain that accompanies it. (For more information, see Diarrhea, *page 354*, and Vomiting, *page 377*.)

Lead poisoning most often occurs in toddlers living in an older house or attending daycare in an older building (built before the mid-1970s) where lead-based paint has been used. Children in this age group may eat small chips of paint. The lead is then stored in their bodies and can create many serious health problems. Parents also should be aware of toys, dishes, decorations, or other products with unacceptable lead content. (Recalls are posted on the US Consumer Product Safety Commission website at cpsc.gov.) Symptoms of lead poisoning include not only abdominal pain, but also constipation, irritability (the child is fussy, crying, difficult to satisfy), lethargy (they are sleepy, don't want to play, have a poor appetite), and seizures. If your child is exposed to lead paint, has eaten paint chips, has been exposed to toys with cracking, peeling, or chipping paint, and has any of the above symptoms, call your pediatrician. They can order a blood test for lead and advise you as to what else needs to be done. For all children, it is a good idea to be tested for lead as early as 9 to 12 months of age, as often there are no symptoms, especially in young infants. (See Lead Poisoning, *page 530*.)

Milk allergy is a reaction to the protein in milk, usually in younger infants, and can produce cramping abdominal pain, often accompanied by vomiting, diarrhea, blood in the stool, and skin rash.

Strep throat is a throat infection caused by bacteria called streptococci, or strep. It occurs frequently in children over 2 years of age. The symptoms and signs include a sore throat, fever, a sandpaper-like rash, and sometimes abdominal pain. Children can also get perianal strep, which is a strep infection around their anus. This can cause anal pain, constipation (because they don't want to stool), and abdominal pain as well. Your pediatrician can examine your child for either type of infection and may swab your child's throat or anus to check for the bacteria. If the results are positive for strep, your child will need to be treated with an antibiotic. (See Sore Throat [Strep Throat, Tonsillitis], *page 480*.)

Celiac Disease

Celiac disease is a problem that causes malabsorption—that is, a failure of the bowels to absorb nutrients. It tends to run in families and is caused by an abnormal immune reaction to gluten (the protein found in wheat, rye, and barley—and sometimes oats, which can be contaminated with gluten) that takes place in the intestine and stimulates the body's immune system to attack and damage the lining of the intestine, preventing nutrients from being absorbed into the system. As a result, food simply passes through the intestines, only partially digested. The result may be crampy abdominal pain, foul-smelling stools, diarrhea, weight loss, irritability, and a continuous feeling of being sick. It can also cause constipation, skin rashes, poor dental enamel, and growth concerns. In many cases, however, there may be no symptoms at all with celiac disease.

Treatment

Once your pediatrician suspects celiac disease, they'll order certain blood tests that can be used to screen for it. However, to make a definitive diagnosis, your pediatrician will refer your child to a pediatric gastroenterologist. This specialist will do a small-bowel biopsy, which entails using an endoscope inserted down the throat to remove a very tiny piece of the intestine for laboratory examination.

If the intestinal lining turns out to be damaged in a way that is suggestive of celiac disease, the doctor will recommend feeding your child a gluten-free diet. This means staying away from wheat, rye, barley, and contaminated oat products. Your pediatrician or gastroenterologist will give you a complete list of foods to avoid, but you also need to carefully check the labels of any foods you purchase, since wheat flour is a hidden ingredient in many items. Because rice and rice products do not contain gluten, they'll probably become a major part of your child's diet. The number of gluten-free products in the grocery stores continues to increase, and some restaurants even have gluten-free menus. Consultation with a dietitian is recommended, as the diet is very strict and must be followed exactly.

Some parents ask if they can just try a gluten-free diet without doing diagnostic testing. This is not recommended for several reasons. First, as stated before, the gluten-free diet in celiac disease is very strict. Few families can adhere rigidly enough to the diet without confidence that the diagnosis is correct. Second, it may take months for symptoms to completely resolve in a patient with celiac disease on a gluten-free diet. Finally, the gluten-free diet will cause both the serum and tissue markers of celiac disease to disappear, making it impossible to diagnose the disease accurately without putting your child back on a gluten-containing diet for several months.

Incidentally, your child may not be able to tolerate the sugar in milk (lactose) for as long as several months after the initial diagnosis is made. In this case, you may be advised to eliminate milk temporarily, as well as gluten products, from their diet. During this time, they might be given milk treated with enzymes to eliminate the lactose (such as lactose-free milk). Extra vitamins and minerals also might be necessary.

If your child does have celiac disease, they must remain on a gluten-free diet for their entire life, completely avoiding wheat, rye, barley, and contaminated oat products. Luckily, this is easier to do now than it was years ago due to the many gluten-free products and recipes available.

(See also Diarrhea, *page 354*; Malabsorption, *page 375*; Anemia, *page 605*.)

Constipation

Bowel patterns vary in children just as they do in adults. Because of this, it is sometimes difficult to tell if your child is truly constipated. One child may go two or three days without a bowel movement and still not be constipated, while another might have relatively frequent bowel movements but have difficulty passing the stool. Or a child's constipation may go unnoticed if they pass a small stool each day, while a buildup of stool develops in their colon. In general, it is best to watch for the following signals if you suspect constipation:

- In a newborn, firm stools less than once a day, though this can be normal in some exclusively breastfed infants (some breastfed babies will stool only once a week)
- In an older child, stools that are hard and compact, with three or four days between bowel movements
- At any age, stools that are large, hard, and dry ("rabbit pellets") and associated with painful bowel movements
- Episodes of abdominal pain relieved after having a large bowel movement
- Blood in or on the outside of the stools
- Soiling between bowel movements

Constipation can occur for several possible reasons, including inadequate fluid intake, not enough dietary fiber, withholding stool, and poor muscle coordination of the pelvic muscles (if the muscles at the end of the large intestine tighten, preventing the stool from passing normally), and, less likely, from celiac or thyroid disease. The longer the stool remains there, the firmer and drier it becomes, making it even more difficult to pass without discomfort. Then, because the bowel movement is painful, your child may actively try to hold it in, making the problem still worse.

Treatment

Mild or occasional episodes of constipation may be helped by the following suggestions.

Constipation due to breast milk is unusual, unless your supply has decreased or your baby is also eating solid food, but if your breastfed infant is constipated, it is probably due to a reason other than diet. Consult your doctor before substituting formula for breast milk. (Keep in mind that the American Academy of Pediatrics recommends breastfeeding and avoiding cow's milk for the first 12 months after birth.)

For infants, ask your pediatrician about giving small amounts of water or prune juice. In addition, for infants older than 6 months, fruits (especially prunes and pears) can often help resolve constipation.

For a toddler or older child who is eating solid foods and has problems with constipation, you may need to add high-fiber foods to their daily diet. These include prunes, apricots, plums, raisins, high-fiber vegetables (peas, beans, broccoli), and whole-grain cereals and bread products. At the same time, cut back on junk food and on cereals or breads that are not high in fiber. Increasing the daily water intake also may help.

In more severe cases, your pediatrician—alone or in consultation with a pediatric gastroenterologist—may prescribe a stool softener, stimulant laxative, or enema. Follow such prescriptions exactly. Although some newer softeners are sold over the counter and are simpler to use than these products used to be, never give your child a stool-loosening medication without first consulting with your child's doctor.

Prevention

Parents should become familiar with their children's normal bowel patterns and the typical size and consistency of their stools. Doing this is helpful in determining when constipation occurs and how severe the problem is. If the child does not have regular bowel movements each day or two, or is uncomfortable when passing stool, they may need help in developing proper bowel habits. This may be done by providing a proper diet and establishing a regular bowel routine.

In a child who is not yet toilet trained, the best way to guard against constipation is to provide a high-fiber diet. Increase the fiber as they get older.

Diarrhea

Normally your child's bowel movements will vary in number, color, and consistency, depending on their age and diet. Breast-fed newborns may have up to twelve small bowel movements a day, but by the second or third month, they may have some days without passing any stool. By age 2, most children will have only one or two large bowel movements a day, but your child can have several smaller ones and still be normal, especially if their diet includes juices or fiber-containing foods, such as prunes or bran.

An occasional loose stool is not cause for alarm. If, however, your child's bowel pattern suddenly changes to loose, watery stools that occur more frequently than usual, they have diarrhea.

Diarrhea often occurs when the inner lining of the intestine is injured. The stools become loose because the intestine does not properly digest or absorb the nutrients from the foods that your child eats and drinks. Also, the injured lining tends to leak fluid. Minerals and salt are lost along with the fluid. This loss can be made even worse if your child is fed food or beverages that contain large amounts of sugar, such as fruit juice or sweetened beverages, since unabsorbed sugar draws even more water into the intestine, increasing the diarrhea.

CAUSES OF DIARRHEA

In young children, the intestinal damage that produces diarrhea is caused most often by viruses such as norovirus and rotavirus. Such viruses are easily transmitted from person to person, so it is very important that your family practices excellent handwashing if a member of the house has a diarrheal illness. Diarrhea caused by bacteria and parasitic infections has decreased in frequency as a result of improvements in public health such as clean drinking water and proper disposal of sewage. Other causes of diarrhea are:

- Food poisoning (from things such as mushrooms, shellfish, or contaminated food)
- Side effects of antibiotics and other oral medications
- Food or milk allergy

- Drinking excessive amounts of fruit juice
- Overflow constipation (when loose stool leaks around an area of constipation)

When a child has diarrhea, the body may lose too much salt and water, leading to dehydration. This can be prevented by replenishing losses due to the diarrhea with adequate amounts of fluid and salt, as described under Treatment (*below*).

The medical term for intestinal inflammation is "enteritis." When the problem is accompanied by or preceded by vomiting, as it often is, there is usually some small-intestine inflammation as well, and the condition is called "gastroenteritis."

The causes of diarrhea are described in the bulleted list Causes of Diarrhea (*page 354*) and include viral or bacterial infections of the intestine. Children with viral diarrheal illnesses often have symptoms such as vomiting, fever, and irritability. (See Vomiting, *page 377*, and *Chapter* 22, Fever.) Their stools tend to be more greenish yellow and have a significant amount of water with them. (If the stools occur very frequently, the child may not have any solid stool at all.) If the stools appear red or blackish, they might contain blood; this bleeding may arise from the injured lining of the intestine or, more likely, simply may be due to irritation of the rectum by frequent, loose bowel movements. In any event, if you notice blood or any other unusual stool color, you should notify your pediatrician.

A rotavirus vaccine is now given routinely to infants starting at 2 months of age. This is a liquid vaccine that is given by mouth in your pediatrician's office. Infants are given the vaccine in a two- or three-dose regimen (depending on the formulation) at 2 months, 4 months, and (if the three-dose regimen is used) 6 months of age. It is very good at preventing diarrhea and vomiting caused by rotavirus. Almost all babies who get rotavirus vaccine will be protected from severe rotavirus diarrhea. However, this vaccine will not prevent diarrhea or vomiting caused by other infections.

Treatment

There are no effective medications for treating viral intestinal infections, which cause most cases of diarrhea in infants. The most important treatment of a young child with vomiting or diarrhea is to keep them adequately hydrated with breast milk, formula, electrolyte solution, or other fluids recommended by your pediatrician. Prescription medications should be used only to treat certain types of bacterial or parasitic intestinal infections, which are much less common in the United States and other developed nations. When such infections are suspected, your pediatrician will ask for stool specimens to be tested in the laboratory; other tests also may be done.

Some studies indicate that probiotics may be beneficial for certain causes of infectious diarrhea and may shorten the duration if started early and given daily. These dietary supplements are believed to help with the digestive process, as well as allergies and vaginal infections, and preventing some illnesses. Other studies, however, have shown no benefit, and confusion remains about what dose and which organisms might help. (See Probiotics and Prebiotics, *page 360*.)

Over-the-counter antidiarrheal medications are not recommended for infants or children. They often worsen the intestinal injury and cause the fluid and salt to remain within the intestine instead of being absorbed. With these medications, your child can become dehydrated without your being aware of it, because the diarrhea appears to stop. Always consult your pediatrician before giving your child any medication for diarrhea.

Mild Diarrhea

If your child has a small amount of diarrhea but is not dehydrated (see Signs and Symptoms of Dehydration, *page 366*), does not have a high fever, and is active and hungry, you may not need to change their diet.

If your child has mild diarrhea and is vomiting, substitute a commercially available electrolyte solution for their normal diet. Your pediatrician will recommend that these solutions be given in small amounts frequently, to maintain normal body water and salt levels, until the vomiting has stopped. In most cases, they're needed for only one to two days. Once the vomiting has subsided, gradually restart the normal diet.

Significant Diarrhea

If your child has a watery bowel movement every one to two hours, or more frequently, and/or has signs of dehydration (see Signs and Symptoms of Dehydration, *page 366*), consult their pediatrician. They may advise you to avoid liquids that are high in sugar (Jell-O, soft drinks, full-strength fruit juices, or artificially sweetened beverages), high in salt (packaged broth), or very low in salt (water and tea). If you are breastfeeding, they will probably have you continue, but in other cases they may recommend only prepared electrolyte solutions, which contain the ideal balance of salt and minerals. (See the table Estimated Amount of Fluid Children Should Drink Daily, *page 359*.)

Remember, if your child has diarrhea, keeping them hydrated is very important. If they show any signs of dehydration (such as decreased wet diapers, no tears, sunken eyes, or sunken fontanelle [soft spot]), call your pediatrician right away and withhold all foods and milk beverages until they give you further instructions. Also contact your doctor if your child looks sick and the symptoms aren't improving with time. Take your child to the pediatrician or nearest emergency department immediately if you think they are moderately to severely dehydrated. In the meantime, give your child a commercially prepared electrolyte solution.

For moderate or severe dehydration, hospitalization is sometimes necessary so that your child can be rehydrated intravenously. In milder cases, all that may be necessary is to give your child an electrolyte replacement solution according to your pediatrician's directions. The table on *page 359* indicates the approximate amount of this solution to be used.

Exclusively breastfed babies are less likely to develop severe diarrhea. If a breastfed infant does develop diarrhea, generally you can continue breastfeeding, giving additional electrolyte solution if your doctor feels this is necessary. Many breastfed babies can continue to stay hydrated with frequent breastfeeding alone.

Once diarrhea is decreasing and your child wants to eat, you can gradually expand the diet with a goal of returning to their usual diet as they can tolerate. Sometimes cow's-milk ingestion worsens diarrhea, so in children over age 1 your pediatrician may recommend holding off on cow's milk or may advise giving lactose-free formula or milk for a period of time.

It is not necessary to withhold food for longer than twenty-four hours, as your child will need some normal nutrition to start to regain lost strength. After you have started giving them food again, their stools may remain loose, but that does not necessarily mean that things are not going well. Look for increased activity, better appetite, more frequent urination, and the disappearance of any of the signs of dehydration. When you see these, you will know your child is getting better.

Diarrhea that lasts longer than two weeks (chronic diarrhea) may signify a more serious type of intestinal problem. When diarrhea persists this long, your pediatrician may want to do further tests to determine the cause and to make sure your child is not becoming malnourished. If malnutrition is becoming a problem, the pediatrician may recommend a special diet or special type of formula.

If your child drinks too much fluid, especially too much juice or sweetened beverages, a condition commonly referred to as toddler's diarrhea could develop. This causes ongoing loose stools but shouldn't affect appetite, affect growth, or cause dehydration. Although toddler's diarrhea is not a dangerous condition, the pediatrician may suggest that you limit the amounts of fruit juice and sweetened fluids your child drinks. Ideally, toddlers and children would drink mainly milk and water.

When diarrhea occurs in combination with other symptoms, it could mean that there is a more serious medical problem. Notify your pediatrician immediately if the diarrhea is accompanied by any of the following:

- Fever that lasts longer than twenty-four hours
- Bloody stools
- Vomiting that lasts more than twelve hours
- Vomited material that is green, blood-tinged, or like coffee grounds in appearance
- A distended (swollen-appearing) abdomen
- Refusal to eat or drink
- Severe abdominal pain
- Rash or jaundice (yellow color of skin and eyes)
- Signs of dehydration such as no urination for more than six hours

ESTIMATED AMOUNT OF FLUID CHILDREN SHOULD DRINK DAILY (DEPENDING ON BODY WEIGHT)		
1 pound = 0.45 kilograms 1 ounce = 30 milliliters		
Body Weight (in pounds)	**Minimum Daily Fluid Requirements (in ounces)***	**Electrolyte Solution* Requirements for Mild Diarrhea (in ounces per 24 hours)**
6–7	10	16
11	15	23
22	25	40
26	28	44
* Note: This is the smallest amount of fluid that a normal child requires. Most children drink more than this.		

If your child has another medical condition or is taking medication routinely, it is best to tell your pediatrician about any diarrheal illness that lasts more than twenty-four hours without improvement, or anything else that really worries you.

Prevention

The following guidelines will help lessen the chances that your child will get diarrhea:

1. Most forms of infectious diarrhea are transmitted by direct hand-to-mouth contact following exposure to contaminated fecal (stool) material. This happens most often in children who are not toilet trained. Promote handwashing after using the toilet or changing diapers and before handling food, as well as other sanitary measures, in your household and in your child's daycare.
2. Do not give your child raw (unpasteurized) milk or

foods that may be contaminated. (See Food Poisoning and Food Contamination, *page 361*.)

3. Avoid unnecessary medications, especially antibiotics.
4. If your child needs to take antibiotics, consider the use of probiotics to potentially prevent antibiotic-associated diarrhea.
5. If possible, breastfeed your child through the first year after birth at a minimum and through age 2 or longer if desired.
6. Make juice and sweet beverages an occasional treat, not a daily source of fluids.
7. Make sure your child has received the rotavirus vaccine, as it protects against the most common cause of diarrhea and vomiting in infants and young children.

(See also Abdominal Pain, *page 348*; Celiac Disease, *page 350*; Malabsorption, *page 375*; and Vomiting, *page 377*.)

PROBIOTICS AND PREBIOTICS

Probiotics are types of "good" bacteria. These living organisms inhabit the intestines and may have beneficial health effects, although the evidence is not yet conclusive. Some studies have shown that foods or infant formula containing probiotics can prevent or even treat diarrhea in children, whether this condition is chronic, acute, or associated with the use of antibiotics. Other studies have found a correlation in children between taking daily probiotics and experiencing fewer illnesses and therefore fewer missed days of school. Some research has shown that giving specific probiotics to newborns can help colonize the gut with beneficial bacteria and actually decrease harmful bacteria later in life. Many studies are currently under way, and ongoing research will provide more guidance on the role of probiotics in newborns and children, such as which ones may help and how much to give your child. Currently there is no standard recommendation to use these products routinely, but if your child has diarrhea or other gastrointestinal issues, talk to your doctor about the use of these organisms.

Probiotics are available in many forms. Many infant formulas are now supplemented with prebiotics and probiotics. Some dairy products such as live active cultured yogurt and kefir contain them, too. So do some miso and tempeh products and soy beverages. Probiotic supplements (powders, capsules, and liquids) are sold in health food stores. Pediatricians are still debating the most appropriate use of these commercial probiotics—for example, what are the best organisms and dosages, how frequently should they be taken, and should they be used at all for preventing or managing certain health conditions?

Foods containing probiotics appear to be safe for most children, although they can cause mild bloating or gas in some cases. If probiotic supplements have been exposed to heat or moisture, the living "good" bacteria may be killed, and thus the products will become useless. For now, if you're interested in trying probiotics, talk to your pediatrician first. (For more information about probiotics, see *page 85*.)

Some doctors recommend that rather than giving your child probiotics, you should consider using prebiotics instead. While probiotics are living bacteria, prebiotics are nondigestible food components—special carbohydrates naturally found in breast milk and other complex sugars and fiber—that promote the growth of beneficial bacteria that are already present in the intestines, thus increasing the number of these good bacteria while also suppressing the growth of unhealthy strains. Breast milk is a good source of prebiotics, as are foods like bran, legumes, barley, certain vegetables such as asparagus, spinach, and onions, and fruits such as berries and bananas.

Food Poisoning and Food Contamination

Food poisoning occurs after eating food contaminated by bacteria. The symptoms of food poisoning are basically the same as those of a stomach virus: abdominal cramps, nausea, vomiting, diarrhea, and sometimes fever. But if your child and other people who have eaten the same food all have the same symptoms, the problem is more likely to be food poisoning than a stomach virus. The bacteria that cause food poisoning cannot be seen, smelled, or tasted, so your child won't know when they are eating them. Sources of food poisoning include eggs, contaminated fish and meat products, and improperly canned foods. Many mushrooms and plants that are poisonous can cause gastrointestinal symptoms. Young children may not care for most of these foods and so will eat very little of them. However, it still is very important to be aware of the risk. If your child has unusual gastrointestinal symptoms and there is any chance they might have eaten contaminated or poisonous foods, call your pediatrician.

Botulism

This is the deadly food poisoning caused by *Clostridium botulinum*. Although these bacteria normally can be found in soil and water, illness from them is extremely rare because they need very special conditions in order to multiply and produce poison. *C. botulinum* grows best without oxygen and in certain chemical conditions, which explains why improperly canned food may be contaminated and low-acid vegetables such as green beans, corn, beets, and peas are most often involved. Honey also can be contaminated and can cause severe illness, particularly in children under 1 year of age. **This is the reason honey should never be given to an infant under the age of 1 year.**

Botulism attacks the nervous system and causes double vision, droopy eyelids, decreased muscle tone, and difficulty in swallowing and breathing. It also can cause vomiting, diarrhea, and abdominal pain. The symptoms develop within eighteen to thirty-six hours and can last weeks to months. Without treatment, botulism can cause death. Even with treatment, it can cause nerve damage.

Campylobacter

One form of infectious food poisoning is caused by the bacterium *Campylobacter*, which a child may ingest when they eat raw or undercooked chicken, or when they drink unpasteurized milk or contaminated water. This infection typically leads to symptoms such as watery (and sometimes bloody) diarrhea, cramps, and fever about two to five days after the germs are consumed in food.

To diagnose a *Campylobacter* infection, your doctor will have a stool specimen analyzed in the laboratory. Fortunately, most cases of this infection run their course without any formal treatment, other than making sure that your child drinks plenty of fluids to replace the fluids lost from diarrhea. When symptoms are severe, however, your pediatrician may prescribe antibiotics. In most cases, your child will be back to normal in about two to five days.

Clostridium perfringens

Clostridium perfringens is a bacterium frequently found in soil, sewage, and the intestines of humans and animals. It usually is transferred by the food handler to the food itself, where it multiplies and produces its toxin. *C. perfringens* often is found in school cafeterias because it thrives in food that is served in quantity and left out for long periods at room temperature or on a steam table. The foods most often involved are cooked beef, poultry, gravy, fish, casseroles, stews, and bean burritos. The symptoms of this type of poisoning, such as vomiting and diarrhea, start eight to twenty-four hours after eating the contaminated food, and can last from one to several days.

Cryptosporidiosis

Cryptosporidiosis is a parasitic infection, usually caught from swimming in or drinking contaminated water. It causes watery diarrhea, low-grade fever, and abdominal pain. Common sources include public pools and drinking fountains. This infection can occur in anyone, but it is of special concern in children who do not have a normal immune system.

E. coli

Escherichia coli is the name for a group of bacteria that normally live in the intestines of children and adults. A few strains of these bacteria can cause food-related illnesses. Undercooked ground beef is a common source of *E. coli*, although raw produce and contaminated water have caused some outbreaks.

Symptoms of an infection typically include diarrhea (which can range from mild to severe and can be bloody) to abdominal pain, and in some cases nausea and vomiting. Some *E. coli* outbreaks have been quite severe and have even caused deaths in rare instances. The optimal treatment for an *E. coli*–related illness is rest and fluids (to counteract dehydration). But if symptoms are more severe, you should have a discussion with your pediatrician.

Salmonella

Salmonella bacteria (there are many types) are another major cause of food poisoning in the United States. The most commonly contaminated foods are raw meat (including chicken), raw or undercooked eggs, unpasteurized milk, and vegetables. Fortunately, salmonella is killed when the food is cooked thoroughly. For vegetables, make sure they are washed thoroughly. Salmonella is also found on some pets, like turtles, other reptiles, and chickens. Your child should always wash their hands after handling one of these pets. Symptoms caused by salmonella poisoning start six to forty-eight hours after eating, may last two to seven days, and may include vomiting and diarrhea, though rarely bloody diarrhea. Although a salmonella infection is usually self-limiting, it can be severe, so if your child appears sick and has a high fever, call your doctor. Children with sickle cell disease or other problems with their spleen will need antibiotics if they have this infection.

Shigellosis

Shigella infections, or shigellosis, are intestinal infections caused by one of many types of shigella bacteria. These bacteria can be transmitted through contaminated food and drinking water, as well as via poor hygiene (in childcare centers, for example). The organisms invade the lining of the intestine and can lead to symptoms such as bloody diarrhea, fever, and cramps.

Shigellosis and its symptoms usually subside after about five to seven days. In the meantime, your child should consume extra fluids and (if your pediatrician recommends it) a rehydrating solution. In severe cases, your doctor may prescribe antibiotics, which can shorten the duration and intensity of the infection. Shigella is one of the few bacterial causes of gastroenteritis that is usually treated with antibiotics. Also, infants and toddlers should not be at daycare until treated or until the infection is completely resolved.

Staphylococcus aureus (Staph)

Staph contamination is one of the leading causes of food poisoning. These bacteria ordinarily cause skin infections, such as pimples or boils, and are transferred when foods are handled by an infected person. When food is left at a specific temperature (100 degrees Fahrenheit [37.8 degrees Celsius])—generally one that is lower than the temperature needed to keep food hot—the staph bacteria multiply and produce a poison (toxin) that ordinary cooking will not destroy. The symptoms begin one to six hours after eating the contaminated food, and the discomfort usually lasts about one day.

Treatment

In most cases of food-borne illnesses, all that's necessary is to limit your child's eating and drinking for a while. The problem will then usually resolve itself. Infants can tolerate three to four hours without food or liquids; older children, six to eight. If your child is still vomiting or their diarrhea has not decreased significantly during this time, call your pediatrician.

Also notify the doctor if your child:

- Shows signs of dehydration (see Signs and Symptoms of Dehydration, *page 366*)
- Has bloody diarrhea
- Has continuous diarrhea with a large volume of water in the stool, or diarrhea alternating with constipation
- May have been poisoned by mushrooms
- Suddenly becomes weak, numb, confused, or restless, and feels a tingling sensation, acts drunkenly, or has hallucinations or difficulty breathing

SIGNS AND SYMPTOMS OF DEHYDRATION (LOSS OF SIGNIFICANT AMOUNTS OF BODY WATER)

The most important part of treating diarrhea is to prevent your child from becoming dehydrated. Be alert for the following warning signs of dehydration, and notify the pediatrician immediately if any of them develop.

Mild to Moderate Dehydration

- Plays less than usual
- Urinates less frequently (for infants, fewer than six wet diapers per day)
- Parched, dry mouth
- Fewer tears when crying
- Sunken soft spot of the head in an infant or toddler
- Loose stools, for dehydration caused by diarrhea; decreased bowel movements, for dehydration caused by other fluid loss (vomiting, lack of fluid intake)

Severe Dehydration (In Addition to the Signs and Symptoms Already Listed)

- Very fussy
- Excessively sleepy
- Sunken eyes
- Cool, discolored hands and feet
- Wrinkled skin
- Urinates only one to two times per day

Tell the doctor the symptoms your child is having, what foods they have eaten recently, and where those foods were obtained. The treatment your pediatrician gives will depend on your child's condition and the type of food poisoning. If they are dehydrated, fluid replacement will be prescribed. Sometimes antibiotics are helpful for specific bacteria. Antihistamines help if the illness is due to an allergic reaction to a food, toxin, or seasoning, although if the reaction or symptoms are severe, call your doctor, as other medications, such as epinephrine, may be required. If your child has botulism, they will require hospitalization and treatment in the intensive care unit.

Prevention

Most food-borne illness is preventable if you observe the following guidelines.

Cleanliness

- Be especially careful when preparing raw meats and poultry. Wash your hands, and all surfaces that have come in contact with the raw meat and poultry, with hot, sudsy water before continuing your preparation.
- Always wash your hands before preparing meals and after going to the bathroom or changing your child's diaper.
- If you have open cuts or sores on your hands, wear gloves while preparing food.
- Do not prepare food when you are sick, particularly if you have nausea, vomiting, abdominal cramps, or diarrhea.

Food Selection, Preparation, and Serving

- Carefully examine any canned food (especially home-canned goods) for signs of bacterial contamination. Look for milky liquid surrounding vegetables (it should be clear), cracked jars, loose lids, and swollen cans or lids. Don't use canned or jarred goods showing any of these signs. Do not even taste them. Throw them away so that nobody else will eat them. (Wrap them first in plastic and then in a heavy paper bag.)
- Buy all meats and seafood from reputable suppliers.
- Do not use raw (unpasteurized) milk or cheese made from raw milk.
- Do not eat raw or undercooked meat.
- Do not give honey to a baby under 1 year of age.
- If your child turns away from a particular food or drink, smell or taste it yourself; you may find that it is spoiled and that it shouldn't be eaten.
- Do not let prepared foods (particularly starchy ones), cooked or cured meats, cheese, or anything with

mayonnaise stay at room temperature for more than two hours.

- Do not interrupt the cooking of meat or poultry to finish the cooking later.
- Do not prepare food one day for the next unless it will be frozen or refrigerated right away. (Always put hot food right into the refrigerator. Do not wait for it to cool first.)
- Make sure all foods are cooked thoroughly. Use a meat thermometer for large items like roasts or turkeys, and cut into other pieces of meat to check if they are done.
- When reheating meals, cover them and reheat them thoroughly.
- You also may want to visit the US Department of Agriculture website, usda.gov, for more information. The department has several helpful pamphlets and newsletters, including topics such as cooking on a grill and preparing holiday turkeys.

Hepatitis

Hepatitis is an inflammation of the liver that, in children, is almost always caused by one of several viruses. In some children it may cause no symptoms, while in others it can provoke fever, jaundice (yellow skin), loss of appetite, nausea, and vomiting. There are multiple forms of viral hepatitis. The most common forms include:

- Hepatitis A. Routine vaccination is recommended for all children at 1 year of age, with a booster dose six to twelve months later.
- Hepatitis B. Routine vaccination is now recommended for all infants at birth, with two booster doses given.
- Hepatitis C. Currently there is no vaccine, but effective treatment is available and curative for infected patients.

Most children in the United States are now vaccinated against hepatitis A, but the infection can be transmitted directly from person to person or through contamination of food or water (such as while swimming or eating in a restaurant or traveling). In a childcare or household setting, the infection can be spread when hands are not washed after having a bowel movement or after changing the diaper of an infected infant. Anyone who drinks water contaminated with infected human feces or who eats raw shellfish taken from polluted areas also may become infected. A child infected with hepatitis A virus may develop no symptoms or will become ill two to six weeks after the virus is transmitted. The illness usually disappears within one month after it begins.

Hepatitis B infection is transmitted during sexual activity, during childbirth, and via contact with infected blood, semen, or other body fluids. In young children, however, it can also be contracted through non-sexual, person-to-person contact, such as at daycare, which is why the hepatitis B vaccine is recommended for all young children.

Risk is greatest from contaminated needles, shared syringes or drug paraphernalia, and sex partners of infected persons; babies may be exposed to the virus in utero. When a pregnant woman has acute or chronic hepatitis B, the infection may transmit to the newborn at the time of delivery. Therefore, all pregnant women should be tested for hepatitis B infection and all newborn babies should be vaccinated against hepatitis B.

Hepatitis C can be acquired by intravenous (IV) drug use, through contaminated needles or, less commonly, through needle injections; by sexual contact with an infected person; and by birth to a person infected with hepatitis C. In the United States, the use of sterile disposable needles and the screening of all blood and blood products has essentially eliminated the risk of transmission of hepatitis B and C in hospitals and doctors' offices.

Infection with the hepatitis C virus commonly produces no symptoms, or only mild symptoms of fatigue and jaundice. In many cases, however, this form of hepatitis becomes chronic and can result in severe liver disease, liver failure, cancer of the liver, and even death later in life. There are antiviral medications available that can cure hepatitis C, and anyone at risk should be tested so that effective treatment may be offered.

Signs and Symptoms

A child could have hepatitis without anyone being aware of it, since many affected children have few, if any, symptoms. In some children the only signs of disease may be malaise and fatigue for several days. In others there will be a fever followed by jaundice (the sclera, or whites of the eyes, and the skin develop a noticeable yellowish color). This jaundice is due to an abnormal increase in bilirubin (a yellow pigment) in the blood, caused by liver inflammation.

With hepatitis B, fever is less likely to occur, although the child may suffer loss of appetite, nausea, vomiting, abdominal pain, and malaise, in addition to jaundice. In children, hepatitis C doesn't always have symptoms.

If you suspect that your child has jaundice, notify your pediatrician. Your child's doctor may order blood tests to determine if hepatitis is causing the problem or if it is due to another condition. You should contact your doctor if vomiting or abdominal pain persists beyond a few hours; if appetite loss, nausea, or malaise (a vague feeling of low energy or feeling sick) continues for more than a few days; or if your child becomes jaundiced. These may be indicators of hepatitis.

Treatment

In most settings, there is no specific treatment for hepatitis. As with most viral infections, the body's own defense mechanisms usually will overcome the infecting agent. Although you do not need to rigidly restrict the diet or activity of your child, you may need to make adjustments depending on their appetite and energy levels. Your doctor may recommend that your child avoid aspirin and ibuprofen (and other non-steroidal anti-inflammatory drugs), but acetaminophen can be used in children with chronic liver disease as long as aggressive hepatitis is not present and your pediatrician has agreed to its use. Also, children on certain medications for long-term illnesses should have their dosages carefully reviewed by the pediatrician to avoid the side effects that might result from the liver's inability to handle the usual medication load.

Medications are available to treat chronic hepatitis B and hepatitis C. If your child's hepatitis becomes a chronic condition, your pediatrician will refer you to a pediatric gastroenterologist or infectious disease specialist to help decide on appropriate management.

Most children with hepatitis do not need to be hospitalized. However, if loss of appetite or vomiting is interfering with your child's fluid intake and posing a risk of dehydration, your pediatrician may recommend that they be hospitalized. You should contact your doctor immediately if your child appears very lethargic, unresponsive, or delirious, as these may mean that their illness is worsening and hospitalization is indicated.

There is no chronic infection following hepatitis A; in comparison, among unimmunized children, chronic hepatitis B occurs more frequently in infants than in older children and adults. A high percentage of infants who are born to mothers with acute or chronic hepatitis B become chronically infected if they are not properly immunized after birth. Children with chronic hepatitis B will need monitoring and medication management to reduce the lifetime risk of liver damage, cirrhosis, and liver cancer.

Prevention

All newborns should be immunized with the hepatitis B vaccine at birth; a second dose should be given at age 1 to 2 months. Two doses of hepatitis A vaccine are recommended for all children between their first and second birthdays (12 to 23 months of age), as well as older children and adolescents who have not yet been vaccinated. In addition, most international travelers, adults employed in certain high-risk occupations, and people with chronic liver disease, among other conditions, should ask their physician about receiving the hepatitis A vaccine. (See the immunization schedule in the Appendix, *pages 696–97.*)

Handwashing before eating and food preparation, as well as after using the toilet, is the most important preventive measure against hepatitis. Children should be taught as young as possible to wash their hands at these times. If your child is in childcare, check to be sure that members of the staff wash their hands after handling diapers and before feeding the children.

If you find out that your child has been exposed to a person with active hepatitis, immediately contact your pediatrician, who will determine if the exposure has placed your child at risk. If there's a risk that the infection might have been passed to your child, the doctor may recommend post-exposure measures such as an injection of gamma globulin or a hepatitis vaccine, depending on which hepatitis virus was involved.

Prior to foreign travel with your child, consult your physician to determine the risk of exposure to hepatitis in the countries you plan to visit and consider vaccination against hepatitis A and B if your family has not yet received it.

Inguinal Hernia

If you notice a small lump or bulge in your child's groin area or an enlargement of the scrotum, you may have discovered an inguinal hernia. This condition, which is present in up to 5 of every 100 children (most commonly in boys), occurs when an opening in the lower abdominal wall allows the child's intestine to squeeze through. An inguinal hernia may be confused with a more benign condition, a communicating hydrocele (see *page 374*).

The testicles of the developing male fetus grow inside the abdominal cavity, moving down through a tube (the inguinal canal) into the scrotum as birth nears. When this movement takes place, the lining of the abdominal wall (peritoneum) is pulled along with the testes to form a sac connecting the testicle with the abdominal cavity. Normally this connection closes before or shortly after birth. Hernia is due to a failure of this normal protrusion from the abdominal cavity to close properly, leaving a space for a small portion of the bowel to later push through into the groin or scrotum.

Most hernias do not cause any discomfort, and you or the pediatrician will discover them only by seeing the bulge either in the groin or in the scrotum. Although this kind of hernia must be treated, it is not an emergency condition. You should, however, notify your doctor, who may instruct you to have your child lie down and elevate their legs. Sometimes this will cause the bulge to disappear. However, your doctor will still want to examine the area as soon as possible.

Rarely, a piece of the intestine gets trapped in the hernia, causing swelling and pain. (If you touch the area, it will be tender.) Your child may have nausea and vomiting as well. This condition is called an incarcerated (trapped) hernia and does require immediate medical attention. Call your pediatrician immediately if you suspect an incarcerated hernia.

Treatment

Even if the inguinal hernia is not incarcerated, it still should be surgically repaired. The surgeon also may check the other side of the abdomen to see if the defect is present there, too, which is very common.

If the hernia is causing pain, it may indicate that a piece of intestine has become trapped, or incarcerated. In that case, consult with your pediatrician immediately. They may try to move the trapped piece of intestine out of the sac. Even if this can be done, the hernia still needs to be surgically repaired soon thereafter. If the intestine remains trapped despite your doctor's efforts, emergency surgery must be performed to prevent permanent damage to the intestine.

Umbilical Hernia

Another common kind of hernia occurs at the umbilicus, or belly button. Weakness of the abdominal wall in that spot may allow part of the intestines to bulge forward, especially when your child strains, such as with laughing, coughing, or using the toilet. Umbilical hernias affect up to 20 percent of children, and unlike inguinal hernias, they are generally harmless. You don't have to do anything for them, and folk remedies like using a belly band or taping a coin over them will not help. For cosmetic reasons, your pediatrician may refer your child to a pediatric surgeon if the hernia has not gone away on its own by age 4 or 5.

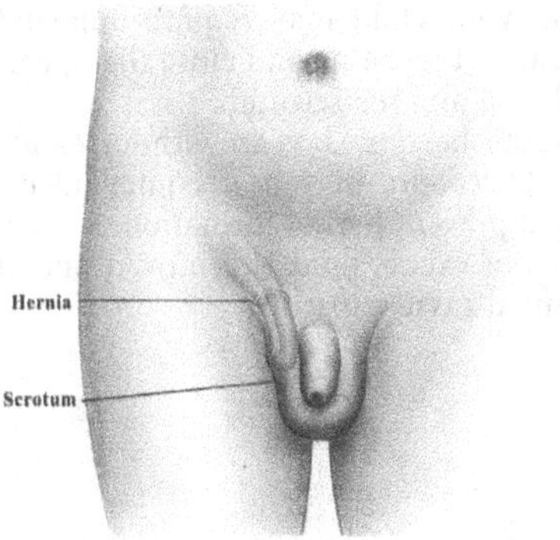

In boys, an internal opening leading to the scrotum allows abdominal contents to slide downward, causing an inguinal hernia. In girls, an inguinal hernia may simply appear as a bulge in the groin area.

Communicating Hydrocele

If the opening between the abdominal cavity and the scrotum has not closed properly and completely, abdominal fluid can pass into and out of the sac around the testes, causing a changing fluid collection called a communicating hydrocele. Many newborns have this problem; however, it usually disappears within one year without any treatment. Although most common in newborns, hydroceles also can develop later in childhood, sometimes with a hernia.

If your child has a hydrocele, they probably will not complain or be bothered by it, but you or your child will notice that one side of the scrotum is swollen. In an infant or young child, this swelling increases with activity or crying but decreases when they are resting or lying down. Sometimes you will not be able to notice any change in size. Your pediatrician may make the final diagnosis by shining a bright light through the scrotum, to show the fluid surrounding the testicle. Your doctor also may order an ultrasound examination of the scrotum if it is very swollen or hard.

If your baby is born with a hydrocele, your pediatrician will examine it at each regular checkup until around 1 year of age. During this time, your child should not feel any discomfort in the scrotum or the surrounding area. But if it seems to be tender in this area or your child has unexplained discomfort in the scrotum with associated nausea or vomiting, call the doctor at once—these are signs that a piece of intestine may have entered the scrotal area along with abdominal fluid. (See Inguinal Hernia, *page 372*.) If this occurs and the intestine gets trapped in the scrotum, your child may require immediate surgery to release the trapped intestine and close the opening between the abdominal wall and the scrotum.

If the hydrocele persists beyond 1 year without causing pain, a simple surgical procedure may be recommended to correct the hydrocele and prevent hernia formation in the future. In this operation, the excess fluid is removed and the opening into the abdominal cavity closed.

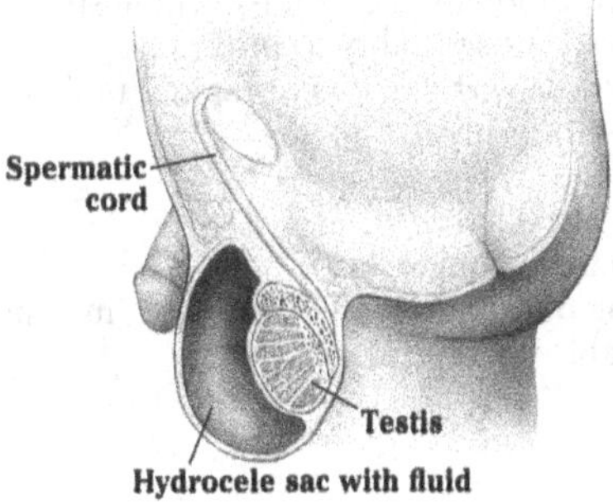

Malabsorption

Sometimes even children who eat a balanced diet suffer from malnutrition. The reason for this may be malabsorption, the body's inability to absorb nutrients from the digestive system into the bloodstream.

Normally the digestive process converts nutrients from the diet into small units that pass through the wall of the intestine and into the bloodstream, where they are carried to other cells in the body. If the intestinal wall is damaged by an infection (from a virus, bacterium, or parasite) or an immune disorder (such as celiac or inflammatory bowel disease), its surface may change so that digested substances cannot pass through. When this happens, the nutrients will be eliminated through the stool.

Malabsorption commonly occurs in a normal child for a day or two during severe cases of stomach or intestinal virus. It rarely lasts much longer, since the surface of the intestine heals quickly without significant damage. In these cases, malabsorption is no cause for concern. However, chronic malabsorption may develop, and if two or more of the following signs or symptoms persist, notify your pediatrician.

Signs and Symptoms

Possible signs and symptoms of chronic malabsorption can include the following:

- Persistent abdominal pain and vomiting
- Frequent, loose, bulky, foul-smelling stools
- Increased susceptibility to infection
- Weight loss with the loss of fat and muscle
- Increase in bruises
- Bone fractures
- Dry, scaly skin rashes
- Personality changes
- Slowing of growth and weight gain (may not be noticeable for several months)

Treatment

When a child suffers from malnutrition, malabsorption is just one of the possible causes. A child might be undernourished because they are not getting enough of the right types of food, or because they have digestive problems that prevent their body from properly digesting food. A combination of these problems might also exist. Before prescribing a treatment, the pediatrician must determine the cause. This can be done in one or more of the following ways:

- You may be asked to list the amount and type of food your child eats.
- The pediatrician may collect and analyze stool samples. In healthy people, only a small amount of the fat or protein consumed each day is lost through the stool. If too much is found in the stool, it is an indication of malabsorption.
- Collection of sweat from the skin, called a sweat test, may be performed to see if cystic fibrosis (see *page 411*) is present.
- In some cases, the pediatrician might request that a pediatric gastroenterologist obtain a biopsy from the wall of the small intestine and have it examined under the microscope for signs of infection, inflammation, or other injury.

Ordinarily, these tests are performed before any treatment is begun, although a seriously sick child might be hospitalized to receive special feedings while their problem is being evaluated.

Once the physician is sure the problem is malabsorption, they will try to identify a specific reason for its presence. When the reason is infection, the treatment usually will include antibiotics. If malabsorption occurs because the intestine is too active, certain medications may be used to counteract this so that there's time for the nutrients to be absorbed.

Sometimes there's no clear cause for the problem. In this case, the diet may be changed to include foods or special nutritional formulas that are more easily tolerated and absorbed.

Vomiting

Because many common childhood illnesses can cause vomiting, you should expect your child to have this problem several times during these early years. Usually it ends quickly without treatment, but this doesn't make it any easier for you to watch. That feeling of helplessness combined with the fear that something serious might be wrong and the desire to do something to make it better may make you feel tense and anxious. To help put your mind at ease, learn as much as you can about the causes of vomiting and what you can do to treat your child when it occurs.

First of all, there's a difference between real vomiting and just spitting up. Vomiting is the forceful throwing up of stomach contents through the mouth. Spitting up (most commonly seen in infants under 1 year of age) is the easy flow of stomach contents out of the mouth, frequently with a burp.

Vomiting occurs when the abdominal muscles and diaphragm contract vigorously while the stomach is relaxed. This reflex action is triggered by the "vomiting center" in the brain after it has been stimulated by any of the following:

- Nerves from the stomach and intestine when the gastrointestinal tract is either irritated or swollen by an infection or blockage
- Chemicals in the blood (e.g., drugs)
- Psychological stimuli from disturbing sights or smells
- Stimuli from the middle ear (as in vomiting caused by motion sickness)

The common causes of spitting up or vomiting vary according to age. During the first few months, for instance, most infants will spit up small amounts of formula or breast milk, usually within the first hour after being fed. It may occur less often if a child is burped frequently and if active play is limited right after meals. This spitting up tends to decrease as the baby becomes older, but it may persist in a mild form until 10 to 12 months of age. Spitting up is not serious and doesn't interfere with normal weight gain. (See Spitting Up, *page 96*.)

Occasional vomiting may occur during the first month. If it appears repeatedly or is unusually forceful, call your pediatrician. It may be just a mild feeding difficulty, but it also could be a sign of something more serious.

Around 2 weeks to 4 months of age, persistent forceful vomiting may be caused by a thickening of the muscle at the stomach exit. Known as hypertrophic pyloric stenosis, this thickening prevents food from passing into the intestines. It requires immediate medical attention. Surgery usually is required to open the narrowed area. The important sign of this condition is forceful vomiting occurring approximately fifteen to thirty minutes or less after every feeding. Anytime you notice this, call your pediatrician as soon as possible.

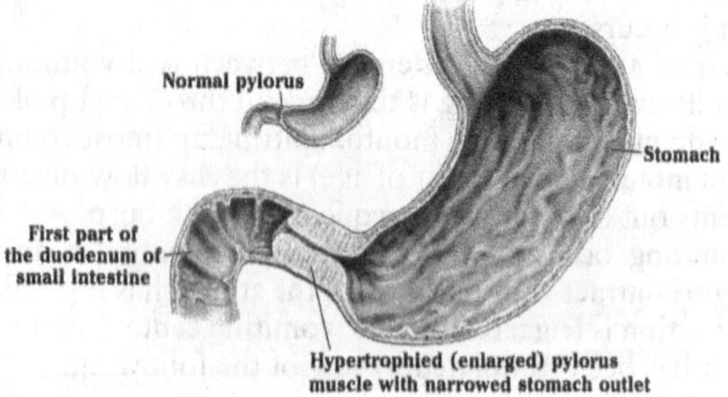

Gastroesophageal Reflux (GER). Occasionally the spitting up in the first few weeks to months after birth gets worse instead of better—that is, even though it's not forceful, it occurs all the time. This happens when the muscles at the lower end of the esophagus become overly relaxed and allow the stomach contents to back up. This condition is known as gastroesophageal reflux (GER). It is important to note that when an infant is growing typically and spitting up, this is most likely normal physiologic spitting up, and it does not require therapy or management. This is certainly not convenient or pleasant for a parent, but it's not bad for the baby. Common ways to treat GER include:

1. Avoid overfeeding or give smaller feeds more frequently.
2. Burp your baby frequently.
3. Leave your infant in a safe, quiet, upright position for at least thirty minutes following feeding.
4. Thicken the breast milk or formula with small amounts of baby cereal as directed by your pediatrician. Some newer formulas, labeled "anti-reflux," are designed with this thickening included.

If these steps are not successful, if your baby isn't gaining weight or growing typically, or if your child is upset by the spitting up or vomiting, your pediatrician may consider starting medication and/or refer you to a pediatric gastrointestinal (GI) specialist.

Infectious Causes. After the first few months after birth, the most common cause of vomiting is a stomach or intestinal infection. Viruses are by far the most frequent infecting agents, but occasionally bacteria and even parasites may be the cause. The infection also may produce fever, diarrhea, and sometimes nausea and abdominal pain. The infection is usually contagious; if your child has it, chances are good that some of their playmates also will be affected.

Viruses are a leading cause of vomiting in infants and young children, with symptoms often progressing to diarrhea and fever. Rotavirus is one of the viral causes of gastroenteritis, but other types of viruses—such as noroviruses and adenoviruses—can cause it as well. Rotavirus has become much less frequent due to the availability of a vaccine that can prevent severe disease. (For more information about gastroenteritis, see *page 349*.)

Occasionally infections outside the gastrointestinal tract will cause vomiting. These include infections of the respiratory system (also see discussions of middle ear infections, *page 471*, and pneumonia, *page 421*), infections of the urinary tract (see *page 591*), and meningitis (see *page 597*). Some of these conditions require immediate medical treatment, so be alert for the following trouble signs, whatever your child's age, and call your pediatrician if they occur:

- Blood or bile (a green material) in the vomit, or vomit that appears to consist of coffee-ground-like material
- Severe abdominal pain
- Strenuous, repeated vomiting
- Swollen or enlarged abdomen
- Lethargy or severe irritability
- Convulsions
- Jaundice
- Signs or symptoms of dehydration (see Signs and Symptoms of Dehydration, *page 366*)
- Inability to drink adequate amounts of fluid
- Vomiting continuing beyond twenty-four hours

Treatment

Most cases are caused by a virus and will get better on their own and stop without specific medical treatment. You should never use over-the-counter or prescription remedies unless they've been specifically prescribed by your pediatrician for your child and for this particular illness.

When there is continued vomiting, you need to make certain that dehydration doesn't occur. "Dehydration" is a term used when the body loses so much water that it can no longer function efficiently (see Signs and Symptoms of Dehydration, *page 366*). If allowed to reach a severe degree, it can be serious and life-threatening. To prevent this from happening, make sure your child consumes enough extra fluids to restore what has been lost through throwing up. If they vomit these fluids, notify your pediatrician.

For the first twenty-four hours or so of any illness that causes vomiting, keep your child off solid foods, and encourage them to sip or drink small amounts of fluids such as electrolyte solution instead of eating. Liquids not only help to prevent dehydration, but also are less likely than solid foods to stimulate further vomiting.

Be sure to follow your pediatrician's guidelines for giving your child fluids. Your doctor will adhere to requirements like those described in the table Estimated Amount of Fluid Children Should Drink Daily, *page 359*).

In most cases, your child will just need to stay at home and receive a liquid diet for twelve to twenty-four hours. Your pediatrician usually won't prescribe a drug to treat the vomiting, but some doctors will prescribe anti-nausea medications for children.

If your child also has diarrhea (see *page 354*), ask your pediatrician for instructions on giving liquids and restoring solids to their diet.

If they can't retain any clear liquids or if the symptoms become more severe, notify your pediatrician. They will examine your child and may order blood and urine tests or imaging tests such as X-rays to make a diagnosis. Occasionally hospital care may be necessary.

Until your child feels better, remember to keep them hydrated, and call your pediatrician right away if they show signs of dehydration. If your child looks sick, if the symptoms aren't improving with time, or if your pediatrician suspects a bacterial infection, they may perform a culture of the stool and treat appropriately.

CHAPTER 13

ASTHMA AND ALLERGIES

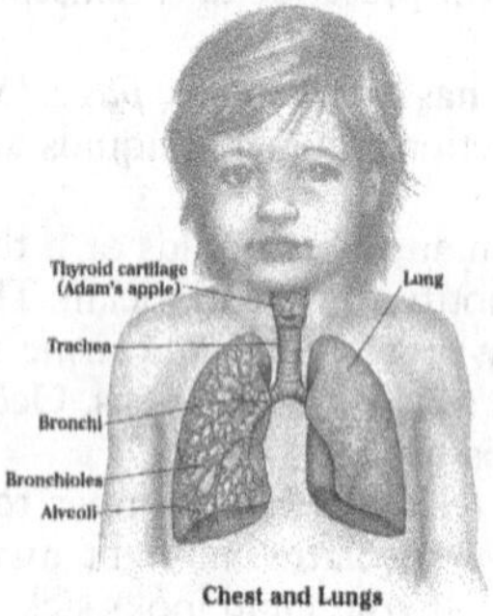

Chest and Lungs

Asthma

Asthma is a chronic disease of the breathing tubes that carry air to the lungs. In the last twenty years, there has been a major increase in the number of people with asthma, especially young children and those living in urban areas. In fact, asthma is now the most common chronic condition of childhood, affecting about 5 million children. We don't know what caused this increase, but some reasons or triggers for asthma or wheezing episodes are air pollution (including exposure to tobacco smoke early in life), exposure to allergens or not enough exposure to allergens, obesity, and respiratory illnesses.

Asthma symptoms can be different for each person, but wheezing is a hallmark sign. Wheezing is the high-pitched sound heard on breathing out that occurs when the breathing tubes in the lungs are narrowed, typically due to inflammation. In asthma, wheezing occurs most often at night or in the early morning. Still, not everyone who wheezes has asthma. Other symptoms of asthma include cough, chest tightness or pressure, shortness of breath, and chest pain. Although no specific test can determine asthma, the diagnosis is often made after a child has had multiple wheezing attacks. Many times, in between attacks children do well, but since they often get colds (a common trigger for wheezing in children), the attacks can be as frequent as every month, particularly in toddlers or children less than 3 years of age who get sick often. If a child has no other allergies—meaning that they do not have eczema or food allergy—and neither parent has asthma, wheezing will likely decrease between 3 and 6 years of age once they outgrow catching frequent colds that often trigger the wheezing. If these children continue to have repeated wheezing attacks, they are diagnosed with asthma.

Every child is unique, and thus it is important to discuss your child's health with your primary physician or specialist. Asthma is such a variable disease that some infants and children may wheeze without much distress while others have such severe wheezing and breathing difficulty that it may create an emergency. In general, most asthma attacks or flare-ups are manageable at home if symptoms are recognized early and treatment initiated as directed by your doctor.

If there is a family history of asthma or allergy, a child who frequently wheezes is likely to continue wheezing for a number of years. However, asthma can also occur in children who are not allergic. It is generally not possible to cure asthma (and only a small percentage of childhood asthma cases are outgrown), but it is possible to control asthma symptoms. Proper treatment reduces wheezing and prevents future attacks. How you breathe starts with what you breathe. Irritants and allergens can cause asthma problems. Irritants are a problem for everyone. Allergens are a problem only if you are allergic to the allergen.

Tobacco smoke is one of the most common asthma triggers. Tobacco smoke exposure increases the risk of wheezing from viral infections and decreases response to some of the most important medications used to control asthma. One of the best things that a family can do to protect a child is to eliminate their exposure to tobacco smoke. Keeping the home and car smoke-free is an important start, but it is difficult to eliminate a child's exposure as long as close family members are smokers. The best thing a family member can do to protect the child would be to stop smoking. Free help with stopping is available from the National Smokers' Helpline at 1-800-QUIT-NOW.

Electronic cigarettes (also called vapes, Juuls, e-hookahs, and other names) are very dangerous, especially to children with asthma. They are not safe to use around children. Their emissions expose children to nicotine as well as a number of irritating, inflammation-producing, and carcinogenic chemicals. Use of fireplaces and burning of incense also can trigger asthma. Other common irritant asthma triggers include strong-smelling household cleaners, insecticides (bug spray), other strong chemicals, paint, air fresheners, and perfumes.

Viral infections—even the common cold—can trigger asthma attacks, especially in young children. It is difficult to keep a child from catching a cold, but you can practice healthy habits by ensuring they get the flu shot (influenza vaccine) every fall and encouraging them to wash their hands frequently.

Allergens—irritants that your child is allergic to—also can trigger asthma. Since asthma is a breathing problem, the common allergens that trigger asthma are the ones that are breathed in. Food allergies would not cause asthma symptoms alone, as the food proteins that are absorbed travel to all parts of the body. Environmental allergy testing can help determine what your child is allergic to.

Common allergens that trigger asthma include:

- House dust mites (microscopic insects that live in house dust and feed on shed skin; pillows and bedding can have high concentrations of house dust mites)
- Cockroaches
- Pet (animal) dander (the shed skin from animals with fur or feathers)
- Pollens (from trees, grasses, or weeds)
- Molds and mold spores (from either water damage in the home or decomposing plant material outside)

Signs and Symptoms

When your child has an asthma flare-up (or "attack"), the major symptom will be a cough or wheeze that gets worse at night, with physical activity, or after contact with an irritant (e.g., cigarette smoke) or an allergen (e.g., animal dander, mold, dust mites, or cockroaches). As the attack progresses, the wheezing actually may decrease, as less air is able to move in and out. The child also may experience shortness of breath, breathe fast, and have retractions, when the chest and neck pull in while they work harder to take in air.

Many children with asthma have chronic symptoms, such as daily (or nightly) cough, cough whenever they exercise, or cough after exposure to pets, dust, or pollen. Your child's doctor will classify their asthma as mild intermittent, mild persistent, moderate persistent, or severe based on how often they need medicine for wheezing, how often symptoms wake them up at night, and how much their breathing interferes with daily activities. Treatments are based on these classifications (see Treatment, *page 386*).

In some children, the physician may hear wheezing (especially when the child blows out hard) even without more obvious signs. Abnormalities may be detected by peak flow testing, pulmonary function testing (PFT), or functional exhaled nitric oxide (FeNO) testing in children old enough to cooperate with this breathing test.

When to Call the Pediatrician

Children with well-controlled asthma can participate in the same activities as other children, including outdoor play and exercise. Watch your child closely when they're outside or exercising, and if symptoms develop or worsen, talk to your pediatrician.

For a child with asthma, you should know the situations that require immediate medical attention. As a rule, call your pediatrician immediately or consider going to the emergency room if:

- Your child has severe trouble breathing and seems to be getting worse, especially if they are breathing rapidly and there is pulling in of the chest wall when they inhale and forceful grunting when they exhale.
- Your child's mouth or fingertips appear blue.
- Your child acts agitated, unusually sleepy, or confused.
- There is any chest pain with breathing.

You also should call your pediatrician without delay if:

- Your child has a fever and persistent coughing or wheezing that is not responding to treatment.

- Your child is vomiting repeatedly and cannot take oral medication or drink fluids.
- Your child has difficulty speaking or sleeping because of wheezing, coughing, or trouble breathing.

Treatment

Asthma always should be treated under your pediatrician's supervision. The goals of treatment are to:

1. Prevent asthma symptoms such as coughing, wheezing, chest tightness, and shortness of breath
2. Allow your child to run and play as hard as they want
3. Prevent serious asthma attacks
4. Control your child's asthma with the smallest amount of medication possible

Preventing severe asthma problems starts by preventing mild asthma problems. Work with your child's doctor to develop an asthma action plan. Like a traffic light, an asthma action plan has green, yellow, and red zones and discusses what to do at each step, including which medications to give. The green zone plan is the action you take every day, even when your child is completely well, to keep your child well. The yellow zone plan is what actions you take when your child has mild asthma symptoms such as beginning to cough. The red zone plan is what actions you follow when your child experiences moderate or severe asthma problems such as fast and hard breathing or inability to speak in a full sentence due to shortness of breath. Work with your doctor to create a written asthma action plan for your child. Asthma action plans should be in a clearly visible and easily accessible place where you live, and a copy should be shared with your child-care provider.

With these goals in mind, your pediatrician will prescribe medication and may refer you to a specialist who can evaluate your child's asthma—a pediatric pulmonologist (breathing specialist) or allergist (allergy specialist). Your doctor also will help you plan your child's specific home treatment program. This will include learning how to use the medicines and treatments that are prescribed and developing a plan to avoid the irritants and allergens that may be causing your child to cough or wheeze.

The medication prescribed for your child will depend on the nature of the asthma. There are two main types of asthma drugs: One type opens the breathing tubes and relaxes the muscles causing obstruction. These quick-relief or rescue medicines are called bronchodilators. The second type is controller or maintenance medications, which are used to treat the airway inflammation (swelling and mucus production).

- Quick-relief or rescue medications are intended for short-term use. If your child has an asthma attack, with coughing and/or wheezing, a rescue medication should be given. Medicines such as albuterol are a common choice. By relaxing the muscle squeezing down around the breathing tubes, these rescue medicines can relieve the tightness in your child's chest and ease their wheezing and feelings of breathlessness. They are prescribed on an as-needed basis. After your child uses a rescue inhaler, breathing will usually improve for a few hours. Rescue inhalers provide a few hours of symptom relief but are not meant to fix the underlying problem. The rescue medication can be given by an HFA-propelled inhaler (HFA = hydrofluoroalkanes)—also known as a puffer—or by nebulizer (see *page 389*).

  It is important to note that if there is no improvement or change after giving the rescue medicine, the child may need further evaluation: The asthma problems may be severe and need stronger medicine, or the problem may not be asthma but something else such as an infection or other lung problem. Should an attack become severe, your doctor may prescribe an additional medication, such as an oral corticosteroid (usually prednisone, prednisolone, or dexamethasone). Oral corticosteroids are powerful medicines that shrink the swelling and inflammation of the breathing tubes. Rescue medications such as albuterol should not be given more than every four hours outside of the healthcare setting. Let your pediatrician know if your child requires a rescue medication more often, as they may need reevaluation.

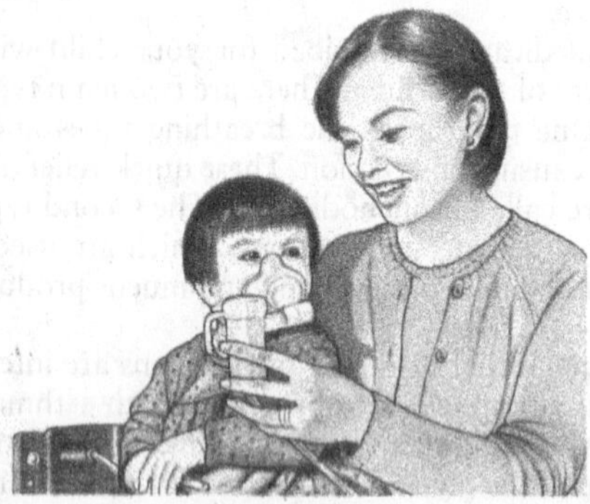

- Controller medications are intended to be used every day. They are designed to control your child's asthma and reduce the number of days and nights that they have asthma symptoms. In general, controller medicines are appropriate for children who have symptoms two or more times a week, who awaken with symptoms more than twice a month, who require two or more oral steroid courses within a year, or who have been hospitalized due to asthma symptoms.

  The most effective controller medication is an inhaled corticosteroid. Inflammation of the breathing tubes typically leads to an asthma reaction. By controlling the inflammation and making the breathing tubes less sensitive, these medications help to prevent asthma symptoms and asthma attacks. Daily use can help to keep your child's breathing regular. There are several different types, but they all work by preventing inflammation in the airway. By making the airways less sensitive to allergens and irritants, these medicines can reduce the number and severity of asthma episodes. Inhaled corticosteroids are administered via inhaler. An inhaler requires using a plastic tube called a spacer or volume holding chamber, which is required to allow the particles to spread out and reach the small areas of the lungs. Without the spacer, most of the medication will travel to the back of the throat and be swallowed instead of inhaled. Not using a spacer can lead to thrush (a yeast infection in the mouth) and, most

> importantly, ineffectiveness of the medication because it does not reach the lungs. Infants and small children use spacers with a mask (small or medium), which needs to be placed on the face with a good seal while the child takes several breaths. Older children can use spacers with a mouthpiece, which requires the child to slowly inhale and hold their breath for ten seconds. After taking an inhaled steroid, it is important for your child to rinse and spit or brush their teeth, as the medicine is important for the lungs but should not stay on the teeth or in the mouth. Another way for a child to receive certain medication is through a dry powder inhaler. These release the medicine without a propellant. Your child must rely on the force of their own inhalation to take in the medicine and get it into their lungs.

Another way to deliver the rescue medication is by nebulizer (sometimes called a breathing machine). The compressor connects by tubing to a device that is like a small cup into which the medication is placed. The compressor converts the liquid into a mist that is then breathed in. For small children, a mask is used (see illustration on *page 388*) and needs to be on the face with a good seal. If there is not a good seal, most of the medication escapes into the air and never reaches the lungs.

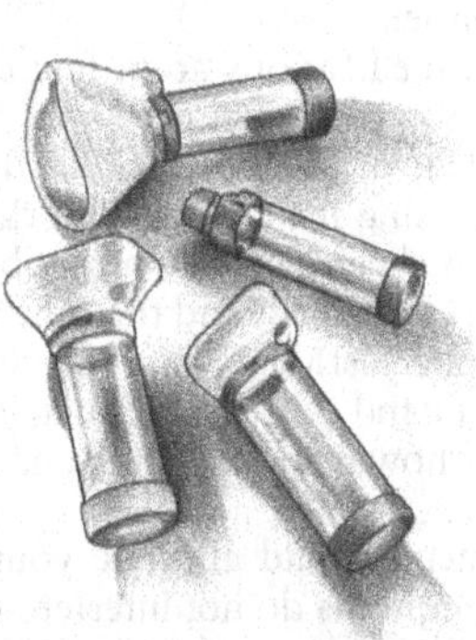

Spacers come in various shapes and sizes.

It is ideal to give the medication when your child is not crying, as crying decreases the amount of medicine that can reach the lungs. This may not always be possible, but over time most children learn to accept the medication. Although the techniques are relatively equally effective, your child may be more cooperative with one over the other. It may appear that the rescue medication (e.g., albuterol) is more effective through a nebulizer, but nebulized doses of albuterol are typically much greater than two puffs delivered through an inhaler. Inhalers are much more portable than nebulizers, and they don't require a power supply, so learning to use an inhaler can help you and your child enjoy more activities outside the home.

Leukotriene receptor antagonists block the activity of chemicals (leukotrienes) that are associated with airway inflammation; they are available only in oral preparations (pill form, granule powder, and chewable tablet). They are not as strong as the inhaled corticosteroid medications, but they can be very helpful when used in combination with an inhaled corticosteroid. Anti-inflammatory medications, inhaled corticosteroids, and/or leukotriene receptor antagonists are recommended for all children with asthma who have persistent symptoms.

As prevention, all these medications work best when used regularly. They can't work as well if they are not taken consistently. Giving your child medicine when they feel well can be challenging; however, having a routine, such as giving the medicine before brushing the teeth, can make taking the medicine daily a lot easier.

Be sure to give medications according to your doctor's directions. Do not stop medicines too soon, give them less often than recommended, or switch to other drugs or treatments without first discussing the change with the doctor. For some children, several medicines may be prescribed at the same time to get the asthma controlled, and then the number of medications is reduced once asthma symptoms are under control. If you do not understand why a particular treatment has been recommended, or how it should be given, ask for an explanation.

Asthma treatment should alleviate your child's symptoms so that asthma symptoms do not interfere with sleep, activity, or sports. If your child is not achieving the goals of treatment, the asthma action plan needs to be reevaluated. Maybe there is an asthma trigger that can be controlled or a problem with how your child takes their medicine, or perhaps your child needs more or different asthma medications. Sometimes when asthma medicines aren't helping, it's a clue that your child has another condition that affects breathing. Your pediatrician will examine your child and check for problems that could be making their asthma worse and consider whether your child needs a referral to an asthma specialist.

Prevention

While you cannot eliminate allergens and other irritants, there are some things that can be done to reduce exposure and lower your child's chances of having asthma symptoms. For example, in your home you can:

- Cover your child's bed mattress and pillow with special allergen-proof encasings to reduce the number of dust mites.
- Wash sheets, blankets, throw rugs, and stuffed animals every week in hot water and dry them in a hot dryer to kill dust mites.
- Limit stuffed animals in your child's room.
- Keep pets out of your child's room if the child is allergic.
- Keep your child out of rooms while you're vacuuming and dusting.
- Consider investing in a high-efficiency particulate air (HEPA) filter to keep the air in your child's room clean.
- Maintain the humidity in your house below 50 percent when possible; dust mites and mold grow best in damp areas.
- Avoid perfumes, scented cleaning products, and other items with scents that could become irritants.
- Reduce mold in your house by repairing leaky plumbing.
- Keep your child away from cigarette, cigar, or pipe smoke, as well as smoke from a fireplace.
- Don't allow anyone to smoke in your home or car.

Eczema

Although many patients and practitioners use the terms "eczema" and "atopic dermatitis" interchangeably, "eczema" is a general term used to describe a group of skin conditions characterized by a red itchy rash. Atopic dermatitis and contact dermatitis are two of the most common types of eczemas in children. Acute eczema may appear as red skin that is dry and peeling or moist and oozing. When eczema is persistent, the skin tends to thicken, darken, and become scaly.

Atopic Dermatitis

Atopic dermatitis is a long-lasting, itchy, inflammatory skin disease. Atopic dermatitis often occurs in infants and children in families with a history of atopic dermatitis, food allergies, asthma, and/or environmental allergies. It also affects adults. Although the cause of atopic dermatitis is not fully understood, there is a strong genetic component that leads to a structural abnormality in the skin barrier. This skin barrier abnormality leads to allergens being presented to the immune system through the skin, which leads to food allergies. Because atopic dermatitis is due to this primary skin barrier dysfunction, it is often the first condition to develop in many children who will go on to develop the other allergic conditions (the "atopic march").

Atopic dermatitis usually develops in three different phases. The infantile phase occurs between several weeks and 6 months of age, with itching, redness, and the appearance of small bumps on the cheeks, forehead, or scalp. The bumps may spread to the trunk and extremities as well. Although atopic dermatitis can be confused with other types of dermatitis, severe itching is typically a prominent feature. In many cases, the rash improves by 2 or 3 years of age.

Contact Dermatitis

Contact dermatitis can occur when the skin encounters an irritating substance or allergen. One form of this problem results from repeated contact with irritating substances such as citrus or other acidic foods, bubble baths, harsh soaps, fragrances, nickel, and wool or rough fabrics. One of the most common irritants is a child's own saliva. Constant drooling or licking the lips can cause an eczematous dermatitis of the lips and the skin around the mouth and neck.

Another form of contact dermatitis develops after contact with substances the child is allergic to. The most common potential allergens are:

- Nickel in jewelry, glasses, braces, snaps on jeans or pants, belt buckles
- Flavorings or additives to toothpastes and mouthwashes
- Glues, dyes, or leather used in the manufacture of shoes
- Dyes used in clothing
- Plants, especially poison ivy, poison oak, and poison sumac (this rash usually appears within several hours after contact, or within one to three days with poison ivy)
- Medications such as antibiotic/antibacterial ointments

Treatment

If your child has a rash that looks like eczema, your pediatrician will need to examine it to make the correct diagnosis and prescribe the proper treatment. In some cases, they may arrange for consultation with a pediatric dermatologist or allergist. Although there is no cure for eczema, it can be controlled and will often go away after several months or years. The most effective treatment is to prevent the skin from becoming dry and itchy and to avoid triggers that cause the condition to flare. To do this:

- Use skin moisturizers regularly and frequently to decrease the dryness and itchiness and improve the skin barrier. Ointments often work better than creams, which often work better than lotions.
- Give your child short baths in lukewarm water. After a bath, rinse twice to remove any residual soap (which might be an irritant). Pat dry, then apply the moisturizing cream or ointment within three minutes of getting out of the bath to lock in the moisture.

- Avoid harsh or irritating clothing (wool or synthetic material). Avoid dyes and fragrances in soap and detergents.
- If there is extreme itching, use cool compresses on the area, followed by the application of prescribed medications.

There are many types of prescription creams and ointments available, so ask your pediatrician to prescribe one that they prefer to control inflammation and itching. These preparations often contain a form of steroid, which is the first line of treatment. These creams or ointments should be used under the direction of your child's doctor. There are important instructions to follow regarding the maximum amount of time you can use some creams and ointments, typically for a maximum of two weeks out of the month. It's important to continue to apply the medications for as long as your pediatrician recommends their use.

In addition to the skin preparations, your child also may take an antihistamine by mouth to help with sleep and to relieve the itching, and may need antibiotics if the skin becomes infected. If your child develops frequent infections, your pediatrician may suggest a very dilute bleach bath, usually made by adding ⅛ to ½ capful of bleach in a regular-size bathtub of water, or a wet wrap for flares on the extremities.

For moderate to severe atopic dermatitis not well controlled by topical therapies, there are new biologic therapies that can be very effective. Talk to your doctor if you think your child has not responded to prescribed treatments.

Treatment of allergic contact dermatitis is similar, but the key is avoiding triggers. Although a little detective work will often help identify the trigger, your pediatric dermatologist or allergist may conduct a series of patch tests. These tests are done by placing small patches of allergens against your child's skin for forty-eight hours. If the skin reacts with redness and itching, that substance should be avoided.

Alert your pediatrician if any of the following occurs:

- Your child's rash is severe and is not responding to home treatment.
- There is any fever or evidence of infection (i.e., blisters, extensive redness, yellow crusts, pain, or oozing of fluid).

Food Allergy

While many foods can cause allergic reactions, true food allergies are less common than you might think. Food allergies are most likely to happen in infants and children, as well as in children with other allergies or whose family members have allergies. When food allergies do occur, they may be in response to any food that contains protein, although particular items are more likely to cause reactions (see the list below). While in many cases food allergies may reveal themselves with mild symptoms, they can be potentially life-threatening.

While any food can trigger a food allergy, several cause the vast majority of cases in children. Cow's milk is among them. Other common foods associated with allergies include:

- Eggs
- Peanuts and tree nuts (such as cashews, walnuts, etc.)
- Soy
- Wheat
- Fish (such as tuna, salmon, and cod) and crustacean shellfish (such as shrimp, crab, and lobster)
- Sesame seeds

If your child has a food allergy, their immune system responds in an exaggerated way to otherwise harmless proteins in foods. When this food is consumed, their immune system manufactures antibodies that attempt to fight off the offending food. In the process, substances called histamines and other chemicals are released that cause allergic symptoms.

Another condition, food intolerance or food sensitivity, occurs more often than true food allergies. Although the terms are often confused and sometimes used interchangeably, food intolerance does not involve the immune system. For example, a child with lactose intolerance (a condition of food sensitivity) is deficient in an enzyme required to digest milk sugar, leading to stomachaches, bloating, and diarrhea. Additionally, acidic foods (such as strawberries and tomatoes) can cause a rash to develop around the mouth, which is evidence of a sensitivity, not a food allergy.

Symptoms

A true food allergy happens when the body reacts against proteins found in foods. The reaction usually happens shortly after a food is eaten. Food allergy reactions can vary from mild to severe and include:

- Skin problems (itchy skin rashes, hives, swelling)
- Stomach problems (nausea, vomiting, diarrhea)
- Breathing problems (sneezing, wheezing, throat tightness)
- Circulation problems (pale skin, light-headedness, loss of consciousness)

HOW ALLERGIES DEVELOP

When an allergy-prone child is exposed to an allergen, their immune system produces an antibody called immunoglobulin E (IgE) in a process called allergic sensitization. The IgE sticks to mast cells in the skin and the linings of the airways and gut. The next time they come in contact with allergens, these cells release chemicals (e.g., histamine and leukotrienes) that cause allergic symptoms. However, the presence of IgE in response to a certain food during blood testing is common and not always indicative of a true food allergy. Additionally, not all food allergies involve IgE; other parts of the immune system may also be involved.

The intensity of the allergic reaction can range from mild to severe. If your child is highly allergic, even trace amounts of the food may trigger a potentially dangerous allergic response called anaphylaxis. Anaphylaxis can develop without warning and can progress rapidly; it must be treated immediately with a prescribed emergency injectable medication (using a device called an epinephrine auto-injector), which should always be with a trained adult near your child. Symptoms of anaphylaxis include:

- Swelling or tingling of the lips, throat, and tongue
- Difficulty breathing

- Wheezing
- A sudden drop in blood pressure, which would make your child look pale, feel lethargic, or lose consciousness
- Turning blue
- Loss of consciousness
- The uvula (the little punching bag at the back of the throat) may deviate in one direction instead of hanging straight
- Two-system involvement (e.g., respiratory symptoms as previously mentioned plus GI symptoms like stomachache or vomiting or diarrhea or skin manifestation like hives)

(See Anaphylactic Reactions: What You Should Do, *page 403*.)

Diagnosis and Management

Because some food allergies can be serious, talk to your pediatrician if you suspect that your child has one. To help make the diagnosis, your pediatrician will review your concerns and may perform some tests or refer you to an allergist, who may recommend additional testing. The presence of a food allergy is usually obvious, like when a child gets hives and lip swelling after eating a walnut. Tests, including a skin prick test and blood tests, can provide more information:

- With the skin prick test (or scratch test), the doctor will prick the skin with drops of the suspicious food allergens on your child's back or forearm. This can result in redness, swelling, and itching at the site, which the doctor will measure after twenty minutes.
- A blood test can measure IgE levels as well. A sample of your child's blood will be drawn and sent to the laboratory for testing.

It is important that your doctor tests your child only for the specific foods that have caused potential reactions. General blood panels are rarely recommended. A positive skin or blood test alone is not sufficient to diagnose food allergy; only an oral food challenge can confirm a food allergy. Your doctor should discuss with you the specifics of your child's diet, including any of your concerns about reactions to particular foods, to know what tests to consider and how to interpret the results.

There is no treatment for food allergies at this time, although research is currently under way and there is hope that in your child's lifetime treatment may be available. Avoidance of what your child is allergic to is currently the only way to avoid food allergy symptoms, including a life-threatening reaction. However, with some foods such as milk, soy, wheat, and eggs, many children will outgrow their food allergy over time. Some children can tolerate certain forms of milk and egg, depending on how it is cooked or processed. Some children can eat baked food with milk and eggs, such as in a muffin, without symptoms of an allergic reaction. In such cases, your pediatrician or allergist may recommend continuing to feed your child a small amount of the food such as egg or milk regularly, as this might help your child outgrow their food allergy. In other cases, your pediatrician or allergist may recommend that you avoid the food your child is allergic to altogether and retest your child in the future to see if they are still allergic. Certain food allergies—like those to peanuts and fish—are less likely to be outgrown. Only 20 percent of children with peanut allergy outgrow it or develop a natural tolerance.

Even once you're successful in keeping allergenic foods out of your refrigerator and off your dining room table, it may be more difficult to keep your child away from those items when they are out of your care. As your child gets older, you'll have to educate them, as well as their friends, grandparents, teachers, childcare workers, and other caregivers, about the importance of avoiding specific foods that could trigger allergy symptoms. Every time you shop, read food labels and look for major allergens to which your child is allergic. Also, when your family is eating in restaurants or traveling, ask questions about the ingredients of menu items. While the waiter may be helpful, confirm the information by speaking with the chef.

As you make adjustments in your child's diet, talk to your pediatrician regularly about compensating for the missing foods and keeping their diet balanced. For example, if your child is allergic to milk, you will need to include other calcium-rich foods (like green leafy vegetables and calcium-fortified drinks) in their diet. If your infant is allergic to formula, refer to *page 84* about choosing an elemental formula.

Prevention

Unless you yourself are allergic to a certain food, there is no need to avoid any foods while pregnant or breastfeeding. All infants are recommended to receive breast milk exclusively for the first four to six months, if possible. Introducing highly allergenic foods, especially peanut and egg protein, as early as 4 months of age or as soon as developmentally appropriate can prevent your child from developing allergies to those foods. Delayed introduction of solid foods has been shown to increase the risk of food allergy. Please talk to your pediatrician if you have concerns about food introduction.

Nasal Allergy/Allergic Rhinitis

If your child's nose starts to run and their eyes become itchy, red, and swollen, but there are no other symptoms of a cold or an infection, they may be having allergic rhinitis. This is a reaction to allergens in the environment. The most common environmental allergens are pollen, dust mites, mold, and animal dander. Like other allergies, this condition tends to run in families. The symptoms may not appear immediately, however. Seasonal respiratory allergies (e.g., to pollen) are quite uncommon in children under age 2 because infants must be exposed to a few pollen seasons to develop allergies.

It is sometimes difficult to tell the difference between a common cold and nasal allergy because many of the symptoms are the same. Here are some of the signs of a possible nasal allergy:

- Sneezing, sniffling, stuffiness; itchy and runny nose (usually clear discharge)
- Tearing; itchy, red, or swollen eyes
- A horizontal crease across the bridge of the nose from frequent wiping (nasal salute)
- Nosebleeds
- Dark rings under the eyes (allergic shiners)
- Mouth breathing because of nasal congestion
- Fatigue (mostly from not sleeping well at night)
- Frequent throat clearing or clucking (rubbing tongue against roof of mouth)

If your child has nasal allergies, potential complications include frequent sinus and ear infections (see Middle Ear Infections, *page 471*). If the allergy causes eye irritation and rubbing, they may be more susceptible to eye infections (see *page 545*). Since chronic allergies also can interfere with sleep, this may also affect school performance in older children.

Common Household Allergens

Pets (Dogs, Cats, Guinea Pigs, Rabbits, and Hamsters)

The best pets for allergenic families are fish and reptiles because they don't cause allergies. While some dog breeds are categorized as "hypoallergenic," in truth all dogs are equally likely to cause allergies, regardless of how much or little they shed.

Mold

Mold grows outdoors in cool, damp, dark places, such as in soil, grass, and dead leaves. Indoors, it's found in cluttered storage areas, recently flooded areas, basement areas, plumbing spaces, and areas with poor ventilation such as closets and attics, as well as pillows and blankets that haven't been aired out in a long time.

House Dust Mites

Many people are allergic to house dust mites, which are found in bedding (pillows, blankets, sheets, and mattresses), upholstery, furniture, and carpet. These mites, which are too small to be seen by the naked eye, thrive in humid environments (humidity greater than 50 percent).

What to Do

If your child is allergic to an animal, it's best not to have that animal in the house. If that isn't possible, keep the animal out of your child's bedroom. Have your child wash their hands and face after playing with a pet, and shower and wash their hair at night before bed so they don't sleep in pet dander. Also, run a HEPA filter in the child's bedroom to remove airborne allergens.

The key to controlling mold is to limit humidity. Avoid using vaporizers, humidifiers, and swamp coolers. A dehumidifier in a damp basement can be helpful. Throughout the house, replace any carpet that's been saturated by a big water spill, or dry it completely. You can destroy mold with several types of disinfectants, but be careful to store them in a safe place (locked in a high cabinet), away from curious toddlers.

The most important measures for reducing exposure to house dust mites should be focused on the bedroom. Put dust-mite-proof covers on mattresses and pillows, and wash sheets and blankets in hot water once a week to remove allergens and kill the mites. It's also helpful to keep the humidity in the home at less than 50 percent to control the growth of mites. If you're remodeling the bedroom, consider removing carpets from the room.

Treatment

Call your pediatrician if your child's nasal allergies start to interfere with sleep or other activities. To prevent or treat allergy symptoms, the doctor can suggest treatment, including prescription and non-prescription antihistamines, nose sprays of various types (including saline), and other medications. In many cases, they will recommend an oral antihistamine; most are now available over the counter, including loratadine, fexofenadine, and cetirizine. For more severe or persistent allergy symptoms, your physician may recommend a prescription or over-the-counter steroid nasal spray that, when used daily, will help prevent nasal allergy symptoms. If your child's eyes are swollen, itchy, and red, your pediatrician may also recommend prescription or over-the-counter allergy eye drops.

The best thing you can do for your allergic child is to remove the sources of allergens from your home, if possible.

Hives/Urticaria

Another allergic type of common rash that is characteristically very itchy, hives (urticaria) looks almost like a raised map of bumps. Hives are red, swollen bumps that tend to move around; individual lesions typically resolve within about twenty-four hours. When the rash remains in the same place for more than twenty-four hours, other diagnoses should be considered.

Among the most common causes of hives are:

- Response to an infection, most commonly a virus
- Foods (most commonly peanuts, tree nuts, egg whites, milk, shellfish, and sesame)
- Medications, either over-the-counter or prescription (such as ibuprofen and antibiotics)
- Bites or stings from bees or other insects

In at least half of cases of acute hives, it is not possible to identify the cause. An episode of acute hives can last up to six weeks before resolving. If hives persist longer than six weeks, they are considered chronic and may need further guidance by your pediatrician or allergist. Foods, medications, and venom stings are generally not responsible for chronic hives (those lasting more than six weeks).

Treatment

Non-sedating oral antihistamine medication should relieve or at least help reduce the itching and appearance of hives. These medications (e.g., loratadine, cetirizine, levocetirizine, fexofenadine) can be obtained without a prescription. You may need to use this type of medication regularly for several days or weeks. These medications are usually given once or twice a day. Applying cool compresses to the area of itching and swelling may help. When these medications aren't helping, your doctor may add medications called H2 blockers (e.g., ranitidine, famotidine, nizatidine, cimetidine) that are more commonly used to reduce stomach acid but are, in fact, another kind of antihistamine.

ANAPHYLACTIC REACTIONS: WHAT YOU SHOULD DO

An anaphylactic reaction is the most serious of allergic reactions and is always an emergency. It is potentially fatal and requires immediate medical attention. If symptoms such as swelling of the face or throat and wheezing occur, administer self-injectable epinephrine and then call 911 or go to the emergency room immediately. When used properly and promptly, self-injectable epinephrine can reverse most serious reactions and allow for time to get to an emergency room for further treatment. In most cases, it reduces symptoms rapidly, but if it doesn't, another injection should be given five minutes later.

To use an auto-injector, you'll press the device against your child's thigh and hold it there for ten seconds. Make sure to ask your doctor or nurse to give you precise instructions and demonstrate its use with a trainer. At the same time, your childcare center should have written instructions on how to recognize and react to a severe allergic reaction that may be life-threatening, and epinephrine should be available to care providers, along with a step-by-step guide and demonstration on how to administer it. Keep in mind that unused medication in these auto-injectors should be replaced at regular intervals, so check the expiration date and replace it as recommended by your doctor.

If your child has an anaphylactic reaction, see your pediatrician afterward, and find out exactly why the reaction happened and how to avoid another one. Your child should also wear a medical identification bracelet if they have had an anaphylactic episode in the past. This bracelet should give information about the allergies that your child has.

If your child is wheezing or having trouble swallowing, seek emergency treatment. The doctor usually will prescribe self-injectable epinephrine to stop the allergic response. Self-injectable epinephrine should be always available for such patients, including at home, in childcare, or at school, in case of such reactions in the future.

Prevention

Your doctor will try to determine what is causing the hives. For example, does it usually happen an hour after eating a specific food? Or after taking a specific medication? Does your child have any other illness symptoms? How quickly does it resolve? Does it start within one hour of eating and resolve quickly (food allergy) or last days to weeks (infection or unknown cause)? Consult your doctor for evaluation and management.

Insect Bites and Stings

Your child's reaction to a bite or sting will depend on their sensitivity to the insect's venom. While most children have only mild reactions, those who are allergic to certain insect venoms can have severe symptoms that require emergency treatment.

In general, bites are usually not a serious problem, but in some cases, stings may be. While it is true that most stings and bites (from honeybees, yellow jackets, hornets, wasps, and fire ants, for example) may cause pain and localized swelling, severe anaphylactic reactions are also possible. Delayed allergic reactions to being bitten by fleas, bedbugs, or mosquitoes are common, and although uncomfortable, they are not life-threatening.

Treatment

Although insect bites can be irritating, they usually begin to disappear by the next day and do not require a doctor's treatment. To relieve the itchiness that accompanies bites by mosquitoes, flies, fleas, and bedbugs, apply a cool compress and calamine lotion or a low-potency topical steroid on the affected areas. Use oral antihistamines to control itch.

If your child is stung by a wasp or bee, this can be more serious. If redness, pain, and itching are present at the site of the sting, this is a local reaction. Soak a cloth in cold water and press it over the area of the sting to reduce pain and swelling. Non-steroidal anti-inflammatory drugs (ibuprofen) may also be helpful. Call your pediatrician if symptoms persist or become difficult to control. Your child may be prescribed an oral steroid if the swelling is significant. If the reaction occurs in another area of the body (or all over the body), this is a systemic reaction and needs immediate medical attention. If there is throat swelling or trouble breathing, administer self-injectable epinephrine and call 911.

INSECT BITES AND STINGS		
Insect/Environment	**Characteristics of Bite or Sting**	**Special Notes**
Mosquitoes		
Water (pools, lakes, birdbaths)	Stinging sensation followed by small, red, itchy mound with tiny puncture mark at center	Mosquitoes are attracted by bright colors, sweet scents, and sweat.
Flies		
Wet areas with standing water or mud	Painful, itchy bumps; may turn into small blisters	Bites often disappear in a day but may last longer.
Fleas		
Cracks in floor, rugs, pet fur	Multiple small bumps clustered together on exposed areas, particularly arms, legs, face	Fleas are most likely to be a problem in homes with pets.
Bedbugs		
Cracks of walls, floors, crevices of furniture, bedding	Itchy red bumps occasionally topped by a blister; usually 2–3 in a row (same as fleas but may affect covered areas)	Bedbugs are most likely to bite at night and are less active in cold weather.

Fire ants		
Mounds in pastures, meadows, lawns, and parks in southern states	Painful, itchy bumps; may turn into small blisters	Fire ants usually attack intruders.
Bees and wasps		
Flowers, shrubs, picnic areas, beaches	Immediate pain and rapid swelling	A few children have severe reactions, such as difficulty breathing and hives/swelling all over the body.
Ticks		
Wooded areas, tall grass, and underbrush	May not be noticeable; hidden by hair or on skin	Don't remove ticks with matches, lighted cigarettes, or nail polish remover. Grasp the tick firmly with tweezers near the head; gently pull the tick straight out.

If your child disturbs a beehive or wasps' nest, get them away from it as quickly as possible. Any disturbance makes other bees and wasps more likely to sting as well. Keep your child's fingernails short and clean to minimize the risk of infection from scratching. If infection does occur, the bite will become redder, larger, and more swollen. In some cases, you may notice red streaks or yellowish fluid near the bite or your child may get a fever. Have your pediatrician examine any infected bite right away because it may need to be treated with antibiotics.

Call for medical help immediately if your child has any of these other symptoms after being bitten or stung:

- Sudden difficulty in breathing
- Weakness, collapse, or unconsciousness
- Hives or itching all over the body
- Extreme swelling near the eyes, lips, or penis that makes it difficult for the child to see, eat, or urinate

It is impossible to prevent all insect bites, but you can minimize the number your child receives by following these guidelines.

- Avoid areas where insects nest or congregate, such as garbage cans, stagnant pools of water, uncovered foods and sweets, and orchards and gardens where flowers are in bloom.
- When you know your child will be exposed to insects, dress them in long pants and a lightweight long-sleeved shirt as well as closed-toe shoes.
- Avoid dressing your child in clothing with bright colors or flowery prints, because they seem to attract insects.
- Don't use scented soaps, perfumes, or hair sprays on your child, because they also are inviting to insects.

Insect repellents are generally available without a prescription, but they should be used sparingly on infants and young children (see *page 663*). The most common insect repellents are DEET (N,N-diethyl-meta-toluamide) and picaridin. DEET is a chemical that can be used with children 2 months of age and older. The AAP recommends that when used on children, repellents should contain no more than 30 percent DEET. The concentrations of DEET vary significantly from product to product—from less than 10 percent to over 30 percent—so read the label of any product you purchase. DEET's effectiveness peaks at a concentration of 30 percent, which is also the maximum concentration currently recommended for children. It is recommended to use the lowest concentration that will last for the needed length of exposure.

In children who consistently get itchy bumps after insect bites, topical treatment and oral antihistamines are of little help. For these children, wearing protective clothing, treating household pets for fleas, and applying insect repellent are the most effective ways to manage the situation. These repellents are effective in preventing bites by mosquitoes, ticks, fleas, chiggers, and biting flies, but they have virtually no effect on stinging insects such as bees, hornets, and wasps. (The table on *pages 405–6* summarizes information about common stinging or biting insects.)

CHAPTER 14

CHEST AND LUNGS

Bronchiolitis

Bronchiolitis is an infection of the small breathing tubes (bronchioles) of the lungs. It is one of the most common diseases of early childhood. (Note: The term "bronchiolitis" sometimes is confused with "bronchitis," which refers to an infection of the larger, more central airways.) Bronchiolitis is caused most commonly by respiratory syncytial virus (RSV), which can be especially common from October or November through March, though other viruses can be responsible.

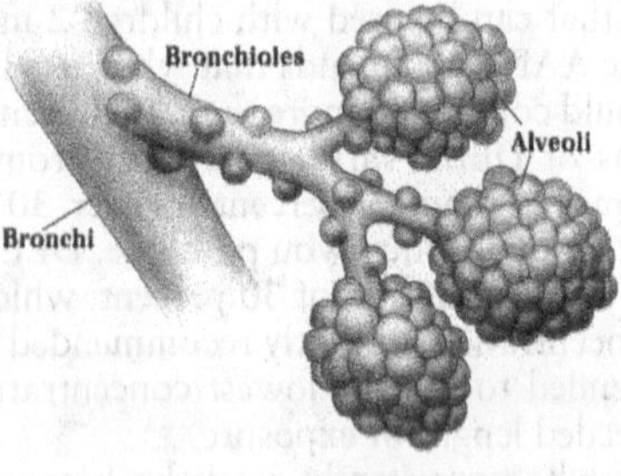

Signs and Symptoms

Almost all children get an RSV infection by the time they are 3 years old. The majority of them develop only an upper respiratory infection (a cold) with a runny nose, mild cough, and sometimes fever. Unfortunately, in a small number of infants, especially those under the age of 1 year, the RSV infection leads to inflammation and swelling of the bronchioles. When this happens, after a day or two the cough becomes more pronounced, and the child begins to breathe more rapidly and with more difficulty.

If your baby shows any of the following signs of breathing difficulty, or if their fever lasts more than three days (or if fever is present at all in an infant under 3 months), call your pediatrician immediately:

- They make a high-pitched whistling sound, called a wheeze, each time they breathe in (inhale) or out (exhale).
- There is drawing in of the skin between and around the ribs and breastbone with each breath.
- They are unable to drink fluids well because they are working so hard to breathe that they have difficulty sucking and swallowing.
- They develop a bluish color around their lips or fingertips. This means the airways are so blocked that not enough oxygen is getting into their lungs and into the blood.

Also call the pediatrician if your child develops any of the following signs or symptoms of dehydration (not enough fluid in the body), which also can appear with bronchiolitis:

- Dry mouth
- Drinking less than their normal amount of fluids
- Not making tears when they cry
- Urinating less often than usual
- Lethargic or not acting as usual (not playing, smiling, or interacting)

Notify your pediatrician as soon as you suspect that your child has bronchiolitis, or if they have any of the following conditions:

- A persistent cough and runny nose (symptoms not improving after a week)
- Any difficulty breathing
- An underlying medical condition such as:
  - —Cystic fibrosis
  - —Congenital heart disease
  - —Bronchopulmonary dysplasia, seen in some infants who were born prematurely or were on a respirator (breathing machine) as newborns

- Low immunity
- Organ transplant
- Cancer for which they are receiving chemotherapy

Treatment

There are no medications to treat bronchiolitis. All you can do during the early phase of the illness is ease your child's cold symptoms. You can relieve some of the nasal stuffiness with a humidifier and salt water (saline) nose drops, with or without gentle nasal suction (aspiration). Coughing is one way for the body to clear the lungs, and normally a cough should not need to be treated with cough suppressant medicine.

If your child has a fever and is over 3 months old, you can give children's acetaminophen (e.g., Tylenol) as instructed on the box, or children's ibuprofen (e.g., Motrin, Advil) if your child is 6 months of age or older. Also, to avoid dehydration, make sure your child drinks lots of fluid during this time. They may prefer clear liquids rather than milk or formula. Because of their breathing difficulty, they also may feed more slowly or eat smaller amounts more frequently. They also may not eat solid foods very well due to decreased appetite. It's usually fine if they eat less solid food while sick as long as they drink enough fluids to avoid dehydration.

In contrast to asthma treatment, no breathing treatments have been shown to help children with bronchiolitis. Your pediatrician may try treatments that open up the lungs (bronchodilators) and steroids (medication inhaled or taken by mouth to decrease inflammation) to see if there is any improvement, but such medications do not prevent hospitalization or change the course of illness in otherwise healthy children with bronchiolitis. If your child is having difficulty breathing, is having trouble feeding, or shows signs of dehydration, take them to the emergency department, where they can receive additional supportive treatment.

Prevention

The best way to protect your child from bronchiolitis is to keep them away from the viruses that cause it. Whenever possible, and especially when your child is an infant, avoid close contact with children or adults who are in the early (contagious) stages of respiratory infections. What produces just a mild cold in an older child or adult can cause breathing problems for an infant. If they are in a childcare center where other children might have the virus, make sure that those who care for them wash their hands thoroughly and frequently. Infants should not be exposed to secondhand smoke, as this can increase the risk of infection.

Previously there was a monthly shot available during RSV season for high-risk infants under 24 months of age to lower their risk of severe RSV infection. Now RSV immunizations are available to be given during pregnancy or during your infant's first year post-birth, depending on how old they will be during RSV season. Some children up to 24 months of age who remain vulnerable to severe RSV disease may also receive an immunization.

Cystic Fibrosis

Cystic fibrosis (CF) is the second-most-common inherited, life-shortening disease of childhood in the United States (second only to sickle cell disease). The overall prevalence is approximately 1 out of every 3,500 live births. Considerable progress has been made in treating cystic fibrosis and its symptoms, although there is still no cure. CF is a disease that changes the secretions of certain glands in the body. It is inherited from parents who carry the gene that causes this disease. For a child to get cystic fibrosis, both parents must be carriers of a genetic abnormality that can cause the disease. Although the sweat glands and the glandular cells of the lungs and pancreas are affected most often, the sinuses, liver, intestines, and reproductive organs also can be involved. In 1989, researchers discovered the most common gene defect that causes CF. Couples planning to have children can undergo genetic testing and counseling to find out if they carry one of the identified abnormal CF genes. They can also receive prenatal testing to detect the gene in the fetus. If both parents are carriers, there are other options available, such as in vitro fertilization (IVF). Talk to your doctor about these alternatives.

Signs and Symptoms

The majority of CF cases are diagnosed within the first two years after birth; in all US states, newborn screenings now include mandatory testing for CF, though not all states test as extensively as others. Therefore, even if the newborn screen was reported as "not suggestive of cystic fibrosis," additional testing is routinely done if there are symptoms of CF present. More than half of CF cases are diagnosed because of repeated lung infections. These infections tend to recur because mucus in the airways is thicker than normal and more difficult to cough out, leading to a persistent cough and potentially pneumonia or bronchitis. Over time, these infections cause damage to the lungs, and are the major cause of death in CF patients in later life. Most children with CF are also deficient in digestive enzymes, making it difficult for them to digest fats and proteins as well as they should. As a result, these children can have large, bulky, foul-smelling stools, accompanied by poor weight gain, if the enzymes are not supplemented (see Treatment, *below*, for more information on enzymes).

To confirm the diagnosis, your pediatrician will order a sweat test to measure the amount of salt your child loses as they perspire. Children with cystic fibrosis have much more salt in their sweat than children who do not have CF. Two or more of these tests may be required to ensure an accurate diagnosis, since the results are not always clearly positive or negative. Often, genetic testing is performed as well, as different abnormal CF genes can indicate the most likely course of the illness in the child. If your child is diagnosed as having the disease, your pediatrician will help you get the additional specialized medical help that is necessary. At a medical center that specializes in treating children with CF, you can find multidisciplinary experts to help your child and family.

Treatment

CF treatment is lifelong and typically requires many visits to a CF center, where your child will be treated by a healthcare team specializing in CF care. Treating the lung infections that develop in children with CF is the most important aspect of your child's care. The goal is to help clear the thick secretions from your child's lungs, which may involve various techniques and medications that help them cough out the sputum more easily. The lung infections themselves are treated with antibiotics. Your child may also be prescribed capsules containing digestive enzymes to be taken with every meal and snack. The amount of enzymes is based on the composition of the diet and the weight of your child. Once the correct amount of enzymes is taken, your child's stool pattern should become more normal and they'll begin gaining more weight. Close observation by your child's primary care physician, the CF center physicians, and the center care team is designed to detect failure to respond to treatment and allow additional therapy.

The majority of children with CF can expect to grow up and lead productive adult lives with continuous treatment according to care guidelines. Balancing the physical and emotional demands created by this disease is hard on both the CF patient and their family, so it is very important that you get as much support as possible. Ask your pediatrician to put you in touch not only with the nearest CF center, but also with CF support groups. The Cystic Fibrosis Foundation can be of help as well (cff.org; 1-800-344-4823). Connecting with other parents is essential to support you, your child, and your family.

Cough

Coughing is almost always an indication of an irritation in your child's air passages. When the nerve endings in the throat, windpipe, or lungs sense the irritation, a reflex causes air to be ejected forcefully through the passageways.

Coughs frequently accompany colds (see *page 468*). When a child has a cold, the cough may be either productive (bringing up mucus) or dry and irritating. The cough may last longer than the accompanying runny nose, up to two to three weeks.

Other respiratory illnesses can produce a cough as well, including bronchiolitis (see *page 408*), croup (see *page 416*), flu (see *page 418*), and pneumonia (see *page 421*). Your pediatrician can often tell by the sound of the cough what may be causing it. For example, an irritation in the larynx (voice box), caused by an illness such as croup, causes a cough that sounds like the bark of a dog or seal, while irritation of the larger airways (bronchi) or the trachea (windpipe) produces a deeper, raspy cough.

In a very young infant, anything more than an occasional cough has to be taken seriously and merits a visit to the pediatrician. If your child has a cough plus a fever and difficulty breathing (the breathing is too fast, too slow, or noisy, or you see a drawing in of the skin between and around the ribs and breastbone when they inhale), they may have a serious infection in the lungs, such as pneumonia. If they have these symptoms, see your doctor immediately.

Allergies and sinus infections can cause a chronic cough because mucus drips down the back of the throat (a condition known as postnasal drip), producing a dry, hard-to-stop cough, particularly at night upon lying down. A child who coughs only while asleep may have asthma (see *page 382*) or gastroesophageal reflux (a condition where the contents of the stomach rise up into the esophagus, causing irritation and cough; see *page 378*).

Here are some cough-related issues that can affect children:

- The most common causes are colds and bronchiolitis, which usually get better in a few days. It is important to watch for signs of breathing difficulties and seek medical help if needed. These signs include not only rapid breathing, especially while asleep, but also drawing in of the skin between and around the ribs and breastbone (sternum).
- Sometimes children cough so hard that they throw up. Usually they vomit liquid and food from the stomach, but there also may be a lot of mucus, especially during a cold or an asthma attack.
- Wheezing is a high-pitched sound during breathing that occurs when there is an obstruction of the airway inside the chest. It is one of the symptoms of asthma, but it also can occur if your child has bronchiolitis, pneumonia, or certain other disorders.
- Children with asthma often cough. Although coughing and wheezing may occur together in children with asthma, they may also only have a cough. This may happen when they are active or playing, or at night. Sometimes their cough can be heard, but the wheezing may be evident only to your doctor when they listen with a stethoscope. The cough and the wheeze usually get better after using asthma medications.

- A cough is commonly worse at night. When your child coughs at night, it may be caused by irritation in the throat or a sinus infection with postnasal drip. Asthma is another major reason for a nighttime cough.

A sudden cough in children can mean that some food or liquid or an object (such as a coin or toy) has "gone down the wrong way" and ended up in the lungs. The coughing is an attempt to clear the airways. However, if coughing continues for more than a few minutes, or if your child is having difficulty breathing, seek medical help right away. Don't put your fingers in your child's mouth to clear the throat because you may push the food or other cause of the obstruction down farther. (See Choking, *page 494*.)

When to Call the Pediatrician

An infant under 2 months of age who develops a cough should be seen by the doctor. For older infants and children, consult your physician immediately if the coughing:

- Makes it difficult for your child to breathe
- Is painful, persistent, and accompanied by whooping, vomiting, or turning blue
- Interferes with eating and sleeping
- Appears suddenly and is associated with a fever
- Begins after your child chokes on food or any other object (see Choking, *page 494*)—though in about 50 percent of cases when a foreign body (food or toy) is inhaled into the lungs, the cough may not develop until a few hours or days later

Your pediatrician will try to determine the cause of your child's cough; most commonly it's due to an upper respiratory virus. When the cough is from a medical problem other than a cold or the flu, such as a bacterial infection or asthma, it will be necessary to treat that condition before the cough will clear. Occasionally when the cause of a chronic cough (lasting longer than four weeks) is not apparent, further tests such as chest X-rays or even testing for tuberculosis may be necessary.

Treatment

Treating a cough depends on its cause. Some people may feel a cool-mist humidifier can help with comfort, especially in dry weather. However, be sure to clean the device thoroughly each morning, as recommended in the manufacturer's manual, so it doesn't become a breeding ground for harmful bacteria or fungi.

Nighttime coughing associated with allergies can be problematic, because they prevent the child (and often the rest of the family) from getting a good night's sleep. Nighttime coughing from asthma is often a sign that asthma treatment is needed or, if the child is already taking asthma medication, that a change in asthma medication is needed. If the night cough is due to asthma, use a bronchodilator or other asthma medication as directed by your pediatrician.

Although cough medicines can be purchased without a prescription, these cough medicines are not effective for children younger than 6 years old and may not help older children either. They may even pose a health risk from serious side effects, especially for children under age 2. As long as your child is over 1 year of age, honey straight from a spoon or diluted in warm water works just as well. (Never give honey to an infant, because it can cause a serious and deadly infection called botulism.)

Croup

Croup is an inflammation of the voice box (larynx) and windpipe (trachea). It causes a barking cough and a high-pitched sound when breathing in (stridor). Croup is usually caused by a virus, most commonly the parainfluenza virus. Other, less common viral causes of croup include the flu, RSV, adenovirus, and enteroviruses. The illness most often is caught from someone who is infected, sometimes from air droplets or from your child's own hand, which they use to transfer the virus into their nose or mouth.

Croup tends to occur in the fall and winter in children between 3 months and 3 years old. Initially your child may develop nasal stuffiness (resembling a cold) and fever. After a day or two, the sound of the cough will turn into something resembling a barking or seal-like cough. The cough tends to become worse at night.

The greatest danger with croup is that your child's airway will continue to swell, further narrowing their windpipe and making it difficult to breathe. As your child tires from the effort of breathing, they may stop eating and drinking. They also may become too fatigued to cough. Some children are particularly prone to getting a croup-like cough whenever they have a respiratory illness.

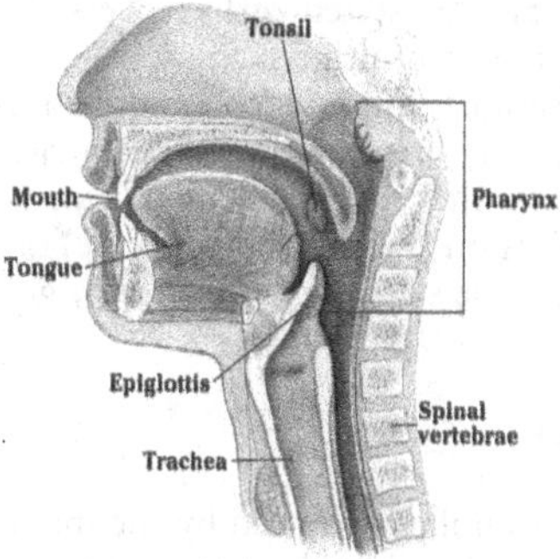

Treatment

If your child has mild croup symptoms, steam up the bathroom by turning on the hot water in the shower. Take your child into the steamy bathroom, close the door, and sit in the bathroom with your child. Inhaling the warm, humidified air should ease their breathing within fifteen to twenty minutes. Or, weather permitting, you can take them outside to breathe in the cool, damp night air. While they are sleeping, use a cool-mist humidifier in their room.

Do not try to open your child's airway with your finger. Their breathing is being obstructed by swollen tissue beyond your reach, so you can't clear it away. They may throw up because of the coughing, but don't try to make them vomit. Pay close attention to your child's breathing. Take them to the nearest emergency room immediately if:

- They seem to be struggling to get a breath.
- They can't speak because of a lack of breath.

- They get excessively sleepy.
- They turn blue when they cough.
- You still hear stridor when your child is calm or resting.

Your pediatrician may prescribe various medications, usually steroids, to help decrease the swelling in the upper airway and throat and make it easier for them to breathe. Steroids will also decrease the amount of time your child has symptoms of croup. Antibiotics are not helpful for croup because the infection is usually caused by a virus. Cough syrups do not help, either. In fact, as stated earlier, over-the-counter cough medicines may pose a health risk.

In the most serious cases, which are quite rare, if your child has a lot of difficulty breathing, your pediatrician may recommend you go to the emergency department for a special breathing medication (racemic epinephrine) or admit them to the hospital until the swelling in the airway gets better.

Influenza (Flu)

Influenza (flu) is an illness caused by the influenza virus. The infection can spread rapidly through communities as the virus is passed from person to person. When someone with the flu coughs or sneezes, the influenza virus gets into the air, and people nearby, including children, can inhale it. The virus also can be spread when a contagious person touches a hard surface, such as a door handle, and then someone else touches the same surface and then their nose, mouth, or eyes. The virus is most likely to be transmitted to other people during the first several days of illness. Flu is most common from fall through spring.

Flu symptoms include:

- A sudden fever, usually above 101 degrees Fahrenheit (38.3 degrees Celsius)
- Chills and body shakes
- Headache, body aches, and being a lot more tired than usual
- Sore throat
- Dry, hacking cough
- Stuffy, runny nose

While influenza may cause some abdominal pain, vomiting, and diarrhea, it does most of its damage in the respiratory system; it should not be confused with viruses that cause what is commonly known as stomach flu.

You may wonder whether your child has a cold or the flu. A child with a common cold (see Colds/Upper Respiratory Infections, *page 468*) usually has a lower fever, a runny nose, and only a small amount of coughing. Children with the flu usually feel much sicker, achier, and more miserable.

Most children get over the flu in about a week or two without any lingering problems. However, you might suspect a complication if their cough and fever persist beyond two weeks.

Children who appear to have the greatest risk of complications from influenza are those with an underlying chronic medical condition, such as heart, lung, or kidney disease, an immune system problem, diabetes, some blood diseases, or a malignancy. Such children should be kept away from anyone showing symptoms suggestive of influenza, such as fever, cough, and runny nose, and your pediatrician may suggest additional precautions.

Treatment

For all children with the flu who don't feel well, lots of tender loving care is in order. Children can benefit from extra bed rest, extra fluids, and light meals. A cool-mist humidifier or vaporizer in the room may add additional moisture to the air and make breathing a little easier.

If your child is uncomfortable because of a fever, acetaminophen or ibuprofen in doses recommended by your pediatrician for their age and weight will help them feel better. (See *Chapter* 22, Fever.) Ibuprofen is approved for use in children 6 months of age and older; however, it should never be given to children who are dehydrated or who are vomiting continuously. It is extremely important never to give aspirin to a child who has or may have the flu. Giving a child aspirin during a viral illness is associated with an increased risk of developing Reye syndrome, a serious disease that affects the liver and brain.

Prevention

Every child 6 months or older (including infants who were born preterm) should get the flu vaccine each year—the vaccine is safe, and it's the best way to prevent the illness. The best time to get the flu vaccine is the late summer or early fall, or as soon as it is available in your community.

Currently there are two types of the vaccine to protect against the flu—an inactivated (killed) vaccine, also called the flu shot, which is given by injection, and a live, attenuated (weakened) influenza vaccine that is sprayed into the nostrils, often called the flu mist. Ask your pediatrician which is preferred for your child. If your child is receiving the flu vaccine for the first time, they will need two doses given at least one month apart.

Everyone should get the flu vaccine annually, but for some people it's especially important. All healthcare personnel and adults who live in the same household as someone with a high risk for flu complications or who care for children under the age of 5 years should receive the flu vaccine yearly. All women who are pregnant, are considering pregnancy, have recently delivered, or are breastfeeding during the flu season should also receive a flu vaccine.

The flu vaccine has few side effects, the most common being redness, soreness, or swelling at the injection site and fever. Although some flu vaccines are produced using chicken eggs, the vaccine itself has been shown to contain minimal egg protein, and many studies have shown that it is safe for people with egg allergy, so all children with presumed egg allergy can safely receive the flu vaccine without any special precautions.

In addition to being vaccinated, here are some tips that will help protect your family from becoming sick:

1. Wash hands often. Use soap and warm water and lather up for at least twenty seconds—about as long as it takes to sing the "Happy Birthday" song two times. An alcohol-based hand sanitizer works well, too. Put enough on your hands to make them all wet, and then rub them together until dry.
2. Teach your child to cover their mouth and nose when coughing or sneezing. Show your child how to cough

into the elbow or upper sleeve (not a hand) or use a tissue.

3. Throw all tissues used for runny noses and sneezes in the trash right away.
4. Wash dishes and utensils in hot, soapy water or the dishwasher.
5. Don't let children share pacifiers, cups, spoons, forks, washcloths, or towels without washing. Never share toothbrushes.
6. Teach your child to try not to touch their eyes, nose, or mouth.
7. Clean doorknobs, toilet handles, countertops, and even toys. Use a disinfectant wipe or a cloth with soap and hot water.

If your child does become ill, antiviral medications to treat some kinds of influenza infection are available by prescription. Antiviral medications work best if started within the first one to two days of showing signs of the flu, so call your pediatrician within twenty-four hours to ask about antiviral medications if your child is at high risk of influenza complications or if your child:

- Has any serious health problem like asthma, diabetes, sickle cell disease, or cerebral palsy
- Is younger than 2 years, but especially if younger than 6 months, as young children are at an increased risk of influenza infection, hospitalization, and serious complications, including death

Pneumonia

The word "pneumonia" refers to an infection of the lung. While such infections were extremely dangerous in past generations, today most children recover from pneumonia if they receive proper medical attention.

Most cases of pneumonia follow a viral upper respiratory tract infection. Pneumonia also can be caused by bacteria. If a viral infection has irritated the airway enough or weakened a child's immune system, bacteria may begin to grow in the lung, adding a second infection to the original one.

Children whose immune defenses or lungs are weakened by other illnesses, such as cystic fibrosis, asthma, or cancer, are more likely to develop pneumonia. Children whose airways or lungs are abnormal in any other way also have a higher risk.

Because most forms of pneumonia are linked to viral or bacterial infections that spread from person to person, they're most common during the fall, winter, and early spring, when children spend more time indoors in close contact with others. The chance that a child will develop pneumonia is not affected by how warmly they are dressed or by air temperature on cold days.

Signs and Symptoms

Like many infections, pneumonia usually produces a fever, which in turn may cause sweating, chills, flushed skin, and general discomfort. The child also may lose their appetite and seem less energetic than normal. Babies and toddlers may seem pale and limp and cry more than usual.

Because pneumonia can cause breathing difficulties, you may notice these other, more specific symptoms, too:

- Cough (see *page 413*)
- Fast, labored breathing
- Drawing in of the skin between and around the ribs and breastbone with each breath
- Flaring (widening) of the nostrils
- Pain in the chest, particularly with coughing or deep breathing
- Wheezing
- Bluish color to the lips or nails, caused by decreased oxygen in the bloodstream

Although the diagnosis of pneumonia usually can be made by a pediatrician on the basis of the signs, symptoms, and examination, a chest X-ray sometimes is necessary to make certain and to determine the extent of lung involvement.

Treatment

When pneumonia is caused by a virus, usually there is no specific treatment other than rest and the usual measures for fever control (see *Chapter 22*, Fever). Coughing is helpful in clearing the excessive secretions caused by the infection. Viral pneumonia usually improves after a few days, although the cough may linger for several weeks.

Because it is often difficult to tell whether the pneumonia is caused by a virus or by bacteria, your pediatrician may prescribe an antibiotic. All antibiotics should be taken for the full prescribed course and at the specific dosage recommended. Your child will feel better after just a few days, and you may be tempted to discontinue medication early, but you should not do so—some bacteria may remain, and the infection might return unless the entire course is completed. Check back with the doctor if your child shows any of the following signs that the infection may be worsening or spreading:

- Fever lasting more than a few days despite using antibiotics
- Fever that goes away and then returns after a few days
- Breathing difficulties
- Increased lethargy and sleepiness
- Evidence of an infection elsewhere in the body: red and swollen joints, bone pain, neck stiffness, vomiting, or other new symptoms or signs

Prevention

Your child should be vaccinated against pneumococcal infections, a bacterial cause of pneumonia. The American Academy of Pediatrics recommends that all children younger than 2 years old receive this immunization (called pneumococcal conjugate). A series of doses needs to be given at 2, 4, 6, and 12 to 15 months of age, at the same time that children receive other childhood vaccines.

If your child did not receive the initial doses at the recommended times, talk to your pediatrician about a catch-up schedule. One dose of pneumococcal conjugate vaccine should be given to all healthy children ages 2 through 5 years who have not previously received their recommended doses before the age of 2 years and to children ages 2 through 18 years with certain underlying medical conditions who have not previously received a dose.

(See also Asthma, *page 382*; Colds/Upper Respiratory Infections, *page 468*; and *Chapter* 22, Fever.)

Tuberculosis

Tuberculosis (TB) is an airborne infection that primarily affects the lungs. While TB is less common than it once was, some groups of children have a higher risk of developing tuberculosis, including:

- Children living in a household with an adult who has active tuberculosis or has a high risk of contracting TB
- Children infected with HIV or another condition that weakens the immune system
- Children born in a country that has a high prevalence of TB
- Children visiting a country where TB is regularly found (endemic) and who have extended contact with people who live there
- Children from communities that generally receive inadequate medical care
- Children living in a shelter or living with someone who has been in jail

Tuberculosis usually is spread when an infected adult coughs the bacteria into the air. These germs are inhaled by the child, who then becomes infected. Children younger than about 10 years with TB of the lungs rarely transmit infection to other people, because they tend to have very few bacteria in their mucous secretions and also have a relatively ineffective cough.

Fortunately, most children exposed to tuberculosis do not become ill. When the bacteria reach their lungs, the body's immune system attacks the bacteria and prevents further spread. However, the child still must be treated to prevent the disease from becoming active. Occasionally, in a small number of children without proper treatment, the infection does progress to disease, causing fever, fatigue, irritability, a persistent cough, weakness, heavy and fast breathing, night sweats, swollen glands, weight loss, and poor growth.

In a very small number of children (mostly those less than 4 years old), the tuberculosis infection can spread through the bloodstream, affecting virtually any organ in the body. This illness requires much more complicated treatment, and the earlier treatment is started, the better the outcome. These children have a much greater risk of developing tuberculous meningitis, a dangerous form of the disease that affects the brain and central nervous system.

If your child has any of the risk factors mentioned earlier, your pediatrician may recommend a test to see whether they have ever been exposed to the illness. The tuberculin skin test can be used in infants under age 1. Your child may need testing if you answer yes to at least one of the following questions:

- Has a family member or contact had tuberculosis disease?
- Has a family member had a positive tuberculin skin test?
- Was your child born in a high-risk country (countries other than the United States, Canada, Australia, New Zealand, or Western European countries)?
- Has your child traveled (had contact with resident populations) to a high-risk country for more than one week?

The skin test is performed in the pediatrician's office by injecting a purified, inactive piece of TB germ into the skin of the forearm. If there has been an infection, your child's skin will gradually swell and redden at the injection site. Your pediatrician must check the skin forty-eight to seventy-two hours after the injection and measure the diameter of the reaction. The test will be able to tell if the bacteria have ever entered the child's body, even if the child has had no symptoms.

If your child's skin test for TB comes back positive, a chest X-ray will be ordered to determine if there is evidence of an active or past infection in the lungs. If the X-ray does indicate the possibility of an active infection, the pediatrician also will search for the TB bacteria in your child's cough secretions or in the stomach. This is done in order to determine the type of treatment needed.

Treatment

If your child's skin or blood test is positive but they do not have symptoms or signs of active tuberculosis infection, they still have the tuberculosis bacteria hiding out in their body and will need to be treated to prevent the bacteria from becoming active and causing symptoms. The medication used for treatment, isoniazid, must be taken by mouth once a day every day for a minimum of nine months (antibiotics for shorter lengths of time may be possible).

For an active tuberculosis infection, your pediatrician or an infectious disease specialist will prescribe three or four medications. You will have to give these to your child every day for six to twelve months. Your child may have to be hospitalized initially for the treatment to be started, although most of it can be carried out at home.

Prevention

If your child has been infected with TB, regardless of whether they develop symptoms, it is very important to attempt to identify the person from whom they caught the disease. Usually this is done by looking for symptoms of TB in everyone who came in close contact with them, including family members and childcare providers, and having TB skin tests or blood tests done. The most common symptom in adults is a persistent cough, especially one that is associated with coughing up blood. Anyone who has a positive skin test or blood test should receive a physical examination, a chest X-ray, and treatment.

When active tuberculosis infection is found in an adult, they should be isolated as much as possible—especially from young children—until treatment is under way. Certain family members who have been in contact with that person, including all children under 5 years old and those with conditions like HIV, usually are also initially treated with isoniazid, regardless of the results of their own skin tests. Anyone who becomes ill or develops an abnormality on a chest X-ray should be treated as having an active case of tuberculosis.

Whooping Cough (Pertussis)

Pertussis, or whooping cough, is caused by bacteria that attack the lining of the breathing passages (bronchi and bronchioles), producing inflammation and narrowing of the airways. Severe coughing is a prominent symptom. Because the child is short of breath, they inhale deeply and quickly between coughs. These breaths frequently make a "whooping" sound—which is how this illness got its common name. The intense coughing scatters the pertussis bacteria into the air, spreading the disease to other susceptible persons.

Many years ago, there were several hundred thousand cases of whooping cough each year in the United States. After the development of a vaccine for pertussis, that figure decreased. But in recent years there has been a rise in the number of cases seen in the United States. As a result, giving the pertussis vaccine to children and their caregivers is more important than ever. Infants under 1 year of age are at greatest risk of developing severe breathing problems and life-threatening illness from whooping cough.

Pertussis often acts like a common cold for a week or two. Then the cough gets worse (rather than better, as usually happens with a cold), and older children may start to have the characteristic "whoop." During this phase (which can last two weeks or more), the child often is short of breath and can look bluish around the mouth. They also may tear up, drool, and vomit. Young infants with pertussis may have episodes where they appear to stop breathing or they begin vomiting after a long bout of coughing. Infants with pertussis become exhausted and develop complications such as susceptibility to other infections, pneumonia, and seizures. Pertussis can be fatal in some infants, but the usual course is for recovery to begin after two to four more weeks. The cough of pertussis, which has also been called the "100-day cough," may not disappear for months, and may return with subsequent respiratory infections.

When to Call the Pediatrician

Pertussis infection starts out acting like a cold. You should consider whooping cough if the following conditions are present:

- The child is a very young infant who has not been fully immunized and/or has been exposed to someone with a chronic cough or the disease.
- The child's cough becomes more severe and frequent, or their lips and fingertips become dark or blue.
- They become exhausted after coughing episodes, eat poorly, vomit after coughing, and/or look "sick."

Treatment

The majority of infants less than 6 months old with whooping cough initially need to be treated in the hospital. In addition, slightly less than half of older babies with the disease are initially treated in the hospital. This more intensive care can decrease the chances of complications. These complications can include pneumonia, which occurs in slightly less than one-fourth of children under 1 year old who have whooping cough.

While in the hospital, your child may need to have the thick respiratory secretions suctioned. Their breathing will be monitored, and they may need to have oxygen administered. Your child will be isolated from other patients to keep the infection from spreading to them.

Whooping cough is treated with an antibiotic that is most effective when given in the first stage of the illness, before coughing spells begin. Although antibiotics can stop the spread of the infection, they cannot prevent or treat the cough itself. Because cough medicines do not relieve the coughing spells, your pediatrician probably will recommend other forms of home treatment to help manage the cough. Let your child rest in bed, and use a cool-mist vaporizer to help soothe their irritated lungs and breathing passages. A vaporizer also will help loosen secretions in the respiratory tract. Ask your pediatrician for instructions on the best position for your child to help drain those secretions and improve breathing. Also ask your doctor whether antibiotics or vaccine boosters need to be given to others in your household to prevent them from developing the disease. Children who have been diagnosed with pertussis should be kept home from daycare until finishing five days of antibiotics.

Prevention

The best way to protect your child against pertussis is with the DTaP vaccine (immunizations at 2 months, 4 months, and 6 months of age, and booster shots at 12 to 18 months and at 4 or 5 years of age or prior to starting school). Parents or family members who will be in close contact with infants younger than 1 year old should also receive the Tdap booster to decrease the risk of passing the infection to the infant. In addition, all women who are pregnant should receive the Tdap vaccine during each pregnancy. This allows mothers to pass on protection against pertussis to their newborns.

CHAPTER 15

CHRONIC HEALTH CONDITIONS

Coping with Chronic (Long-Term) Health Problems

We tend to think of childhood as a carefree and healthy time of life, but some children face chronic health problems during these early years. What distinguishes a chronic health problem from an acute health problem is that the acute problem is expected to resolve in a relatively short time frame and the child will return to their typical level of health. An acute health problem could mean an injury or a fracture that will heal, or an infection such as pneumonia, from which your child will recover completely. There are also many conditions that the child will outgrow without any treatment or intervention. For example, a child with bed-wetting or intoeing will usually outgrow such health issues by school age.

In contrast, a chronic health problem is usually expected to last a year or more and requires ongoing medical attention for management. For example, a child with asthma may require inhalers every day to prevent an asthma attack. Parents should take steps to reduce exposure to irritants and allergens in the child's environment, and will need to learn about asthma, the treatment plan, and what to do if the child has an asthma attack. The child will need to visit their primary care doctor, specialist, or both several times throughout the year. Parents also need to learn how to navigate the healthcare system so that their child gets the treatment they need. Finally, parents need to help their child cope with the chronic condition emotionally and physically, and to be able to help themselves and other family members cope as well. You could substitute diabetes, autism spectrum disorder, juvenile idiopathic arthritis, or any other number of diagnoses, and the challenges would be very similar.

The information that follows is aimed at helping parents and caregivers deal with the emotional and practical challenges of caring for a child who has a long-term health condition, special healthcare need, or disability. (The specific medical treatment of many chronic conditions is discussed elsewhere, under the names of those conditions; see the Index.)

Some long-term health conditions in children are relatively mild, and some children with chronic health conditions will be able to enjoy good health due to the success of ongoing medical treatment. Regardless, any type of long-lasting condition, special healthcare need, or disability is stressful for both the child and their family. It is important to be able to manage all of these aspects and take care of yourself in the process.

Learning about your child's chronic condition is a slow process, and it can be very frustrating at times; occasionally you may feel alone with these challenges. Rest assured that you are not alone. Your reactions, grief, and frustrations are normal, and your journey will be filled with many highs and lows; you will meet other parents on the same journey; and you will have many victories. Also remember that your child is still your child—they are not, and should not be, defined by the medical condition.

Receiving the Diagnosis of a Chronic Condition in Your Child

All parents, from the time they find out they are expecting a child, start out assuming the child will be healthy. You may have found out about your child's condition during pregnancy, in the newborn nursery, or afterward when you noticed that something was not quite right about your child's health. Regardless of when your child was diagnosed, being given the diagnosis of a chronic condition can cause a parent to feel sadness, fear, guilt, or grief at losing the expectation of a healthy child. This is a normal reaction and an adjustment that all parents of a child with a chronic condition endure.

You may feel that your hopes and expectations for your child have been replaced by fear of the unknown. You may think: "What will happen to my child in two years? Five? Ten? Will the condition get better or worse? How am I going to manage all of these medications? Will I have to take time off from work? How much pain will my child have? Will my insurance cover all the costs?" You may never forget the day that you were given the diagnosis for your child. It's a lot of information to absorb, and it takes time to process it all.

This may be a brand-new world for you, with a lot to learn in a relatively short period of time. There may be highs and lows, flares and periods of quiet, denial and fear of the unknown. There may be days when you think you are the only parent with a child who has special needs, and you may wonder if anyone else knows how you feel. All of this can take a toll on your own well-being and health, which in turn can affect how you take care of your child. Recognizing these emotions will help you learn how to care for your child, your family, and yourself.

If your child is born with a serious medical problem or develops a chronic medical condition during their first years, you may face some of the following stressors and decisions:

- The realization that your child is not perfectly healthy may lead to feelings of disappointment and guilt, and fear for the child's future. In trying to deal with these feelings, you may find yourself struggling with unexplained emotional swings ranging from hopefulness to depression and anxiety.
- It can help to select and work with a team of medical and community partners who can help your child and work with you in shared decision-making.
- You may be faced with learning about a new diagnosis and understanding your child's prognosis.
- You may face decisions about treatment or surgery.
- You may have to be responsible for giving your child certain medications, guiding them in usage of special equipment, or performing special therapies.
- You will be called on to provide the time, energy, money, and emotional commitment necessary for your child to receive the treatment and coordinated care they need.
- You will need to learn how to access appropriate services and information.
- In adapting your life to meet your child's needs without neglecting other family members, you may face many difficult choices, some of which may require compromise solutions.

Navigating the Healthcare System

Parents of children with chronic conditions routinely describe navigating the healthcare system as one of their biggest challenges. Depending on your child's condition, you may be dealing with a few extra doctor visits per year, or you could be working with multiple specialists, pharmacies, therapists, insurance companies, and home healthcare agencies and personnel as well as hospitalizations. All of this may sometimes seem overwhelming and take up a great deal of time. Empowering yourself with information about your child's condition is a necessary start to learning how to navigate the healthcare system as effectively as possible.

You know your child and their needs better than anyone else. Read about your child's condition, ask questions of your child's doctors and nurses, and talk with other parents. The information you learn—and particularly the answers to questions that you don't know to ask in the early stages—will help you engage with your child's doctors in making decisions. Healthcare and developmental outcomes are improved when the parents are part of the decision-making process and knowledgeable about the child's condition. Keep a notebook with questions, and make sure they are answered. If you see something at home that concerns you, call your pediatrician, specialist, or medical provider, or use the patient portal of your health system's electronic health record; do not assume that you have to wait until the next scheduled appointment. Your healthcare team will depend on and respect the information parents and caregivers provide them to make the right medical decision for your child.

It's best to make sure your child has a "medical home" that includes physical, behavioral, and dental/oral healthcare providers. The American Academy of Pediatrics defines a medical home as care that is accessible, continuous, comprehensive, family-centered, coordinated, compassionate, and culturally effective. The medical home model of care means that the medical care team, child, and family work in partnership together to meet all the child's special needs. At a minimum, ensure that your child has regularly scheduled visits with their doctors to actively manage the child's condition; this will help keep your child as healthy as possible. It is essential that you and your family have a strong relationship with your child's primary care physician, who will help oversee all aspects of care. It is also helpful to select one medical person as the overall coordinator of your child's medical care. This person may be someone in your pediatrician's office or another health professional who is closely involved with your child's treatment. It should be someone who knows your family well, fosters shared decision-making, values you as an equal team member, makes you feel comfortable, and is willing to spend time answering questions, partnering with you, and working with other doctors and therapists involved in your child's care. Many primary care offices, healthcare systems, and insurance companies provide a care manager, often a nurse or social worker, who is knowledgeable about your child's condition, your child's care team, and the community services, equipment, medications, and other resources they require.

Keep track of and manage what goes on at home to ensure that you can carry out the medical care recommendations, and that your child gets good nutrition and all their medications as recommended. Make sure that your child's medical care needs are met proactively—that is, everyone works to keep your child healthy and ensure they do not get sicker due to a complication of the chronic health problem. Many children with chronic healthcare conditions have relatively long periods in which those conditions are well controlled; at other times, the condition may flare up. Your goal is to keep the condition under control and learn the signs and symptoms of a flare so you can intervene early and prevent complications, whether those are emergency department visits, hospital admissions, or even long-term consequences to your child.

Be sure that you include dental/oral health and behavioral health providers in your team to ensure optimal health for your child. Chronic medical conditions can add challenges when it comes to dental health, but pediatric dentists are usually equipped to help you address those challenges.

Parent support groups will have meetings (either online or in person), offer online groups and listservs, and provide literature and emotional support. Learn about the options for treatment, including those that your doctor may not know about or is not familiar with. Regardless of whether those options are what you decide to choose, information enables you to take control of the treatment plan and have the knowledge to make the right decision for your child and family.

Getting Help for Your Child

There are many ways that you can help with a chronic condition. You can start by making sure that your child gets to all of their doctor appointments on time. If you must miss a doctor's appointment, call the doctor's office right away and get it rescheduled—preferably before you miss the appointment. That way, your child's doctors can help you manage the medical condition before there is a disease flare. If you find that you are unable to give your child their medications because of scheduling conflicts, financial barriers to filling the prescription, or your child's refusal, call your provider or healthcare team. Doctors will give you advice on how to help your child accept the regimen, or they may be able to propose an alternative treatment plan. It is important that you let your child's doctors know what is going on at home and if something needs to be changed.

Where We Stand

When children have a chronic, serious illness or disability, their parents may turn to complementary or alternative therapies, wanting to try everything and anything to help their child. These treatments often are used in addition to the care their child is receiving from their pediatrician or other medical practitioner. In most cases, parents use these complementary or alternative therapies even though they are happy with traditional medical care; however, in some cases, parents may turn to them when they become frustrated with the limitations on what mainstream medicine can offer their child.

If you've made the decision to seek alternative therapies for your child's care, involve your pediatrician in the process. In most cases, such therapies work best when used in combination with traditional or integrative medical care. In fact, pediatricians trained in integrative medicine are specially trained in combining conventional (standard) therapies such as medications and surgery with complementary therapies that have been shown to be safe and effective, such as acupuncture and meditation. In addition, your doctor may be able to help you better understand these therapies, whether they have scientific merit, whether claims about them are accurate or exaggerated, and whether they pose any risks to your child's well-being. Keep in mind that an alternative treatment does not always mean a safe one, and your pediatrician can help you determine whether there is a risk of interactions with your child's other medications.

The American Academy of Pediatrics has encouraged pediatricians to evaluate the scientific merits of alternative therapies, determine whether they might cause any direct or indirect harm, and advise parents on the full range of treatment options. If you decide to use a complementary or alternative therapy, your pediatrician or integrative medicine physician may be able to assist in evaluating your child's response to that treatment.

Good nutrition and growth are at the root of helping a child with chronic healthcare needs. Some children with a chronic health condition have difficulty eating and swallowing. It is especially important for your child to be offered a good, healthy diet. If necessary, a parent or caregiver can work with the doctors or nutritionists to make sure your child is not gaining too little weight or too much. Some children with difficulty swallowing will cough or retch with feeds. If that is the case, you may also need to work with an occupational therapist or speech and language pathologist, who can focus on helping your child learn to swallow with less difficulty to avoid inhaling food particles into the lungs.

Not all of your child's chronic needs will be medical, of course. They may require community supports such as special schooling, counseling, or other therapy. Many children with chronic conditions can attend daycare or school. Some children may be in private daycare; others may be in a center-based learning center specifically for children with disabilities. It is important that you speak with your child's teachers and caregivers about the medical needs. Specifically, you should let your child's teachers and caregivers know what the medical condition is, medications or therapies that are needed during the day, and warning signs about which you need to be called.

School nurses may be available to help you and your child manage any medical condition.

Your family may need outside financial or governmental assistance. The team that coordinates your child's medical care also should provide some guidance in obtaining this extra help, but the best way to make sure you and your child get the services and support needed is to learn about the resources and regulations that apply to special services for children with chronic healthcare needs. You also should find out what you can do if the services received do not meet your child's needs. Family Voices (familyvoices.org) is one organization that helps families connect with needed resources.

Focus on emotional state and well-being. Help your child adapt to their chronic condition. You should offer your child every opportunity to enjoy typical activities and participate to the extent that it is medically safe to do so. That means going to the park to run and play if they are able, making friends, and attending school. As your child gets older, they will become increasingly aware of the medical treatments and the sense of being "different," regardless of whether there is any actual physical disability or appearances. Many children may not talk about their feelings but will act out in different ways, including throwing tantrums, having a short fuse, or being sad. Meeting other children with a chronic condition can help. It is also important to acknowledge your child's feelings and help caregivers and teachers understand how your child is coping so they can help. Many children and families benefit from counseling or therapy to help cope with these unique stresses.

CHAPTER 16

DEVELOPMENTAL DISABILITIES

It's natural to compare your child with others their age. Each child, however, has their own unique rate of development, so some learn certain skills faster than others. Sometimes, when a child is slightly delayed, they may simply need a little more time to catch up to other peers. If your child seems especially behind or different from their peers, however, it's important to let their pediatrician know. Significant developmental issues should be identified as soon as possible so that early intervention can help ensure that the child reaches their full developmental potential.

Chapters 5 through 9 of this book can give you a better idea of what skills your child should have by certain ages. If you notice something that doesn't seem right or if your child loses a skill they had previously gained, make sure your pediatrician knows. Developmental disabilities that can be identified during childhood include intellectual disability, language and learning disorders, attention-deficit/hyperactivity disorder, cerebral palsy, autism spectrum disorder, and sensory impairments such as vision and hearing impairments. (Some pediatricians include epilepsy in this category, but some children who have epilepsy develop typically.)

Within each developmental disability there is a range of mild to severe that may impact daily functioning just a little bit or a lot. Also, some children may have more than one disability, each requiring different types of support. Your pediatrician and medical home will be integral to helping you navigate any medical and other support if your child has a developmental disability.

The AAP recommends that all children have developmental surveillance at all well-child visits and developmental screening with an approved standardized instrument at 9, 18, and 30 months. If your child fails the developmental screening examination and/or there are parental concerns, your child should have a complete medical and developmental evaluation, including a consultation with a developmental-behavioral pediatrician, child neurologist, geneticist, or pediatric rehabilitation medicine physician, all of whom are specialists trained in evaluation, diagnosis, and care planning for children with disabilities. Your pediatrician will refer you to the most appropriate professional for further assessment. Doing this will give your pediatrician the information they need to determine whether a true disability exists and, if so, how it should be managed. Your physician may recommend additional evaluation by a physical, speech and language, or occupational therapist. Early intervention services are typically recommended for children under the age of 3 with developmental delays/disabilities or medical conditions that place children at high risk for delay or disability. You don't need a referral from a doctor for an evaluation by an early intervention specialist (ages birth to age 3 years), but your pediatrician is often available to help you arrange these consultations. These evaluations may be available through the public early intervention system for your county if your child is under 3 years of age.

Most states also offer special early intervention programs for infants and toddlers. For children under 3, such intervention may be provided in your home.

The families of children with diagnosed disabilities also need special support and education. Families often worry about how they can help their child once a developmental disability is identified. To understand how your child can make developmental progress, each member of your family should be educated about the child's developmental condition and counseled about how to help them develop new skills. One of the most important tenets of early intervention, in fact, is to teach parents appropriate therapeutic techniques that can be practiced and utilized even outside therapy sessions.

If your child is diagnosed with a developmental disability, you may find yourself feeling overwhelmed. Where will you find care? Does your home need modifications? How will this process affect their education, your career, other children in the home? The questions may seem endless. Support is all around you, however, and your pediatrician can help you in starting to find answers. Look for family support networks (organizations like Family Voices, familyvoices.org, can help). Take time to talk with family members and caregivers, including your pediatrician, about what outcomes your family most values and what sort of interventions might work best for your particular situation (this process is called shared decision-making). Remember that you may be relying on any number of experts to help your child, but you are the best expert in the world on your own child's specific needs.

Autism Spectrum Disorder

Autism spectrum disorder (ASD), commonly referred to as autism, affects a child's behavior, social skills, and communication abilities. Both "ASD" and "autism" are used to describe the same condition. Autism is a lifelong condition and can impair the way an individual interacts with others. Although there is a range of symptoms with varying levels of severity, from mild differences in social awareness to severe disabilities in relating to and communicating with others, the scientific consensus now is that autism spectrum disorder is a single diagnosis that results from many different causes. The diagnosis of ASD can be further modified by indicating whether a child has an additional language disorder and/or intellectual disability and whether there is a known neurogenetic condition associated with or predisposing to autism.

The social symptoms associated with ASD are typically seen in the first year after birth (although they may be subtle). Children may have difficulty with non-verbal communication, such as use of gestures, pointing, making eye contact, and imitation. If you are concerned that your child is delayed in any of the milestones noted in this book, be sure to bring this up with your pediatrician at your infant's next checkup, or schedule a separate appointment to discuss your concerns.

Autism affects children of all races, ethnicities, and socioeconomic groups. It occurs about four times more often in boys than in girls and is diagnosed in nearly one of every forty-four children in the United States. Although autism was once thought of as relatively rare, the number of children identified as having this diagnosis has risen in recent years. This increase in reported cases is likely due in part to a greater awareness of autism's signs and symptoms on the part of parents, teachers, and pediatricians, which means that more children are being diagnosed. In addition, some children who are diagnosed as having autism today might have been classified in the past as having a different diagnosis, like intellectual disability; this would also contribute to the increase in numbers.

As noted, autism is a diagnosis that describes a spectrum of symptoms. Likely there are many different underlying reasons for these symptoms, so in most individual cases the exact cause of autism remains unclear. Studies of families, including those with twins, have shown that genetics plays an important role in autism. Researchers are also studying factors in the environment that may interact with genes to increase a child's risk of developing symptoms of autism. Better awareness leads to diagnosis in children with milder symptoms. This allows for treatment, which has been shown to help, especially when started earlier in life.

Some parents have been concerned about a possible link between autism and certain childhood immunizations. Numerous studies have now examined the claim that childhood vaccines cause autism, and they have effectively ruled out any link between vaccines and autism. In fact, in 2010, the original researchers claiming a link between vaccines and autism admitted to falsification of data and fraudulent research. The changes in the brain that lead to autism start in the womb, long before the baby is born and receives any vaccines. If you have questions about vaccines for your child, talk to your pediatrician, who can provide scientifically confirmed information about the safety of vaccines and the important benefits of vaccinating your child.

Diagnosis

Typically, the earlier that therapies are started after diagnosis, the better the response. Therefore, if your child has shown delays in developing language, has difficulties with social communication, or has unusual behaviors, talk to your pediatrician. Other early signs should raise concerns and should be evaluated for a potential diagnosis. Contact your doctor if your child is not doing the following activities by 12 months:

- Plays games with you, like pattycake
- Uses simple gestures, like waving bye-bye
- Says "mama," "dada," or another special name
- Understands "no" (pauses briefly or stops when you say it)

Further signs and symptoms can be found at the Centers for Disease Control and Prevention website, cdc.gov/ncbddd/actearly.

If you observe signs like these in your child or are concerned about other aspects of their language and social development, let your pediatrician know—and the earlier, the better. In fact, as soon as the diagnosis of autism is suspected, treatment should begin, even before a diagnosis is conclusively made. Children with other types of delays may have some of these symptoms as well, but these other developmental diagnoses also benefit from intervention, so getting your child evaluated is important even if you are not concerned about autism.

Where We Stand

The American Academy of Pediatrics encourages doctors to be aware of the signs of ASD, and to be on the lookout for these signs during every well-child visit.

At the same time, the Academy urges parents to always let their pediatricians know of any concerns they may have about their child's behavior and development. The AAP recommends autism-specific screening when children are 18 and 24 months of age; the sooner an intervention program is started, the better. However, children should be evaluated at any age if a parent or professional has concern about the possibility of ASD. If ASD is suspected or diagnosed, parents should seek a referral for early intervention and local specialists (like speech therapy or behavioral intervention to promote social skills). Public early intervention programs are specific for children from birth to 3 years of age. Above the age of 3, a referral should be made to your school district. Parents should make an effort to become as familiar as possible with available treatments and programs in their community and support their child in learning the skills needed to be successful in the least restrictive educational setting.

Unfortunately, no laboratory test is available to diagnose autism, nor, as we have seen, does a single set of symptoms always characterize it. If your pediatrician is concerned about ASD but the symptoms are unclear or more complex, they should refer you to a team of healthcare specialists with expertise in ASD (developmental pediatricians, neurologists, child psychiatrists, child psychologists, etc.) who can clarify whether the collection of symptoms is consistent with ASD. As part of the diagnostic process, your child's play behavior will be observed, as will their interactions with their caregivers. The physician will take a detailed history, conduct a physical examination, and perhaps order laboratory tests to look for medical conditions that can cause symptoms associated with autism. The diagnostic process should also include evaluation of your child's language and cognitive ability using standardized testing. Children with language delays should always be evaluated to make sure they can hear normally.

To help make the diagnosis, start with your pediatrician. Pediatricians are trained to identify the most common symptoms associated with ASD. Your pediatrician may refer you to a specialist in ASD, typically found in major medical centers. You can also call your state's public early childhood system or school district to request a free evaluation, without a doctor's referral, to find out if your child qualifies for intervention services. Check out cdc.gov/FindEI to help find available resources.

Treatment

There is no known cure for autism spectrum disorder, but there are effective treatments that improve many of the difficulties associated with ASD. A child diagnosed with ASD will need specialized services aimed at the management of the specific findings associated with their ASD. Early treatment will likely improve the ability of a child with autism to function more independently.

Cerebral Palsy

Children with cerebral palsy (CP) have abnormal development of or damage to the area of the brain that controls movement, posture, and muscle tone. About 1 to 4 children per 1,000 have CP. About half of children with cerebral palsy have typical intelligence, even though they have difficulty with motor control and movement. The condition causes different types of motor difficulties, which can vary from quite mild and barely noticeable to profound. Depending on the severity of the problem, a child with cerebral palsy may have clumsy movement patterns, or they may be unable to walk. Some children have weakness and poor motor control of one arm and one leg on the same side of the body (called hemiparesis), some have difficulties with both their legs (diplegia), and some have problems with control of both upper and lower extremities (quadriplegia). In some children the muscle tone generally is increased (called spasticity or hypertonia), while in others it is very low (called hypotonia), and in some it is mixed. Muscles with increased tone feel stiff and may be difficult to move, while muscle with decreased tone may feel floppy and have excessive flexibility. While many children with cerebral palsy have no trouble understanding language, they may have difficulty in coordinating the mouth movements needed to produce speech.

Cerebral palsy is caused by malformation of or damage to the brain. Often the damage occurs before birth, while the brain is being formed, but occasionally it occurs during delivery or after birth. Premature birth is associated with an increased risk of cerebral palsy due to the fragility of the developing brain. Other causes of cerebral palsy include underlying genetic or metabolic abnormalities, in-utero stroke, congenital infections, and abnormal formation or development of certain parts of the brain. A baby also can get cerebral palsy from very severe jaundice after birth, or later on in infancy from an injury or illness affecting the brain.

Although parents often look for an explanation as to why this happened, a report by the American Academy of Pediatrics and the American College of Obstetricians and Gynecologists concluded that most cases of cerebral palsy are not the result of events during labor and delivery, such as an insufficient supply of oxygen (hypoxia).

Signs and Symptoms

The signs and symptoms of cerebral palsy vary tremendously because there are many different types and degrees of motor problems. The main clue that your child might have cerebral palsy is a delay in achieving the motor milestones listed in

Chapters 5 through 9 of this book. Here are some specific warning signs.

In a Baby over 2 Months

- Their head lags when you pick them up while they're lying on their back, and they have poor head control in sitting.
- They feel stiff.
- They feel floppy.
- When held cradled in your arms, they seem to overextend their back and neck—constantly acting as if they are pushing away from you.
- When you pick them up, their legs get stiff and they cross, or "scissor."

In a Baby over 9 Months

- They are not yet able to sit without support.
- They use one side of the body more than the other, such as crawling in a lopsided manner, pushing off with one hand and leg while dragging the opposite hand and leg.
- They hop on their knees but do not crawl on all fours.
- They do not walk independently by 18 months of age.

If you have any concerns about your child's development, talk to your pediatrician right away. Because children's rates of development vary widely, it is sometimes difficult to make a definite diagnosis of mild cerebral palsy right away. Often a consultation with a developmental pediatrician, pediatric neurologist, or pediatric rehabilitation medicine physician will assist in the diagnosis. Your pediatrician will refer you to the appropriate professional. Your child will also be referred to a physical and/or occupational therapist for additional assessment of their motor skills. An MRI (magnetic resonance imaging) scan of the head should be done in all children with cerebral palsy to determine whether a brain abnormality exists. Additional genetic or metabolic testing is sometimes needed as well. Even when a firm diagnosis is made during these early years, it often is difficult to predict how severe the motor problems will be in the future.

Treatment

If your pediatrician suspects that your child has cerebral palsy, you may be referred to an early intervention program. These programs are staffed by early childhood educators; physical, occupational, and speech and language therapists; nurses; social workers; and medical consultants. In such a program, your child will get therapies specifically targeting their needs and you'll learn how to better help your child. You will be taught by a physical and/or occupational therapist what exercises to do with your infant, what positions are most comfortable and beneficial to them, and how to help with specific problems such as feeding difficulties. Sometimes medications such as baclofen or botulinum toxin type A are used to minimize the spasticity or decrease muscle tightness in the legs or arms, though medication for spasticity is not typically recommended for younger children. Older children may be treated with implantable baclofen pumps or have surgical procedures to decrease spasticity or treat problems with the hips or spine. You may receive information about adaptive equipment that can help your child participate in everyday activities and position them so they can use their hands better in play. Special equipment may include customized utensils to make eating easier, adapted bath or potty chairs, pencils that can be held more easily, braces or orthotics for the legs and ankles, wheelchairs, and walkers. These adaptations allow children to be more independent and participate with peers and within the community. Through support groups, you also can meet parents of other children with similar disabilities and share experiences, concerns, and solutions.

The most important thing you can do for your child is to help them develop skills, become resilient, and gain positive self-esteem. Encourage them to perform the tasks they are capable of and practice more challenging tasks so that they learn to do them with as little assistance as possible. The professionals at early intervention centers can help you evaluate your child's abilities and teach you how to reach appropriate goals. You may be offered advice about other types of therapies besides those provided by the conventional therapy team. Discuss any non-standard therapies with your pediatrician before trying them.

A number of organizations are available to help parents

learn more about how best to take care of their child with cerebral palsy. These include United Cerebral Palsy (ucp.org), the Cerebral Palsy Foundation (yourcpf.org), and the Cerebral Palsy Research Network (cprn.org).

Associated Problems

Intellectual Development Disorder

It has been estimated that more than half of children with cerebral palsy have global developmental delays that include thinking and problem-solving. Many children with cerebral palsy also are diagnosed with intellectual development disorder, while others have average intellectual abilities. (See also Intellectual Development Disorder, *page 464*.)

Autism

About 7 to 8 percent of children with cerebral palsy will also be diagnosed with having autism spectrum disorder. If you have concerns about your child's play, social, or communication skills, ask your pediatrician about the possibility of autism.

Seizures

Four out of every ten people with cerebral palsy have or will develop seizures. The seizures may not start until later in childhood. Fortunately, these seizures often can be controlled with anti-seizure medications (see *page 604*).

Eating and Digestive Difficulties

Many children with cerebral palsy experience difficulties with eating and digestion. Children who have problems with the muscles in their face or mouth may need more help learning to chew or swallow food safely. Constipation and reflux are very common and are thought to be associated with abnormalities in the muscles that control the gastrointestinal tract. These problems can affect continence (learning to control the bowel and bladder function). Some children require minor dietary changes or fiber supplements, while others need prescription medications or more intensive support for healthy digestion and/or continence.

Vision Difficulties

Because the injury to the brain often affects eye muscle coordination, more than three out of four children with cerebral palsy have vision difficulties. Some of the vision issues include strabismus (eyes not properly aligned; see *page 550*), amblyopia (decreased vision in one eye that may cause turning in or out), or cortical visual impairment (where the brain can't understand what the eyes are seeing). It is extremely important to have your child's eyes checked regularly by your pediatrician and a pediatric ophthalmologist. Many of these vision difficulties can be corrected if identified and treated early, but if left untreated they may worsen and may even cause permanent vision loss.

Joint Contractures

In children with spastic forms of cerebral palsy, it is often difficult to prevent contracture, a loss of range of motion of a stiff joint, caused by the unequal pull of one muscle over the other. Possible problems that may result include scoliosis (curvature of the spine) or dislocation of the hips. Some children with asymmetry of their muscle tone may have differences in the size of the affected arm or leg, or contractures of joints.

A physical therapist, developmental pediatrician, or pediatric rehabilitation medicine physician can teach you how to stretch the muscles to try to prevent the onset of contracture. Sometimes braces, splints, casting, or medication may be used to improve joint mobility and stability. In some situations, orthopedic surgery is performed as part of contracture management.

Dental Problems

Many children with cerebral palsy have a greater risk of developing oral diseases. This can mean more gingivitis (gum disease) and cavities. One reason may be that it is difficult for them to brush their teeth. However, they also have more enamel defects than other children, which may make their teeth more susceptible to decay. In addition, some medications such as seizure or asthma medications may contribute to cavity formation. Because of the special skills needed to monitor their dental needs, families often seek out pediatric dentists with training in caring for children with chronic needs.

Hearing Loss

Some children with cerebral palsy have a complete or partial hearing loss as part of the injury or illness that caused the damage to the brain. All babies in the United States are screened for hearing loss before leaving the nursery, but if you find that your baby does not blink or startle at loud noises by 1 month, is not turning their head toward a sound by 3 to 4 months, or is not saying words by 12 months, discuss it with your pediatrician. The results of newborn hearing screening should be reviewed and follow-up hearing evaluation should be obtained along with formal speech and language testing. (See also Hearing Loss [Hearing Impairment], *page 458*.)

Problems with Spatial Awareness

Over half the children with cerebral palsy affecting one side of the body have challenges sensing the position of their arm, leg, or hand on the affected side. (For example, when a child's hands are relaxed, they cannot tell whether their fingers are pointing up or down without looking at them.) If this problem exists, the child may limit use of the involved hand, even if the motor disability is minimal. They might act as if it is not there. Physical or occupational therapy can help them learn to use the affected parts of their body despite this disability.

Congenital Abnormalities

Congenital abnormalities are caused by problems during the fetus's development before birth. About 3 of every 100 babies born in the United States have congenital abnormalities.

There are five categories of these abnormalities, grouped according to the cause.

Chromosome Abnormalities

Chromosomes carry the genetic material inherited from one generation to the next in the egg and sperm. Normally, twenty-three chromosomes come from the father and twenty-three from the mother. The genes carried on the chromosomes provide the instructions for how the body is made and determine a child's characteristics.

When a child does not have the normal forty-six chromosomes, or when pieces of the chromosomes are missing or duplicated, there may be problems in the development and function of organs, including the brain. Down syndrome (trisomy 21) is an example of a condition that can occur when a child is born with an extra chromosome.

Single-Gene Abnormalities

Sometimes the chromosomes are normal in number, but one or more of the genes on them are abnormal. Some of these genetic abnormalities are inherited from a parent who also has that abnormality. This is known as autosomal dominant inheritance. Each child has a one in two chance of inheriting this gene from the parent. Examples include achondroplasia and Marfan syndrome.

Other genetic problems can be passed to the child only if both parents carry the same gene. Cystic fibrosis, Tay-Sachs disease, and spinal muscular atrophy are all examples of disorders inherited in this fashion. In these cases, neither parent has the disorder, but each carries one gene for it, and the disorder results when the child inherits the abnormal gene from both parents. Each child has a one in four chance of inheriting this gene from both parents and being affected. This is known as autosomal recessive inheritance.

A third type of genetic abnormality is called sex-linked and generally is passed on to boys only, although the abnormality runs on the mother's side of the family. Girls may carry the abnormal gene that causes these disorders on one of their X chromosomes but not show the actual disease because they have an extra X chromosome with a normal gene. Because boys have only one X chromosome, if they inherit an abnormal gene on the X chromosome, they will have the disorder. (Examples of this problem include hemophilia, fragile X syndrome, color blindness, and the common forms of muscular dystrophy.) When the mother is a carrier of one of these genes, each of her sons has a one in two chance of inheriting this gene.

The fourth type of genetic abnormality is of the mitochondria, which are the parts of the cell that make energy. Mitochondrial DNA is inherited from the mother only. Mitochondrial diseases may cause a wide variety of problems, including seizures, developmental delays, hearing and vision abnormalities, or kidney and intestinal problems.

Conditions During Pregnancy That Affect Development

Some infections, illnesses, and conditions that affect the mother during pregnancy, particularly during the first nine weeks, can cause serious congenital abnormalities—Zika, German measles, and cytomegalovirus, for example. That is why infections and other disorders such as diabetes are screened for during pregnancy. In many cases, working closely with your physician, getting recommended vaccines, and following strict management protocols can help decrease complications during pregnancy and later problems for your baby. Other things that can affect your baby during development are alcohol consumption, illegal drugs, particular medications, and certain chemicals that can pollute air, water, and food, like mercury, lead, and dioxin. Always check with your doctor before using any medication or nutritional supplement while you are pregnant.

Combination of Genetic and Environmental Problems

Spina bifida and cleft lip and palate are types of congenital abnormalities that may occur when there is a genetic tendency for the condition combined with exposure to certain environmental influences, toxins, chemicals (alcohol, cigarette smoke, etc.), or vitamin deficiencies (folic acid, etc.) within the womb during critical stages of the pregnancy. Women are prescribed prenatal vitamins containing folic acid even while they are planning to become pregnant, to help prevent the fetus from having spina bifida.

Unknown Causes

Most congenital abnormalities have no known cause. If you and your family have had one child with congenital abnormalities or developmental problems without a known cause, ask your pediatrician or obstetrician for a referral to a geneticist or genetic counselor. They can review with you your risk for having another child with similar problems.

When Your Child Has a Congenital Disorder

Despite advances in prenatal diagnostics, such as ultrasound, many families learn their baby has a congenital abnormality only after they are born. It is very important to ask the doctors caring for your baby to explain everything so that you understand what is happening with them and so that you can enlist the support of friends and family. Siblings need to be informed about the condition of the baby in words that are appropriate to their developmental level. Once a diagnosis is made, many families find it very helpful to be put in contact with family support groups for that disorder.

Congenital Conditions

Congenital abnormalities are so diverse and require such different types of treatment that it would be impossible to discuss them all in this section. Instead, we will look only at the medical management of two conditions: Down syndrome and spina bifida. However, clinical symptoms accompanying congenital conditions might include global developmental delay or intellectual disability, cerebral palsy, sensory impairment, or autism spectrum disorder; in these cases, the evaluations and interventions described for those clinical conditions would apply.

Down Syndrome

Approximately 1 out of every 700 babies is born with Down syndrome. Fortunately, through prenatal testing, Down syndrome can often be detected prenatally. Down syndrome is caused by the presence of an extra chromosome. One result of this extra chromosome is a typical appearance that includes up-slanted eyes with extra folds of skin at the inner corners, flattening of the bridge of the nose, a tongue that looks larger in the setting of a small mouth, and a decrease in the muscle and ligament tone of the body.

Most children with Down syndrome will have mild to moderate intellectual disability and will benefit from early intervention services, which can be started in infancy. However, it is important to remember that children with Down syndrome are more like other children than they are different. Children with Down syndrome can form deep and meaningful relationships with others, can learn in special education and inclusive classrooms, and can participate in community activities and sports. Many can be employed competitively or in a workshop setting and can live independently or in a group home setting as adults.

Children with Down syndrome are at higher risk for a number of medical conditions. Congenital heart disease is common in children with Down syndrome, so your doctor will arrange for an ultrasound of the heart (echocardiogram) shortly after birth. These children may also get frequent ear infections, which can affect their hearing and speech over time. Children with Down syndrome may be born with problems with the gastrointestinal tract or with other organ systems; these can usually be found by exam and by monitoring how the baby eats and moves their bowels.

Many children with Down syndrome are shorter and weigh less than average for their age when they are infants. However, older children with Down syndrome may struggle with excess weight gain. More than half have vision and hearing impairments. Many will develop sleep apnea, so all children with Down syndrome should have a sleep study by the time they start school. Some children with Down syndrome will develop hypothyroidism, which can lead to decreased metabolism, weight gain, and slowed behavior. Children with Down syndrome are also at higher risk for loosening of the ligaments that provide neck stability and connect the vertebral column to the base of the skull, although this is rare. If these ligaments are too loose, overextension (bending backward) of the neck can occur, causing serious spinal injury. For this reason, caution should be taken with contact sports that could place a child at increased risk of spinal cord injury, such as football, soccer, and gymnastics. Medical procedures like surgeries and even X-rays can also put the spine at risk if the child is not positioned appropriately. A physician must perform an examination and obtain radiographs of the neck before the child participates in specific sports.

In 2022, the American Academy of Pediatrics published health supervision guidelines for children and adolescents with Down syndrome. These guidelines can be used by families and by pediatricians to ensure all the unique medical needs for children with Down syndrome are met.

Spina Bifida

Spina bifida occurs when the tissue surrounding the spinal cord fails to close properly during early fetal development. There are many different subtypes of spina bifida. The most common form, spina bifida occulta, occurs when the spinal bones don't close but there are no problems with the nerves, as they are protected by the spinal column. Most people with spina bifida occulta don't even know they have it. Another form is meningocele, in which a sac of fluid that protects the spinal cord pushes out between the opening in the spinal bones, but no spinal nerve tissue is involved. A third type is myelomeningocele, in which the protruding sac of fluid also contains parts of the spinal nerves and spinal cord. Most of the time when people say spina bifida, they are referring to myelomeningocele, so that is what this section will discuss.

Spina bifida is often caused by an interaction between genes and the environment. A parent who has one child with spina bifida has a greater chance (1 out of 100) of having another. This increased frequency appears to be due to some combined effect of heredity and environment. One factor we know of is inadequate intake of folic acid during very early pregnancy, so supplements including this vitamin are recommended for all women of childbearing age, preferably starting before pregnancy begins, to minimize the risk for spina bifida in the fetus. Ultrasound examination can usually identify spina bifida during pregnancy, and blood tests done on the mother can help to identify an increased risk of having a baby with spina bifida. Knowing that a baby will have spina bifida allows the family to plan for delivery at a medical center that offers specialty care. At some centers with experts in high-risk maternal-fetal medicine and specialist surgeons, pregnant women may choose to be evaluated for fetal surgery (surgery done while the fetus is still in the womb), which is not a cure but may lessen the impact of the condition in some children.

Where We Stand

In an effort to reduce the prevalence of spina bifida, the American Academy of Pediatrics endorses the recommendation of the US Public Health Service that all women capable of becoming pregnant consume 400 mcg per day of folic acid (a B vitamin). Folic acid helps to prevent neural tube defects (NTDs), which include spina bifida. Although some foods are fortified with folic acid, it is not possible for women to meet the 400 mcg goal through a typical diet. Thus, an Academy policy statement recommends a daily multivitamin tablet that contains folic acid in the recommended dose. Studies show that if all women of childbearing age met these dietary requirements, 50 percent or more of NTDs could be prevented.

Women who are at high risk for an NTD-affected pregnancy (for example, because of a previous NTD-affected pregnancy, having diabetes mellitus, or taking anti-seizure medications) are advised to discuss their risk with their doctor. This includes possible treatments with very high doses of folic acid (4,000 mcg per day), beginning one month before becoming pregnant and continuing throughout the first trimester. As the doctor will explain, however, women should not attempt to achieve this very high dose of folic acid by taking multivitamin supplements (because then they may receive too much of other vitamins), and should follow the advice of the physician.

A newborn with spina bifida has a sac protruding from the spine that contains spinal fluid and a portion of the spinal cord. These are the nerves that control the lower part of the body. On the first or second day after birth, surgery must be performed to close the opening in the spine. Unfortunately, little can be done to repair the damaged nerves, but a lot can be done to help children be as functional as possible. Most babies with spina bifida have several other medical complications. These include:

Hydrocephalus. Up to nine out of ten children with spina bifida eventually develop hydrocephalus, or increased fluid in and around the brain. The increase occurs because the path through which the fluid ordinarily flows is blocked. This condition is serious and must be treated surgically. Signs of hydrocephalus can include that the baby's head is growing more rapidly than expected, a bulging fontanelle (soft spot), or symptoms of irritability, lethargy, or seizures. The condition is confirmed by a computed tomography (CT) scan, magnetic resonance imagery (MRI) scan, or ultrasound scan of the head. If the condition exists, surgery will be required to relieve fluid buildup by placement of a shunt to remove the fluid.

Latex Allergies. People with spina bifida are more likely to be allergic to latex, likely because of early surgeries and latex sensitization. Allergic reactions can vary from mild to very severe. All children with spina bifida should take precautions to avoid latex. Children with latex allergies should have an emergency care plan in place should an allergic event occur. You can reduce the chances that your child will acquire this sensitivity by avoiding exposure to latex. But be aware that many infant products contain latex (bottle nipples, pacifiers, teething toys, changing pads, mattress covers, and some diapers). If your child does have a latex allergy, make sure you have an anaphylaxis plan (see *page 403*).

Muscle Weakness or Paralysis. Because the congenital abnormality of the spinal cord impacts the development of nerves connecting the brain to the lower limbs, the muscles in the legs may be very weak or not function at all in children with spina bifida. Because they may not be able to move their feet, knees, or hips, they may be born with contractures of these joints (shortening or tightening of the joints or muscles). Surgery can be performed to correct some of these contractures, and the muscle weakness can be helped with physical therapy and bracing. Depending on the level of the spinal lesion, children with spina bifida may be able to walk independently or with walkers. Many use wheelchairs, however.

Bowel and Bladder Problems. Often the nerves that control bowel and bladder function do not work properly with spina bifida. As a result, these children are more likely to develop urinary tract infections and can have urine back up from the bladder and damage the kidneys. Your pediatrician will refer your child to a urologist, who will monitor your child's bladder function and determine if they need to have urine drained through a catheter to protect their kidneys. These children are prone to urinary tract infections, which might cause fever or abdominal or back pain.

Bowel control may be a problem because of the lack of nerve control of the rectum. Careful dietary management to keep the stools soft, including stool softeners, suppositories, or enemas, may be recommended to help with bowel management.

Educational and Social Problems. Seven out of ten children with spina bifida have developmental and learning disabilities requiring some educational supports for learning needs. Issues of health and wellness, including weight control, physical activity, and social inclusion, are particularly important to the long-term physical, emotional, and social well-being of children with spina bifida.

Parents of a child with spina bifida need more than one physician to manage their child's medical care. In addition to the basic care your pediatrician delivers, this condition requires a team approach that involves neurosurgeons, orthopedic surgeons, urologists, developmental-behavioral pediatricians, rehabilitation experts, physical therapists, psychologists, and social workers. Many medical centers run special spina bifida clinics, which offer the services of all these health professionals in one location. Having all members of the team together makes it easier for everyone to communicate and usually provides better access to information and assistance when parents need it.

Resources

Information and support for parents of children born with congenital conditions are available from various organizations.

Centers for Disease Control and Prevention (CDC)
1-800-232-4636
cdc.gov

March of Dimes
1-888-663-4637
marchofdimes.org

The National Down Syndrome Congress
1-800-232-NDSC (6372)
ndsccenter.org

The Spina Bifida Association
1-800-621-3141
spinabifidaassociation.org

United Cerebral Palsy
1-800-872-5827
ucp.org

Hearing Loss (Hearing Impairment)

Although hearing loss can occur at any age, hearing difficulties that are present at birth or that develop during infancy and the toddler years can have serious developmental consequences if unrecognized and untreated. This is because normal hearing is needed to understand spoken language and then, later, to produce clear speech. Consequently, if your child experiences hearing loss during infancy or early childhood, immediate attention is required. Even a temporary but significant hearing loss during this time can make it very difficult for the child to learn spoken language or speech patterns. Sometimes parents will see their child respond to a loud noise and be reassured that their child is not deaf. However, subtle or mild losses in hearing may not be obvious but will still negatively impact language development.

Most children experience mild hearing loss when fluid accumulates in the middle ear from congestion, colds, or ear infections. This hearing loss is usually only temporary; normal hearing commonly returns once the congestion or infection subsides and the Eustachian tube (which connects the middle ear to the throat) drains the remaining fluid into the back of the throat. In many children, perhaps one in ten, fluid stays in the middle ear following an ear infection (see *page 471*) because of problems with the Eustachian tube. Children with this problem don't hear as well as they should and sometimes develop speech delays. Much less common is the permanent kind of hearing impairment that always impacts normal speech and language development. Permanent hearing impairment varies from mild or partial to complete or total deafness.

There are two main kinds of hearing loss or impairment: conductive and sensorineural. When a child has a conductive hearing loss, there may be an abnormality in the structure of the outer ear canal or middle ear, there may be a large amount of cerumen (wax) lodged in the ear canal, or there may be fluid in the middle ear that interferes with the transfer of sound.

By contrast, a sensorineural hearing loss is caused by an abnormality of the inner ear or the nerves that carry sound messages from the inner ear to the brain. The loss can be present at birth or occur anytime thereafter. Even without a family history of deafness, the cause is frequently genetic, with parents and other family members often unaffected because each parent is only a carrier for a hearing loss gene; because future children have an increased risk of being hearing impaired, genetic counseling is recommended. Or if the mother had rubella (German measles), cytomegalovirus (CMV), toxoplasmosis, or another infectious illness that affects the inner ear during pregnancy, the fetus could have been infected and may lose hearing as a result. Some infections cause hearing loss in early childhood. The problem also may be due to a malformation of the inner ear.

Hearing loss must be diagnosed as soon as possible, so that your child isn't delayed in learning language—a process that begins the day they are born. The American Academy of Pediatrics recommends that before a newborn infant goes home from the hospital, they undergo a formal hearing screening. In fact, every state and territory in the United States now has an Early Hearing Detection and Intervention (EHDI) program, which mandates that all newborns be screened for hearing impairment before they are discharged from the hospital. If your newborn's screen is abnormal, make sure your pediatrician knows; a follow-up screen should be performed as soon as possible.

While it is very reassuring when an infant passes their newborn hearing screen, some children develop hearing loss over time. At any time during your child's life, if you and/or your pediatrician suspect that your child has hearing loss, insist that a formal hearing evaluation be performed promptly. (See Hearing Loss: What to Look For on *page 461*.) Some family doctors, pediatricians, and well-baby clinics can test in the office for hearing loss or fluid in the middle ear, a common cause of hearing loss. If a problem is detected, your child may be referred to an audiologist (hearing specialist) and/or ear, nose, and throat doctor (ENT; otolaryngologist).

If your child is under 6 months of age, is unable to cooperate with or understand a hearing examination, or has significant developmental delays, they may be given one of two available tests, which are like the tests performed during newborn hearing screenings. They are painless and can take anywhere from five to sixty minutes.

- The auditory brainstem response (ABR) test measures how the brain responds to sound during deep sleep. Clicks or tones are played into the baby's ears through soft earphones, and electrodes placed on the baby's head measure the brain's response. This allows the doctor to test your child's hearing without having to rely on their cooperation. ABRs are performed during a natural sleep in infants under 3 or 4 months old. Older babies and toddlers need to be sedated to undergo an ABR.
- The otoacoustic emissions (OAE) test measures sound waves produced by the ear. A tiny probe is placed just inside the baby's ear canal, which then measures the response when clicks or tones are played into the baby's ear. Babies and young children usually do not need to be napping or sedated for an OAE test, as it is a brief screening exam. This can be done at any age.

Behavioral audiometry, or conditioned response audiometry, can be performed with a cooperative baby as young as 6 months old. A combination of visual and auditory stimuli is provided, and the test can determine frequency-specific (although not ear-specific) hearing levels in infants and toddlers.

Formal behavioral audiometry can determine hearing levels as well as eardrum function in each ear. This is performed using soft earphones that send sounds and words to the ear and is typically well tolerated by children ages 3 to 5 years old.

Not all these tests may be available in your immediate area, but the consequences of undiagnosed hearing loss are so serious that your doctor may advise you to travel to where the tests and potential treatment can be offered. Certainly, if these tests indicate that your baby may have a hearing problem, your doctor should recommend a more thorough hearing evaluation as soon as possible to confirm whether your child's hearing is impaired. Even mild hearing loss can still affect overall hearing and should be properly diagnosed and treated.

HEARING LOSS: WHAT TO LOOK FOR

Here are the signs and symptoms that should make you suspect that your child has a hearing loss and alert you to call your pediatrician:

- Your child doesn't startle at loud noises by 1 month or turn to the source of a sound by 3 to 4 months of age.
- They don't notice you until they see you.
- They concentrate on gurgling and other vibrating noises that they can feel, rather than experimenting with a wide variety of vowel sounds and consonants. (See Language Development on *pages 196, 209*, and *234*.)
- Their speech is delayed or hard to understand, or they don't say single words such as "dada" or "mama" by 12 to 15 months of age.
- They do not say three or more words besides "mama" or "dada" by 18 months of age.
- They do not put two to three words together at 2 years of age.
- Their speech is not understandable 50 percent of the time by 2½ years of age.
- They don't always respond when called. (This is usually mistaken for inattention or resistance, but it could be the result of a partial hearing loss.)
- They seem to hear some sounds but not others. (Some hearing losses affect only high-pitched sounds; some children have hearing loss in only one ear.)

- They seem not only to hear poorly but also to have trouble holding their head steady or are slow to sit or walk unsupported. (In some children with sensorineural hearing loss, the part of the inner ear that provides information about balance and movement of the head is also damaged.)

Also, any child being evaluated for possible autism spectrum disorder or delay in language development should undergo a hearing evaluation.

Treatment

Treating hearing loss will depend on its cause. If it is a mild conductive hearing loss due to fluid in the middle ear, the doctor may simply recommend that your child be retested in a few months to see whether the fluid has cleared by itself. Medications such as antihistamines, decongestants, and antibiotics are ineffective in clearing up middle ear fluid.

If there is no improvement in hearing over a three-month period, and there is still fluid behind the eardrum, the doctor may recommend a referral to an ENT specialist. If the fluid persists and there is sufficient (even though temporary) conductive hearing impairment from the fluid, the specialist may recommend draining the fluid through ventilating tubes. These are surgically inserted through the eardrum. This is a minor operation and takes about fifteen minutes, but your child must receive a general anesthetic for it to be done properly, so your child usually will spend part of the day in a hospital or an outpatient surgery center.

Even with the tubes in place, future infections can occur, but the tubes help reduce the amount of fluid and decrease your child's risk of repeated infection. If the cause for the hearing loss was purely the fluid, the tubes will improve hearing.

If conductive hearing loss is due to a malformation of the outer or middle ear, a hearing aid may restore hearing to normal or near-normal levels. However, a hearing aid will work only when it's being worn. You must make sure it is on and functioning at all times, particularly in a very young child. Reconstructive surgery may be considered when the child is older.

Early placement of hearing aids for infants with hearing loss is important to give them awareness of sound and language. Early exposure to either aural (spoken) or visual (sign) language has a very positive impact on language development. In children with mild to moderate sensorineural hearing loss, hearing aids can improve hearing so much that most can develop normal speech and spoken language.

Should your child have severe or profound hearing loss in both ears and receive little or no benefit from hearing aids, they could be a candidate for cochlear implants. Cochlear implants have been approved by the Food and Drug Administration for children since 1990. If your family is considering an implant for a child whose hearing loss occurred at birth, outcomes for developing useful speech and hearing are better with early (ideally by 1 year of age) rather than late (over 3 years old) implantation. Therefore, it is extremely important to seek out early and efficient evaluation and treatment of hearing loss. Most children with typical development and early implantation coupled with intensive therapy after the surgery can develop good to excellent hearing and can be supported in a mainstream educational setting; almost all children with cochlear implants gain better awareness of sounds in their environment.

Parents of children with sensorineural hearing loss usually are most concerned about whether their child will learn to talk. The answer is that although optimally timed cochlear implantation will greatly improve the chances of learning spoken language, not all may learn to speak clearly. However, all children with hearing loss can be taught to communicate. Some children learn to lip-read well, while others never fully master the skill. However, speech is only one form of communication. For children in whom hearing aids or cochlear implants cannot offer enough improvement in hearing to develop spoken language, or for those families who have chosen not to pursue spoken language, sign language is another mode of communication that can be learned. If your child is learning sign language, you and your immediate family also must learn it. This way you will be able to teach, praise, comfort, and laugh with them. You should encourage friends and relatives to learn signing, too. Written language is very important as well, because it is the key to educational and future career success.

Intellectual Development Disorder

The term "intellectual development disorder" (IDD) is used when a child's intelligence and adaptive behavior, which covers many everyday social and practical skills, are significantly below average and affect the way they learn, develop new skills, and participate in the world around them. The more severe the disability, the more delayed a child's skills will be in comparison to their chronological age.

The diagnosis of IDD no longer relies on an IQ measurement below 70, which used to be the standard definition. Now specialists who diagnose this condition tend to focus more on assessing adaptive behavior, as this correlates most with functioning and levels of independence. Generally, lower intellectual functioning correlates with more difficulties in different areas of adaptive functioning. This includes conceptual skills (language, literacy, time, number concepts), practical skills (personal care skills, travel and transportation, schedules/routines, safety, use of money), and social skills (interpersonal skills, gullibility, ability to follow rules).

Signs and Symptoms

Generally, the more severe the degree of intellectual disability, the earlier you will notice the signs. It may be difficult to predict in young children who have delays in both language and problem-solving skills what their level of function might be as they develop.

When a baby is late in developing basic motor skills (e.g., holding their head up by themselves by 3 to 4 months or sitting unsupported by 7 to 8 months), there also may be some associated intellectual development disorder. However, this is by no means always the case. Nor does typical motor development guarantee normal intelligence. Some children with mild to moderate degrees of intellectual development disorder have normal physical development. In such cases, the first sign of IDD may be a delay in language development or in learning simple imitation skills, such as waving bye-bye or playing pattycake.

In many cases of mild disability, the young child may reach developmental milestones at typical times. Later, when they begin preschool or school, they may have difficulty performing academic skills at their grade level. They might have trouble completing puzzles, recognizing colors, or counting when their classmates already have mastered these tasks. Remember, however, children do develop at very different rates, and problems in school are often not a sign of intellectual development disorder. In fact, specific learning disabilities—which are not the same as IDD—are often diagnosed only when a child has more difficulty learning than would be expected for the child's overall intelligence level. The key is watching a child's trajectory over time. Children with learning disabilities can often close the gap with their peers with the help of targeted interventions, although other learning disabilities, like dyslexia, can remain lifelong. When a child doesn't seem to be catching up, then an intellectual development disorder should be considered.

Early developmental delays also can be caused by disorders such as hearing loss, vision problems, learning disabilities, or lack of experience due to environmental challenges. Formal testing can be done closer to kindergarten age.

When to Call the Pediatrician

If you are concerned about a delay in your child's development, call your pediatrician, who will review your child's overall development and determine whether it is appropriate for their age. If the pediatrician is concerned, they will probably refer you to a pediatric developmental specialist, a pediatric neurologist, or a multidisciplinary team of professionals for further assessment. Children under 3 years of age should be referred to the public early intervention program, and children over 3 years of age should be referred to your school district for formal testing.

Treatment

Young children and toddlers who demonstrate delays across many areas of development may be suspected to have an intellectual development disorder. Early support for optimal development might include speech therapy, occupational therapy, and physical therapy. Special education programs through the public school can be started after the third birthday. In general, the main treatment for children with IDD is supportive therapy and education with a goal of achieving their optimal developmental potential. Children with IDD often benefit from life-skills and vocational training through the end of high school and can often qualify for public school education through 21 years of age. Many are capable of graduating with diplomas, though some are better suited to graduate with a certificate.

Intellectual development disorder has a range of impact, with symptoms that can be mild, moderate, or severe in degree. Adults with mild IDD may develop the academic or trade skills for community employment, often read at a fourth- to sixth-grade level, and can frequently live independently with some minor supervision. However, with increasing functional impairment, there is a greater likelihood that the person will need supports for daily needs and employment. People with severe to profound IDD are often dependent upon others for care and supervision through adulthood and will require thoughtful planning for the transition to adulthood.

In the past, people with IDD often were forced to live in large residential facilities. The goal is now for adults with IDD to live with their families, in their communities, or in small supported living units with meaningful work options. (For more information, visit the American Association on Intellectual and Developmental Disabilities, aaidd.org/home, and the CDC, cdc.gov.)

Prevention

Preventable causes of intellectual development disorder include alcohol consumption by the mother during pregnancy and other fetal exposures. Women planning to become pregnant should consult with their obstetricians regarding support they may need to have the healthiest possible pregnancy.

While an increasing number of genetic causes for IDD can be identified, early screening can only prevent symptoms due to metabolic disorders such as phenylketonuria (PKU) and hypothyroidism. Currently there are 116 treatable inborn errors of metabolism, which may account for 5 percent of IDD cases. If these conditions are detected soon after birth through standard screening tests performed in the hospital nursery, they can be treated. Other examples of conditions that can cause IDD if not detected and treated early in life include lead poisoning, infections in the newborn period, hydrocephalus (excess fluid causing increased pressure in the brain; see *page 456*), and epilepsy (seizures).

Genetic testing for other causes (single-gene mutations, chromosome abnormalities) may not provide an opportunity for treatment or prevention, but it may offer insights into other ways to help children with intellectual development disorder. Many times, a specific genetic cause is associated with other medical problems. If your doctor knows about an underlying genetic cause for your child's IDD, they can provide early evaluation for those problems. One example is fragile X syndrome, which is one of the most common causes of heritable IDD. Children with fragile X syndrome may also have problems with their heart or kidneys, even though some of these problems don't present until a child is older. Sometimes, an underlying genetic cause may also be important for understanding the risk of having additional children with the same genetic change. For example, with fragile X syndrome, there is a 50 percent likelihood for each boy in the family to be born with the syndrome. If you are interested in understanding whether your child's IDD has an underlying genetic cause, or if you would like to discuss the likelihood of your future children also having an IDD, ask your child's pediatrician about genetic counseling or a referral to a genetic specialist.

Consult your pediatrician, local advocacy organizations, and other reputable professionals to find out what programs (Special Olympics, Best Buddies, etc.) are available in your community. Professional assistance can be extremely helpful. In the long run, however, you and your family members will be your child's most important advocates. Along with your child's teachers and therapist, you can set realistic objectives for your child and encourage them to reach these objectives. Assist them, if necessary, but let them do as much as possible on their own. You and your child will feel most rewarded when they reach a goal by themselves.

CHAPTER 17

EARS, NOSE, AND THROAT

Colds/Upper Respiratory Infections

Your child probably will have more colds, or upper respiratory infections, than any other illness. In the first two years alone, most children have around eight to ten colds. And if your child spends time in a childcare setting, or if there are school-age children in your house, they may have even more, since colds spread easily among children who are in close contact with one another. That's the bad news, but there is some good news, too: Most colds go away by themselves and do not lead to anything worse.

Colds are caused by viruses, which are extremely small infectious particles (much smaller than bacteria). A sneeze or a cough may directly transfer a virus from one person to another. The virus also may be spread indirectly, when someone infected with the virus transfers some of the virus particles onto their hand by coughing, sneezing, or touching their nose. They then touch a surface such as a toy or doorknob, and a healthy person touches it after, or they may touch the healthy person's hand directly. This healthy person touches their newly contaminated hand to their own nose, introducing the infectious agent to a place where it can multiply and grow—the nose or throat. Symptoms of a cold soon develop. The cycle then repeats itself, with the virus being transferred from this newly infected child or adult to the next susceptible one, and so on.

Once the virus is present and multiplying, your child will develop the familiar symptoms and signs:

- Runny nose (first, a clear discharge; later, a thicker, often colored one)
- Sneezing
- Mild fever (101–102 degrees Fahrenheit [38.3–38.9 degrees Celsius]), particularly in the evening
- Decreased appetite
- Sore throat and, perhaps, difficulty swallowing

- Cough
- On-and-off irritability
- Slightly swollen glands in the neck

If your child has a typical cold without complications, the symptoms should disappear gradually in seven to ten days.

Treatment

An older child with a cold usually doesn't need to see a doctor unless the condition becomes more serious. If they are 3 months old or younger, however, call the pediatrician at the first sign of illness. With a young baby, symptoms can be misleading, and colds can quickly develop into more serious ailments, such as bronchiolitis (see *page 408*), croup (see *page 416*), or pneumonia (see *page 421*). For a child older than 3 months, call the pediatrician if you notice any of the following:

- The nostrils are widening with each breath, there is drawing in of the skin between and around the ribs and breastbone as the child inhales, your child is breathing rapidly, or there are any other signs of difficulty breathing.
- The lips or nails turn blue.
- Nasal mucus persists for longer than fourteen days.
- A daytime cough lasts more than ten days.
- They have pain in their ear (see Middle Ear Infections, *page 471*) or persistent fussiness or crying.
- Their temperature is higher than 102 degrees Fahrenheit (38.9 degrees Celsius).
- They are excessively sleepy or cranky.

Your pediatrician may want to see your child, or they may ask you to watch them closely and report back if they don't improve each day and are not completely recovered within one week from the start of their illness.

Unfortunately, there's no cure for the common cold. Antibiotics may be used to combat bacterial infections, but they have no effect on viruses, so the best you can do is to make your child comfortable. Make sure they get extra rest and drink a lot of fluids. If they have a fever or are uncomfortable, give them single-ingredient acetaminophen or ibuprofen. Ibuprofen is approved for children 6 months of age and older; however, it should never be given to children who are dehydrated or who are vomiting repeatedly. (Be sure to follow the recommended dosage for your child's age and the time interval for repeated doses.)

It's important to note that the American Academy of Pediatrics' position is that over-the-counter cough medicines are not effective for children younger than 6 years old; in fact, they can have potentially serious side effects. In addition, keep in mind that coughing clears mucus from the lower part of the respiratory tract, and ordinarily there's no reason to suppress it.

If your infant is having trouble breathing or drinking because of nasal congestion, clear their nose with saline (salt water) nose drops or spray, which are available without a prescription. This can then be followed by suction with a bulb syringe every few hours, or before each feeding and before bed. For the nose drops, use a dropper that has been cleaned with soap and water and rinsed well with plain water. Place two drops in each nostril fifteen to twenty minutes before feeding, and then immediately suction. Never use nose drops that contain any medication, since too much of the medication can be absorbed and cause problems in an infant. Only use normal saline nose drops.

When using the suction bulb, remember to squeeze the bulb part of the syringe first, gently stick the rubber tip into one nostril, and then slowly release the bulb. This slight amount of suction will draw the clogged mucus out of the nose and should allow your child to breathe and suck at the same time once again. You'll find that this technique works best when your baby is under 6 months of age. As they get older, they'll fight the bulb, making it difficult to suction the mucus, but the saline drops will still be effective. Alternatively, there are nasal aspirators on the market powered by battery or by parents' oral suction.

Placing a cool-mist humidifier or vaporizer in your child's room also will help keep nasal secretions more liquid and make them more comfortable. Set it close to them (but safely beyond their reach) so that they get the full benefit of the additional moisture. Be sure to clean and dry the humidifier thoroughly each day as recommended in the manufacturer's manual to prevent bacterial or mold contamination. Hot-water vaporizers are not recommended since they can cause serious scalds or burns.

Prevention

If your baby is under 3 months old, the best way to prevent colds is to keep them away from anyone who has a cold. This is especially true during the winter, when many of the viruses that cause colds are circulating in larger numbers. A virus that causes a mild illness in an older child or an adult can cause a more serious one in an infant. If your child is in childcare and would be in contact with children who have colds and it is convenient for you to keep them away from them, do so.

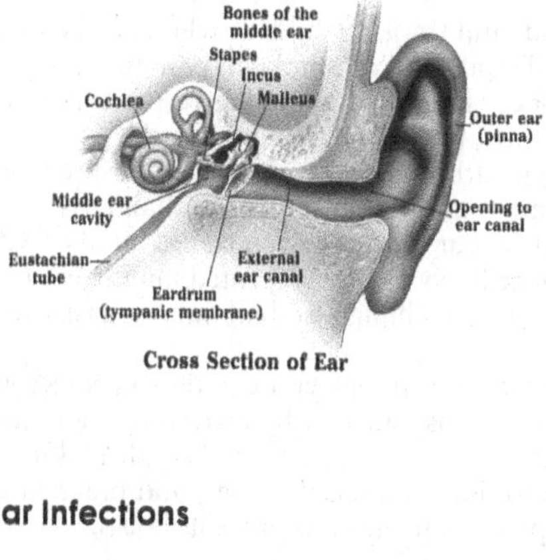

Cross Section of Ear

Middle Ear Infections

During your child's first few years, there's a good chance that they'll get a middle ear infection. At least 70 percent of the time, middle ear infections occur after colds that have weakened the body's ability to prevent bacteria from entering the middle ear. Doctors refer to this middle ear infection as acute otitis media.

Middle ear infections are one of the most prevalent treatable childhood illnesses, occurring most often in children between 6 months and 3 years of age. Two-thirds of all children have at least one ear infection by their second birthday. It's a particularly common problem among young children because they are more susceptible to colds and because of the length and shape of their tiny Eustachian tubes, which normally ventilate the middle ear.

Children under 1 year of age who spend time in childcare programs tend to get more middle ear infections than those cared for at home, primarily because they are exposed to more viruses. Also, infants who self-feed from a bottle when lying on their backs are susceptible to ear infections, as this way of feeding may allow small amounts of formula to enter the Eustachian tube. Two things may explain the fact that by the time your child reaches school age, their likelihood of getting a middle ear infection will decrease: The growth of their middle ear structures reduces the likelihood of fluid blockage, and the body's defenses against infection improve with age.

Several other factors may place children at a higher risk of middle ear infections:

- Secondhand smoke. Children who breathe in secondhand tobacco smoke have a markedly increased risk of ear infections as well as respiratory infections, bronchitis, pneumonia, and asthma.
- Gender. Although researchers are not sure why, boys have more middle ear infections than girls.
- Heredity. Ear infections can run in families. Children are more likely to have repeated middle ear infections if a parent or a sibling also had numerous ear infections.

There are certain things you can do to protect your infant from ear infections, such as breastfeeding, not smoking and not allowing smokers around your child, making sure your child is up to date on their vaccines, and practicing good hygiene and proper nutrition to prevent illness.

Signs and Symptoms

Middle ear infections are usually painful, but not always. A child old enough to talk will tell you that their ear hurts; a younger child may pull at their ear and cry. Babies with ear infections may cry even more during feedings, because sucking and swallowing cause painful pressure changes in the middle ear. A baby with an ear infection may have trouble sleeping. Fever is another warning signal: Ear infections sometimes (about a third of the time) are accompanied by elevated temperatures ranging from 100.4 to 104 degrees Fahrenheit (38–40 degrees Celsius). In addition, children may appear off balance or clumsy because the fluid or infection in the middle ear may affect their sense of balance (vestibular system).

You might see blood-tinged yellow fluid or pus draining from the infected ear. This kind of discharge means that the eardrum has developed a small hole (called a perforation). This hole usually heals by itself without complications, but you will want to describe the discharge to your pediatrician.

You also may notice that your child does not hear well. This occurs because the fluid behind the eardrum interferes with sound transmission. But the hearing loss is usually temporary; normal hearing will be restored once the middle ear is free of fluid. Occasionally, when ear infections recur, fluid may remain behind the eardrum for many weeks and continue to interfere with hearing. If you feel your child's hearing is not as good as it was before their ear became infected, consult your pediatrician. Good hearing is important for proper speech development, so if your child is having any speech delay, ask your pediatrician if a referral for a hearing test or a consultation with an ear, nose, and throat doctor (ENT; otolaryngologist) or an audiologist (hearing specialist) would be appropriate. Even when there's no speech delay, if your child has had middle ear fluid in both ears for more than three months, or in one ear for more than six months, referral for a hearing test is important.

Middle ear infections are most common during the cold and flu season of winter and early spring. When your child complains of moderate or severe pain in their ear during the summer, especially when you touch or pull on the ear, they could be suffering from an infection of the outer ear canal, called swimmer's ear. Swimmer's ear is essentially an infection of the skin lining the inside of the outer ear canal. Although this may temporarily affect hearing, it poses no risk of long-term hearing loss. Swimmer's ear can be extremely painful and should be treated.

ANTIBIOTIC OVERUSE

Antibiotics are an important treatment in managing bacterial infections such as severe ear infections and strep throat. But infections caused by viruses will not improve with antibiotics. That is why the common cold, certain types of mild ear infections, and most sore throats do not require an antibiotic. When an antibiotic is prescribed, the goal is to make sure that the antibiotic is specific for the type of bacteria causing the infection and that it is given for the right length of time.

If antibiotics are used when they are not needed—or if patients do not take the drug consistently—new strains of bacteria may develop. When that happens, antibiotics eventually may stop working and the infections they're designed to treat will no longer be curable using these medications, because the bacteria have become resistant to them. In addition, antibiotics can produce side effects, including allergic reactions and a potentially serious form of antibiotic-associated diarrhea.

Here are three important points to keep in mind if your child has an infection, to make sure your child gets the right kind of antibiotic and only when it's necessary:

- Ask your pediatrician if the infection causing your child's illness is caused by bacteria. Antibiotics work only against bacterial illnesses, not those caused by viruses. So while these medications may be appropriate for treating severe ear infections, you should not ask your pediatrician for a prescription for antibiotics to treat your child's colds and flu (as well as many sore throats and coughs), which are viral infections.
- If an antibiotic is not necessary because your child has a viral infection, ask what other measures are recommended to help with your child's symptoms. For children with mild ear infections, your child's doctor may recommend pain medicine to treat ear pain while the infection clears on its own.
- If your child's doctor prescribes an antibiotic for an ear infection or other bacterial infection, ask how to follow up if your child's condition worsens or has not improved in forty-eight to seventy-two hours. Make sure that your child takes the prescribed antibiotic exactly as your doctor instructs. And don't give your child antibiotics that have been prescribed for another family member or for another illness. If your child develops an itchy rash, hives, or watery diarrhea while taking antibiotics, notify your child's doctor.

Treatment

Whenever you suspect an ear infection, call your pediatrician. In the meantime, try to make your child more comfortable. If they have a high fever, cool them using the procedures described in *Chapter 22*, Fever. Give acetaminophen or ibuprofen in the dose appropriate for their age to help decrease the pain. (Do not give aspirin to your child; it has been associated with Reye syndrome, a serious disease that affects the liver and brain.)

If there's a fever, the doctor will examine your child to determine whether there are any other problems. To treat middle ear infections, the doctor will recommend steps to ease pain and may prescribe an antibiotic. For swimmer's ear or a middle ear infection with perforation, antibiotic ear drops may be prescribed as well.

An antibiotic is one of the treatment options for ear infections. If one is recommended, your doctor will specify the schedule for giving it to your child; it usually includes dosing once, twice, or three times a day. It's important to follow the medication schedule precisely. If an antibiotic is prescribed by an urgent care or emergency department doctor, let your pediatrician know so that they can check the dose and make a note in your child's chart.

As the infection begins to clear, some children experience a sense of fullness or popping in the ears; these are normal signs of recovery. There should be clear signs of improvement and disappearance of ear pain and fever within two days.

When your child starts feeling better, you may be tempted to discontinue the medication—but don't. Some of the bacteria that caused the infection still may be present, and stopping the treatment too soon may allow them to multiply again and permit the infection to return with full force. Your pediatrician may want to see your child after the medication is finished, to check if any fluid is still present behind the eardrum, which can occur even if the infection has been controlled. This condition (fluid in the middle ear), known as otitis media with effusion, is extremely common: Five out of every ten children still have some fluid three weeks after an ear infection is treated. In nine out of ten cases, the fluid will disappear within three months without additional treatment. Also, this fluid accumulation may be caused by something other than an ear infection, such as swollen adenoid tissue in the upper throat that interferes with drainage; for that reason, seeing a doctor is especially important to determine the cause of and best care for the problem.

Occasionally an ear infection won't respond to the first antibiotic prescribed. If your child continues to complain of significant ear pain and still has a high fever for more than two days after starting an antibiotic, call your pediatrician. To determine if the antibiotic is working, your doctor may examine your child and take another look at your child's eardrum. Sometimes the antibiotic may need to be changed, or another antibiotic added. In more severe or persistent cases, an antibiotic shot or shots may be needed to treat the infection. If none of those options works, your pediatrician may refer you to an ENT specialist for another exam. In rare cases, the ENT may take a sample of the fluid from the ear by inserting a needle through the eardrum. This will help determine the specific cause of the infection and assist in determining treatment. In very rare instances, a child may be hospitalized so that antibiotics can be given intravenously and the ear can be drained surgically.

Should a baby with an ear infection be kept home? Not unless they have a fever, are in serious pain, or feel or look sick. If they're feeling well, and if medication can be given before and after childcare (or perhaps by a school nurse), they can go to childcare. If your child's eardrum has ruptured, they'll be able to engage in most activities, although they may not be permitted to swim until the ear is dry and healed. Ordinarily, there's no reason to prevent them from flying in an airplane, although they may have some discomfort from the pressure change. Pain medication and drinking fluids during takeoff and landing can help prevent and ease discomfort.

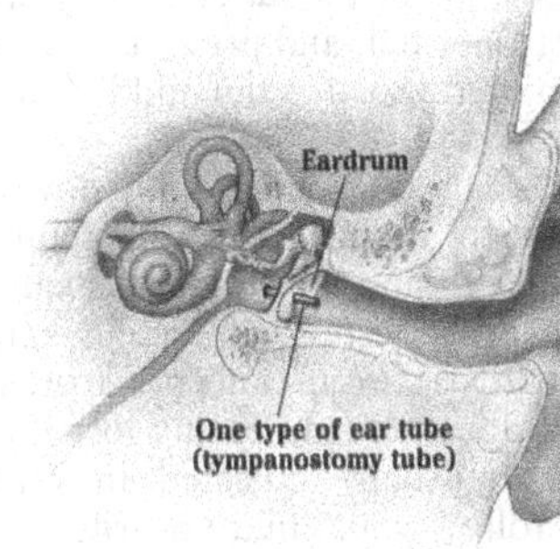

Prevention

Occasional ear infections cannot be prevented. In some children, ear infections may be related to seasonal allergies, which also can cause congestion and block the natural drainage of fluid from the ear to the throat. If your child seems to get ear infections more frequently when their allergies flare up, mention this to your pediatrician, who may suggest additional testing or recommend nasal saline spray, antihistamines, or a nasal allergy spray.

If your baby is being bottle-fed, hold their head higher than their stomach during feedings. Doing this keeps the Eustachian tubes from becoming blocked. Keep your baby away from cigarette smoke and vape emissions, as children exposed to secondhand tobacco smoke have more ear infections—and more respiratory infections, bronchitis, pneumonia, poor lung function, and asthma—than children who aren't exposed to smoke. In addition, careful handwashing can help protect your baby from illness and subsequent ear infections. Breastfeeding is also associated with fewer ear infections in children. Pacifier use after the age of 6 months is associated with ear infections as well, so it may be a good idea to stop pacifier use, especially if your baby is prone to ear infections.

And what about children who recover from one ear infection only to get another shortly thereafter? If your child continues to have ear infections, and continues to have hearing loss, they will be referred to an ENT, who may recommend that tiny ventilation tubes (sometimes called tympanostomy tubes or pressure-equalizing [PE] tubes) be inserted in the eardrum under anesthesia. While the tubes are in place, they usually restore hearing to normal, and prevent fluid and harmful bacteria from becoming trapped in the middle ear, where they can cause another infection.

Ventilation tubes are used less commonly now than in past decades, but they are still useful in certain circumstances. An ENT specialist will take a careful history and examine the ears and also perform hearing testing in a child before placing tubes. In children with recurrent infections or a history of fluid in the ears and documented hearing loss for more than three months, tubes are usually indicated. In other cases, the ENT specialist may follow your child's hearing and examination every three to six months over time before deciding on surgery. If the placement of ventilation tubes is proposed for your child, discuss their specific problem with your child's specialist and pediatrician so you fully understand the advantages and disadvantages.

Keep in mind that although ear infections are bothersome and uncomfortable, they are usually minor and clear up without causing any lasting problems. Most children stop getting ear infections by the time they are 4 to 6 years old.

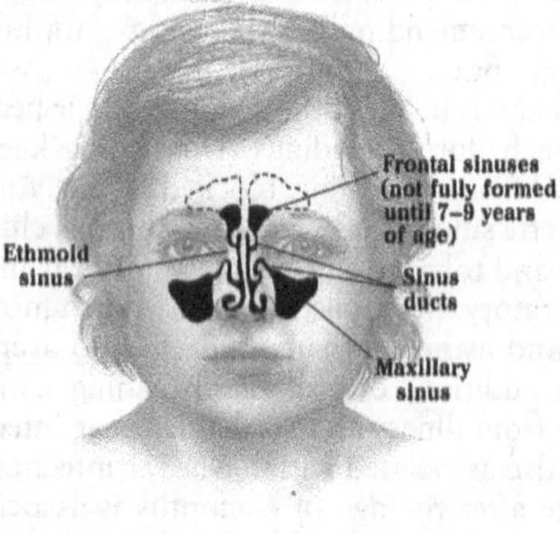

Herpes Simplex

Oral herpes is a common viral disease of childhood. This condition produces sores (cold sores), blisters (fever blisters), and swelling of the inside of the mouth and lips. Oral herpes is highly contagious and is spread by direct contact, frequently by kissing. Most infants are protected by their mothers' antibodies up to about age 6 months, but they become susceptible after that.

When the virus is transmitted to a child for the first time, the child is said to have primary herpes. This may cause pain, swelling, and reddening of the gums and an increase in saliva, followed a day or two later by blisters inside the mouth. When the blisters break, they leave sore areas that take several days to heal. The child also may develop a fever and headache, act irritably, lose their appetite, and have swollen lymph glands for a week or so. Many children, however, have such mild symptoms that no one realizes they have the virus.

Once a child has had primary herpes, they become a carrier of the virus. This means that the virus, usually in an inactive state, remains within their system. However, during episodes of stress (including other infections), injury to the mouth, sunburn, allergies, and fatigue, the virus can become reactivated, producing what's called recurrent herpes. This condition is usually milder than the primary infection, and usually doesn't occur until later in childhood or adulthood. Cold sores and fever blisters are the symptoms of recurrent herpes.

Treatment

If your child complains of symptoms resembling those of herpes, consult your pediatrician. Primary herpes is not a serious illness, but it can make your child uncomfortable. The treatment, which should be aimed at reducing this discomfort, includes:

- Bed rest and sleep.
- Plenty of cold fluids, including non-acidic drinks like water, milk, and apple juice.
- Acetaminophen if there's fever or excessive discomfort.
- Mouth rinse or gargles prescribed by your pediatrician. These medications may contain a painkiller that will numb the areas affected by the mouth sores. Carefully follow the directions for these preparations.
- A soft, bland, but nutritious diet.
- Antiviral medication (such as acyclovir or a similar type of drug) that may be prescribed by your pediatrician in some severe cases. If started early in the illness, this will

stop the virus from multiplying, but it will not prevent reactivation after the medication is stopped. It is important to keep in mind that antiviral medication will likely decrease symptom duration only by a day or so and may not make your child feel immediately better.

Occasionally a child infected with primary herpes refuses to drink fluids because of the associated mouth pain. Such a child must be hospitalized if they show signs of dehydration. Never use any creams or ointments containing steroids (cortisone) on mouth sores if there is the slightest suspicion that the sores are due to herpes, as these preparations can make the viral infection spread.

Prevention

Direct contact is required to spread the herpes virus, so you should not let anyone with herpes blisters or sores kiss your child. People with a history of oral herpes often shed the virus in their saliva even when they have no sores. In general, to prevent spread of germs, discourage individuals from kissing your baby or child directly on the lips. Also, try to discourage your child from sharing eating utensils with other children or touching a water fountain with their mouth. (This is more easily said than done.) If your child has active open primary herpes cold sores, keep them home to prevent other children from getting this infection from them.

Sore Throat (Strep Throat, Tonsillitis)

The terms "sore throat," "strep throat," and "tonsillitis" often are used interchangeably, but they don't mean the same thing. Tonsillitis refers to tonsils that are inflamed. Strep throat is an infection caused by a specific type of bacteria, group A beta-hemolytic *Streptococcus*. When your child has strep throat, the tonsils are usually very inflamed, and the inflammation may affect the surrounding part of the throat as well. Most sore throats result from viruses, which may cause inflammation only of the throat around the tonsils and not of the tonsils themselves.

In infants, toddlers, and preschoolers, the most frequent

cause of sore throats is a viral infection. No specific medicine is required when a virus is responsible, and the child should get better over a seven- to ten-day period. Often children who have sore throats due to viruses also have a cold at the same time. They may develop a mild fever, too, but they generally aren't very sick.

One particular virus (called Coxsackie), seen most often during the summer and fall, may cause the child to have a somewhat higher fever, more difficulty swallowing, and a sicker overall feeling. If your child has a Coxsackie infection, they also may have one or more blisters in their throat and on their hands and feet (and so Coxsackie is often called hand, foot, and mouth disease).

Infectious mononucleosis can produce a sore throat, often with marked tonsillitis; however, most young children who are infected with the mononucleosis virus have few or no symptoms.

Strep throat is caused by a bacterium called *Streptococcus pyogenes*, or group A streptococcus. Strep throat is most common among school-age children and adolescents, peaking at 7 to 8 years of age. Children over 3 years of age with strep may have an extremely painful throat, fever over 102 degrees Fahrenheit (38.9 degrees Celsius), swollen glands in the neck, and pus on the tonsils. Strep throat does not cause a cough, runny nose, hoarseness (changes in the voice that make it sound raspy), or conjunctivitis (also called pinkeye). These symptoms suggest that a virus is the cause of the illness instead. It's important to be able to distinguish strep throat from a viral sore throat because strep infections are treated with antibiotics.

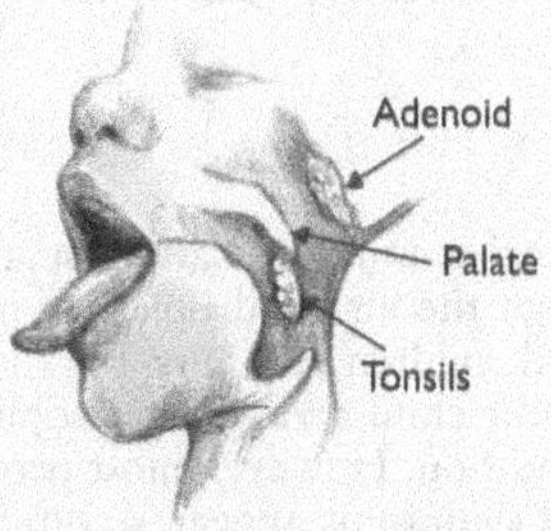

Diagnosis and Treatment

If your child has a sore throat that persists (not one that goes away after their first drink in the morning), whether or not it is accompanied by fever, headache, stomachache, or extreme fatigue, you should call your pediatrician. That call should be made even more urgently if your child seems extremely ill, or if they have difficulty breathing or extreme trouble swallowing (causing them to drool). This may indicate a more serious infection.

If your pediatrician is concerned that your child may have strep throat, they may want to perform a swab of the back of the throat and tonsils to test for bacteria. Most pediatric offices perform rapid strep tests that provide findings within minutes. If the rapid strep test is negative, your doctor may confirm the result with a culture, which can take two days to complete. A negative test means that the infection is presumed to be due to a virus. In that case, antibiotics (which work against bacteria, not viruses) will not help and need not be prescribed.

If the test shows that your child does have strep throat, your pediatrician will prescribe an antibiotic to be taken by mouth or by injection. If your child is given the oral medication, it's very important that they take it for the full course, as prescribed, even if the symptoms get better or go away. If a child's strep throat is not treated with antibiotics, or if they don't complete the treatment, the infection may worsen or spread to other parts of their body, leading to conditions such as abscesses of the tonsils or kidney problems. Untreated strep infections also can lead to rheumatic fever, a disease that affects the heart. However, rheumatic fever is rare in the United States and in children under 5 years old.

Prevention

Most types of throat infections are contagious, being passed primarily through the air on droplets of moisture or on the hands of infected children or adults. For that reason, it makes sense to keep your child away from people who have symptoms of this condition. However, most people are contagious before their first symptoms appear, so often there's no practical way to prevent your child from contracting the disease. In the past when a child had several incidents of sore throat, their tonsils might have been removed in an attempt to prevent further infections. But this operation, called a tonsillectomy, is recommended today only for the most severely affected children. Even in difficult cases, where there is repeated strep throat, antibiotic treatment is usually the best solution.

CHAPTER 18

EMERGENCIES

The information in this chapter, such as first-aid procedures for the choking child and cardiopulmonary resuscitation (CPR), is constantly evolving. Visit HealthyChildren.org and ask your pediatrician or other qualified health professional for the latest information on these procedures. It is rare for children to become seriously ill with no warning signs. Based on your child's symptoms, you should usually contact your child's pediatrician for advice. Timely treatment of symptoms can prevent an illness from getting worse or turning into an emergency.

At the same time, take steps before an emergency occurs to prepare for such an event if it should happen (see Emergency Contact Information, *page 485*). Also read the description of how to assemble a first-aid kit (*page 499*). For the CPR guidelines chart, see the Appendix, *page 703*.

Many emergencies involve sudden injuries. These injuries are often caused by the following:

- Motor-vehicle impacts (involving passengers or pedestrians) or other sudden impacts, such as bicycle accidents, falling TVs or furniture, or falls from heights such as a window
- Poisoning (if the child is not seriously ill, call Poison Help first, 1-800-222-1222)
- Burns or smoke inhalation
- Choking
- Drowning (including non-fatal events) in a swimming pool, bathtub, etc.
- Sports accidents
- Firearms or other weapons
- Electric shock

Other emergencies can result from illnesses or medical conditions. Often you can tell that an emergency is happening if you observe that your child has any of the following symptoms:

- Strange behavior, including becoming more withdrawn and less alert
- Increasing difficulty with breathing
- Skin or lips that look blue or purple (or gray for darker-skinned children)
- A cut or burn that is large or deep
- Bleeding that does not stop
- Rhythmic jerking and loss of consciousness (a seizure)
- Unconsciousness
- A head injury followed by confusion, a bad headache, vomiting, or any change in consciousness
- Very loose or knocked-out teeth, or other major mouth or facial injuries
- Increasing or severe persistent pain
- Decreasing responsiveness when being spoken to

EMERGENCY CONTACT INFORMATION

Keep the following phone numbers and addresses handy by programming them into your cellphone and the phone of anyone who cares for your child. You can also post them on your refrigerator or near other phones and insert a copy in your wallet.

- Your cellphone number
- Home or caregiver's phone number and address
- Phone number of a nearby relative, trusted neighbor, or friend
- Your pediatrician's contact information
- Your dentist's contact information
- Emergency medical services (ambulance) (911 in most areas)
- Police (911 in most areas)
- Fire department (911 in most areas)
- Poison Help (1-800-222-1222)
- Hospital

It is important that everyone who cares for your child, including care providers and sitters, knows where to find emergency phone numbers. If you have 911 service in your area, make sure your older children and your sitter know to dial 911 in case of an emergency. Be certain that they know your home address and your phone number, since an emergency operator will ask for or confirm this information. Always leave another phone number and the address where you can be located. You should also make sure your sitter knows about any medications your child takes and any food and medication allergies they may have. Those caring for your child (including you and your spouse and family) also should take a CPR class.

Remember, for a medical emergency, always call 911 first, then your child's pediatrician. If your child is seriously ill or injured, it may be safer for your child to be transported by emergency medical services (an ambulance).

Call your child's pediatrician or Poison Help (1-800-222-1222) at once if your child has swallowed or come in contact with a suspected poison or any medication you did not intend for them to ingest, even if your child has no signs or symptoms. You should not make your child vomit (do not give them syrup of ipecac, make them gag, or give them salt water) unless specifically instructed to by Poison Help or your pediatrician, as vomiting can cause further injury to your child's body.

Always call for help if you are concerned that your child's life may be in danger or your child is seriously hurt.

In Case of a True Emergency

- Stay calm.
- If your child is unresponsive and is not breathing, and you know how, start CPR (cardiopulmonary resuscitation). (For information on CPR, see the Appendix, *page 703*.)
- If you need immediate help, call 911. For example, if your child is having trouble breathing, is having a seizure, or is unresponsive, dial 911. If you do not have 911 service in your area, call your local emergency ambulance service or county emergency medical service. Otherwise, call your child's pediatrician's office and state clearly that you have an emergency.
- If there is bleeding, apply continuous pressure to the site with a clean cloth.
- If your child is having a seizure, place them on a carpeted floor with their head turned to the side, and stay with your child until help arrives. Do not put

anything in their mouth. Your child can bite down while unaware of their actions. Turning the child's head to the side will help the tongue move to the side, which will help open their airway.

After you arrive at the emergency department, make sure you tell the emergency staff the name of your child's pediatrician, who will work closely with the emergency department and can provide them with additional information about your child. Bring any medication your child is taking and their immunization record with you to the hospital. Also bring any suspected poisons or medications your child might have taken. If your child has a medically complicated condition, it's a good idea to keep a notebook/folder on their medical history, including information such as dates of and types of surgeries.

In the event of a car crash, the driver or other adults in the car may be unconscious or otherwise unable to give first responders information about the child. To help ensure that your child can be identified and treated promptly, consider attaching a sticker to your child's car safety seat with their name, date of birth, parents' names and phone numbers, and any other information you think might be important to emergency personnel (e.g., special healthcare needs or severe allergies). Place the sticker in a spot where first responders will be able to find it but where it is not easily visible from outside the car. Many police and fire departments, hospitals, and health departments keep a stock of preprinted stickers for this purpose, or you can make your own.

Bites

Animal Bites

Keep your child safe around animals, including family pets. Review Safety Around Animals, *page 341*. Many parents assume that children are most likely to be bitten by unknown or wild animals, but in fact most bites are inflicted by animals the child knows, including the family pet. Although the injury often is minor, biting does at times cause serious wounds, facial damage, and emotional problems.

As many as 1 percent of all visits to pediatric emergency centers during the summer months are for human or animal bite wounds. An estimated 4.7 million dog bites, 400,000 cat bites, 45,000 snake bites, and 250,000 human bites occur annually in the United States. About six in ten of those bitten by dogs are children.

Treatment

If your child is bleeding from an animal bite, apply firm, direct, continuous pressure to the area for five minutes or until the bleeding stops. Then wash the wound gently with soap and water and consult your pediatrician. Animal bites to the face, head, and neck (which are common in small children) can be serious, and your child will need to be examined by an emergency health provider.

If the wound is very large, or if you cannot stop the bleeding, continue to apply pressure, and call your pediatrician to find out where to take your child for treatment. If the wound is so large that the edges won't come together, it probably will need to be sutured (stitched). Although this will help reduce scarring, in an animal bite it increases the chance of infection, so your doctor may prescribe antibiotics or choose not to suture the wound.

Contact your pediatrician whenever your child receives an animal bite that breaks the skin, no matter how minor the injury appears. The doctor will need to check whether your child has been adequately immunized against tetanus (see the immunization schedule in the Appendix, *pages 696–97*) or might require protection against rabies. Both diseases can be spread by animal bites.

Rabies is a viral infection that can be transmitted by an infected animal through bites or scratches. It causes a high fever, difficulty swallowing, seizures, paralysis, and ultimately death. Fortunately, rabies in humans is rare today, with an average of two to three deaths each year in the United States; the decline in recent years is due to the availability of animal control and vaccination programs, as well as effective human rabies vaccines and immunoglobulin treatments. Nevertheless, because the disease is so serious, your pediatrician will carefully evaluate any bite for the risk of contracting this disease. Bites from wild animals—especially bats but also skunks, raccoons, coyotes, and foxes—are much more dangerous than those from tame, immunized (against rabies) dogs and cats. Avoid contact with the animal, and call animal control to evaluate any dead animal for rabies and dispose of it.

Your pediatrician or the emergency department physicians who evaluate your child will determine if the risk of contracting rabies is high; if so, they will refer your child to receive immunoglobulin and a rabies vaccine series to prevent them from contracting the disease. If the animal that bit your child is a healthy dog or cat, the animal should be observed for ten days, and treatment for your child should be started only if the animal shows signs of rabies.

As noted earlier, an animal bite, even when it doesn't cause rabies, can become infected. Notify your pediatrician immediately if you see any of the following signs of infection:

- Pus or drainage coming from the bite
- The area immediately around the bite becoming swollen and tender (it normally will be red for two or three days, but this in itself is not cause for alarm)
- Red streaks that appear to spread out from the bite
- Swollen glands above the bite

(See also Safety Around Animals, *page 341*.)

Your pediatrician may recommend antibiotic therapy for a child who has:

- Moderate or severe bite wounds
- Puncture wounds, especially if the bone, tendon, or joint has been penetrated
- Facial bites
- Hand and foot bites
- Genital area bites

For very severe or deep bites, an X-ray may be needed to make sure that the bite has not penetrated the bone or a joint. If that happens, there is a much higher risk of infection and a child may need surgery to decrease that risk.

Children who have a weakened immune system or have no spleen often receive antibiotic treatment for a bite. Your pediatrician may recommend a follow-up visit to inspect any wound for signs of infection within forty-eight hours. Many children who have been bitten by dogs may also show signs of traumatic stress in the weeks and months after the incident, long after the physical wound has healed. These children may feel fear, including anxiety about being bitten again, especially when they see or hear about another dog. They may withdraw, or cling to their parents. They may resist going outside to play, have trouble sleeping, have nightmares, and wet the bed.

To help the healing process, be attentive to what your child is saying and feeling. Give them extra attention, particularly when you sense that they need it. Some children with traumatic stress may require treatment by a mental health professional.

Human Bites

Children often experience a human bite from a sibling or a playmate. If your child is bitten by another person, call your pediatrician immediately to describe the severity of the injury. Doing this can be especially important if the biter's teeth pierced your child's skin or if the injury is large enough to require stitches. Bites that occur over the knuckles of the hand (commonly known as fight bites) are at extremely high risk of infection and should be evaluated in the emergency department.

Be sure to wash the bite carefully with cool water and soap right away to help prevent infection. For a bite that barely breaks the skin, such as a cut or scrape, a good washing with soap and water, followed by bandaging and close follow-up, is all that is needed. For more serious bites, your pediatrician should evaluate the wound. Your pediatrician will also check your child's tetanus and hepatitis B vaccine status, and assess the risk for other infections.

Burns

Burns are divided into three categories, according to their severity. First-degree burns are mild and cause redness and perhaps slight swelling of the skin (like most sunburns). Second-degree burns are painful and cause blistering and considerable swelling. Third-degree burns lack sensation and may appear white or charred and cause serious injury, not just to the surface but also to the deeper skin layers.

There are many different causes of serious burns in children, including sunburn, scalds from hot water or other liquids, and those due to fire, electrical contact, or chemicals. All of these can cause permanent injury and scarring to the skin and important organs such as the eyes, mouth, and genitalia.

Treatment

Your immediate treatment of a burn should include the following:

1. As quickly as possible, soak the burn in cool water. Don't hesitate to run the water over the burn long enough to cool the area and relieve the pain immediately after the injury. Do not use ice on a burn, as it may delay healing. Also, do not rub a burn; it can increase blistering.
2. Cool any smoldering clothing immediately by soaking with water, then remove any clothing from the burned area unless it is stuck firmly to the skin. In that case, cut away as much clothing as possible.
3. If the injured area is not oozing, cover the burn with a sterile gauze pad or a clean, dry cloth.
4. If the burn is oozing, cover it lightly with sterile gauze if available and immediately seek medical attention. If sterile gauze is not available, cover burns with a clean sheet or towel.
5. Do not put butter, grease, mustard, or powder on a burn. All these so-called home remedies actually can make the injury worse.

For anything more serious than a superficial burn, or if redness and pain continue for more than a few hours, consult a physician. All children with electrical burns and burns of the hands, mouth, or genitals should receive immediate medical attention. Chemicals that cause burns also may be absorbed through the skin and cause other symptoms. Call Poison Help (1-800-222-1222) or your pediatrician after washing off all the chemicals. (For treatment of a chemical contact to a child's eye, see Poison in the Eye, *page 516*.)

If your physician thinks the burn is not too serious, they may show you how to clean and care for it at home using medicated ointments and dressings. Under the following circumstances, however, hospitalization may be necessary:

- If the burns are third-degree
- If 10 percent or more of the body is burned
- If the burn involves the face, hands, feet, or genitals; involves a moving joint; or is circumferential (goes completely around the part of the body)
- If the child is very young or fussy, and therefore too difficult to treat at home

When treating a burn at home, watch for any increase in redness or swelling or the development of a bad odor or discharge. These can be signs of infection, which will require medical attention.

Prevention

Chapter 11, Keeping Your Child Safe, provides ways to safeguard your child against fire and scalding at home. For added protection, here are a few more suggestions:

- Install smoke detectors (and carbon monoxide detectors) in hallways outside bedrooms, the kitchen, the living room, and near the furnace, with at least one on every floor of the house. Test them every month to be sure they work. It is best to use alarms that have ten-year long-life batteries, but if these are not available, change batteries at least annually on a specific date that you'll remember (such as January 1 of each year). Smoke alarms are coming on the market with new technologies that make them more sensitive to flaming and smoldering fires and less prone to nuisance alarms caused by cooking heat or steam. This may give you more time to evacuate in case of a fire. Consider investing in new alarms if yours are several years old.
- Practice home fire drills. Make sure every family member and others who care for your children in your home know at least two ways to leave any area of the home safely in case of a fire.
- Have several working fire extinguishers readily available, and familiarize yourself with how to use

them. Place fire extinguishers around the home where the risk of fire is greatest, such as in the kitchen, in the furnace room, and near the fireplace.

- Teach your children to crawl to the exits if there's smoke in the room. (They will avoid inhaling the smoke by staying below it.)
- Purchase a safety ladder if your home has a second story, and teach your children how to use it. If you live in a high-rise building, teach your children the locations of all exits and make sure they understand never to use the elevator in a fire. (It can become trapped between floors or open on a floor where the fire is burning.)
- Agree on a family meeting point outside the house or apartment so you can make certain everyone has gotten out of the burning area.
- Teach your children to stop, drop, and roll on the ground if their clothing catches fire.
- Avoid smoking indoors.
- Do not leave food cooking on the stove unattended.
- Lock up flammable liquids in the home. It is best to store them outside the home, out of children's reach, and away from heat or ignition sources.
- Lower the temperature of your water heater so the temperature at the faucet is no more than 120 degrees Fahrenheit (48.9 degrees Celsius) to prevent hot-water scalds and burns.
- Don't plug appliances or other electrical equipment into extension cords if they place too much amperage or load on the cord, thus creating a potentially unsafe situation.
- Keep matches and lighters away from children, locked up and out of reach.
- Avoid all fireworks, even those meant for consumer use.
- Keep lit candles out of reach of children.

Cardiopulmonary Resuscitation (CPR) and Mouth-to-Mouth Resuscitation

CPR can save your child's life if their heart stops beating or if they have stopped breathing for any reason, such as drowning, poisoning, suffocation, smoke inhalation, or choking. Become familiar with the CPR instructions in the Appendix (*page 703*). However, reading about CPR is not enough to teach you how to perform it. The American Academy of Pediatrics strongly recommends that all parents and anyone who is responsible for the care of children should complete a course in basic CPR and treatment for choking.

This training is especially vital if you own a swimming pool or live near water, such as a lake or community swimming pool or spa. Contact your local chapter of the American Heart Association or the American Red Cross to find out where and when certified courses are given in your community. Most of the classes teach basic first aid, CPR, and emergency prevention, along with what to do for a choking infant or child.

Choking

Choking occurs when a person inhales something other than air into the windpipe or when food or other objects block the windpipe. Among children, choking often is caused by liquid that "goes down the wrong way." The child will cough, wheeze, gasp, and gag until the windpipe is cleared, but this type of choking rarely results in serious health problems.

Choking becomes life-threatening when a child swallows or inhales an object—often food—that blocks airflow to the lungs. This is an emergency that calls for immediate first aid. For specific and complete choking/CPR instructions, familiarize yourself with the chart in the Appendix (*page 703*), and take a course on CPR for children. A child who begins to breathe by themselves within two or three minutes after a choking incident probably will not suffer any long-term damage. The longer the child is deprived of oxygen, however, the greater the risk of permanent injury.

Occasionally a choking episode is followed by persistent coughing, gagging, wheezing, excessive salivation, or difficulty in swallowing or breathing. If this occurs, it may mean that an object is still partially blocking the airway—possibly in the lower breathing tubes. In this case, the object can cause continued breathing difficulty, irritation, and possibly pneumonia. See your pediatrician or go to the emergency department if any symptoms persist, so that further tests, such as chest X-rays, can be done. If they show that your child has inhaled something, admission to the hospital may be needed for a procedure to remove the object. Any choking incident that lasts more than a few seconds warrants medical attention.

THE HAZARDS OF BUTTON AND COIN BATTERIES AND MAGNETS

Two choking and swallowing hazards deserve special attention: batteries (button batteries, lithium coin batteries) and rare-earth magnets. The small circular batteries found in a variety of portable electronic devices can form acid that quickly erodes a hole in the airway or intestinal tract. If you suspect your child has swallowed or inhaled one of these batteries, seek care immediately. While waiting for help, you can give your child 2 teaspoons of honey at ten-minute intervals, as long as they are at least 1 year of age. This may help prevent damage while the battery remains stuck. Batteries that no longer can power a device still hold enough charge to be dangerous, so when you change batteries, always wrap the old batteries in tape and dispose of them promptly.

Likewise, the extra-strong little magnets used in toys, containers, and electronics can stick together when swallowed, cutting off circulation in the intestines and causing life-threatening complications. If you have any concern your child may have swallowed one of these magnets, get them care right away.

Prevention

Choking is a significant danger for children, especially until age 5. Objects such as small balls or marbles, balloon fragments, small parts from toys, and coins can cause choking, but food is responsible for most incidents. You must be particularly watchful when children around the age of 1 are sampling new foods. Here are some additional suggestions to prevent choking:

- Don't give young children hard, smooth foods (e.g., peanuts, raw vegetables) that must be chewed with a grinding motion. Children don't master that kind of chewing until around age 4, so they may attempt to swallow the food whole. Do not give whole peanuts or other nuts to young children. When your child does start to eat peanuts (and you know they don't have an allergy to peanuts), watch them very closely while they are chewing and give only one nut at a time.

- Don't give your child round, firm foods (like hot dogs, grapes, and carrot sticks) unless they are chopped completely. Cut them lengthwise and then into bite-size pieces (no larger than ½ inch [1.25 cm]), and encourage your child to chew thoroughly.
- Do not give your child compressible foods like marshmallows or fruit snacks until at least 4 years of age.
- Supervise mealtimes for your infant or young child. Only permit eating while your child is seated and supervised, never while playing or running. Teach your child to chew and swallow their food before talking or laughing.
- Chewing gum is a choking hazard for young children.

Foods that pose particular risk include hot dogs; hard, gooey, or sticky candy or vitamins; grapes; and popcorn.

Because young children put everything into their mouths, small non-food objects are also responsible for many choking incidents. Look for age guidelines in selecting toys, and follow the manufacturer's recommended ages, especially for children younger than 3 years. Also be aware that certain objects have been associated with choking, including uninflated or broken balloons, baby powder, items from the trash (e.g., eggshells, pop-tops from beverage cans), safety pins, coins, marbles, small balls, pen or marker caps, magnets, and small button or coin-type batteries (see *page 495*).

If you're unsure whether an object or food item could be harmful, you can purchase a standard small-parts cylinder at juvenile products stores that you can use to determine whether an object is small enough to choke a child.

Cuts and Scrapes

Your child's natural curiosity and eagerness are likely to produce some scrapes and cuts along the way. Their reaction may be far more severe than the actual damage. In most cases, good treatment will require little more than cleansing the injury, protecting it, and providing plenty of reassurance (and perhaps a kiss on the minor bump or bruise).

Cuts, Lacerations, and Bleeding

A cut or laceration is a wound that breaks through the skin and into the tissues beneath. The deeper the cut, the more likely there are to be problems, such as bleeding and the possibility of damage to nerves and tendons. The following simple guidelines will help you prevent serious bleeding and other problems, such as scarring, when your child gets a cut:

1. Apply pressure. Almost all active bleeding can be stopped by applying direct pressure with clean gauze or cloth over the site for five to ten minutes. The most common mistake is interrupting the pressure too early to peek at the wound. Doing this may result in more bleeding or the buildup of a clot that can make it harder to control the problem with further pressure. If bleeding starts again after five minutes of continuous pressure, reapply pressure and call your doctor for help. Do not use a tourniquet or tie-off on an arm or leg unless you are trained in its use, since this can cause severe damage if left on too long. However, if the cut is on an extremity, you can elevate the arm or leg to help decrease bleeding.
2. Stay calm. The sight of blood can be frightening, but this is an important time to stay in control. You'll make better decisions if you are calm, and your child will be less likely to get upset by the situation. Remember, by using direct pressure you will be able to control bleeding from even the most severe lacerations until help can arrive. Relatively minor cuts to the head and face will bleed more than cuts to other parts of the body

because of the greater number of small, superficial blood vessels.

3. Seek medical advice for serious cuts. No matter how much (or how little) bleeding occurs, call your doctor if the laceration is deep (all the way through the skin and into the tissue below) or more than ½ inch (1.25 cm) long. Deep cuts can severely damage underlying muscles, nerves, tendons, and joints even if on the surface the wound does not appear serious. Long lacerations and those on the face, chest, and back are more likely to leave disfiguring scars. In these situations, if the wound is properly closed, the scar probably will be much less apparent. In some circumstances, a skin adhesive (a glue-like substance) may be used to close the wound. If in doubt about whether stitches, adhesives, or staples are needed, call your doctor right away for advice, as it's important for repair to occur within eight to twelve hours of the injury.

   You should be able to treat short, minor cuts yourself as long as the edges come together by themselves or can be brought together with the aid of a butterfly bandage, and if there is no numbness beyond the wound and no reduction in sensation or movement. (A butterfly bandage is a strip of adhesive with ends that flare. It's used to keep the edges of a cut together during the healing process.) However, have your doctor examine your child if there is any possibility that foreign matter, such as dirt or glass, is trapped in the cut. Any injury that you cannot manage should be seen by your pediatrician or emergency medical services as soon as possible to maximize healing. Your child may not like to let you examine a laceration thoroughly because of the pain involved. The pediatrician, however, can use a local anesthetic if necessary to ensure a thorough exam. The doctor may also use topical skin adhesives.

4. Clean and dress the wound. If you feel comfortable handling the problem, wash the wound with plain water and examine it carefully to be sure it is clean. Apply an antibiotic ointment, then cover it with a sterile dressing. It's easy to underestimate the extent or severity of a cut, so even if you choose to treat it yourself, don't hesitate to call your pediatrician for advice. If any redness, swelling, or pus appears around the wound, or

if bleeding recurs, consult your physician as soon as possible. Antiseptics such as iodine and alcohol are not necessary and increase your child's discomfort, so do not use them on cuts. If your child's immunizations are current, tetanus shots are not necessary after most abrasions and lacerations. However, if your child is not up to date on their tetanus booster or it is time for a booster dose, your pediatrician may recommend that one be given.

FIRST-AID SUPPLIES FOR YOUR HOME AND CAR

You should prepare a first-aid kit for your home as well as one for each of your cars. The kit should contain:

- Fever- or pain-reducing medication: acetaminophen or a non-steroidal anti-inflammatory medication such as ibuprofen
- Antihistamine for allergic reaction
- Antibiotic ointment
- Prescription medications that anyone in your family takes
- Sterile adhesive bandages (in various sizes)
- Gauze pads
- Medical tape
- Scissors
- Tweezers
- Soap or another cleansing agent
- Petroleum jelly or another lubricant
- Moistened towelettes
- Thermometer

Scrapes

Most minor injuries in young children are scrapes, or abrasions, which means that the outer layers of skin literally have been scraped off. If the abrasion covers a large area, it may appear to be very bloody, although the actual amount of blood lost is small. The area should be rinsed first with cool water to flush away debris and then washed gently with warm water and soap. Avoid using iodine and other antiseptic solutions. They have little protective value and can add to the pain and discomfort.

If left alone, most abrasions scab over quickly, and formerly this was thought to be the best natural remedy. But scabs slow the healing process and can lead to more scarring. Treat large or oozing scrapes with an antibiotic ointment and then cover them with a sterile (germ-free) dressing. These can be obtained at your local pharmacy, in the form of either an adhesive bandage or a separate gauze pad that is held in place by rolled gauze or adhesive tape. Some dressings are made of certain non-stick materials that are less likely to adhere to the raw surface of a wound. Antibiotic ointment also helps prevent the dressing from sticking to the healing wound surface. The purpose is to prevent the injury from becoming infected while healing occurs. It is best to keep the bandage in place, except for dressing changes, until the wound heals. Take care that dressings around such areas as fingers or toes are not so tight as to interfere with circulation.

Examine the wound daily during the dressing change, or whenever it becomes dirty or wet. If a bandage sticks when you try to remove it, soak it off with warm water. Most wounds require a dressing for only two or three days, but your child may be reluctant to stop applying bandages that quickly, because small children tend to regard bandages as badges or medals. There is no harm in leaving the area loosely covered as long as the bandage is kept dry and clean and the wound is checked daily.

Call your pediatrician if you can't get a wound clean or if you notice drainage or pus, increasing tenderness or redness around the site, or fever. These are signs that the wound may be infected. If necessary, the doctor can use a local anesthetic to prevent severe pain while cleaning out dirt and debris that you are not able to remove. If the wound is infected, they may prescribe antibiotics in the form of an oral medicine or else an ointment or a cream.

Prevention

It is almost impossible for a curious and active child to avoid some scrapes and minor cuts, but there are things you can do to decrease the number your child will have and to minimize their severity. Keep potentially dangerous items like sharp knives, easily breakable glass objects, and scissors out of their reach. When your child gets old enough to use knives and scissors themselves, teach your child how to handle them properly and insist that they be used safely. At regular intervals, make a safety check of your house, garage, and yard. If you find objects that are potentially dangerous because your child is older and can get into them, store them securely out of their reach.

(See also *Chapter 11*, Keeping Your Child Safe.)

Dental Trauma

As children become more mobile and have increasing stumbles and falls, tooth injuries may occur. Most injuries are minor and will heal on their own, but there are some dental situations where you should reach out to your pediatrician or pediatric dentist, such as if a tooth is knocked out, is pushed into the gum, or appears loose or wiggly after trauma.

If a tooth is knocked out of the mouth, retrieve it and handle the tooth carefully. Do not scrub it. Rinse it under cool water and place it in a glass of milk. Then call a pediatric dentist or your pediatrician for additional instructions. These will differ depending on whether the tooth is a primary ("baby") or permanent tooth. If a tooth is pushed into the gum, this is a situation for which you should ask for help from your pediatrician or dentist. Call a pediatric dentist or your pediatrician for additional instructions.

If a tooth is loose from trauma, have the child avoid hard foods for twenty-four hours, and if the tooth remains loose, call a pediatric dentist.

Drowning

Drowning is a leading cause of death among children, including infants and toddlers. Most infant drownings occur in bathtubs and buckets. Toddlers between 1 and 4 years old most commonly drown in swimming pools. However, many children in this age group drown in ponds, rivers, and lakes. Children older than 5 years old are more likely to drown in rivers and lakes, but this varies from one area of the country to another. It is important to know that children can drown in even 1 inch of water, such as a bathtub or toilet. When a child is rescued before death, the episode is called a non-fatal drowning.

What You Should Do

Without putting yourself in harm's way, get your child out of the water immediately, then check to see if they are breathing on their own. If they are not breathing, begin CPR immediately (see the Appendix, *page 703*). If someone else is present, send them to call for emergency medical help (911), but don't spend precious moments looking for someone, and don't waste time trying to drain water from your child's lungs. Concentrate instead on giving your child rescue breathing and CPR until they are breathing on their own. While you are doing CPR, it is very likely your child will vomit some of the swallowed water. Only when the child's breathing has resumed should you stop and seek emergency help. Call 911 if you haven't already. Once the paramedics arrive, they will administer oxygen and continue CPR if necessary.

Any child who has come close to drowning should be given a complete medical examination, even if they seem all right. If they stopped breathing, inhaled water, or lost consciousness, they should remain under medical observation for at least twenty-four hours to be sure there is no damage to the respiratory or nervous system. A child's recovery from a non-fatal drowning depends on how long they were deprived of oxygen. If your child was underwater only briefly, they are more likely to recover completely. Longer periods without oxygen can cause damage to the lungs, heart, or brain. A child who doesn't respond quickly to CPR may have more serious problems, but it's important to keep trying, because sustained CPR has revived children who have appeared lifeless or who have been immersed in very cold water for lengthy periods.

Prevention

For newborn infants and all children under 5 years of age (and older children who are not strong swimmers), parents and caregivers should never—not even for a moment—leave children alone or in the care of another child while in or near bathtubs, pools, spas, or wading pools, or near irrigation ditches or other open bodies of water. With children of this age, use touch supervision; that means that a supervising adult should be within an arm's length of the child, with full attention focused on the child at all times, when they are in or near water. The supervising adult should not be engaged in distracting activities, such as using a phone, reading, socializing, or tending to household chores. If you are hosting a pool party, hire or designate an adult lifeguard so that a supervising adult always has eyes on the water in case of emergency.

Home swimming pools should be surrounded by a fence that is not connected to the house, to prevent a child from getting to the pool from the house. There is no substitute for a four-sided, non-climbable fence that is at least 4 feet (1.2 m) high, with a self-closing, self-latching gate that opens away from the pool. Parents, caregivers, and pool owners should know CPR, should be able to swim, and should keep a phone and equipment approved by the US Coast Guard (life preservers, life jackets, shepherd's crook) at poolside.

Toddlers, children with intellectual disabilities, and children with seizure disorders are particularly vulnerable to drowning, but all children are in danger if unsupervised in or near water. Even a child who knows how to swim may drown a few feet from safety. Remember, children should be supervised at all times. Swimming lessons should not be considered as "drownproofing" your child. (For more information, see Water Safety, *page 338*.)

Electric Shock

When the human body comes in direct contact with a source of electricity, the current passes through it, producing what's called an electric shock. Depending on the voltage of the current and the length of contact, this shock can cause anything from minor discomfort to serious injury and even death. Young children, particularly toddlers, experience electric shock most often when they bite into electrical cords or poke metal objects such as forks or knives into unprotected outlets or appliances. These injuries also can take place when electric toys, appliances, or tools are used incorrectly, or when an electric current makes contact with water in which a child is sitting or standing. Christmas trees and their lights are a seasonal hazard.

What You Should Do

If your child comes in contact with electricity, always try to turn the power off first. In many cases you'll be able to pull the plug or turn off the switch. If this isn't possible, consider an attempt to remove the live wire—but not with your bare hands, which would bring you in contact with the current yourself. Instead, try to cut the wire with a wood-handled ax or well-insulated wire cutters, or move the wire off the child using a dry stick, a rolled-up magazine or newspaper, a rope, a coat, or another thick, dry object that won't conduct electricity.

If you can't remove the source of the current, try to pull the child away. Again, do not touch the child with your bare hands when the child is attached to the source of the current, since their body will transmit the electricity to you. Instead, use a non-conducting material such as rubber or those described previously to shield you while freeing them. (Caution: None of these methods can be guaranteed safe unless the power can be shut off.)

As soon as the current is turned off (or the child is removed from it), check the child's breathing, skin color, and ability to respond to you. If the child's breathing or heartbeat has stopped or seems very rapid or irregular, immediately use CPR (see the Appendix, *page 703*) to restore it and have someone call for emergency medical help. At the same time, avoid moving the child needlessly, since such a severe electrical shock may have caused a spinal fracture.

If the child is conscious and it seems the shock was minor, check them for burned skin, especially if their mouth was the point of contact with the current. Call 911. Electric shock can cause internal organ damage that may be difficult to detect without a medical examination. For that reason, all children who receive a significant electric shock should see a doctor. In the pediatrician's office, any minor burns from the electricity will be cleansed and dressed. The doctor may order laboratory tests to check for signs of damage to internal organs. If the child has severe burns or any sign of brain or heart damage, they will need to be hospitalized.

Prevention

The best way to prevent electrical injuries is to use outlet covers that are not a choking hazard, make sure all wires are properly insulated, tuck wires away from your child's reach, and provide adult supervision whenever children are in an area with potential electrical hazards. Small appliances are a special hazard around bathtubs, sinks, or pools. (See also *Chapter 11*, Keeping Your Child Safe.)

Fingertip Injuries

Children's fingertips get smashed frequently, usually getting caught in closing doors. Either the child is unable to recognize the potential danger or they fail to remove their hand quickly enough before the door is shut. Fingers also sometimes get crushed when children play with a hammer or other heavy object, or when they're around a car door. Because fingertips are exquisitely sensitive, your child will let you know immediately that they've been injured. Usually the damaged area will be blue and swollen, and there may be a cut or bleeding around the cuticle. The skin, tissues below the skin, and the nail bed—as well as the underlying bone and growth plate—all may be affected. If bleeding occurs underneath the nail, it will turn black or dark blue, and the pressure from the bleeding may be painful.

Home Treatment

When the fingertip is bleeding, wash it with soap and water, and cover it with a soft, sterile dressing. An ice pack or a soaking in cold water may relieve the pain and minimize swelling. If the swelling is mild and your child is comfortable, your doctor may recommend that you allow the finger to heal on its own. But be alert for any increase in pain, swelling, redness, or drainage from the injured area beginning twenty-four to seventy-two hours after the injury. These may be signs of infection, and you should notify your pediatrician. When there's excessive swelling, a deep cut, or blood under the fingernail, or if the finger looks as if it may be broken, call your doctor immediately. Do not attempt to straighten a fractured finger on your own.

Professional Treatment

If your doctor suspects a fracture, they may order an X-ray. If the X-ray confirms a fracture—or if there's damage to the nail bed, where nail growth occurs—a consultation with a hand surgeon may be necessary. A fractured finger may need to be straightened and set under local anesthesia. An injured nail bed also must be repaired surgically to minimize the possibility of a nail deformity developing as the finger grows. If there's considerable blood under the nail, the pediatrician may drain it by making a small hole in the nail, which should relieve the pain.

Although deep cuts may require stitches or skin glue, often all that's necessary are sterile adhesive strips (thin adhesive strips similar to butterfly bandages). A fracture underneath a cut is considered an open fracture and is susceptible to infection in the bone. In this case, antibiotics will be prescribed. Depending on your child's age and immunization status, the doctor also may order a tetanus booster.

Firearms

According to the CDC, firearm injury is now the leading cause of death for children in the United States. Most firearm deaths of young children are classified as homicide deaths, but accidental firearm injuries also occur. It is important to note that firearm injury has a very high case fatality rate, meaning that when a firearm is fired, death is common. Around 25 percent of firearm injuries result in death, compared to only 4 percent of accidental poisonings.

What You Should Do

If a child has been shot, call 911, or ask someone nearby to call. Ensure that the firearm has been secured or is no longer a danger, and then apply lifesaving measures, including applying direct pressure to wounds, applying a tourniquet (see the organization Stop the Bleed, stopthebleed.org, for training), or beginning CPR. Once emergency responders arrive, they will take over and transport the child to the nearest trauma center. Those surviving a firearm injury can be left with lasting physical injuries, ongoing medical care needs, and psychological trauma. The best approach is to prevent the firearm injury.

Prevention

To prevent firearm deaths, you can take action by doing the following.

Secure Your Firearms.

When not under an authorized user's active control, all firearms should be kept locked away from children by using one or more of the following: trigger lock, cable lock, gun safe, or firearm cabinet safe. Firearms should never be left unattended (e.g., left on the top of a nightstand, resting in a purse or bag, left in a drawer, or stored in a closet or attic).

Ask About Safe Firearm Storage.

If your child is visiting another home for any length of time, ask about firearm storage. Given that firearm injury is the leading cause of death for children of all ages, parents and other caregivers should check before allowing their children to spend any time in another home.

Avoid Alcohol and Drug Use.

No authorized user should ever have a firearm under their active control when they have been drinking or using impairing drugs.

Know the Limits of Training.

All adults in a home with firearms should take a firearm safety training course. Firearm owners should understand that teaching children about firearm safety is not an effective method of preventing firearm injuries. Children do not have the level of brain development required to understand the risk of firearms.

Report Family Violence.
Women are most often the victims of firearm violence in the home, along with children. Seek help by reaching out to your local domestic violence hotline or call the National Domestic Violence Hotline at 1-800-799-7233. They can help you navigate options for you and your children, including the use of laws in many states that authorize the removal of firearms from abusers.

Fractures/Broken Bones

Although the term "fracture" may sound serious, it is just another name for a broken bone. Fractures are the fourth-most-common injury among children under 6 years of age. Falls cause most of the fractures in this age group, but the most serious bone breaks usually result from car crashes.

A broken bone in a child is different from one in an adult, because young bones are more flexible and have a thicker covering, which makes them better able to absorb shock. Because children's bones are still growing, the bones have tremendous potential to repair themselves, so perfect alignment is often not necessary. Many fractures can be treated non-operatively. They usually just need to be kept free of movement, most often using a molded cast or splint.

Often children's fractures are either greenstick fractures, in which the bone bends like green wood and breaks only on one side, or torus fractures, in which the bone is buckled, twisted, and weakened but not completely broken. A fracture with plastic deformation is a bone that is bent but not broken and is relatively common among children as well. Complete fractures, in which the bone breaks all the way through, also occur in children.

Because your child's bones are still growing, they are vulnerable to an additional type of fracture that does not occur in adults. This involves damage to the growth plates at the ends of the bones, which regulate future growth. If this part of the bone does not heal properly after the fracture, the bone may grow at an angle or more slowly than the other bones in the body. Unfortunately, the impact on the bone's growth may not be visible for a year or more after the injury, so these fractures must be followed carefully by an orthopedist or sports medicine specialist for twelve to eighteen months to make sure no growth damage has occurred. Fractures that involve injury to the growth plate sometimes need surgery to minimize the risk of future growth problems.

Fractures around the elbow often cause the arm to heal abnormally, resulting in a crooked position. Many require surgery to minimize this risk. Children with fractures near the elbow may be referred to an orthopedic specialist.

Signs and Symptoms

It's not always easy to tell when a bone is broken, especially if your child is too young to describe what they are feeling. Ordinarily with a fracture, you will see swelling and your child will clearly be in pain and unable—or unwilling—to move the injured limb. However, just because your child can move the limb doesn't necessarily rule out a fracture. Often with a fracture there is tenderness at one spot where the fracture is when you press along the limb. Anytime you suspect a fracture, notify your pediatrician immediately. If the limb is crooked, you should seek immediate treatment for your child at the emergency department or urgent care.

Home Treatment

Until your child can be seen in the pediatrician's office, emergency room, or urgent care center, use an improvised sling or rolled-up newspaper or magazine as a splint to protect the injury from unnecessary movement. If you think your child may have a broken bone, do not give them anything to eat or drink (even pain medication) before going to the doctor in case they need to be sedated with general anesthesia to fix the fracture. For older children, you can use a cold pack or a cold towel, placed on the injury site, to decrease pain. Extreme cold can cause injury to the delicate skin of babies and toddlers, so do not use ice with children this young.

If your child has broken their leg, do not try to move them yourself. Call 911 for an ambulance; let the paramedics supervise their transportation and make the child as comfortable as possible. If part of the injury is open and bleeding, or if bone is protruding through the skin, place firm pressure on the wound (see Cuts, Lacerations, and Bleeding, *page 497*), then cover it with clean (preferably sterile) gauze. Do not try to put the bone back underneath the skin. After this injury has been treated, be alert to any fever, which may indicate that the wound has become infected.

Professional Treatment

After examining the break, the doctor will order X-rays to determine the extent of the damage. If the doctor suspects that the bone's growth plate is affected, or if the bones are out of line, an orthopedic consultation will be necessary. Because children's bones heal rapidly and well, a plaster or fiberglass cast, or sometimes just an immobilizing splint, is all that is needed for most minor fractures. For a displaced fracture, where the bones aren't aligned properly, an orthopedic surgeon may have to realign the bones. This may be done without surgery, with an orthopedic surgeon manipulating the bones until they're straight (closed reduction), and then applying a cast. If the break is more severe, your child may need to be given medication in the emergency department for them to set the fracture, or your child may need to be sedated under general anesthesia in the operating room. After the reduction, a cast will be used until the bone has healed, which usually takes less time than adult bones require. The nice thing about young bones is that they don't have to be in perfect alignment for them to remodel as they grow. Your orthopedist may order periodic X-rays while the bone is healing, just to make sure they are aligning properly.

Usually casting brings rapid relief or at least a decrease in pain. Your child may experience pain for the first two to three days after the injury or after setting or surgery. It is important to elevate the broken limb for the first two to three days to decrease the swelling. Typically, pain can be treated with over-the-counter medications, as well as activities to distract your child from the pain. If your child has an increase in pain, numbness, or pale or blue fingers or toes, call your doctor immediately. These are signs that the extremity has swollen and requires more room within the cast. If the cast is not adjusted, the swelling may press on nerves, muscles, and blood vessels, which can produce permanent damage. To relieve the pressure, the doctor may split the cast, open a window in it, or replace it with a larger one.

Also let the doctor know if the cast breaks or becomes very loose, or if the plaster or fiberglass gets wet and soggy. Without a proper, secure fit, the cast will not hold the broken bone in position to mend correctly. Often, bones that have been broken will form a hard knot, known as a callus, at the site of the break during the healing process. Especially with a broken collarbone, this may look unsightly, but there is no treatment for this, and the knot will not be permanent. The bone will remodel and resume its normal shape in a few months.

Head Injury/Concussion

It's almost inevitable that your child will hit their head every now and then, especially when they're a toddler—falling off playground equipment or a bed, for example. These blows may upset you, but your anxiety is usually worse than the bump. Most head injuries are minor, causing no serious problems. Even so, it's important to know the difference between a head injury that warrants medical attention and one that needs only a comforting hug.

By definition, a concussion is a hard strike to the head resulting in temporary confusion or a change in behavior, and sometimes is accompanied by a loss of consciousness. Particularly if a child has significant memory loss, disorientation, altered speech, visual changes, seizure, or nausea and vomiting after a head injury, call 911 and contact your pediatrician. In fact, if your child experiences head trauma with persistent pain or any other symptoms, your child should be examined by a doctor.

Treatment

If a child's head injury has been mild, they'll remain alert and awake after the incident, and their color will be normal. They may cry out due to momentary pain and fright, but the crying should last no more than ten minutes and then they'll go back to playing as usual.

If the injury seems minor and there's not a significant cut (one that's deep and/or actively bleeding) that might require immediate medical attention or possibly stitches (see Cuts and Scrapes, *page 497*), you may be able to treat your child at home. Just wash the cut with soap and water. If there's a bruise, apply a cold compress. This will help minimize the swelling if you do it in the first few hours after the injury. Even in these cases, however, it may be wise to call your pediatrician and explain the circumstances and your child's condition.

Even after only a minor head injury, you should observe your child for twenty-four to forty-eight hours to see if they develop any signs that the injury was more severe than it first appeared. Although it's very rare, children can develop a serious brain injury after a seemingly minor bump on the head that causes no immediate obvious problems. If your child develops any of the following symptoms, be sure to consult your pediatrician immediately or seek prompt attention from the nearest emergency room:

- Your child seems excessively sleepy or lethargic during their usual wakeful hours, or you cannot awaken them from sleep at night. It is normal for children to seem tired or less active after a head injury, but this should improve within a few hours; seek medical attention if it doesn't.
- Your child vomits or has a headache that won't go away (even with acetaminophen). Headache and vomiting occur commonly after head trauma, but they are usually mild and last only a few hours. (Small children may not be able to let you know they have a headache, so they may cry or be inconsolable.) Vomiting that occurs more than four to six hours after the head trauma is less common, so call your doctor or take your child to the emergency department for an evaluation.
- Your child is persistently or extremely irritable. With an infant who cannot tell you what they're feeling, irritability may indicate a severe headache.
- Any significant change in your child's mental abilities, coordination, sensation, or strength warrants immediate medical attention. Worrisome changes would include weakness of arms or legs, clumsy walking, slurred speech, crossed eyes, or difficulty with vision.
- Your child becomes unconscious again after being

awake for a while, or they have a seizure (convulsion) or start to breathe irregularly.

If your child loses consciousness at any time after hitting their head, notify the pediatrician. If your child doesn't awaken within a few minutes, they need immediate medical attention. Call 911 for help while you follow these steps:

1. Move your child as little as possible. If you suspect that they might have injured their neck, do not attempt to move them. Changing the position of the neck might make the injuries worse. One exception: Move them if they are in danger of being injured further where they are (e.g., on a ledge or in a fire), but try to avoid bending or twisting the neck.
2. Check to see if your child is breathing. If not, perform CPR (see the Appendix, *page 703*).
3. If your child is bleeding severely from a scalp wound, apply direct pressure with a clean cloth over the wound.
4. After calling 911, wait for the ambulance's arrival rather than taking your child to the hospital yourself.

Loss of consciousness following a head injury may last only a few seconds or as long as several hours. If you find the child after the injury happened and you are not sure if they lost consciousness, notify the pediatrician.

Most children who lose consciousness for more than a few minutes will be observed in the emergency department, and some may be hospitalized overnight for observation. Hospitalization is essential for children with severe brain injury and irregular breathing or convulsions. Fortunately, with modern pediatric intensive care, some children who have suffered serious head injury—and even those who have been unconscious for several weeks—eventually may recover completely.

Poisoning

About 2.2 million people swallow or have contact with a poisonous substance each year. More than half of these poison exposures occur in children under 6 years of age. Most children who are poisoned are not permanently harmed, particularly if they receive immediate treatment. If you think your child has been poisoned, stay calm and act quickly. You should suspect poisoning if you ever find your child with an open or empty container of a toxic substance, especially if they are acting strangely. Be alert for these other signs of possible poisoning:

- Unexplained stains on their clothing
- Burns on the lips or mouth
- Unusual drooling, or odd odors on their breath
- Unexplained nausea or vomiting
- Abdominal cramps
- Difficulty in breathing
- Sudden behavior changes, such as unusual sleepiness, irritability, or jumpiness
- Seizures or unconsciousness (only in very serious cases)

POISON-PROOFING YOUR HOME

- Store drugs and medications in a medicine cabinet that is locked or in a locked medication box that is out of reach. Do not keep toothpaste, soap, or shampoo in the same cabinet. If you carry a purse, keep potential poisons out of your purse, and keep your child away from other people's purses.
- The best way to keep your child safe from substances like marijuana edibles is not to have them in your home. However, if you do, store these products securely out of reach, as you would medications. Avoid buying edibles that look like real candies. Teach your kids to ask permission first before eating food they find. This gives a chance for an adult to make sure the food is safe to eat.
- Buy and keep medications in their own containers with child safety caps. (Remember, however, that these caps are child-resistant, not childproof, so keep the containers in a locked cabinet.) Dispose of all expired or unused medicines. Many pharmacies and municipalities accept leftover medications and will dispose of them safely.
- Do not take medicine in front of small children; they may try to imitate you later. Never tell a child that a medicine is candy to get them to take it.

- Check the label every time you give medication, to be sure you are giving the right medicine in the correct dosage. Mistakes are most likely to occur in the middle of the night, so always turn on the light when handling any medication.
- Read labels on all household products before you buy them. Try to find the safest ones for the job and buy only what you need to use immediately.
- Store hazardous products in locked cabinets that are out of your child's reach. Do not keep detergents and other cleaning products under the kitchen or bathroom sink unless they are in a cabinet with a safety latch that locks every time you close the cabinet. (Most hardware stores and department stores sell these safety latches.) Detergent products packaged in single-load packets or "pods" offer convenience but often resemble candy or gummy treats and are tempting for children to put in their mouth. This can make them violently ill very quickly and lead to serious breathing or stomach problems, coma, and even death. It is best to use traditional liquid or powder detergent products until all children in the household are at least 6 years of age. If you do use concentrated detergent packets, keep them locked up out of sight and reach of children.
- Never put poisonous or toxic products in containers that were once used for food, especially empty drink bottles, cans, or cups.
- Always open the garage door before starting your car, and never run the car in a closed garage. Be sure that coal, wood, or kerosene stoves are properly maintained. If you smell gas, turn off the stove or gas burner, leave the house, and then call the gas company.
- Post the Poison Help number, 1-800-222-1222, near every telephone in your home and in your cellphone contacts, along with other emergency numbers. Be sure that your childcare provider and anyone else caring for your child knows when and how to use these numbers.

Keep in mind that these guidelines should apply not only to your home but also to any other settings where your child visits, including the homes of grandparents and babysitters.

Treatment

If there's an emergency and you cannot find the Poison Help number, dial 911 or directory assistance and ask for the number. Keep the Poison Help number in your cellphone (1-800-222-1222). Poison Help will provide the immediate information and guidance you need. These centers are staffed twenty-four hours a day with experts who can tell you what to do without delay. (Anytime your child has been exposed to a poison of any kind, you should notify your pediatrician as well.) The immediate action you need to take will vary with the type of poisoning. Poison Help can give you specific instructions if you know the particular substance your child has swallowed. However, carry out the following instructions before calling them.

(For more information about poisoning, see Food Poisoning and Food Contamination, *page 361*.)

Poison in the Eye

Flush your child's eye by holding their eyelid open and pouring a steady stream of lukewarm water into the inner corner. A young child is sure to object to this treatment, so get another adult to hold them while you rinse the eye. If that's not possible, wrap them tightly in a towel and clamp them under one arm so that you have one hand free to hold the eyelid open and the other to pour in the water.

Continue flushing the eye for fifteen minutes. Then call Poison Help, 1-800-222-1222, for further instructions. Do not use an eye cup, eye drops, or ointment unless Poison Help tells you to do so. If there is any question of continued pain or severe injury, seek emergency assistance immediately.

Poison on the Skin

If your child spills a dangerous chemical substance on their body, remove their clothes and rinse the skin with lukewarm—not hot—water. If the area shows signs of being burned, continue rinsing for at least fifteen minutes, no matter how much your child may protest. Then call Poison Help, 1-800-222-1222, for further advice. Do not apply ointments or grease.

Poisonous Fumes

In the home, poisonous fumes are most likely to be produced by an idling automobile in a closed garage; leaky gas vents; wood, coal, or kerosene stoves that are improperly vented or maintained; or space heaters, ovens, stoves, clothes dryers, or water heaters that use gas. Regardless of whether you have any of these appliances, you should have carbon monoxide detectors in your home, since carbon monoxide has no odor. If your child is exposed to fumes or gases from these or other sources, get them into fresh air immediately. If they are breathing, call Poison Help, 1-800-222-1222, for further instructions. If your child has stopped breathing, start CPR (see the Appendix, *page 703*), and don't stop until they breathe on their own or someone else can take over. If you can, have someone call 911 for emergency medical help immediately; otherwise, try one minute of CPR and then call for emergency assistance.

Swallowed Poison

First, get the poisonous substance away from your child. If your child still has some in their mouth, make them spit it out, or remove it with your fingers. Keep this material along with any other evidence that might help determine what they swallowed.

Next, check for these signs:

- Severe throat pain
- Excessive drooling
- Breathing difficulty
- Seizures
- Excessive drowsiness

If any of these are present, or if your child is unconscious or has stopped breathing, start emergency procedures such as CPR and get medical help immediately by calling 911. Take the poison container and remnants of material with you to help the doctor determine what was swallowed. Vomiting may be dangerous, so do not make your child vomit—even if the label on the container suggests it—as this may cause further damage. Strong acids (e.g., toilet bowl cleaner, bleach) or strong alkalis (e.g., lye, drain or oven cleaner, or dishwasher detergent) can burn the throat, and vomiting will only increase the damage by bringing these fluids back up into the esophagus and throat. Syrup of ipecac is a drug that was used in the past to make children vomit after they swallowed a poison; although this may seem to make sense, it is no longer considered a good poison treatment. If you have syrup of ipecac in your home, properly dispose of it and throw away the container. Do not make a child vomit by other means either, such as making them gag or giving them salt water. Instead, you may be advised to have your child drink milk or water.

If your child is not showing these serious symptoms, call Poison Help, 1-800-222-1222, which will direct your call to your regional poison center. The person answering the phone will need the following information to help you:

- Your name and phone number.
- Your child's name, age, and weight. Also be sure to mention any serious medical conditions your child has or medications they are taking.
- The name of the substance your child swallowed. Read it off the container, and spell it if necessary. If ingredients are listed on the label, read them, too. If your child has swallowed a prescription medicine and the drug is not named on the label, give the center the name of the pharmacy and its phone number, the date of the prescription, and its number. Try to describe the color and shape of the tablet or capsule and mention any imprinted numbers on it. If your child swallowed another substance, such as a part of a plant, provide as full a description as possible to help identify it.
- What time your child swallowed this poison (or when you found them), and the amount you think they swallowed.

If the poison is extremely dangerous, or if your child is very young, you may be told to take them directly to the nearest emergency department for medical evaluation. Otherwise, you will be given instructions to follow at home.

Prevention

Young children, especially those between ages 1 and 3, are commonly poisoned by things in the home such as medications—even those sold over the counter—and illegal drugs, cleaning products, plants, cosmetics, pesticides, paints, solvents, antifreeze, windshield wiper fluid, gasoline, kerosene, and lamp oil. This happens because tasting and mouthing things is a natural way for children to explore their surroundings, and because they imitate adults without understanding what they are doing.

Keep all poisons, medications, and toxins high out of children's sight and reach. The best way to prevent poisonings is to store all toxic substances in a locked cabinet where your child cannot possibly get to them, even when you are not directly watching them. Also, supervise them even more closely whenever you're visiting a store or a friend or relative's home that has not been childproofed. (See also *Chapter 11*, Keeping Your Child Safe.)

CHAPTER 19

ENVIRONMENTAL HEALTH

All children are potentially exposed to environmental toxins in the world in which we live. But while you can't protect your child from every environmental hazard that exists, whether indoors or out, you can prevent their exposure to some and decrease cumulative risk of exposure to others.

Air Pollution

The outdoor air contains several substances that could be harmful to children. One of the most worrisome is ground-level ozone, which is a colorless gas that is created when nitrogen oxides interact with volatile organic compounds. These compounds are released by cars and industry, and react with sunlight to make ozone. Ground-level ozone is the main ingredient in smog. Ozone concentrations are likely to be at the highest, unhealthiest levels in the summer on warm, sunny days, peaking in the mid- to late afternoon. Ozone can be present at high levels in the winter, too. It can travel by wind, resulting in rural areas being affected by ozone as well. Because children spend more time playing outdoors than adults and are therefore more likely to experience increased exposure, they are particularly vulnerable to ozone's effects, with breathing difficulties most likely to occur in children with asthma. Children also have increased exposure to air pollution because they breathe more rapidly than adults and inhale more pollutants per pound of body weight.

Multiple health harms also occur to fetuses and children from particulate matter, especially those that are very tiny (called PM2.5), from power plants, vehicle exhaust, or forest fires. Wood-burning stoves and gas cookstoves in our homes also produce particulate matter and other air pollutants harmful to health. Breathing PM2.5, by children and those who are pregnant, has been linked to preterm birth, small-for-age babies, and neurodevelopmental harms.

Other air pollutants that can cause harm include carbon

monoxide, particulate matter released from cars and industry, and sulfur dioxide. Not all chemicals in our air are regulated by the Environmental Protection Agency. Parents and caregivers should pay attention to air alerts in the media or should assess data online before sending children out to play. Children with asthma or other chronic diseases can be greatly affected by poor air quality and should be kept indoors when air quality alerts show danger.

Prevention

To protect your child from air pollution, limit their playtime outdoors when local agencies have issued health advisories or smog alerts—particularly if your child has a respiratory problem like asthma. When wildfire smoke is present, limit outdoor time in accordance with the AirNow.gov chart (airnow.gov/). Refer to this webpage when needed to find out when it's best to keep your kids indoors. Newspapers and TV news programs also provide information about the air quality in the community.

To reduce the air pollution from automobiles on smoggy days, keep your car in the garage and use public transportation or car pools instead. Do not use gasoline-powered lawnmowers on high-pollution days, and limit their use at other times. Turn off the car rather than letting it idle while you wait, as idling increases air pollution. Work with local, state, and national governments to enforce and tighten air pollution laws and regulations.

Exposure to indoor air pollution should be minimized if possible. HEPA filters in homes can help remove air pollution from indoor and outdoor sources. Weatherization of homes can decrease the amount of outdoor pollution entering the home.

Asbestos

Asbestos is a natural fiber that was widely used as a spray-on material for fireproofing, insulation, and soundproofing in schools, homes, and public buildings from the 1940s through the 1970s. It does not pose health risks unless it deteriorates and becomes crumbly, at which point it can release microscopic asbestos fibers into the air. When asbestos fibers are inhaled, they can cause chronic health problems to the lungs, throat, and gastrointestinal tract, including a rare type of chest cancer (called mesothelioma) that can occur as long as five decades after asbestos exposure.

Today, schools are mandated by law to either remove asbestos or otherwise ensure that children are not exposed to it. However, it is still in some older homes, especially as insulation around pipes, stoves, and furnaces, as well as in walls and ceilings.

Prevention

Follow these guidelines to keep your child safe from asbestos:

- If you think there may be asbestos in your home, have a professional inspector check for it. State agencies have the most up-to-date listings of accredited professionals in your area. To locate your state's asbestos contact, go to epa.gov/asbestos/state-asbestos-contacts.
- Do not let your youngster play near any exposed or deteriorating materials that could contain asbestos.
- If asbestos is found in your home, it may be acceptable to leave it there if it is in good condition. But if it is deteriorating, or if it might be disturbed by any renovations you're planning, have a properly accredited and certified contractor remove the asbestos, which must be taken off in a safe manner. Again, ask your state's asbestos contact for information on finding a certified contractor in your community.

Carbon Monoxide

Carbon monoxide is a toxic gas that is a by-product of appliances, heaters, and automobiles that burn gasoline, natural gas, wood, oil, kerosene, and propane. It has no color, no taste, and no odor. It can become trapped inside your home if appliances are not working efficiently; if a furnace, stove, or fireplace has a clogged vent or chimney; or if a charcoal grill is used in an enclosed area. Carbon monoxide also might enter your home when an automobile is left running in an attached garage. During power outages and storms, using electrical generators indoors increases the risk for carbon monoxide poisoning. These appliances should remain outdoors.

When your child breathes carbon monoxide, it harms the ability of their blood to transport oxygen. Although everyone is at risk for carbon monoxide poisoning, it is particularly dangerous for children because they breathe faster and inhale more carbon monoxide per pound of body weight. Carbon monoxide poisoning of those who are pregnant can also be very dangerous to fetal development. Symptoms may include headaches, nausea, shortness of breath, fatigue, confusion, and fainting. Persistent exposure to carbon monoxide can lead to personality changes, memory loss, severe lung injury, brain damage, and death.

Prevention

You can reduce your child's risk of carbon monoxide poisoning by:

- Buying, installing, and periodically checking the function of carbon monoxide detectors in your home, particularly near the bedrooms, or near a furnace or woodstove
- Never leaving your car running in an attached garage (even if the garage door is open)
- Never using a charcoal or propane grill, hibachi, or portable camping stove indoors or in an enclosed area
- Never using a fuel-burning electric generator inside your home, and even when using a generator outdoors, never running it near an open window or a fresh air intake vent for your home
- Scheduling an annual inspection and servicing of oil and gas furnaces, woodstoves, gas ovens and ranges, gas water heaters, gas clothes dryers, and fireplaces
- Never using your non-electric oven to heat your kitchen or your house

Drinking Water

Children drink much more water for their size than adults. Most of this water comes from the tap, and the quality of this water is regulated by standards instituted by Congress, included in the Safe Drinking Water Act of 1974. Subsequent laws have set drinking water standards for chemicals that were known to be in some water supplies.

Today the drinking water in the United States is among the safest in the world, although problems can occur from time to time. Violations in water safety standards are most likely to occur in small systems that serve fewer than 1,000 people. Also, keep in mind that private wells are not federally regulated and should be tested for nitrates and other environmental toxins if appropriate.

PLASTICS (BISPHENOL A [BPA] AND PHTHALATES)

Breastfeeding is the safest and most important way to nourish your baby. Many food and liquid containers, including some baby bottles, are made of polycarbonate, or have a lining that contains the chemical bisphenol A (BPA). BPA is used to harden plastics, keep bacteria from contaminating foods, and prevent cans from rusting. Other synthetic chemicals, called phthalates, are used in soft, flexible plastics. BPA and phthalates can leach from products and into the environment after repeated use, heating (such as during microwave cooking), and cleaning.

There are concerns over the possible harmful effects that BPA and phthalates may have on humans, particularly on infants and children. For example, animal studies have shown effects on endocrine function in animals related to BPA and phthalate exposure. BPA acts as a weak estrogen in animals and perhaps in humans, too.

Risk Reduction

As research continues, concerned parents can take the following precautionary measures to reduce babies' exposure to BPA and phthalates:

- Avoid clear plastic baby bottles or containers with the recycling number 7 and the letters "PC" imprinted on them. Many contain BPA, although newer bottles should be BPA-free.
- Consider using certified or identified BPA-free plastic bottles.
- Glass bottles can be an alternative, but be aware of the risk of injury to you or your baby if the bottle is dropped or broken.
- Because heat may cause the release of BPA and phthalates from plastic, do not heat polycarbonate bottles or other plastic food containers in the microwave, and do not wash polycarbonate bottles or other plastic food containers in the dishwasher.
- Breastfeeding is another way to reduce potential exposure to unwanted chemicals. The AAP recommends exclusive breastfeeding for about six months. Breastfeeding should be continued thereafter as long as it is mutually desired by mother and infant.
- Many parents are concerned about BPA in dental sealants or fillings. Science shows that the exposure to BPA in these dental materials is very minimal, and fears over BPA should not prevent your child from receiving necessary dental care.

The drinking water standards for lead are not health-based standards. Thus, the federal action level for lead, at 15 parts per billion (ppb), may result in elevated blood lead levels if that water is the only source of liquid. This can be very important for infants who are bottle-fed with reconstituted formula. The American Academy of Pediatrics recommends that lead in water be as low as possible (a maximum of 1 ppb) in drinking water, including school drinking fountains. Pipes connecting from water mains to homes, and pipes within homes, have been made with lead. In addition, before 1986 lead solder was typically used inside homes with copper pipes, and fixtures were made with brass with high lead content. Water companies often use corrosion control measures to decrease the amount of lead that enters water from the pipes. Recent events have shown this may not occur to the extent it should. Also, water treatment facilities are not responsible for the pipes in homes and leading up to the homes, which may also be lead.

Flushing the lines before use for an appropriate amount of time together with using cold water rather than hot water may decrease the amount of lead exposure.

The addition of fluoride to municipal water supplies has resulted in a substantial decrease in dental caries in children. There can be too much fluoride in water, though, and care is needed to not let it get too high. However, science shows that fluoride in tap water is a safe and effective way to promote the development of healthy teeth and help prevent cavities. In many communities, tap water is better for children to drink than bottled water due to the fluoride that is added. Children who do not have access to fluoridated tap water may be at higher risk for cavities, and finding a dental home by 1 year of age is especially important for these children. Fluoridated tap water is safe to drink for those who are pregnant and is also safe to mix with formula for an infant.

Contaminants in drinking water that can cause illness in the immediate or longer term include germs, nitrates, synthetic chemicals, metals, radioactive materials, and by-products of the disinfecting process. In some communities, bottled water is being used or recommended due to contamination in the drinking water supply. It is important to note that while bisphenol A and phthalates may not be used in the manufacturing of plastics, other chemicals used to make plastic serve the same functions. These "regrettable substitutes" have resulted in less knowledge about what chemicals have entered our bodies from plastics.

Although bottled water can be purchased in markets, most brands are just tap water that has been bottled for sale. Bottled water is generally much more expensive than tap water, and unless there are known contamination problems in your community's water supply, it is not necessary. Fluoride is not typically added to bottled water, and additional fluoride treatments may be needed for children who drink bottled water regularly. In summary, be careful about using bottled water with children on a regular basis.

Prevention

To ensure that your child is consuming safe drinking water, you can check the water quality by contacting the county health department, the state environmental agency, or the Environmental Protection Agency's Safe Drinking Water Hotline (1-800-426-4791). Local water companies are mandated to report what is in the water on an annual basis. Well water should be tested yearly.

Other guidelines include:

- Use cold water for cooking and drinking. Contaminants can accumulate in water heaters.
- If you are concerned about the quality of your plumbing, run the faucet each morning prior to using the water for cooking or drinking. Contact your local water utility to find out how long to run the water in your home. This will flush the pipes and lower the likelihood that contaminants will end up in the water you consume.
- Have well water tested for nitrates before giving it to infants under 1 year of age.
- Drinking water that may be contaminated with germs should be boiled and then allowed to cool before drinking. Boil for no more than one minute. However, it is important to remember that boiling water only kills bacteria and other germs; it does not remove toxic chemicals. If you don't like the taste or smell of your tap water, filters made with activated carbon will remove the odd taste or smell. Such filters will also remove undesirable chemicals without removing fluoride needed to prevent tooth decay.

In the United States, more than 23 million families rely on private, unregulated wells for water to drink, cook with, and bathe in. Private wells, while convenient, also risk contamination from chemicals, germs, and minerals and require regular testing and maintenance to ensure the safety of everyone who relies on them. Daycares, schools, and vacation rentals may also rely on wells. If your child will be drinking well water in any setting, use the following tips to ensure it's safe:

- If you're buying a new home with a well, the builder should provide the results of coliform, nitrate, inorganic (total dissolved solids, iron, manganese, magnesium, calcium, chloride), fluoride, radon, perfluoroalkyl and polyfluoroalkyl substances, arsenic, chlorinated hydrocarbons, and lead testing. If the home is near agricultural operations, then additional testing for pesticide residues is important. If the home site is near natural gas extraction (fracking) operations, then chemical tests of the well water, including testing for benzene, should be performed. If the well was shock-chlorinated after drilling, it should be retested for coliforms after some period of time as recommended by the local health department or agricultural extension agent. Have the builder or agent provide a site plan with the well, its water lines, and the septic tank and field.

- If you're renting or leasing a home with a well, the well and septic field should be included in any general home inspection. If this cannot be performed, families should arrange for well inspection and testing as previously described and have the septic tank located and inspected to determine if it needs to be pumped. If there are filters, softeners, or other devices in the water supply lines, determine from the seller or landlord what they are treating and the maintenance needs for the equipment.
- If you're vacationing at a home with a well, the water source should be tested each season. Every well should be tested, and there are procedures for properly shutting down and restarting a water system that is only in use for part of the year. For a short stay, if the quality of the well water cannot be ensured, it may be safer and more convenient to use commercially available bottled water for drinking and cooking.
- For an existing home with a well, the well should be examined every spring to make sure that there are no mechanical problems. Well water should be tested annually for coliforms and nitrate. Testing more than once per year may be warranted in the following special situations: (1) someone in the household is pregnant or nursing; (2) there are unexplained illnesses in the household; (3) neighbors find a dangerous contaminant in their well water (in which case the homeowner's well should be tested for that specific contaminant); (4) there is a change in the odor or taste of the well water; (5) there is a chemical spill in the proximity of the well; (6) there are new fracking operations, underground chemical storage tanks, or other commercial/industrial

concerns in the vicinity that may pose a hazard of groundwater contamination; (7) there was a significant repair or replacement in the well; or (8) there was a flooding event or another disaster resulting in possible well contamination.

- Additional testing may be indicated if there is any damage to the well from a fallen tree, a flood, a fire, or similar circumstances, if there are concerns about elevated nitrate levels in the area, if there are any questions about the integrity or sealing of the well, or if a household member becomes sick with an intestinal illness from *E. coli* or *Giardia lamblia.*

Fish

Fish is a protein-rich food that is healthy for both children and adults. It contains a good type of fat (omega-3 fatty acids), as well as nutrients such as vitamin D. It also is low in saturated fat. At the same time, a lot of attention has focused on the contaminants that may be in fish and that could pose health risks.

One of the most widely discussed contaminants is mercury, which at high levels can be toxic. It gets into oceans, rivers, lakes, and ponds, and can end up in the fish we eat. Mercury in bodies of water like lakes and streams—some of it discharged from industrial plants—can be converted by bacteria into mercury compounds such as methylmercury. As a result, certain predatory fish (including shark and swordfish) can contain high quantities of mercury, which when consumed can have a serious negative effect on the nervous system of a developing fetus or young child.

Other environmental pollutants have been found in fish and other foods, including polychlorinated biphenyls (PCBs) and dioxins. PCBs are chemicals that were manufactured primarily for use as fire retardants and in electrical transformers; they were banned in the United States in the late 1970s. However, they have remained in the environment in water, soil, and air, and have been found in fish. PCBs have been associated with thyroid problems, lowered IQ, and memory impairment in young children.

Dioxin is another pollutant that has been detected in fish. It is the by-product of burning certain chemicals and can interfere with the developing nervous system and other organs, particularly when the exposure is long-term. Fortunately, PCBs and dioxins have decreased significantly in recent years.

Prevention

Certain types of fish and shellfish are lower in mercury, including canned light tuna, salmon, shrimp, cod, flatfish, scallops, and pollock. These are the best choices of fish and shellfish for your child to consume. Nevertheless, you should limit your child's intake of even these safer selections to two to three servings per week. On average, a serving is about 1 ounce for children ages 1 through 3; for children ages 4 through 7, a serving is 2 ounces. Government agencies are recommending that young children reduce their intake of certain fish that may contain high levels of mercury. Specifically, young children should not consume king mackerel, swordfish, shark, halibut, sablefish, and tilefish.

For information about the safety of fish and shellfish caught in your area, contact state and local health departments. For current advisories issued by states, territories, or tribes, visit the advisory website of each state, territory, or tribe at fishadvisoryonline.epa.gov/Contacts.aspx. The health department in your state can provide any advisories issued about the presence of other toxins in fish in your area.

Lead Poisoning

Lead poisoning is caused most often by touching and then mouthing dusty toys, chips of old paint, or contaminated dirt; by breathing lead in the air; or by drinking water from pipes lined, made from, or soldered with lead or piped through lead-containing brass fixtures. There also may be lead in hobby materials such as stained glass, paints, solders, bullets, and fishing weights. It might be in miniblinds manufactured outside the United States prior to July 1997. If you buy new miniblinds, look for those that have a label that says "new formulation" or "non-leaded formula." Lead also might be in food cooked or stored in some imported ceramic dishes. Do not serve acidic substances (e.g., orange juice), hot/warm food, or liquids in these dishes, since this can cause the lead from the dishes to leach into the food. Although food cans with soldered seams could add lead to the food inside them, these cans generally have been replaced by seamless aluminum containers in the United States.

Where We Stand

Lead causes serious damage to children's brains even at low levels of exposure, and the effects are difficult to overcome. The American Academy of Pediatrics supports widespread lead screening of children, as well as funding programs to remove lead hazards from the home, learning, and play environments. Primary prevention is the only way to combat lead poisoning. Knowing the environment where your child will live, learn, and play and removing the source of lead before your child encounters it will prevent lead exposure and the adverse effects that result from it.

Parents may work in places where lead is used, such as battery plants, shooting ranges, or oil fields, and dust or lubricants that contain lead may come home on clothes, cars, and hair. Parents should shower and change clothes at work. Any work clothes should be laundered separately.

Other sources of lead can include candy, ethnic remedies, and alternative sources of medicine from countries like Mexico, as well as some spices, cosmetics, items used for worship, and Ayurvedic treatments from India, the Middle East, and Southeast Asia. More recently in the United States, lead has been found in charcoal-containing toothpaste and infant teething bracelets. Avoid toothpastes that are not ADA approved. Infant teething bracelets and necklaces may also present a choking and strangulation hazard, so potential lead contamination is yet another reason to avoid their use; better alternatives include a frozen banana, a teething ring, or a cold, wet, clean washcloth to chew on. Recalls and warnings about lead-contaminated products are available on the Consumer Product Safety Commission (cpsc.gov) and FDA (fda.gov) websites.

Lead was an allowable ingredient in house paint before 1978 and so may be on the walls, door jambs, and window frames in many older homes. The EPA's Federal Lead Disclosure Rule outlines requirements for informing renters and buyers about the possibility of lead paint existing in a pre-1978 residential property. As the paint ages, it chips, peels, and comes off in the form of dust. Toddlers may be tempted by such bite-size pieces and will taste or eat them out of curiosity. Even if they don't intentionally eat the material, the dust can get on their hands and into their food. Sometimes the lead-containing finish has been covered with other layers of newer, safer paints. This can give you a false sense of reassurance, however, since the underlying paint still may chip or peel off with the newer layers and fall into the hands of toddlers.

There is no safe level of lead in the human body. Although there has been a decline in high lead levels in children's blood, somewhere between 500,000 and 1 million children in the United States have unacceptably high levels. Living in a city, being poor, being an immigrant, and being African American or Hispanic are all risk factors that increase the chances of having an elevated blood lead level. But even children living in rural areas or who are in well-to-do families still can be at risk.

In a child who continues consuming lead, the substance will accumulate in the body. Although it may not be noticeable for some time, ultimately it can affect many areas of the body, including the brain. Lead poisoning can cause learning disabilities and behavioral problems. Very high levels will likely cause the most severe problems, but the extent of damage for any individual child cannot be predicted. Lead also can cause stomach and intestinal problems, loss of appetite, anemia, headaches, constipation, hearing loss, and even short stature. Iron deficiency increases the risk for lead poisoning in children, which is why these two disorders are often found together in children. (See Abdominal Pain, *page 348*.)

Prevention

If your home was built after 1977, when federal regulations restricted the amount of lead in paint, the risk of having dangerous amounts of lead in the dust, paint, or soil of your residence is low. However, if your home is older, the likelihood of having dangerous amounts of lead there can be very high, especially for the oldest homes (those built before 1960). This is because of the myriad of other sources that may contain lead. It is imperative that you assess your home and goods for the possibility of lead contamination. If you think your home may contain lead, clean up any paint dust or chips using water. During this cleanup, if you add a detergent to the water, it will help bind the lead into the water. Also, keeping surfaces (floors, window areas, porches, etc.) clean may lower your child's chance of being exposed to lead-containing dust. Older windows are of particular concern, since paint on wood frames frequently is damaged and the action of opening and closing windows can produce lead-containing dust. Do not vacuum the chips or dust using a regular vacuum because that will spread the dust through its exhaust hole. The National Center for Healthy Housing, the EPA, and many state agencies suggest a HEPA vacuum as an effective tool for removing lead paint chips. It's also a good idea to have your child leave their shoes at the door and wash their hands often, particularly before they eat.

Another step is to identify surfaces in your home with lead-contaminated paint, or areas with dangerous amounts of lead in the dust or dirt. A home inspection is necessary to do this, and you can get help from your local or state health department to find a lead inspector in your area.

Diagnosis and Treatment

Children who have lead poisoning rarely show any physical symptoms. However, learning and behavior problems from lead may show up in the preschool child, or they may not show up until the child reaches school age. At that point, children need to learn more complicated tasks like reading or arithmetic and may have trouble keeping up with classwork. Some may even seem overly active or inattentive due to the effects of the lead. For this reason, the only sure way to know if your child has been exposed to excessive lead is to have them tested. In fact, a blood test for lead around ages 1 to 2 years is recommended for all children. The CDC's advisory committee now recommends performing interventions for children who test at 3.5 µg/dL or higher. This recommendation dropped the level for action from 10 µg/dL to 3.5 µg/dL.

ORGANIC FOODS

The US Department of Agriculture has established a certification program that requires farmers to meet government guidelines for growing and processing foods before the "organic" label can be attached to them. When foods like fruits, vegetables, and grains are organic, they are grown in soil fertilized with manure and compost, and without the use of synthetic pesticides, herbicides, dyes, or waxes; these standards prohibit the use of non-organic ingredients for at least three years before crops are harvested. Organically produced meats must be raised free of growth hormones or antibiotics.

But does it really make a difference to buy organic? Are these foods actually safer and more nutritious—and are they worth the premium prices often charged for them? Several studies have examined whether health risks can be reduced by limiting or eliminating exposure to pesticides. These pesticides are sprayed on crops to safeguard them from insects and molds, and their residue can be left on fruits and vegetables and then later consumed. But the fact is that any risk to children and adults when eating these foods is minimal. The traces of pesticides found on produce are usually much lower than the safety levels established by government agencies.

To complicate the issue of whether to buy organic, even organic foods may not be completely chemical-free. Although they haven't been treated with synthetic pesticides, small amounts of these chemicals can be carried by the wind or water and end up on organic crops. Similar concerns surround other chemicals as well, such as nitrates; the levels of nitrates in organically grown plant foods vary from one producer to another and are dependent on factors like the season in which they're grown, the geographic location, and the post-harvest processing.

No matter what you decide, don't let any concerns about chemicals keep you from feeding your children a healthy diet rich in fruits, vegetables, whole grains, and low-fat dairy products, whether those are conventional or organic foods. In fact, there are greater risks in not making fruits and vegetables part of your child's meals, compared with any hazards posed by pesticides or herbicides.

So, are organic foods more nutritious for your child? Bear in mind that there is no convincing evidence that the nutritional content of organic foods differs in any significant way from conventional foods—in other words, there's no persuasive research showing that organic foods are more nutritious or even tastier than conventional foods. Remember that foods labeled as organic may still be unhealthy for other reasons, such as fruit snacks or juices that contain a lot of sugar and may cause dental cavities and that are less healthy than fresh fruits and vegetables. However, if you have easy access to organic foods in local farmers' markets or stores, and their higher prices fit into your budget, there is certainly little downside to choosing organic items.

The most common screening test for lead poisoning uses a drop of blood from a finger prick. If the results of this test indicate that a child has been exposed to excessive lead, a second test will be done using a larger sample of blood obtained from a vein in the arm. This test is more accurate and can measure the precise amount of lead in the blood.

Children who are found to have elevated blood lead levels should receive an assessment of their home to evaluate the source. At higher levels, the child may need to stay in a lead-safe home while the original home is assessed and remediated. In rare instances, they may require treatment with a drug that binds the lead in the blood and greatly increases the body's ability to eliminate it. When treatment is necessary, usually oral medicines are used on an outpatient basis. Much less frequently, the treatment may involve hospitalization.

Some children with lead poisoning require more than one course of treatment. Unfortunately, standard treatments for lead-poisoned children produce only a short-term or marginal lowering of the child's body lead levels and do not lower the child's chance of developing lead-related behavioral or learning problems. Children who have had lead poisoning will need to have their physical health, behavior, and academic performance monitored for many years and should receive special schooling and therapy to help them overcome learning and behavior problems.

The best treatment for lead poisoning is prevention. If you are considering the purchase of an older home, have it tested first by the health department or a commercial lead testing firm. In the same way, children who spend time in older buildings for daycare or other reasons may be at risk.

Pesticides/Herbicides

Pesticides and herbicides are used in a variety of settings, including homes, schools, parks, lawns, gardens, and farms. While they may kill insects, rodents, and weeds, many are toxic to people when consumed in food and water.

More research is needed to determine the short- and long-term effects of pesticides and herbicides on humans. Although some studies have found connections between some childhood cancers and an exposure to pesticides, other studies have not reached the same conclusions. Many pesticides disrupt the nervous system of insects, and research has shown that they have the potential to damage the neurological system of children.

Prevention

Try to limit your child's unnecessary exposure to pesticides or herbicides. To reduce such exposure:

- Minimize using foods in which chemical pesticides or herbicides were used by farmers.
- Wash all fruits and vegetables with water before your child consumes them.
- For your own lawn and garden, use non-chemical pest control methods whenever possible. If you keep bottles of pesticides in your home or garage, make sure they're out of the reach of children to avoid any accidental poisoning.
- Consider that children and adults who eat organic foods have lower levels of pesticide metabolites in their system, so choose organic (when possible) to decrease your family's risk.
- Avoid routinely spraying homes or schools to prevent insect infestations.
- Consider integrated pest management, which focuses on the use of baits and blocking the sources of entry.

Radon

Radon is a gas that is a product of the breakdown of uranium in soil and rock. It also may be in water, natural gas, and building materials.

High levels of radon are found in homes in many regions of the United States. It makes its way into homes through cracks or openings in the foundation, walls, and floors, or occasionally in well water. It does not cause health problems immediately upon inhalation. Over time, however, it can increase the risk of lung cancer and some other forms of cancer. In fact, next to cigarette smoking, radon is thought to be the most common cause of lung cancer in the United States.

Prevention

To reduce your child's risk of radon exposure:

- Ask your local health department whether radon levels are high in your community.
- Have your home tested for radon, using an inexpensive radon detector. (Hardware stores sell these detectors.) A certified laboratory should analyze the results of this test.
- If the levels are too high in your home, call the Radon Fix-It Hotline at 1-800-644-6999; this is a good resource for information on reducing the radon risk in your home.

Smoke Exposure

According to the Centers for Disease Control and Prevention, almost 38 percent of children ages 3 to 11 years old live in a household with at least one person who smokes cigarettes. Secondhand (or environmental) cigarette smoke is exhaled smoke from burning tobacco or smoke from the mouthpiece end or filter of a cigarette, cigar, or pipe. If you or others in your home use cigarettes, pipes, or cigars, your child is being exposed to this smoke. Tobacco smoke contains thousands of chemicals, some of which have been shown to cause cancer, heart disease, and other illnesses, including respiratory infections, bronchitis, and pneumonia. Children exposed to cigarette smoke also have a greater likelihood of developing ear infections and asthma, and they may have a more difficult time getting over colds. They are more susceptible to headaches, sore throats, hoarseness, irritated eyes, dizziness, nausea, lack of energy, and fussiness. For these reasons, many parents have designated their homes as non-smoking areas.

Thirdhand smoke exposure is usually defined as the smoke, residual nicotine, and other chemicals that tobacco smoke leaves behind on clothes, furniture, carpets, a person's hair, and their skin after a cigarette has already been extinguished. Newer tobacco products, including e-cigarettes and vaping devices, can also cause harm through secondhand exposure to aerosols. E-cigarette aerosols can contain substances that harm the body, such as cancer-causing chemicals and tiny particles that reach deep into the lungs.

If a parent or caregiver smokes around a newborn, the baby has a greater risk of dying from sudden infant death syndrome (SUID/SIDS). In addition, babies can be exposed to nicotine and dangerous chemicals from cigarettes through breast milk.

One other important point: The risk of fires is increased when you smoke in your home. Children can suffer burns if they find and play with a lit cigarette or with matches or a lighter. According to a 2006 Surgeon General's report, there is no risk-free level of tobacco exposure. One study showed that when just one cigarette was smoked in a bedroom with a closed door, two hours were needed for particulates in the air to return to a threshold lower than harmful levels; even after that time, thirdhand smoke is still a risk.

E-cigarettes

While e-cigarettes don't have the same second- and thirdhand smoke exposure profile as conventional tobacco products, they are also dangerous to children. The aerosols generated by e-cigarettes are inhaled and then exhaled by the user, and some of the generated aerosols may be discharged directly into the surrounding environment and deposited on surface areas. Children can be exposed to these second- and thirdhand aerosols in a manner similar to that of second- and thirdhand cigarette smoke. Known toxic substances and carcinogens have been found in e-cigarette emissions.

Marijuana Use

Current data are insufficient to assess the effects of exposure of infants to maternal marijuana use during breastfeeding. As a result, maternal marijuana use while breastfeeding is discouraged. Because the potential risks of infant exposure to marijuana metabolites are unknown, women should be informed of the potential risk of exposure during lactation and encouraged to abstain from using any marijuana products and avoid secondhand marijuana smoke exposure.

Prevention

As your child grows, keep in mind that you are a role model. If your child sees you smoking or using an electronic cigarette, vape product, or marijuana, they may want to try it as well.

Unintentional exposures to and poisonings from e-cigarette solutions containing nicotine have increased dramatically in the United States since 2011. The Child Nicotine Poisoning Prevention Act of 2015, which was enacted nationally in January 2016, requires containers of liquid nicotine to be in child-resistant packaging; nonetheless, the National Poison Data System continues to receive thousands of reports of exposure to e-cigarette liquid nicotine yearly. In addition, the lithium-ion batteries used in e-cigarettes have exploded, leading to burns and fires.

To reduce your child's exposure to environmental tobacco smoke, here are some additional steps you can take:

- If you or other family members smoke or use electronic cigarettes, stop! If you've been unable to stop, talk to your doctor. There are a number of medications available that can help you quit tobacco use. Contact 1-800-QUIT-NOW (1-800-784-8669) or smokefree.gov for free help to assist you in stopping smoking.
- Don't allow anyone to smoke or vape in your home or your car, particularly when children are present. It's important to know that harmful chemicals can be

brought into the house or car on the clothes of people who have smoked or vaped. Your home and car should always remain smoke-free.
- Store matches, lighters, e-cigarettes (including solution or other parts), and cigarettes out of reach of children.
- When selecting a babysitter or childcare provider, make it clear that no one is permitted to smoke or vape around your child. In addition, nobody should leave your child unattended to go outside to smoke or vape.
- When you're in public places with your child, ask others not to smoke or vape around you and your child.

CHAPTER 20

EYES

Your child relies on the visual information they gather to help them develop throughout infancy and childhood. If they have difficulty seeing properly, they may have problems in learning and relating to the world around them. For this reason, it is important to detect eye deficiencies as early as possible. Many vision problems can be corrected if treated early but become much more difficult to care for later.

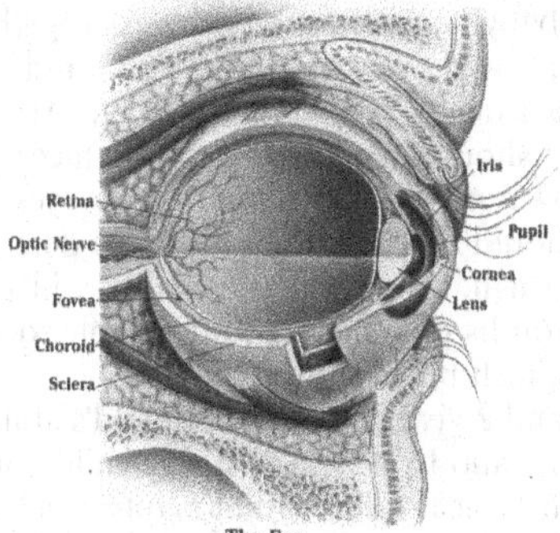

The Eye

Your infant should have their first eye examination at your first visit with your pediatrician. Routine vision checks then should be part of every visit to the pediatrician's office. If your family has a history of serious eye diseases or abnormalities, your pediatrician may refer your baby to an ophthalmologist (an eye specialist with a medical degree) for an early examination and follow-up visits if necessary.

If a child is born prematurely, they will be checked for a vision-threatening condition called retinopathy of prematurity (ROP), especially if they required oxygen over a prolonged period during their early days after birth. The risk is greater in premature infants with a birth weight of less than 3⅓ pounds (1,500 g). This condition may not be prevented even with ideal neonatal care, but in many cases, if detected early, it can be treated successfully. All neonatologists are aware of potential problems resulting from ROP and will let parents know about the necessity for evaluation by an ophthalmologist. Parents also should be told that all premature children are at greater risk for developing astigmatism, nearsightedness, and strabismus (these eye conditions are described later in this section) and that they therefore should be screened regularly throughout childhood.

How much does a newborn baby see? Even during the early weeks after birth, an infant can see light and shapes and can detect movement. Distance vision remains quite blurry, with the optimal viewing length being 8 to 12 inches (20.3 to 30.4 cm), which is roughly the distance from their eyes to yours as you are nursing or feeding your baby.

Until your baby learns to use both eyes together, their eyes may "wander," or move randomly. This random movement should be decreasing by 2 to 3 months of age. Around 3 months old, your baby should be able to focus on faces and close objects and follow a moving object with their eyes. By 4 months of age, they should be using their vision to detect various objects close to them, which they probably will reach for and grasp. By 6 months old, they should be able to visually identify and distinguish between objects.

Between 1 and 2 years of age, your child's ability to see will develop rapidly, and by ages 3 to 5, the child with normal vision will reach typical adult visual acuity levels. By the time your child is 10, their visual system will be fully mature. At this point, many early-onset eye and vision problems may no longer be able to be reversed or corrected. Therefore, early detection and treatment of eye problems in children is so important that your pediatrician will examine your baby's eyes at every routine physical examination.

Vision Screening Recommendations

Vision screening is a very important factor in identifying vision-threatening conditions. Regular eye checks during pediatric visits are done to determine if your baby's eyes are developing normally. The American Academy of Pediatrics recommends that children be screened at each well-child visit.

1. In the newborn nursery. Pediatricians should examine all infants prior to their discharge from the nursery to check for infections (*page 545*) and ocular defects, cataracts (*page 544*), and congenital glaucoma. If a problem is suspected, a pediatric ophthalmologist should see the newborn. All children with multiple medical problems or with a history of prematurity should be examined by an ophthalmologist.
2. By the age of 6 months. Pediatricians should screen infants to check for ocular alignment (eyes working together) and the presence of any eye disease.

Your pediatrician may use a newer method for screening vision, especially in younger children, called photoscreening, in which a specially designed camera is used to help detect potential abnormalities with your child's vision. These devices are an accepted method for screening infants and children, especially for those who are either too young or otherwise unable to have their vision reliably tested with a symbol or letter eye chart.

When to Call the Pediatrician

As noted above, vision screening is a very important factor in identifying vision-threatening conditions. These routine eye checks can detect hidden eye problems, but occasionally you may notice obvious signs that your child is having trouble seeing or that their eyes are not normal. Notify the pediatrician if your child shows any of the following warning signs:

- A white appearance of the pupil (a condition called leukocoria) in one or both eyes
- Persistent (lasting more than twenty-four hours) redness, swelling, crusting, or discharge in their eyes or eyelids
- Excessive tearing
- Sensitivity to light, especially a change in the child's light sensitivity
- Eyes that look crooked or crossed, or that don't move together
- Head consistently held in an abnormal or tilted position
- Frequent squinting

- Drooping of one or both eyelids
- Pupils of unequal size
- Continuous eye-rubbing
- Eyes that "bounce" or "dance"
- Inability to see objects unless they hold them close
- Eye injury (see *page 546*)
- Cloudy cornea

Depending on the symptoms your child displays, your pediatrician probably will check for vision difficulties and/or some of the other problems discussed in the remainder of this chapter.

Amblyopia

Amblyopia, or lazy eye, is a common eye problem (affecting about 2 out of 100 children) that develops when a child has one eye that doesn't see well and they use the other eye almost exclusively. In general, this problem must be detected as early as possible to treat and restore normal vision in the affected eye. If this situation persists for too long (past 7 to 10 years of age), vision is often lost permanently in the unused eye.

Once an ophthalmologist diagnoses the problems in the weaker eye, your child may need to wear a patch over the "good" eye for periods of time. This forces them to use and strengthen the eye that has become "lazy." Patching therapy will be continued for as long as necessary to bring the weaker eye up to its full potential and maintain it there. This could take weeks, months, or even a few years. As an alternative to the patch, the ophthalmologist might prescribe eye drops to blur the vision in the good eye, thereby stimulating your child to use the amblyopic eye.

Cataracts

Although we usually think of cataracts as affecting elderly people, they also may be found in infants and young children and are sometimes present at birth. A cataract is a clouding of the lens (the transparent tissue inside the eye that helps bring light rays into focus on the retina). While rare, congenital cataracts are nonetheless a leading cause of visual loss and blindness in children.

Cataracts in children need to be detected and treated early so their vision can develop more appropriately. A cataract usually shows up as a white discoloration in the center of the child's pupil. If a baby is born with a cataract that blocks most of the light entering the eye, the affected lens must be removed surgically to permit the baby's vision to develop. Most pediatric ophthalmologists recommend that this procedure be performed during the first month after birth. After the clouded lens is removed, the baby must be fitted with a special contact lens or with an eyeglass correction. At the age of about 2 years, the placement of a lens implant within the eye is recommended. In addition, visual rehabilitation of the affected eye will almost always involve use of a patch on the opposite eye until the child's eyes are fully mature (at about age 10 years).

Occasionally a child will be born with a small pinpoint cataract that will not initially impede visual development. These tiny cataracts often do not require treatment; however, they need to be monitored carefully to ensure that they do not become large enough to interfere with normal vision development.

In many cases, the cause of cataracts in infants cannot be determined. Cataracts may be attributed to a tendency inherited from parents; they may result from trauma to the eye; or they may occur because of viral infections such as German measles and chickenpox or an infection from other microorganisms, such as those that cause toxoplasmosis and Zika. To protect the unborn child from cataracts and from other serious disorders, pregnant women should take care to avoid unnecessary exposure to infectious diseases. In addition, as a precaution against toxoplasmosis (a disease caused by parasites), pregnant women should avoid handling cat litter or eating raw or improperly cooked meat, both of which may contain the organism that causes this disease.

Eye Infections

If the white of your child's eye and the inside of their lower lid become red, they probably have a condition called conjunctivitis. Also known as pinkeye, this inflammation, which can be painful and itchy, usually signals an infection, but may be due to other causes, such as irritation from smoke or fumes, an allergic reaction, or (rarely) a more serious condition. It's often accompanied by tearing and discharge, which is the body's way of trying to heal or remedy the situation.

If your child has a red eye, they need to see the pediatrician as soon as possible. Eye infections typically last seven to ten days. The doctor will make the diagnosis and prescribe necessary medication if it is indicated. Never put previously opened medication or someone else's eye medication into your child's eye. It could cause serious damage.

In a newborn baby, serious eye infections may result from exposure to bacteria or viruses during pregnancy or during passage through the birth canal—which is why all infants are treated with antibiotic eye ointment or drops in the delivery room. Such infections must be treated early to prevent serious complications. Eye infections that occur after the newborn period may be unsightly, because of the redness of the eye and the yellow discharge that usually accompany them, and they may make your child uncomfortable, but they are rarely serious. If your pediatrician feels the problem is caused by bacteria, antibiotic eye drops are the usual treatment. Viral causes of conjunctivitis do not respond to antibiotics, but antibiotic eye drops may still be used if a bacterial infection is suspected.

Eye infections can be very contagious. Except to administer drops or ointment, you should avoid direct contact with your child's eyes or drainage from them until the medication has been used for several days and there is evidence of clearing of the redness. Carefully wash your hands before and after touching the area around the infected eye. If your child is in a childcare or nursery school program, you should keep them home until the pinkeye is no longer contagious, usually twenty-four hours after starting drops and/or discharge and redness have disappeared. Your pediatrician will tell you when you can safely send them back to childcare or nursery school.

Eye Injuries

When dust or other small particles get in your child's eyes, the cleansing action of tears usually will wash them out. If that fails to occur, or if a serious injury affecting the eye takes place, call your pediatrician, or take your child to the nearest emergency department after heeding the following emergency guidelines.

PREVENTING EYE INJURIES

Nine out of ten eye injuries are preventable, and almost half occur around the home. To minimize the risk of such injuries in your family, follow these safety guidelines:

- Keep all chemicals out of reach and separate from medications. That includes detergents, ammonia, spray cans, superglue, and all other cleaning fluids.
- Choose your child's toys carefully. Newer toys must meet a standard that prevents any sharp or pointed parts, but if you have any vintage, antique, or other old toys, they should be kept out of sight and out of reach at least while your child is too young to understand their danger. Avoid letting your child walk or play with metal straws, pointy pencils, and other sharp or pointy items that could injure an eye.
- Keep your child away from darts, pellet guns, and BB guns.
- Keep your child away from power lawnmowers and trimmers, which can hurl stones or other objects.
- Don't let your child near you when you're lighting fires or using tools. If you want them to watch you hammer nails, make them wear protective goggles. You should wear goggles as well, for your own safety and to set a good example for your child.
- Tell your child not to look directly into the sun, even with sunglasses. Doing so can cause severe and permanent eye damage. Never allow a child to look directly at an eclipse of the sun or at a laser pointer.
- Never allow your child near fireworks of any kind. The American Academy of Pediatrics encourages children and their families to enjoy fireworks at public fireworks displays rather than purchasing fireworks for home use. In fact, the Academy would support a ban on public sales of all fireworks.

Black Eye

To reduce swelling, apply a cold pack wrapped in a towel to the area for ten to twenty minutes. Then consult the doctor to make sure there is no internal damage to the eye or the bones surrounding the eye.

Chemicals in the Eye

Flush the eye extensively with lots of water (a quart to a half gallon [1 to 2 liters]), making sure you get the water into the eye itself. Then take the child to the emergency department. (See also *page 516.*)

Cut

Minor cuts usually heal quickly and easily, but a deep cut requires emergency medical attention and probably will need stitches. (See Cuts and Scrapes, *page 497.*) Cuts on the border of the eyelids by the eyelashes, or near the tear duct openings, can be of special concern. If the cut is located in these areas, call your pediatrician right away for advice on how to handle the situation.

Large Particle in the Eye

If there's a particle in the eye that won't come out with tears or by flushing with water, or if your child is still complaining of pain after an hour, call your pediatrician. The doctor will remove the object or, if necessary, refer you to an ophthalmologist. Sometimes such particles cause scratches on the cornea (corneal abrasions), which are quite painful but heal rapidly with proper treatment. Corneal injuries also can be caused by blows or other injuries to the eye.

Eyelid Problems

Droopy eyelid (ptosis) may appear as a weak or heavy upper lid; if it is very slight, it may be noticed only because the affected eye appears somewhat smaller than the other eye. Ptosis usually involves only one eyelid, but both may be affected. Your baby may be born with ptosis, or it may develop later. Ptosis may be partial, causing your baby's eyes to appear slightly asymmetrical, or total, causing the affected lid to cover the eye completely. If the ptotic eyelid covers the entire pupillary opening of your child's eye, or if the weight of the lid causes the cornea to assume an irregular shape (astigmatism), it will threaten normal vision development and must be corrected as early as possible. If vision is not threatened, surgical intervention, if necessary, is usually delayed until the child is 4 or 5 years of age or older, when the eyelid and surrounding tissue are more fully developed and a better cosmetic result can be obtained.

Most birthmarks and growths involving the eyelids of the newborn or young child are benign; however, because they may increase in size during the first year, they sometimes cause parents to become concerned. Most of these birthmarks and growths are not serious and will not affect your child's vision. However, any irregularity should be brought to the attention of your child's pediatrician so that it can be evaluated and monitored.

Some children will develop lumps and bumps on their lids that can impair development of good eyesight. In particular, a blood vessel tumor called a capillary or strawberry hemangioma can start out as a small swelling and rapidly enlarge. It may enlarge over the first year after birth, and then start to shrink without any treatment over the next few years. If it becomes large enough, it can interfere with your baby's development of good vision in the affected eye and will need to be treated. Because of their potential to cause vision problems, any rapidly enlarging lumps or bumps around either eye should be evaluated by your pediatrician and perhaps an ophthalmologist as well.

A child might also be born with a flat, purple-colored lesion on their face called a port-wine stain, because of its resemblance to a dark red wine. If this birthmark involves the eye, especially the upper lid, the child may be at risk for development of glaucoma (a condition where pressure increases inside the eyeball) or amblyopia (weak vision). Any child born with this birthmark needs to be examined by an ophthalmologist shortly after birth.

Small dark moles, called nevi, on the eyelids or on the white part of the eye itself rarely cause any problems or need to be removed. Once they have been evaluated by your pediatrician, these marks should cause concern only if they change in size, shape, or color.

Small, firm, flesh-colored bulges underneath your child's eyebrows are usually dermoid cysts. These cysts are noncancerous tumors that usually are present from birth. Because they tend to increase in size during early childhood, their removal is preferred in most cases before they rupture under the skin and cause inflammation.

Two other eyelid problems—chalazae and hordeola (styes)—are common but not serious. A chalazion is a cyst resulting from a blockage of an oil gland. A hordeolum, or stye, is a bacterial infection of the cells surrounding the sweat glands or hair follicles on the edge of the lid. Call your pediatrician regarding treatment of these conditions. They probably will tell you to apply warm compresses directly to the eyelid for twenty or thirty minutes three or four times a day until the chalazion or stye clears. The doctor may want to examine your child before prescribing additional treatment, such as an antibiotic ointment or drops.

Once your child has had a stye or chalazion, they may be more likely to get them again. When they occur repeatedly, it's sometimes necessary to perform lid scrubs to reduce the bacterial colonization of the eyelids and open the glands and pores in the eyelids.

Impetigo is a very contagious bacterial infection that may occur on the eyelid. Your pediatrician will advise you on how to remove the crust from the lid and will prescribe an antibiotic eye ointment and oral antibiotics. (See Impetigo, *page 656*.)

Strabismus

Strabismus is a misalignment of the eyes caused by an imbalance in the muscles controlling the eye. This condition makes it impossible for the eyes to focus on the same point at the same time. Strabismus occurs in about 4 out of 100 children. It may be present at birth (infantile strabismus), or it may develop later in childhood (acquired strabismus). Strabismus can develop if your child has another visual impairment, sustains an eye injury, or develops cataracts. Always report the sudden onset of strabismus to your pediatrician immediately. Although very rare, it may indicate the development of a tumor or other serious nervous system problem. In all cases, it is important to diagnose and treat strabismus as early in your child's life as possible. If a turned eye is not treated early, the child may never develop the ability to use both eyes together (binocular vision), and if both eyes are not used together, it is common for one to become "lazy," or amblyopic (see *page 544*). Amblyopia often coexists with strabismus and must be treated separately with patching or the use of eye drops in the opposite eye.

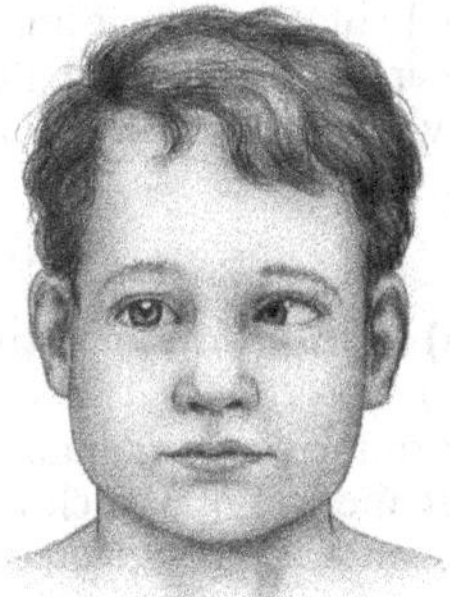

Left eye turning inward

It is important to note that a newborn baby's eyes commonly and normally wander. Within a few weeks, babies learn to move their eyes together, and strabismus should disappear within a few months. However, if this intermittent wandering continues, or if your baby's eyes don't turn in the same direction (if one turns in, out, up, or down), the baby needs to be evaluated by your pediatrician, and often a pediatric ophthalmologist as well.

If your child is born with strabismus and it does not resolve on its own in a few months, it's important for their eyes to be realigned as soon as possible so they can focus them together on a single object. Eye exercises alone cannot accomplish this, so the treatment usually involves eyeglasses or surgery. If your child needs an operation, this surgery is frequently done between 6 and 18 months of age. The operation is usually safe and effective, although it's not uncommon for a child to need more than one procedure. Even after surgery, your child still may need glasses.

Some children look as if they have strabismus because of the way their faces are structured, but in fact their eyes may be well aligned. These children often have a flat nasal bridge and broad skin folds alongside the nose (epicanthus), which can distort the appearance of the eyes, making these children appear cross-eyed when they really aren't. This condition is called pseudostrabismus. The child's vision is not affected, and, in most cases, as the child grows and the nasal bridge becomes more prominent, the child loses the appearance of crossed eyes.

Because of the importance of early diagnosis and treatment of a true misalignment (or true strabismus), if you have any suspicion that your baby's eyes may not be perfectly aligned and working together, you should bring it to the attention of your pediatrician, who can best determine whether your baby has an actual problem.

Tear (or Lacrimal) Production Problems

Tears play an important role in maintaining good eyesight by keeping the eyes wet and free of particles, dust, and other substances that might cause injury or interfere with normal vision. The lacrimal system maintains the continuous production and circulation of tears, and depends on regular blinking to propel tears from the lacrimal gland across the surface of the eye, finally draining through the tear ducts and into the nose.

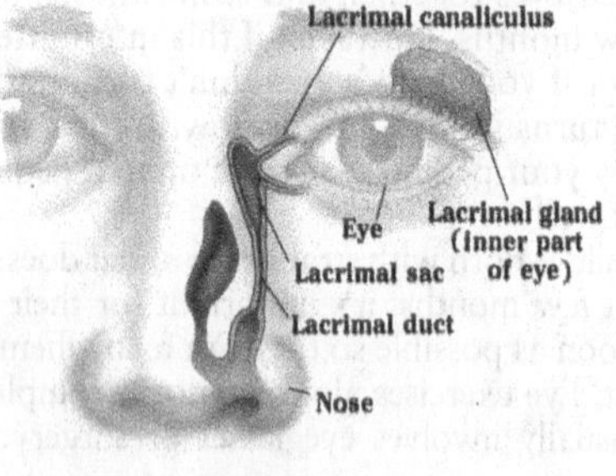

This lacrimal system develops gradually over the first three or four years. Thus, while a newborn will produce enough tears to coat the surface of the eyes, it may be several months after birth before they cry real tears.

Blocked tear ducts, which are very common among newborns and young babies, can cause the appearance of excessive tearing in one or both eyes, because the tears run down the cheek instead of draining through the duct and into the nose. In newborns, blocked tear ducts usually occur when an internal membrane covering them fails to disappear around birth. Your pediatrician will demonstrate how to massage the tear duct. They'll also show you how to clean the eye with moist compresses to remove all secretions and crusting. Until the tear duct finally opens, the sticky mucous discharge may not go away. Since this is not typically a true infection or pinkeye, antibiotics are usually not necessary or helpful.

Sometimes a persistent membrane (or even a small cyst) can cause a blocked tear duct that does not resolve on its own or with massaging. When this occurs and the methods described above are unsuccessful, the ophthalmologist may decide to probe open the blocked tear duct surgically. Rarely, this procedure must be repeated more than once.

Vision Difficulties Requiring Corrective Lenses

Astigmatism

Astigmatism is an uneven curvature of the surface of the cornea and/or lens. If your child has an astigmatism, vision both near and far may be blurred. Astigmatism can be corrected with either glasses or contact lenses, and, like farsightedness, may cause amblyopia if one eye is affected more than the other.

Farsightedness

This is a condition in which the eyeball is shorter than ideal to allow for best focusing, causing difficulty focusing on near objects. Most infants are born farsighted but can compensate for small amounts of it on their own. As they grow, their eyeballs get longer and the farsightedness diminishes. Glasses or contact lenses rarely are needed unless the condition is excessive. If your child has eye discomfort or frequent mild headaches related to prolonged reading, they may be suffering from a severe degree of farsightedness and should be examined by your pediatrician or pediatric ophthalmologist. Excessive farsightedness also may lead to crossed eyes (see Strabismus, *page 550*) and amblyopia (see *page 544*), both of which require treatment in addition to glasses.

Nearsightedness

The inability to see distant objects clearly is the most common visual problem in young children. This inherited trait occasionally is found in newborns, especially premature infants, but it more often develops after 6 to 9 years of age.

Contrary to popular belief, reading too much, reading in dim light, or poor nutrition cannot cause or affect nearsightedness. That said, recent research shows that increasing the amount of time a child spends outdoors can reduce the risk of developing myopia and/or slow its progression. Usually, nearsightedness is the result of an eyeball that is longer in shape, causing the image to be focused improperly. Less frequently, it is due to a change in the shape of the cornea or lens.

The treatment for nearsightedness is corrective lenses—either eyeglasses or contact lenses. Keep in mind that when your child grows, so do their eyes, so they may need new lenses as often as every six to twelve months. Nearsightedness usually changes rapidly for several years and then stabilizes during or after adolescence.

CHAPTER 21

FAMILY ISSUES

Adoption

If you are about to adopt or have just adopted a child, you are likely experiencing a mix of emotions. Along with excitement and delight, you also may feel some anxiety and apprehension. These are emotions common to all parents, regardless of whether a child joins their family by birth or by adoption. Choosing an understanding, supportive, and collaborative pediatrician will be helpful as you begin your new job as a parent. Even before a child joins your family, a pediatrician can discuss with you your feelings about impending parenthood. Whether you are adopting a child internationally or domestically, a pediatrician will also be able to address any medical issues that may arise.

Once your child is home with you, schedule a visit to a pediatrician as soon as possible. Similar to an initial newborn exam, this initial post-adoptive visit can provide an opportunity to ask any questions you have about your child's physical and mental health and development. Schedule future exams as required by the child's age and medical needs. Many families find that they benefit from additional visits with their pediatrician during the first year or so to help address concerns that may arise as parents and child start to develop a relationship.

In addition to the typical challenges of parenting, adoptive parents also face several issues and questions that non-adoptive parents do not.

Where We Stand

Increasing numbers of children have been adopted by gay or lesbian individuals or couples in recent years. In some states this has stimulated political debate and public policy change. A strong and growing body of scientific literature reveals that children who grow up with one or two gay or lesbian parents will develop emotionally, cognitively, socially, and sexually just as well as children whose parents are heterosexual. Parents' sexual orientation is much less important than having loving and nurturing parents.

The American Academy of Pediatrics recognizes the diversity of families. We believe that children who are born to, or adopted by, one member of a gay or lesbian couple deserve the security of two legally recognized parents. Therefore, we support statutory and legal means to enable children to be adopted by the second parent or co-parent in families headed by gay and lesbian couples. The AAP supports the principle that gender identity and sexual orientation should not affect an individual's right to adopt or foster a child.

Child Abuse and Neglect

Child abuse, also known as child maltreatment (a term that encompasses both abuse and neglect), is common. Child maltreatment is defined as "behavior toward a child that is outside the norms of conduct and entails a substantial risk of causing physical or emotional harm." The types of child maltreatment generally recognized are physical abuse, sexual abuse, and neglect, including emotional maltreatment. It is important to understand and reduce the risks of abuse for your child and familiarize yourself with the signs of abuse. Recent statistics show that there are about 4 million reports of suspected child maltreatment, involving almost 7 million children, per year. The highest rate of child abuse is in babies less than 1 year of age, and 25 percent of victims are less than 3. There is considerable overlap among children who are abused, with many suffering a combination of physical abuse, sexual abuse, and/or neglect. Most cases reported to child protection agencies involve neglect, followed by physical and sexual abuse.

According to the nonprofit organization Prevent Child Abuse America, "Child neglect occurs when children's basic needs are not adequately met, resulting in actual or potential harm. Basic needs include adequate food, clothing, education, health care, nurturing and emotional support, and housing." Child neglect can include physical neglect (failing to provide food, clothing, shelter, or other physical necessities); emotional neglect (failing to provide love, comfort, or affection); medical neglect (failing to provide needed medical care); educational neglect (failing to give access to education); or supervisory neglect (failing to appropriately supervise). Psychological or emotional abuse results from all the above but also can be associated with verbal abuse, which can harm a child's self-worth or emotional well-being.

Physical abuse occurs when a child's body is injured because of hitting, kicking, shaking, burning, or other show of force. One study suggests that about one in twenty children has been physically abused in their lifetime. Sexual abuse is any sexual activity that a child cannot comprehend or give consent to. It includes acts such as fondling, oral-genital contact, genital and anal intercourse, exhibitionism, voyeurism, and exposure to pornography. Studies have suggested that up to one in five girls and one in twenty boys have been sexually abused before the age of 18. More than 90 percent of child sexual abuse victims know their abuser, and most of the abuse occurs within the family, which may make it difficult for a child to disclose the abuse. Teach your child that it is not okay for adults to touch them if they do not want them to or if it makes them feel uncomfortable, and teach them to always tell a trusted grown-up if something like that happens.

Child maltreatment is more likely in households where parents are depressed or have other mental health issues or untreated substance use disorder or who themselves are victims of intergenerational trauma, neglect, or domestic violence. Parents who do not have the social supports or the modeling of strong parenting behaviors may not be attuned to their children's needs and may struggle to develop attentive parenting behaviors. Such situations reduce parents' abilities to be strong caregivers.

Signs and Symptoms

It is not always easy to recognize when a child has been abused. Children who have been maltreated are often afraid to tell anyone, fearing they will be blamed or that no one will believe them. Sometimes they remain quiet because the person who abused them is someone they love very much, or because of fear, or both. Some children simply don't understand that what has happened to them is wrong. Children who have not learned the correct terms for private body parts may lack the language to describe what happened.

Parents may overlook signs and symptoms of abuse because it is hard to believe it could happen or they are fearful of repercussions. A child who has been abused needs special support and treatment as early as possible. The longer children continue to be abused or are left to deal with the situation on their own, the harder it is for them to be able to heal and develop optimally physically and mentally.

Parents should always be alert to any unexplainable changes in the child's body or behavior. While physical abuse may cause certain physical injuries, acute and chronic stressful situations including child abuse and neglect may result in a child being anxious and fretful. There are no behaviors that specifically relate to a particular type of child abuse or neglect. Here is a short list of physical signs that may indicate a child has experienced abuse or neglect:

- Non-mobile infant with any injury
- Bruises to the torso, ears, or neck in a child less than 4 years of age
- Any injury (bruise, burn, fracture, or abdominal, chest, or head injury) that is not consistent with the way the injury is said to have happened, that cannot be adequately explained, or that is inconsistent with the child's developmental capabilities
- The child discloses abuse or neglect
- Failure to gain weight (especially in infants) or sudden dramatic weight gain
- Genital pain, bleeding, or discharge
- A sexually transmitted infection and/or disease

Getting Help

If you suspect your child has been abused, get help immediately through your pediatrician, a school social worker, or the local child protection agency. Physicians are legally obligated to report all suspected cases of abuse or neglect to state authorities. Your pediatrician will also examine your child to detect and treat any medical injuries or conditions, recommend a therapist, and provide necessary information to investigators. The doctor also may testify in court if necessary to obtain legal protection for the child or criminal prosecution of the person suspected of perpetrating the abuse or neglect.

If they have been abused, your child will benefit from services including mental health professionals, speech and other therapists, and/or a developmental or behavioral pediatrician depending on the child and situation. You and other members of the family may be advised to seek counseling so that you'll be able to provide the support and comfort your child needs. If someone in your family is responsible for the abuse, a mental health professional may be able to help that person as well.

If your child has been abused, you may be the only person who can help them get the help that they need. Many times this is a complicated process due to multiple family dynamics, especially if the abuser is still emotionally or financially involved with the family. Discuss the situation with a professional, such as your pediatrician, teacher, school social worker, or religious leader, who can then assist and support you through this process. Failure to report can also make it appear you are failing to protect your child and decreases your child's chance for optimal physical and mental health. In any case of abuse or neglect, the child's safety is of primary concern. They need to be in a safe environment free of the potential for continuing abuse and neglect.

Preventing Abuse and Neglect

The major reasons for physical and psychological maltreatment of children within the family are parental feelings of isolation, stress, and frustration. Parents need support and as much information as possible to raise their children responsibly. They need to learn how to cope with their own feelings of frustration and anger without venting them on children. They also need the companionship of other adults who will listen and help during times of crisis. Support groups through local community organizations often are helpful first steps to diminish some of the isolation or frustration parents may be feeling.

If you are worried about your health or how everyday stressors may be affecting the relationship with your child, talk with your primary care physician. They can assess your health and either connect you with community resources or treat/refer you to a physician who can provide you with the necessary healthcare.

Parents who were themselves abused as children are in particular need of support. Confronting, addressing, and healing parental mental and emotional health takes uncommon courage and insight, but this is often the best way to reduce the chances that past abuse will be passed on to the next generation of children.

Personal supervision of and involvement in your child's activities are the best ways to prevent physical and sexual abuse outside the home. Any school or childcare program you select for your child should allow unrestricted and unannounced parental visits without prearrangement. Parents should be allowed to help in the classroom on a volunteer basis and be informed about the selection of or changes in staff members. Parents should pay careful attention to their child's reports about and reactions to their experiences at childcare and school. Always investigate if your child tells you they've been maltreated or if they undergo a sudden unexplained change in behavior.

Separation and Divorce

Every year more than 1 million children in the United States are involved in a parental divorce or separation. Even those children who lived with parental conflict and unhappiness for a long time may find the changes that follow separation and divorce more difficult than anything they have experienced before. At the very least, the child must adjust to living apart from one parent or, if in shared custody, to dividing their life between two homes. Because of financial changes, they also may have to move to a different home and a different neighborhood. A parent who stayed at home before now may have to go to work. Even if the parent doesn't have to go to work, the stress and depression that often accompany divorce may make some parents less attentive to and loving with their children.

No one can predict specifically how separation or divorce will affect your child. A child's response will depend on their own sensitivity, the quality of their relationship with each of their parents, and the parents' ability to work together to meet their child's emotional needs during this time. It also will depend to some extent on their child's age and on the resiliency or vulnerability that their child's previous life experiences have given the child.

Some children have serious and lasting psychological aftereffects from a separation or divorce, but many others do well once the initial impact has been experienced and coped with and the child and other family members have learned how to successfully adapt and support each other with their new life circumstances.

How Parents Can Help the Child

If your child is younger than 2 years, you can't get messages across very well with words. You will have to convey them through your actions. When you are with your child, try to put your own issues and worries aside and concentrate on their needs. Keep the daily routine as consistent as possible, and do not expect them to make any other major changes (e.g., toilet training, moving from a crib to a bed, or, if avoidable, adjusting to a new care provider or home arrangement) during this transitional period. In the beginning, try to be understanding and patient if your child's behavior regresses, but if this regression continues even after the separation or divorce is completed and your life has settled back into a regular routine, ask your pediatrician for advice.

(See also Single-Parent Families, *page 564*; Stepfamilies, *page 567*.)

Sibling Rivalry

If you have more than one child, you almost certainly will have to deal with some amount of sibling rivalry. Competition between children in a family is natural. All children want parental affection and attention, and each child believes they should receive all of yours. Your child does not want to share you with their sibling, and when they realize they have no choice in the matter, they may become jealous, possibly even violent, toward their sibling.

Sibling rivalry between younger children tends to be most troublesome when the age difference is from one and a half to three years. This is because the preschool child is still very dependent on their parents and has not yet established many secure relationships with friends or other adults. However, even when the spread is as much as nine years or more, the older child still needs parental attention and affection. If they feel they are being left out or rejected, they likely will blame the baby. In general, the older the child, the less jealousy they will feel toward their younger sibling. The jealousy is often most intense for preschoolers when the sibling is a newborn.

What to Expect

You may notice the first signs of sibling rivalry even before your younger child is born. As the older one watches you preparing the nursery or buying baby equipment, they may demand gifts for themselves. They may want to wear diapers again or drink from a bottle "like the baby." If they sense that you're preoccupied with the baby, they may misbehave or act out to get your attention.

This unusual or regressive behavior may continue after the baby is home. Your older child may cry more frequently, become increasingly clingy and demanding, or simply withdraw. They may imitate the baby by asking for their old baby blanket, sucking on a pacifier, or even demanding to nurse. School-age children often appear very interested in and affectionate toward the baby but may be aggressive or misbehave in other ways to get attention. Among all siblings, the demand for attention is usually greatest when the parents are actively and intimately involved with the baby—for example, during breastfeeding or bath time.

As your younger child gets older and becomes more mobile, quarrels will erupt over the older child's toys and other possessions. The toddler will go straight for what they want, without caring who owns it, while your preschooler will guard their own territory jealously. When the toddler intrudes on this space, the older child usually reacts strongly.

How Should Parents React?

It is important not to overreact to jealousy between your children, especially if the older child is a preschooler. Feelings of resentment and frustration are understandable—no child wants to give up the spotlight of parental affection. It takes time for a child to discover that their parents don't love them any less because they have a second child.

If your older child starts imitating the baby, do not ridicule or punish them. You can indulge them briefly by allowing them to drink from a bottle or climb into the crib or play yard, but only once or twice at the most, and don't reward this behavior by giving them extra attention. Make it clear that they do not have to behave like a baby to gain your approval, love, or affection. Praise them when they act "grown-up," and give them plenty of opportunities to be a "big brother" (or "big sister" or "big kid"). If you intentionally try to catch them displaying desired behaviors, it should not take long for them to realize that they benefit more by acting maturely than by behaving like a baby.

If your older child is between 3 and 5 years old, try to minimize conflicts over space by guaranteeing some secure, protected area. Separating their private possessions from shared ones will help reduce arguments. It is natural for parents to compare their children, but do not do this in front of them. Each child is special and should be treated as such. Comparisons inevitably make one child feel inferior to the other. A statement such as "Your sister is always so much neater than you," for example, will make a child resent both you and their sister, and actually may encourage them to be messy.

When your children get into an argument, usually the best strategy is to stay out of it. Left alone, they probably will settle it peacefully. If you get involved, you may be tempted to take sides, making one child feel triumphant and the other betrayed. Even if they bring their fight to you, try to be impartial and tell them to settle it peacefully on their own. Instead of blaming either one, explain that they're both responsible for creating the dispute and for ending it. Doing so encourages them to problem-solve together, a social skill that will serve them well in the future.

Obviously, you must intervene if the situation becomes violent, especially if the older child might harm the younger one.

In this case you must first protect the younger child. Make sure the older child understands that you will not tolerate any abusive behavior. If the age difference is large or if there is any reason to suspect that violence may erupt, supervise them closely when they are together. Preventing aggressive behavior is always better than punishment, which all too often increases rather than decreases the older child's feelings of rivalry.

It is important to spend time separately with each child. Even as little as ten to fifteen minutes daily of one-on-one time without electronics, doing an activity your child chooses, often makes a huge difference. Finding the right balance of attention is not always easy, but if your older child's acting out is becoming extreme, it could be a signal that they need more of your time. If the older sibling remains extremely aggressive, or if you feel that you don't know how to handle the situation, consult your pediatrician, who can determine whether this is normal sibling rivalry or a problem that requires special attention. The pediatrician also can suggest ways to ease the tensions. If necessary, they will refer you to a qualified mental health professional.

Single-Parent Families

Single-parent families are becoming more common. Most children of separation and divorce spend at least some years in single-parent households. Another increasingly large group of children live with single parents who were never married or involved in a long-term relationship. A smaller number of children have widowed parents.

From a parent's viewpoint, there are some benefits to being single. You can raise your child according to your own beliefs, principles, and rules, with no need for conflict or resolving differences. Single parents often develop closer bonds with their children. When a father is the single parent, he may become more nurturing and more active in his child's daily life than some fathers in two-parent households. Children in single-parent households may become more independent and mature because they have more responsibility within the family.

Single parenthood is not easy, for parents or for children. If you can't arrange or afford childcare, finding and holding a job may be difficult. (See *Chapter 10*, Childcare.) Without another person to share the day-in, day-out job of raising the child and maintaining the household, you may find yourself so busy that you become socially isolated. When you are under stress, the child may sense and share this stress. You can easily become too tired and distracted to be as emotionally supportive or consistent about rules and discipline as you would like to be. This can lead to distress and behavior problems for the child. Some single parents worry that the lack of a same-sex parent may deprive their child of a potential role model.

PARENTING IN MILITARY FAMILIES

Being a parent in the military can present unique challenges, particularly in times of deployment or military conflict, when the stresses of being away from a child can be difficult for the entire family. Young children may demonstrate a number of behaviors in response to being separated from a parent, such as clinginess to the other parent and/or a caregiver, regressive behaviors (e.g., bed-wetting after having been toilet trained), anxiety over new people or circumstances, and being quiet and pulling away from others.

If you're the parent remaining at home with your child, try to keep things as normal as possible, including maintaining usual daily routines. Answer questions as honestly as possible (keeping in mind their level of understanding) and reassure them that the deployed parent is fine and doing well. Try to maintain as much communication as possible with the absent parent, letting your child communicate by phone, letter, email, or videoconferencing. If your child seems to be in particular distress, talk with your pediatrician, who might make a referral to a mental health professional. Also, there is a website for all military spouses to access mental health services, regardless of location, at MilitaryOneSource.mil.

The AAP's Deployment and Military Medical Home Resources webpage has been designed to support youth in military families, other family members, and the professionals caring for this population. Please spend some time on the site to learn more about what military pediatricians and other youth-serving professionals are doing to help these children and adolescents every day: aap.org/en/patient-care/military-families-and-deployment/.

Here are some suggestions that may help you meet your own emotional needs while providing your child with the guidance they need:

- Take advantage of all available resources in finding help in caring for your child. Use the guide to childcare in *Chapter 10*.
- Maintain your sense of humor as much as possible. Try to see the positive or funny side of everyday surprises and challenges.
- For your family's sake as well as your own, take care of yourself. See your doctor regularly, eat properly, and get enough rest, exercise, and sleep.
- Set a regular time when you can take a break without your child. Relax with friends. Go to a movie. Pursue hobbies. Join groups. Do things that interest you. Pursue a social life of your own.
- Do not feel guilty because your child has only one parent. There are plenty of families in the same situation. You didn't "do it to them," and you don't need to penalize yourself or spoil them to make amends.
- Do not look for problems where none exist. Many children grow up very well in single-parent homes, while others have problems in two-parent homes. Being a single parent does not necessarily mean you'll have more problems or have more trouble resolving them.
- Set firm but reasonable limits for your children, and do not hesitate to enforce them. Children feel more secure and develop responsible behavior better when limits are clear and consistent. Expand these limits as the child demonstrates the ability to accept increased responsibility.
- Find some time each day to spend with your child—playing, talking, reading, helping with homework, or watching television.
- Praise your child often, showing genuine affection and unconditional, positive support.
- Create as large a support network for yourself as possible. Keep active lists of relatives, friends, and community services that can help with childcare. Establish friendships with other families who will let you know of community opportunities (sports leagues,

cultural events, etc.) and are willing to exchange babysitting.

- Talk to trusted relatives, friends, and professionals such as your pediatrician about your child's behavior, development, and relationships within the family.

Stepfamilies

A single parent's remarriage or new partnership can be a blessing for the parent and child alike, restoring the structure and security that were lost through divorce, separation, or death. Benefits may include additional love and companionship for a parent as well as the children. Often a stepparent becomes another adult role model and may take on some responsibilities of the former spouse or partner. In addition, there may be financial benefits from having another caregiver in the house.

In an atmosphere of mutual respect between biological parents and stepparents, the child is more likely to have the benefits of stepfamilies mentioned in the preceding paragraph. The child again has the opportunity of living in a household with two parents. The remarried parent often is happier and thus better able to meet the child's needs. As the child gets older, their relationship to the stepparent may give them additional support, skills, and perspectives. These benefits, together with the economic advantages of the stepfamily situation, may give the child a broader range of opportunities.

Twins and Other Multiples

Having twins (or other multiples, such as triplets) means much more than simply having two or more babies at once, and the challenges go beyond having twice or three times the work or pleasure. Twins and other multiples quite frequently are born earlier than single-born babies and so tend to be smaller than the average newborn; you may need to consult your pediatrician more frequently than you would with a single baby. It is possible that after birth your multiples may need extra time in the hospital's neonatal intensive care unit (NICU). Feeding twins and other multiples, whether by breast or bottle, also requires some special strategies, and the pediatrician and lactation consultant can provide advice and support. There may be added financial pressures on the family as well, requiring more diapers, clothing, food, car safety seats, and dozens of other items—and perhaps needing a larger family car or even a larger home.

Some researchers have attributed much of an increase in multiple births to the more frequent use of infertility treatments and procedures such as in vitro fertilization. In vitro fertilization may involve implanting more than one fertilized egg into the uterus, while using infertility drugs can stimulate the ovaries to release two or more eggs.

This section is written primarily with twins in mind, but most of the same information and guidelines apply to triplets and higher-order multiple births. (For more information on multiples, check out *Raising Twins: Parenting Multiples from Pregnancy Through the School Years*, 3rd edition, by Shelly Vaziri Flais [Chicago: American Academy of Pediatrics, 2019].)

Raising Multiples

You should care for your healthy multiples just like any other infants. From the very beginning, it is important that you recognize that your babies are separate individuals. If they are identical, it is easy to treat them as a "package," providing them with the same clothing, toys, and quality of attention. But as similar as they may appear physically, emotionally, behaviorally, and developmentally, they are two different people, and in order to grow up happy and secure as individuals, they need you to support their differences. As one twin explained, "We're not twins. We're just brothers who have the same birthday!"

Identical twins come from the same egg, are always the same sex, and look very much alike. Fraternal twins come from two separate eggs that are fertilized at the same time. They may or may not be the same sex. Whether identical or fraternal, all twins have their individual personalities, styles, and temperaments. Both identical and fraternal twins may become either competitive or interdependent as they grow. Sometimes one twin acts as the leader and the other as the follower. Whatever the specific quality of their interaction, most twins develop a very intense relationship early in life simply because they spend so much time with each other.

If you also have other children, your twin newborns may prompt more than the usual sibling rivalry. They will require a large amount of your time and energy and will attract a great deal of extra attention from friends, relatives, and strangers on the street. You can help your other children accept, and perhaps even take advantage of, this unusual situation by offering them "double rewards" for helping with the new babies and encouraging even more involvement in the daily baby care chores. It also becomes even more essential that you spend some special time each day alone with your other children, reading books or doing their favorite activities.

You may find that your twins do not develop in the same pattern as do other children their age. Some twins seem to "split the work," with one concentrating on motor skills while the other advances in social or communication abilities. Because they spend so much time together, many twins communicate better with each other than with other family members or friends. They learn how to read each other's gestures and facial expressions, and occasionally they even have their own verbal language that no one else can understand—this is particularly true of identical twins. This unique developmental pattern does not represent a problem, but it does make it very important to separate your twins on a regular basis and expose them individually to other playmates and learning situations.

Twins are not always happy about being apart, especially if they have established strong play habits and preferences for each other's company. For this reason, it is important to begin separating them occasionally as early as possible. If they resist strongly, try a gradual approach, using very familiar children or adults to play with them individually but in the same room or play area. Being able to separate will become increasingly important as the twins approach school age. In preschool most twins can stay together in the same room, but many elementary schools prefer twins to be in separate classes.

As much as you appreciate the individual differences between your twins, you no doubt will have certain feelings for them as a unit. There is nothing wrong with this, since they do share many similarities and are themselves bound to develop a dual identity—as individuals and as twins. Helping them understand and accept the balance between these two identities is one of the most challenging tasks facing you as the parent of twins.

TRANSPORTING YOUR NEWBORN MULTIPLES

In many cases, infant twins and higher-order multiples are smaller and weigh less than the average newborn. When bringing your babies home from the hospital and for subsequent trips in the car, keep the same guidelines in mind for choosing and using car safety seats. That means choosing rear-facing car safety seats and relying on them until your babies have outgrown the rear-facing weight or height limit for their seats, which will likely be well past the second birthday. Rear-facing-only seats have carrying handles and may be sold with a base that can stay in your car. Convertible seats are larger than rear-facing-only seats and can be used both rear-facing and forward-facing, so some parents choose to use a convertible seat from birth.

But here's a very important point to keep in mind if your babies were born prematurely: Rear-facing convertible car seats may be too large to fit your preemies appropriately. Before your newborns are discharged from the hospital, make sure they are tested to determine if they can ride safely while reclining in a car safety seat. The hospital calls this the "car seat test." If they have certain medical issues related to breathing or heart rate, they may not be able to ride in a semi-reclined position. In these instances, preemies should lie flat when they're riding in a car, and you will need a crash-tested car bed. (In most cases, the car bed will be purchased through the hospital, and your babies should be tested in the car beds before being sent home.) Always use the harnesses and buckle that are part of the car beds, and install the beds lengthwise in the backseat; position your babies so their heads are toward the center of the car. After they've had additional time to grow bigger and stronger, your babies should be tested again in their car safety seats to make sure they are ready to make the switch to a regular semi-reclined rear-facing seat.

Your pediatrician can advise you on how to cope with the special parenting challenges with twins. They also can suggest helpful reading material or refer you to organizations that help parents with multiples. It is enormously helpful to connect with other families who are experiencing similar challenges to yours. One organization to look for in your area may be Multiples of America, which has local chapters nationally.

At the same time, take care of yourself, and get as much rest as possible. Many parents find that raising twins and other multiples is much more physically demanding and emotionally stressful than having just one baby. So make an effort to catch up on your own sleep whenever you can. If you have a partner, take turns with who's going to handle the middle-of-the-night feedings and who will bathe and feed the babies. Consider having one parent take the "early shift" of nighttime feeds and a second caregiver take the "late shift," affording you both a longer stretch of sleep. If your budget can afford it, get some extra help for routine tasks like bathing the newborns and grocery shopping—or ask friends and family members for assistance. An extra set of hands, especially when there are more than twins, even for just a few hours a week, can make an enormous difference, and can give you not only more time to enjoy your babies, but also more time for yourself.

CHAPTER 22

FEVER

Your child's normal temperature will vary with age, activity, and the time of day. Infants tend to have higher temperatures than older children, and everyone's temperature is highest between late afternoon and early evening and lowest between midnight and early morning. Ordinarily, a rectal reading of 100.4 degrees Fahrenheit (38 degrees Celsius) and higher indicates fever. When other sites are used for temperature taking, such as oral (mouth), tympanic (ear), and temporal artery (side of forehead), you should still generally use 100.4 degrees or more as the cutoff for a true fever, while axillary (underarm) measurements may have a lower cutoff. A rectal reading is the gold standard for infants, especially those under 3 months of age. Whenever you think your child has a fever, take their temperature with a thermometer. (See Best Ways to Take a Temperature on *page 574*.) Feeling the skin (or using temperature-sensitive tape, also referred to as "fever strips") is not accurate, especially when the child is experiencing a chill.

By itself, fever is not an illness. Rather, it is a sign or symptom of sickness. In fact, usually it is a positive sign that the body is fighting infection. Fever stimulates certain defenses, such as the white blood cells, which attack and destroy invading bacteria and viruses. The fever may be important in helping your child fight the infection. However, fever is often associated with discomfort. It increases their need for fluids and makes their heart rate and breathing rate faster.

Fever may accompany any infection. This includes respiratory illnesses such as croup or pneumonia, ear infections, influenza (flu), colds, and sore throats. Fever may occur with infections of the bowel, blood, urinary tract, or brain and spinal cord (meningitis), and with most viral illnesses.

In children between 6 months and 5 years, fever can rarely trigger seizures (febrile seizures are also called febrile convulsions). These febrile seizures tend to run in families and usually happen during the first few hours of a febrile illness. Children may look "peculiar" for a few moments, then stiffen, twitch, and roll their eyes. They will be unresponsive for a short time, and their skin may appear to be a little darker than usual during the episode. The entire febrile seizure usually lasts less than one minute, and may be over in a few seconds, but it can seem like a lifetime to a frightened parent. Although it is uncommon, a febrile seizure can last for up to fifteen minutes. It is reassuring to know that febrile seizures almost always are harmless—they do not cause brain damage, nervous system problems, paralysis, intellectual disability, or death—although they should be reported promptly to your pediatrician. If your child is having trouble breathing or the febrile seizure does not stop within fifteen minutes, call 911.

Children younger than 1 year old at the time of their first simple febrile seizure have approximately a 50 percent chance of having another such febrile seizure, while children over 1 year of age when they have their first febrile seizure have about a 30 percent chance of having a second one. Nevertheless, febrile seizures rarely happen more than once within a twenty-four-hour period. Although many parents worry that a febrile seizure will lead to epilepsy, keep in mind that epileptic seizures are not caused by a fever, and children with a history of fever-related seizures have only a slightly higher likelihood of developing epilepsy by age 7. Ironically, working extra hard to control fevers does not prevent future febrile seizures, so do not go to extremes trying to keep a child's temperature down just because they had a febrile seizure in the past.

Treating a Febrile Seizure (Convulsion)

If your child has a febrile seizure, take the following steps immediately to prevent injury:

- Place them on the floor or bed away from any hard or sharp objects.
- Turn their head to the side so that any saliva or vomit can drain from their mouth.
- Do not put anything into their mouth; they will not swallow their tongue.
- Call your pediatrician.
- Call 911 if the febrile seizure lasts longer than five minutes.

What Type of Thermometer Is Best?

The American Academy of Pediatrics does not recommend mercury thermometers because these glass thermometers may break, and as their mercury vaporizes it can be inhaled, resulting in toxic exposure. The following are better choices:

- Digital electronic thermometers can measure temperatures in your child's mouth, armpit, or rectum. As with any device, some digital thermometers are more accurate than others. Follow the manufacturer's instructions carefully, and be sure the thermometer is calibrated as recommended by the manufacturer.
- Ear (tympanic) thermometers are another acceptable choice. Their accuracy depends on the ability of the beam emitted by the device to reach the eardrum. Thus, some of these devices may not be as reliable because of earwax or a small or curved ear canal. For that reason, most pediatricians prefer that parents use digital electronic thermometers.
- Temporal artery thermometers are also available. They use an infrared scanner to determine the temperature of the temporal artery, which runs across the forehead just below the skin. They are most useful in children 3 months and older, although recent research shows that they are reliable in babies younger than 3 months as well. They also are simple to use, even while your child is asleep.

BEST WAYS TO TAKE A TEMPERATURE

There are several ways to take your child's temperature. A digital thermometer (which shows the temperature in numbers in a small window) reads the body temperature when its sensor, located in the tip of the thermometer, touches the part of the body where it is used—in the mouth, under the arm, or in the rectum. A tympanic (ear) thermometer or a temporal artery thermometer can also be used. (See above for more information about different types of thermometers.) Whatever approach you use, clean the thermometer as directed—usually with lukewarm soapy water or rubbing alcohol—before each use, and then rinse with cool water. There's no need to add or subtract a degree depending on the device used or how the temperature was taken.

Here are some other guidelines to keep in mind:

- To take the temperature in your child's bottom (rectally), turn on the digital thermometer and then put a small amount of lubricant, such as petroleum jelly, on the end of the thermometer that will be inserted into your baby. Place your child across your lap or on something firm, either face-up or face-down. (If they're face-down, put one hand on their back; if they're face-up, bend your child's legs to their chest, resting your free hand on the back of their thighs.) Then gently insert the small end of the thermometer into your child's bottom (or rectum), putting it in about ½ inch to 1 inch (1–2 cm). Hold the thermometer in place for about one minute or until the device signals that it's done (by beeping or lighting up). Remove it and read the number.
- Taking a rectal or oral temperature is more accurate than taking it under your child's arm. Also, in your household, label one digital thermometer "oral" and another one "rectal." Don't use the same thermometer in both places.
- Tympanic (ear) and temporal artery (side of forehead) thermometers are increasingly popular among parents and healthcare providers, and appear to be quite accurate when used correctly.

When to Call the Pediatrician

If your child is 3 months or younger and has a rectal temperature of 100.4 degrees Fahrenheit (38 degrees Celsius) or higher, call your pediatrician immediately. This is an absolute necessity. The doctor will need to examine the baby to rule out any serious infection or disease.

You also may need to notify the doctor if your child is between 3 and 6 months and has a fever of 101 degrees Fahrenheit (38.3 degrees Celsius) or greater, or is older than 6 months and has a temperature of 103 degrees Fahrenheit (39.4 degrees Celsius) or higher. Such a high temperature may indicate a significant infection or dehydration, which may require treatment. However, in most cases, your decision to call the pediatrician for an older child's fever should depend on associated symptoms, such as a sore throat, an earache, a cough, an unexplained rash, or repeated vomiting or diarrhea. Also, if your child is very fussy or sleeping more than usual, call your doctor. In fact, your child's activity level tends to be a more important indicator than the height of the fever. Again, fever in and of itself is not a sickness; it is a sign of sickness.

If your child is over 1 year of age, is eating and sleeping well, and has playful moments, there usually is no need to call the doctor immediately. If a high fever (as defined earlier) persists for more than twenty-four hours, however, it is best to call even if there are no other complaints or findings.

HEAT-RELATED ILLNESS

A rare but serious problem that is easily confused with fever is heat-related illness, or heatstroke. This is caused not by infection or internal conditions, but by surrounding heat. It can occur when a child is in a very hot place—for example, a hot beach in midsummer or an overheated closed car on a summer day. Leaving children unattended in closed cars is the cause of several deaths a year; never leave an infant or child unattended in a closed car, even for a few minutes. Heatstroke also can occur if a baby is overdressed in hot, humid weather. Under these circumstances, the body temperature can rise to dangerous levels (above 105 degrees Fahrenheit [40.5 degrees Celsius]) and must be reduced quickly by removing some of the clothing, cool-water sponging, fanning, and removal to a cool place. Call 911. Children experiencing heatstroke must be taken to the emergency department right away. Heatstroke is an emergency condition.

If your child becomes delirious (acts frightened, "sees" objects that are not there, talks strangely) while they have a high fever, call your pediatrician, particularly if this has not occurred before. These unusual symptoms probably will disappear when the temperature returns to normal, but the doctor may want to examine your child and determine that the symptoms are not caused by something more serious, such as an inflammation of the brain (encephalitis) or of the membranes covering the brain and spinal cord (meningitis).

Home Treatment

Fevers generally do not need to be treated with medication unless your child is uncomfortable. Even higher temperatures are not in themselves dangerous or significant unless your child has a chronic disease. If your child has a history of a fever-related seizure, treating the fever with medication has not been shown to be an effective strategy to prevent this kind of febrile seizure. It is more important to watch how your child is behaving. If they are eating and sleeping well and have periods of playfulness, they probably don't need any treatment. You should also talk with your pediatrician about when to treat your child's fever. A good time to do this is at well-child visits. When your child has a fever and seems to be quite bothered by or uncomfortable from it, you may treat it with the following approaches.

Medication

Several medications can reduce body temperature by blocking the mechanisms that cause a fever. These antipyretic agents include acetaminophen, ibuprofen, and aspirin. All three of these over-the-counter drugs appear to be equally effective at reducing fever. However, because aspirin may cause or be associated with a serious disease called Reye syndrome, the American Academy of Pediatrics does not recommend using aspirin to treat a fever in children. Acetaminophen can be given without a doctor's advice once your child is older than 3 months, and ibuprofen can be given to children older than 6 months of age. However, if your child has a disease affecting their liver, ask your doctor if acetaminophen is safe to use. Similarly, if your child has kidney disease, an ulcer, or other chronic illness, ask your doctor first if ibuprofen is safe. If your child is dehydrated or vomiting, ibuprofen should be given only under the supervision of a doctor due to risk of kidney damage.

Ideally, the doses of acetaminophen and ibuprofen should be based on a child's weight, not age. (See the dosage charts on *page 579.*) However, the dosages listed on the labels of acetaminophen bottles (which usually are calculated by age) are generally safe and effective unless your child is unusually light or heavy for their age. Keep in mind that at too-high doses of acetaminophen, a toxic response in the liver can develop, although it happens only rarely. When a toxic reaction does occur, the symptoms may include nausea, vomiting, and abdominal discomfort.

As a general guideline, read and follow the instructions on the manufacturer's label when using any medication. Following the instructions is important to ensure that your child receives the proper dosages, and only use the measuring device that comes with the medication you are using. Also, other over-the-counter medications, such as cold and cough preparations, may contain acetaminophen, and using more than one acetaminophen-containing product can result in a dangerously high dosage; read all medication labels to ensure that your child is not receiving multiple doses of the same medicine. Also, as a general rule, do not give a child under 3 months old either acetaminophen or any other medication without the advice of your pediatrician.

Some parents have tried alternating between giving acetaminophen and ibuprofen when their child is running a fever. This approach, however, can theoretically cause medication errors—"Which medicine am I supposed to give them next?"—and could lead to potential side effects. So if your child is uncomfortable with a fever, choose which medicine to give, and then give it according to the dosing recommendations and only if your child still needs it. Either ibuprofen or acetaminophen is effective in reducing fever and making your child feel better. Always consult your doctor before changing the dose schedule or using these medicines in combination.

Also keep in mind that over-the-counter cough and cold medicines should not be given to infants and children under 6 years of age because of potentially serious side effects. Furthermore, studies have shown that these cough and cold products are not effective in treating the symptoms of young children and may even pose health risks.

ACETAMINOPHEN DOSAGE CHART		
Dosages may be repeated every four hours but should not be given more than five times in twenty-four hours. (Note: Use only a syringe or accurate measuring device that measures in milliliters [ml], not household teaspoons, which can vary in size.) Read the label to make sure you are using the right product.		
Age*	**Weight****	**Infant/Children's Oral Suspension (160 mg per 5 ml)**
6–11 mos.	12–17 lbs. (5.5–7.7 kg)	2.5 ml
1–2 yrs.	18–23 lbs. (8.2–10.5 kg)	3.75 ml
* Age is provided as a convenience only. Dosing for fever should be based on current weight.		
** Weight given is representative of the age range.		

IBUPROFEN DOSAGE CHART			
Dosages may be repeated every six to eight hours but should not be given more than four times in 24 hours. (Note: Use only a syringe or accurate measuring device that measures in milliliters [ml], not household teaspoons, which can vary in size.) Read the label to make sure you are using the right product.			
Age*	**Weight****	**Infant Drops (50 mg per 1.25 ml)**	**Children's Suspension (100 mg per 5 ml)**
6–11 mos.	12–17 lbs. (5.5–7.7 kg)	1.25 ml	2.5 ml
1–2 yrs.	18–23 lbs. (8.2–10.5 kg)	1.875 ml	3.75 ml
* Age is provided as a convenience only. Dosing for fever should be based on current weight.			
** Weight given is representative of the age range.			
Aspirin should only be used in special circumstances as recommended by your pediatrician for specific rare conditions.			

Other Treatment Suggestions for Fever

- Keep your child's room and your home comfortably cool, and dress your child lightly.
- Encourage your child to drink extra fluid or other liquids (water, diluted fruit juices, commercially prepared oral electrolyte solutions, soup, Popsicles, etc.).
- If the room is warm or stuffy, place a fan nearby to keep cool air moving.
- Your child does not have to stay in their room or in bed when they have a fever. They can be up and about the house but should not run around and overexert themselves.
- If the fever is a symptom of a highly contagious disease (e.g., chickenpox or the flu), keep your child away from other children, elderly people, or people who may not be able to fight infection well, such as those with cancer.
- Do not give your child a cold bath or use rubbing or other alcohol to bring down the temperature. These measures can cause low body temperature (hypothermia), which is dangerous, as opposed to the fever itself, which is not. In addition, alcohol and other substances can be absorbed through your child's skin and lead to dangerous poisoning or intoxication.

CHAPTER 23

GENITAL AND URINARY SYSTEMS

Blood in the Urine (Hematuria)

If your child's urine has a red, orange, or brown color, it may contain blood. When the urine specifically contains red blood cells, doctors use the medical term "hematuria" to describe this condition. Many things—such as a physical injury, inflammation, or an infection in the urinary tract or kidney—can cause it. Hematuria also is associated with some general medical problems, such as defects of blood clotting, hereditary conditions, or immune system abnormalities.

Sometimes there may be such small amounts of blood in the urine that you cannot see any color change, although it may be detected by a urine test performed by the pediatrician. In some cases, the reddish color is not associated with hematuria at all, and may be due to something your child has eaten or swallowed. Beets, blackberries, red food coloring, phenolphthalein (a chemical sometimes used in laxatives), Pyridium and phenazopyridine (medicines used to relieve bladder pain), and rifampin (a medication used to treat tuberculosis) may cause the urine to turn red or orange. Newborns will also sometimes have a red-orange powdery-looking substance in their diaper called urate, but usually only in the first few days after birth. Anytime you are not certain that one of these substances is responsible for the change in the color of your child's urine, call your pediatrician. When blood in the urine is accompanied by protein (albumin), it is usually due to nephritis, or inflammation of the filtering membranes of the kidney. Your doctor may recommend further tests to distinguish among several different kinds of nephritis.

Treatment

Your pediatrician will ask you about any possible injury, foods, or health symptoms that might have caused the change in urine color. Helpful information may include the presence or absence of pain with urination that could indicate a urinary tract infection. The color of the urine (bright red versus brown) as well as the timing of blood in the urine stream can help to localize where in the urinary tract blood is coming from (i.e., blood throughout the whole stream, versus just at the end of the stream). Your pediatrician will perform a physical exam, checking particularly for any increase in blood pressure, tenderness in the kidney area, or swelling (particularly of the hands or feet or around the eyes) that might indicate kidney problems. They also will conduct tests on a sample of urine and may order blood tests or imaging studies (such as an ultrasound scan or X-rays) or perform other examinations to check your child's kidneys, bladder, and immune system. If none of these reveals the cause of the hematuria and it continues to occur, your pediatrician may refer you to a children's kidney specialist, who will perform additional tests. (Sometimes these tests include examining a tiny piece of kidney tissue under the microscope, a procedure known as a biopsy. This tissue may be obtained by surgery or by performing what's called a needle biopsy.)

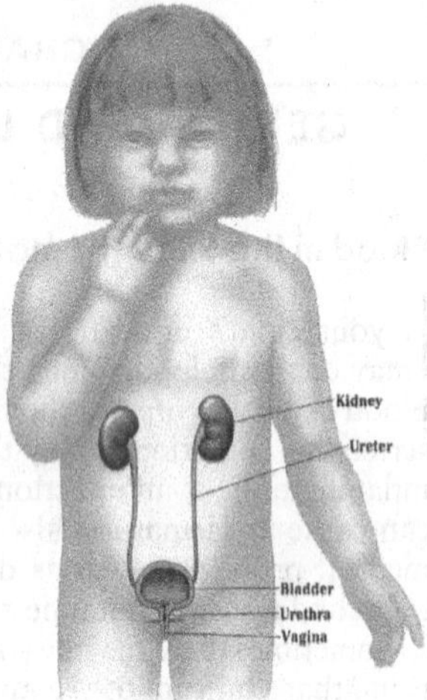

Genitourinary system

Once your pediatrician knows more about what is causing the hematuria, a decision can be made about whether treatment is necessary. Often no treatment is required, indicating that there is nothing to worry about. Occasionally medication is used to suppress the inflammation that is the hallmark sign of nephritis. Whatever the treatment, your child will need to return to the doctor regularly for repeat urine and blood tests and blood pressure checks. This is necessary to make sure that they aren't developing chronic kidney disease, which can lead to kidney failure.

Occasionally hematuria is caused by kidney stones, high urine calcium levels, irritation of the urethra (urethritis), or, rarely, an abnormality of the urinary tract that could require surgery. If this is the case, your pediatrician will refer you to a pediatric urologist (a bladder and kidney surgeon) who can perform such procedures.

Circumcision

Circumcision is a common procedure performed in many male infants. It involves removing the foreskin covering the tip of the penis. There are benefits and risks to circumcision, and you should discuss them with your pediatrician or obstetrician and your spouse or partner before your baby is born. Although it is not routinely recommended for all male newborns, there may be cultural, religious, medical, and other reasons you may decide that it is appropriate for your child. The choice to circumcise or not to circumcise is completely that of the parent, as circumcision is not necessary to have a healthy child; however, current data have shown that the medical benefits at least balance and may outweigh the risks.

Hydronephrosis

Hydronephrosis is a condition in which there is dilation of the kidney that can be seen on an ultrasound. This can be caused by a structural difference in your child's urinary tract or by something temporary, like a kidney stone.

Diagnosis

Most children with hydronephrosis do not have pain. This condition is usually found on a prenatal ultrasound (in 1 to 3 percent of all pregnancies), but it can also be diagnosed in children who get a kidney ultrasound because of abdominal pain or recurrent urinary tract infections.

Hydronephrosis that is diagnosed prenatally has three primary causes:

1. Transient/physiologic hydronephrosis. This problem goes away on its own over time without causing any

problems for your baby or child. This is the most common cause of hydronephrosis diagnosed prenatally.

2. Vesicoureteral reflux. This is an abnormal backflow of urine from the kidneys to the bladder. It doesn't cause symptoms in many children but can increase the risk for urinary tract infection and even cause kidney damage in some cases.
3. Obstruction. Some babies are born with a block in the urinary tract (like posterior urethral valve) that can cause backup of urine into the kidney. This can increase the risk for urinary tract infections and cause kidney damage over time.

Some causes of hydronephrosis, such as a kidney stone, may cause pain in the back, abdomen, or groin. A pediatric urologist or nephrologist may order other blood or imaging tests to identify the causes of hydronephrosis.

Treatment

Mild cases of hydronephrosis can be watched and may improve as your child grows older without causing any problems. Your child may need to see a pediatric urologist or nephrologist and have an occasional kidney ultrasound to monitor the kidneys. More severe cases may require more frequent ultrasounds, other tests, or surgery.

Hypospadias and Chordee

In male babies, the opening through which urine passes (the urethral meatus) is located at the tip of the penis. A condition known as hypospadias is an abnormality in penile development in which this opening is on the underside of the penis. There also may be an abnormal downward bending of the penis called chordee, which may cause sexual problems in adulthood. The meatus may direct the urinary stream downward and cause the stream to spray, making standing to urinate difficult or impossible.

Treatment

After detecting hypospadias or chordee in your newborn, your pediatrician probably will advise against circumcision until after consultation with a pediatric urologist or surgeon. This is because the foreskin may be used for future surgical repair, and circumcision may make that repair more difficult.

Mild hypospadias may require no treatment, but treatment for moderate or severe forms may include surgical repair. Most children with hypospadias undergo outpatient surgery after 6 months of age, but each family should decide for themselves if the risks of anesthesia and surgery are in the best interests of their child. It may help to discuss with a multidisciplinary health team, and other families or older patients who have been through similar surgeries, to consider timing and impact of each procedure. Often, hypospadias and chordee can be repaired in conjunction with circumcision in one procedure. In severe cases, more than one operation may be needed to repair the condition completely. Surgery can impact appearance of the penis, urinary stream, and adult sexual functioning. The goal of surgery is to allow your child to urinate normally, have normal sexual function as an adult, and have an acceptable cosmetic result.

Labial Adhesions

Ordinarily the lips of skin (labia) surrounding the entrance to the vagina and urethra are separated. Sometimes they grow together to partially or completely block the opening. This condition, called labial adhesions (sticking together of labia), may occur in the early months after birth or later on if there is constant irritation and inflammation in the diaper area. Usually, labial adhesions do not cause symptoms, but sometimes they can lead to difficulty with urination and increase a child's susceptibility to urinary tract infections. If the vaginal opening is significantly blocked, urine and/or vaginal secretions will sometimes build up behind the obstruction.

Treatment

If the opening of your child's vagina appears to have closed or looks partially blocked, notify your pediatrician. They will examine your child and advise you whether any treatment is necessary. Most such adhesions require no treatment and resolve on their own as the child gets older. In general, if your child is not having symptoms like dribbling incontinence (wetting) after urination or urinary tract infections, no treatment is needed.

Treatment options for labial adhesions include watchful waiting or observation, treatment with estrogen cream applied a few times daily at home, or manual separation of the adhesions in the office or the operating room with the use of numbing medication.

If estrogen cream is needed, your doctor will instruct you on exactly how and where to apply the cream. Good hygiene, such as giving your child daily sitz baths, is also important in the treatment and prevention of labial adhesions. You may want to apply a lubricant like petroleum jelly along the edges to prevent them from sticking back together. It is important to keep in mind that the estrogen cream may result in temporary changes in the appearance of the hymen (tissue at the opening of the vagina) or withdrawal bleeding (like a period). These will resolve after discontinuation of the estrogen cream. As the adhesion opens up, the area may take on a bruised appearance that can be mistaken for trauma. This also will go away.

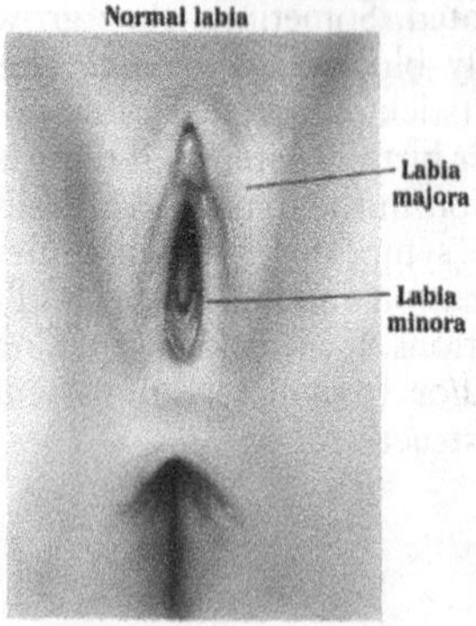

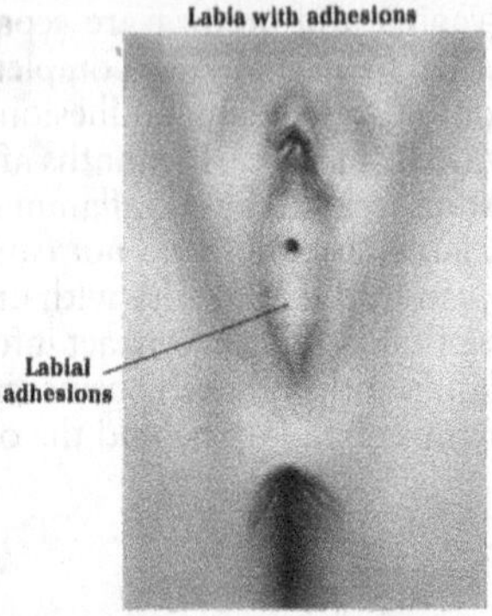

Meatal Stenosis

Sometimes, particularly in those who are circumcised, irritation of the tip of the penis causes scar tissue to form around the urethral meatus, making it smaller. This narrowing, called meatal stenosis, may develop at any time during childhood, but is most commonly found between ages 3 and 7. Children with meatal stenosis have a narrowed and abnormally directed urinary stream. The stream is directed upward (toward the ceiling), making it difficult to urinate into the toilet without pushing the penis down between the legs. Your child may take longer to urinate and have difficulty emptying their bladder completely.

Treatment

If you notice that your child's urinary stream is very small or narrow or is difficult to aim in the toilet, if they strain to urinate, or if they dribble or spray urine, discuss it with your pediatrician. Meatal stenosis is not a serious condition, but it should be evaluated to see if it needs treatment. If an operation is needed, this surgery is very minor. Your child will have some minor discomfort after the procedure, but this should disappear after a very short period.

Posterior Urethral Valve

Urine leaves the bladder through a tube called the urethra. For boys, the urethra passes through the penis. Rarely, a small membrane forms across the urethra early in pregnancy, and it can block the flow of urine out of the bladder. This problem, posterior urethral valve, can have life-threatening consequences by causing blockage of normal urine flow, thus interfering with development of the bladder and kidneys. If there is abnormal kidney development in utero, there can also be abnormal development of the lungs.

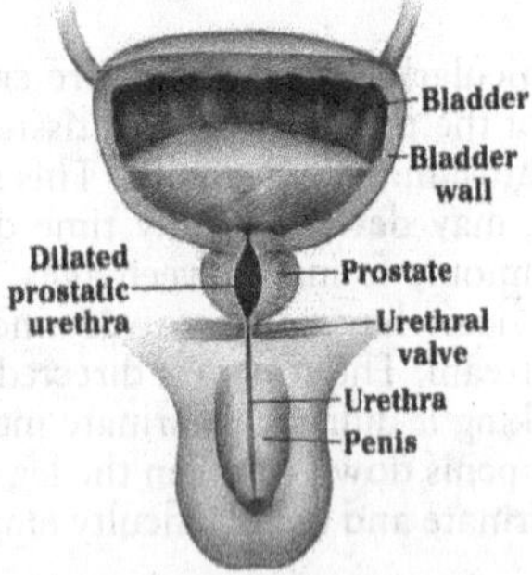

The severity of posterior urethral valve can vary widely. Most cases are diagnosed before birth with a screening ultrasound. This condition may be suspected in pregnancies with boys if there appears to be a decrease in the amount of amniotic fluid. Consulting a pediatric urology specialist is always advisable before the baby is born. In boys who are not diagnosed before birth with posterior urethral valve, sometimes the newborn exam may reveal that the baby's bladder is distended and enlarged. Other warning signals include a continual dribbling of urine and a weak stream during urination. Sometimes, posterior urethral valve is diagnosed in the first year when the boy develops a urinary tract infection with fever and poor feeding. If you notice these symptoms, notify your pediatrician at once.

Posterior urethral valve requires immediate medical attention to prevent serious urinary tract infections and damage to the kidneys. The urine can back up through the ureters (the tubes between the bladder and the kidneys), creating pressure that can damage the kidneys.

Treatment

If your child has posterior urethral valve, your pediatrician may pass a small tube (catheter) into the bladder to relieve the obstruction temporarily and allow the urine to flow out of the bladder. They will obtain imaging of the bladder and kidneys. Your pediatrician will consult with a pediatric urologist, who may recommend surgery to remove the obstructing valve and prevent further infection or damage to the kidneys or urinary system. Bloodwork will be done to look at the level of kidney function, and a pediatric nephrologist will likely be consulted as well. Some children with posterior urethral valve retain normal kidney function, but some children may require dialysis or kidney transplantation.

Testicular Torsion

Testicular torsion is a rare but serious event in which the testicle twists and cuts off its blood supply. This puts the testicle at risk for permanent damage. This can happen in boys of all ages, even before a baby is born. The cause of testicular torsion is not known.

Diagnosis

The most common symptom of testicular torsion is sudden, severe pain of the testicle. Younger children can have a harder time expressing their pain and may complain only of abdominal pain. The testicle may be firm and tender, and the scrotum may be enlarged. If a child is complaining of testicular/scrotal pain that lasts longer than 30 minutes, they should be seen urgently in the emergency department. An ultrasound of the scrotum and testicles may be used to check for blood flow to the testicle.

Treatment

The treatment for testicular torsion is an urgent surgery to untwist the testicle. Once the testicle is untwisted, both testicles may be anchored in the scrotum with stitches to lower the chances of either testicle twisting again. Unfortunately, the testicle may need to be removed if it was twisted for a prolonged period and does not survive.

Undescended Testicles (Cryptorchidism)

During a pregnancy, a boy's testes develop in their abdomen. As they near birth, the testes descend through a tube (the inguinal canal) into the scrotum. In a small number of boys, especially those who are premature, one or both testicles fail to descend by the time of birth. In many of these boys, descent will occur during the first few months after birth. In some, however, this does not happen.

Most boys will have a normal retraction of the testes under certain situations, such as while sitting in cold water (i.e., the testes "disappear" temporarily up into the inguinal canal) or when being examined by your pediatrician. However, in general, when the child is warm and relaxed, testes should be low in the scrotum. The cause of most cases of undescended testicles is unknown.

If your child has undescended testicles, their scrotum may be small and appear underdeveloped. If only one testicle is undescended, the scrotum may look asymmetrical (full on one side, empty on the other). If the testicles sometimes are in the scrotum and at other times (e.g., when the child is cold or excited) are absent and located above the scrotum, they are said to be retractile. This condition usually self-corrects as a child grows older.

Rarely, the undescended testicle may be twisted, and in the process, its blood supply may be stopped, causing pain in the inguinal (groin) or scrotal area. If this situation is not corrected, the testicle can be damaged severely and permanently. If your child has an undescended testicle and complains of pain in the groin or scrotal area, call your pediatrician immediately. Undescended testicles should be reevaluated at each regular checkup. If they do not descend into the scrotum by 6 months of age, treatment should be considered. The diagnosis is made by physical exam, and imaging studies like ultrasound may or may not be needed.

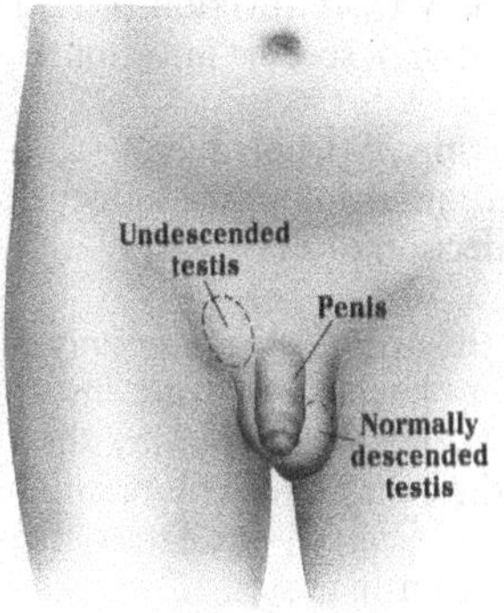

Treatment

Undescended testicles are treated with surgery to bring the testicle into the proper location in the scrotum. Many children with true undescended testes will also have an inguinal hernia (see *page 372*), and the hernia will be repaired at the same time that the undescended testis is surgically moved to the scrotum. If your child's undescended testicle is allowed to remain in that position for more than two years, they may have a higher-than-average risk of being unable to have biological children (infertility). This is especially true if both testes are undescended. Undescended testes are also at higher risk of developing testicular tumors in adult life. The risk is small but is still present even after the testis is surgically brought into the scrotum. Therefore, it is important that children with an undescended testis be taught the importance of testicular self-exam when they are going through puberty.

Urinary Tract Infections

Urinary tract infections are common among young children, particularly girls. They generally are caused by bacteria that enter through the urethra. In infants, they may also rarely be caused by bacteria carried through the bloodstream to the kidneys from another part of the body. As the bacteria move through the urinary tract, they may cause an infection in various locations. Urinary tract infection (UTI) is a general term used for all the following specific infections:

- Cystitis: infection of the bladder
- Pyelonephritis: infection of the kidney
- Urethritis: infection of the urethra

The bladder is the area most commonly infected. Usually, cystitis is caused by bacteria that get into the urinary tract through the urethra. The urethra is very short in girls, so bacteria that live on the skin, in the colon, and in the vagina can get into the bladder easily. Fortunately, these bacteria normally wash out when urinating.

Cystitis can cause lower abdominal pain, vomiting, tenderness, pain during urination, frequent urination, blood in the urine, recurrence of day- or nighttime wetting in a previously toilet-trained child, and a low-grade fever. Infection of the kidneys (pyelonephritis) will cause more general abdominal pain and a higher fever, but it may or may not cause frequent and painful urination. In general, urinary tract infections in infants and young children (up to 2 years of age) may have few recognizable signs or symptoms other than a fever; they also have a greater potential for causing kidney damage than those occurring in older children.

Urinary tract infections must be treated with antibiotics as quickly as possible, so you should notify your pediatrician promptly if you suspect your child has developed one. This is especially the case for infants, in whom an unexplained high fever (that is, not explained by a respiratory infection or diarrhea) may be the only indicator of a urinary tract infection. If your infant has a fever with no other symptoms for more than three days, make sure to talk to your pediatrician, as an evaluation may be indicated.

Diagnosis/Treatment

When a urinary tract infection is suspected, particularly in a child with symptoms, your pediatrician will measure their blood pressure (since an increase in blood pressure can be a sign of a related kidney problem) and examine them for lower abdominal tenderness that might indicate a UTI. An examination of the genitals may be performed to rule out a yeast infection or genital irritation. Your doctor will want to know what your child has been eating and drinking, because certain foods can irritate the urinary tract, causing symptoms similar to those of an infection. Constipation (infrequent or hard-to-pass stools) can also cause symptoms similar to those of a UTI.

Your pediatrician also will want a urine sample from your child for analysis. In infants and toddlers who are not toilet trained, the pediatrician may start with a special bag over the genitals designed to catch urine. If this urine appears possibly infected, however, then urine must be collected by using a catheter to confirm the diagnosis. In toilet-trained children, the urine can be collected by the "clean catch" method. First, you'll use soap and water or special wipes provided by your pediatrician to cleanse the urethral opening (with an uncircumcised penis, hold the foreskin back). Then allow your child to start to urinate, but wait just a moment before you start to collect the sample in the special container provided by the doctor. In this way, any bacteria around the outside of the urethral opening will be washed away by the early urine voided and won't contaminate the specimen. In rare cases, a doctor may perform a suprapubic tap, in which a small needle is inserted through the skin of the lower abdomen into the bladder. The urine that is collected will be examined for any sign of blood cells or bacteria, and special tests (cultures) will be done to identify the bacteria. An antibiotic will be started if an infection is suspected, although depending on what the results of the culture show, the particular antibiotic may need to be changed.

In agreement with guidelines for the treatment of UTI in infants and children (up to age 24 months), your pediatrician may prescribe antibiotics for a total of seven to fourteen days. Prompt treatment is important to eliminate the infection and prevent its spread, and also to reduce the chances of kidney damage. It is important to take the full course of antibiotics, even if the discomfort resolves after a few days of treatment. Otherwise, the bacteria may grow again, causing further infection and more serious damage to the urinary tract.

The American Academy of Pediatrics recommends that imaging tests (such as ultrasound, X-rays, or renal scans) may be done in children depending on their age and how many urinary tract infections they have had. Some imaging studies may not be necessary following a first urinary tract infection if prenatal ultrasound studies have adequately visualized the structure of the infant's urinary tract. Your pediatrician may conduct other tests to check the functioning of the kidneys. If any of these examinations indicate an anatomical abnormality of the bladder, ureters, or kidneys that should be corrected, your doctor will recommend that your child see a pediatric urologist or nephrologist.

CHAPTER 24

HEAD, NECK, AND NERVOUS SYSTEM

Head Tilt (Torticollis)

Head tilt is a condition that causes a child to hold their head or neck in a twisted or otherwise abnormal position. They may lean their head toward one shoulder and, when lying on their stomach, always turn the same side of their face toward the mattress. This can cause their head to flatten on one side and their face to appear uneven or out of line. If not treated, head tilt may lead to permanent facial deformity or unevenness and to restricted head movement.

Most cases of head tilt are associated with a condition called torticollis, although in rare instances a head tilt can be due to other causes such as hearing loss, misalignment of the eyes, reflux (a flowing back of stomach acid into the esophagus), a throat or lymph node infection, or, very uncommonly, a brain tumor.

Acquired Torticollis (Due to Injury or Inflammation)

This is more likely to occur in older children, up to the age of 9 or 10. This type of torticollis usually results from an inflammation of the throat caused by an upper respiratory infection, a sore throat, an injury, or some unknown factor. The swelling, for reasons still not known, causes the tissue surrounding the upper spine to loosen, allowing the vertebral bones to move out of normal position. When this happens, the neck muscles go into spasm, causing the head to tilt to one side. Onset of this condition is typically sudden and very painful.

Congenital Torticollis

By far the most common cause of head tilt among children under age 5 is congenital torticollis. This condition commonly occurs due to positioning while the baby is still in the womb and rarely may occur during birth (particularly breech and difficult first-time deliveries). Whatever the cause, this condition usually is detected in the first six to eight weeks after birth, when the pediatrician notices tightness in one of the muscles of the neck. About half the time there may be a small lump in the muscle. The affected muscle is the sternocleidomastoid muscle, which connects the breastbone, head, and neck. Later the muscle contracts and causes the head to tilt to one side and look toward the opposite side.

Unlike muscular torticollis, ocular torticollis occurs when the infant tilts the head in order to correct misalignment of the eyes. In these cases, the abnormal head position will not be present during sleep, and it will be possible to manually tilt the head toward either shoulder without resistance.

Treatment

Each type of head tilt requires different treatment. It is very important to seek such treatment early so that the problem is corrected before it causes permanent deformity. Your pediatrician will examine your child's neck and may refer you to a pediatric orthopedist or to a physical or occupational therapist, and/or may order X-rays of the area in order to identify the cause of the problem. X-rays or ultrasound of the hip also may be ordered, as some children with congenital muscular torticollis also have an abnormality known as developmental dysplasia of the hip. If the doctor decides that the problem is congenital muscular torticollis, you will learn an exercise program to stretch and massage your child's neck muscles. The doctor will show you how to gently move your child's head in the opposite direction from the tilt. You'll need to do this several times a day, very gradually extending the movement as the muscle stretches.

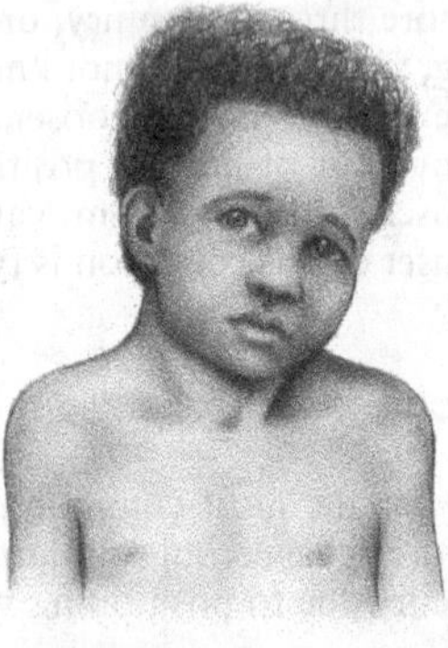

When your child sleeps, it is best to place them on their back, with their head positioned opposite from the direction of the tilt. In rare instances, your pediatrician may suggest adjustments to their sleep position. When they are awake, position them so those things they want to look at (windows, mobiles, pictures, and activity) are on the side in the opposite direction from the tilt. In that way, they'll stretch the shortened muscle while trying to see these objects. Your pediatrician may also recommend placing them on their stomach while awake and turning their face away from the affected side. These simple strategies cure this type of head tilt in the vast majority of cases, preventing the need for later surgery. (Your pediatrician may refer your child to a physical therapist to help work on this condition.)

If the problem is not corrected by exercise or position change, your pediatrician will refer you to a pediatric neurologist or orthopedist. If there is a concern that the head position is caused by misalignment of the eyes, the pediatrician may refer you to a pediatric ophthalmologist. Rarely, it may be necessary to lengthen the involved muscle surgically when the child is no longer an infant. If your child's head tilt is caused by something other than congenital muscular torticollis and the X-rays show no spinal abnormality, other treatment involving rest, a special collar, gentle stretching, massage, traction, application of heat to the area, medication, or, rarely, further imaging or surgery may be necessary. For treating torticollis due to injury or inflammation, your doctor may recommend applying heat, as well as using massage and stretching to ease head and neck pain. Your pediatrician can refer you to a specialist for a definitive diagnosis and treatment program.

Meningitis

Meningitis is an inflammation of the tissues that cover the brain and spinal cord and typically is caused by a viral or bacterial infection. The inflammation sometimes affects the brain itself, in which case it is called encephalitis. With early diagnosis and proper treatment, a child with meningitis has a reasonable chance of a good recovery, though some forms of bacterial meningitis develop rapidly and have a high risk of complications.

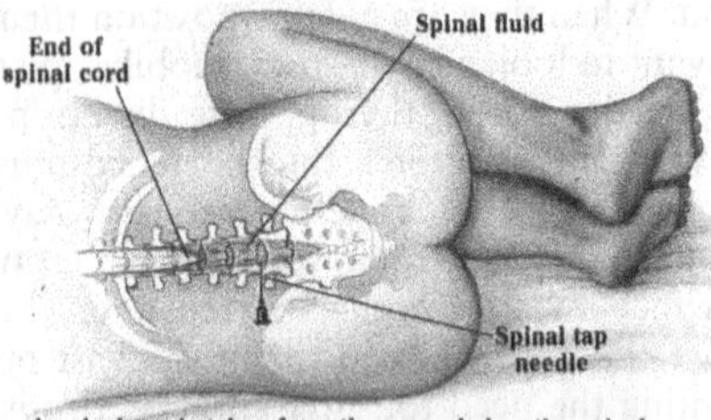

A spinal tap is taken from the space below the spinal cord so that the needle will not touch the spinal cord.

Thanks to vaccines that protect against serious forms of bacterial meningitis, today most cases of meningitis are caused by viruses. The viral form is usually not as serious, except in infants less than 3 months of age and with certain viruses such as herpes simplex, which also cause dangerous encephalitis. While herpes meningitis requires aggressive treatment with antiviral medications, other viral infections do not require antivirals, and children usually recover on their own.

Bacterial meningitis is a very serious disease. It occurs rarely in countries with universal and successful vaccination programs, but when it does occur, children under the age of 2 years are at greatest risk.

The bacteria that cause meningitis often can be found in the mouths and throats of healthy children, but this does not necessarily mean that these children will get the disease. That doesn't happen unless the bacteria get into the bloodstream and spread to the brain.

We still don't understand exactly why some children get meningitis and others don't, but we do know that certain groups of children are more likely to get the illness. These include the following:

- Babies, especially those under 2 months of age (because their immune systems are not well developed, the bacteria can get into the bloodstream more easily)
- Children with recurrent sinus infections

- Children with recent serious head injuries and skull fractures
- Children who have just had brain surgery

With prompt diagnosis and treatment, seven out of ten children who get bacterial meningitis recover without any complications. However, bear in mind that meningitis is a potentially fatal disease, and in about three out of ten cases, it can lead to serious nervous system problems, deafness, seizures, paralysis of the arms or legs, or learning difficulties. Because meningitis progresses quickly, it must be detected early and treated aggressively. Therefore, it's important for you to notify your pediatrician immediately if your child displays any of the following warning signs:

If your child is less than 3 months old: A fever, decreased appetite, listlessness, or increased crying or irritability warrants a call to your doctor. At this age, the signs of meningitis can be very subtle and difficult to detect. It's better to call early and be wrong than to diagnose it too late to treat.

If your child is 2 months to 2 years old: This is the most common age for meningitis. Look for symptoms such as fever, vomiting, decreased appetite, excessive crankiness, or excessive sleepiness. (Their cranky periods might be extreme, and during sleepy periods it might be impossible to arouse them.) Seizures along with a fever may be the first signs of meningitis, although most brief, generalized (so-called tonic-clonic) convulsions in this age group turn out to be simple febrile seizures, not meningitis. (See Seizures, Convulsions, and Epilepsy, *page 602*.) A rash also may be a symptom of this condition.

Treatment

If your pediatrician is concerned that your child may have meningitis, they will send you to the hospital for evaluation, including to check for a bacterial infection with a blood test and to obtain some spinal fluid by performing a spinal tap, or lumbar puncture (LP). An LP involves inserting a special needle into your child's lower back to draw out spinal fluid. This is a safe technique in which fluid is sampled from the bottom of the sac surrounding the spinal cord. Signs of infection in this fluid will confirm that your child has meningitis. In the case of bacterial meningitis, they will need to be admitted to the hospital for intravenous antibiotics and fluids and for careful observation for complications. For bacterial meningitis, intravenous antibiotics may be necessary for seven to twenty-one days, depending on the age of the child and the bacteria identified. If prolonged antibiotics are needed, your child may be able to continue receiving medication at home. Most children with viral meningitis improve within seven to ten days without antibiotics. Children will typically recover at home with rest, fluids, and over-the-counter pain medications, although some might need to be treated in the hospital.

Prevention

Some types of bacterial meningitis can be prevented with vaccines, especially those against Hib (*Haemophilus influenzae* type b) and pneumococcus.

Mumps

Mumps is a viral infection that usually causes swelling of the salivary glands (the glands that produce the digestive juices in the mouth). Thanks to the MMR (measles, mumps, and rubella) vaccine, given at 12 to 15 months with a booster at age 4 to 6 years, most children in developed countries will never get this disease. The American Academy of Pediatrics recommends that if your child has not been immunized with the MMR vaccine in early childhood as suggested, your child (18 years old and younger) should be given two doses of MMR vaccine, separated by four weeks.

While the administration of the MMR vaccine is very important, if a child has not been immunized, the parent should know how to identify mumps and distinguish it from similar ailments. The parotid gland, located in front of the ear at and above the angle of the jaw, is the one most often affected by mumps. The swelling can be on one or both sides of the face. However, other salivary glands in and around the face may be involved. Symptoms normally last seven to ten days. Not all children with mumps appear swollen, as some have a milder case. Anyone who has the virus in their system, whether symptoms were mild or severe, will become immune to it and be protected for life.

The mumps virus is transmitted when an infected individual coughs droplets containing the virus into the air or onto their hands. A nearby child can inhale these particles, and the virus can pass through their respiratory system into their bloodstream, finally settling in their salivary glands. At this point, the virus usually causes swelling of the glands along the side of one or both cheeks.

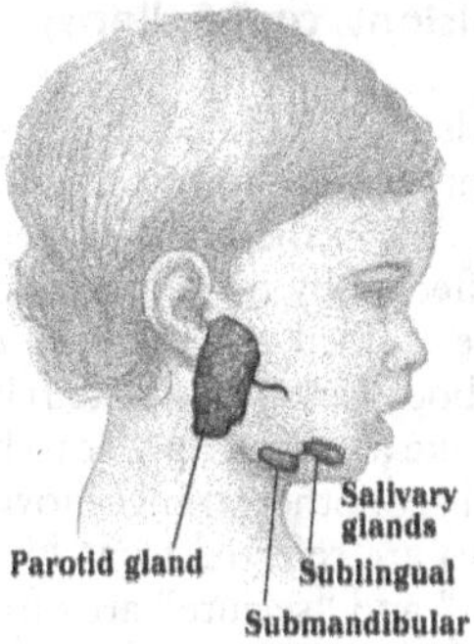

Other symptoms of mumps may include swelling and pain in the joints and, in boys, swelling of the testes. In extremely rare cases, the virus can cause swelling of the ovaries in girls or swelling of the brain in boys or girls.

It's important to note that salivary gland swelling can be caused by infections other than mumps. This explains why some parents are convinced that their children have had the disease more than once. If your child has been immunized or already has had mumps and their cheeks become swollen, consult your pediatrician to determine the cause.

Treatment

There is no specific treatment for mumps, aside from making the child as comfortable as possible with rest, lots of fluids, and acetaminophen for fever. Although a child with the disease may not be too eager to take fluids, you should keep a glass of water or juice (but not citrus juice) nearby, and encourage them to take frequent sips. Sometimes a warm compress over the swollen gland will give some short-term relief.

If your child's condition worsens, or if they develop complications such as painful testes, severe abdominal pain, or extreme listlessness, contact your pediatrician right away. Complications are extremely rare, but the doctor will want to examine your child to see if they need more extensive medical treatment.

Seizures, Convulsions, and Epilepsy

Seizures are sudden temporary changes in consciousness, physical movement, sensation, or behavior caused by abnormal electrical impulses in the brain. Depending on what parts of the brain are affected by the abnormal electrical activity, a seizure may cause sudden stiffening of the body, rhythmic shaking, isolated body jerks, complete relaxation of the muscles (which can make a person appear to be paralyzed temporarily), staring spells, or other strange movements or behaviors. Sometimes seizures are referred to as "fits" or "spells." The terms "convulsion" and "seizure" are often used interchangeably, although not all seizures involve convulsions.

A seizure that involves the whole body (sometimes called a generalized tonic-clonic seizure and previously called grand mal seizure) is the most dramatic type of seizure, causing rapid, forceful movements of both arms and legs and loss of consciousness. By contrast, absence seizures (previously called petit mal seizures) appear as brief staring episodes lasting for a few seconds. These may be so subtle that they aren't noticed until they begin affecting schoolwork and are mistaken for inattentiveness. Seizures that involve only a part of the brain are called focal seizures (previously called partial seizures) and can cause twitching or jerking of one part of the body or other behaviors. About 10 percent of children will experience a seizure at some point during childhood, but only 3 percent will go on to have epilepsy.

Febrile seizures (seizures that occur in association with fever) occur in 3 or 4 out of every 100 children between 6 months and 5 years of age, but most often around 12 to 18 months old. A febrile seizure is usually a brief whole-body convulsion after which the child will return to normal. They often run in families. Most children with febrile seizures will outgrow them by 5 years of age. However, a very small number of affected children will go on to develop epilepsy, with seizures occurring even when a fever is not present.

The term "epilepsy" is used to describe seizures that occur repeatedly over time without an acute illness (like fever) or another trigger. Sometimes the cause of the recurring seizures is known, and sometimes it is not.

Some children experience sudden episodes that might masquerade as or imitate seizure but are really not. Examples include breath holding, fainting (syncope), daydreaming spells, facial or body twitching (myoclonus), and unusual sleep disorders (night terrors and sleepwalking). They may occur just once or may recur over a limited time period. Again, although these episodes may resemble epilepsy or true seizures, they are not, and they require quite different treatment.

Treatment

Most seizures are brief and stop on their own and do not require immediate medical treatment. If your child is having a seizure, lay them on their side so they will not choke if they vomit, move away items that could cause injury, and stay with them until the seizure stops.

If the seizure does not stop within five minutes or is severe (difficulty breathing, choking, blueness of the skin, having several in a row), call 911 for emergency medical help. Do not leave your child unattended. After the seizure stops, call the pediatrician immediately and arrange to meet in the doctor's office or go to the nearest emergency department. If your child has known epilepsy and is already taking a medication to prevent seizures, call your doctor, since the dosage may need to be adjusted.

If your child has a fever, the pediatrician will check to see if there is an infection. If there is no fever and this was your child's first seizure, the doctor will try to determine other possible causes by asking if there is a family history of seizures or if your child has had any recent head injury. They may ask if there was any exposure to bright strobe lighting either in the home or on a video screen. They will examine your child and may order blood tests or testing with an electroencephalogram (EEG), which measures the electrical activity of the brain. In some cases, your child may require imaging of the brain using computed tomography (CT) or magnetic resonance imaging

(MRI). Sometimes a spinal tap will be performed to obtain a specimen of spinal fluid that can be examined for some causes of seizures such as meningitis, an infection of the covering of the brain (see *page 597*). The pediatrician is likely to consult a pediatric neurologist, a pediatrician who specializes in disorders of the nervous system.

If a child has had a febrile seizure, some parents may try controlling fever using fever-reducing medications (acetaminophen, ibuprofen) or lukewarm baths. However, these approaches do not prevent future febrile seizures, but only make the child more comfortable. If a bacterial infection is present, your doctor will probably prescribe an antibiotic. If a serious infection such as meningitis is responsible for the seizure, your child may need to be hospitalized for further treatment. Also, when seizures are caused by abnormal amounts of sugar, sodium, or calcium in the blood, hospitalization may be required so that the cause can be found and the imbalances corrected.

If epilepsy is diagnosed, your child usually will be placed on an anti-seizure medication. When the proper dosage is maintained, the seizures are often well controlled. Your child may need to have their blood checked periodically after starting some medications to make certain there is an adequate amount of medication in their system and that it has no effects on the health of the liver or bone marrow. Depending on the type of epilepsy they have, some children may benefit from other treatments such as surgery, devices, or dietary therapies to help control seizures. In addition to a daily anti-seizure medication, some children may benefit from a seizure rescue medication, which is a medication that parents or caregivers can administer at home or school if a child has a prolonged seizure or a cluster of seizures.

As frightening as seizures can be, many individuals with epilepsy can have their seizures controlled with medication, and many children have fewer seizures as they get older or even outgrow their epilepsy. Unfortunately, a great deal of misunderstanding and confusion about seizures still exists, so it is important that your child's friends and teachers become educated about their condition. (If you need additional support or information, consult with your pediatrician or contact your local or state branch of the Epilepsy Foundation, epilepsy.com; 1-800-332-1000.)

CHAPTER 25

HEART AND BLOOD

Anemia

Blood contains several different types of cells. The most numerous are the red blood cells, which absorb oxygen in the lungs and distribute it throughout the body. These cells contain hemoglobin, a red protein that carries oxygen to the tissues and carries away carbon dioxide (the waste material). Anemia can be either an acute or a chronic condition in which a decreased amount of hemoglobin is available in the red blood cells or there is a reduced number of red blood cells in the blood itself, making the blood less able to carry the amount of oxygen necessary for all the cells in the body to function and grow.

Anemia may occur for any of the following reasons:

1. The production of red blood cells is too slow.
2. Too many red blood cells are destroyed.
3. There is not enough hemoglobin within the red blood cells.
4. Too much blood is lost from the body.

Many cases of anemia are treatable. Young children most commonly become anemic when they fail to get enough iron in their diet, particularly during periods of rapid growth. Iron is necessary for the production of hemoglobin. This iron deficiency causes a decrease in the amount of hemoglobin in the red blood cells.

An infant may get iron-deficiency anemia if they are primarily breastfed and do not begin a form of iron supplementation by 6 months of age or if they start drinking cow's milk too early (before 12 months of age), particularly if they are not given an iron supplement or healthy food that contains enough iron. Cow's milk contains very little iron, and the iron it does have is not easily absorbed. Furthermore, cow's milk can interfere with the absorption of iron from other foods. Large amounts of cow's milk given to an infant or toddler can irritate the bowel and cause small amounts of blood loss. This results in a decrease in the number of red blood cells, which can cause anemia. Finally, drinking too much milk may limit a child's interest in other foods that are rich in iron, placing them at risk for iron-deficiency anemia. Infants shouldn't drink any cow's milk, and toddlers should limit their milk intake to no more than 16 to 24 ounces (480–720 ml) a day. Other nutritional deficiencies, such as a lack of folic acid, can cause anemia as well, but such causes are rare. Premature babies are prone to anemia and should start iron supplementation at two weeks after birth.

Anemia can also be a result of a chronic condition that will need ongoing treatment and follow-up by your child's doctor. It may be caused by blood loss, such as a child losing blood in their stool in amounts tiny enough that it can't be seen. It may also be caused by hemolytic anemia, where red blood cells are prone to being easily destroyed because of changes in the shape of the cells, disturbances on their surface, or other abnormalities. Certain enzyme deficiencies can alter the function of red blood cells and increase the chances they will die or be destroyed early, causing anemia. A severe condition called sickle cell anemia involves an abnormal structure of hemoglobin (see Sickle Cell Disease, *page 616*). This disorder can be dangerous and is associated with frequent episodes of pain and worsening anemia, often requiring repeated hospitalizations. Fortunately, it is now tested for in the newborn screen in all states.

Disorders called thalassemias are inherited blood conditions in which the child has an abnormally low number of red blood cells or not enough hemoglobin. This is due to a decreased ability to make healthy red blood cells and the fact that the red blood cells are more likely to be destroyed. Children with thalassemia can develop anemia, sometimes severe cases. Although some cases of thalassemia have no symptoms, more moderate to severe cases can cause lethargy, jaundice, a poor appetite, slow growth, and an enlarged spleen.

Signs and Symptoms

In some cases, the anemia develops so slowly over time that symptoms aren't noticed. More typically, though, anemia causes the skin to be mildly pale, usually most apparent as a decreased pinkness of the lips, the lining of the eyelids (conjunctiva), and the nail beds (pink part of the nails). Anemic children also may be irritable, mildly weak, or easily tired. Those with severe anemia may have shortness of breath, rapid heart rate, and swelling of the hands and feet. If the anemia continues, it may interfere with normal growth. Children with hemolytic anemia may have episodes of jaundice (skin and eyes turn yellow), although many newborns are mildly jaundiced for reasons that don't involve anemia.

Your child's pediatrician will check their hemoglobin at 12 months and may do so again at 24 months, and periodically if there are any concerns in youth who menstruate. But if your child shows any of these symptoms or signs, or if you suspect they are not getting enough iron in their diet, consult your pediatrician. A simple blood test can diagnose anemia in most cases.

Some children are not anemic but still are deficient in iron. Some children with low iron have no symptoms at all, but those who do may have a decreased appetite and be irritable, fussy, and inattentive, and may develop sleep problems. Iron deficiency may result in developmental delays or poor school performance, even in children who are not anemic. These problems may improve when the children are given iron. Other signs of iron deficiency that may be unrelated to anemia include a tendency to eat unusual things, such as ice, dirt, clay, and cornstarch. This behavior, called pica, can be stressful for families but is generally not harmful unless the material eaten is toxic (e.g., contains lead). Usually the behavior improves after the iron deficiency is treated and as the child becomes older, although it may persist longer in children who are developmentally delayed.

Treatment

Since there are so many different types of anemia, it is very important to identify the cause before any treatment is begun. Talk to your child's pediatrician before starting any vitamins, iron, or other nutrients or over-the-counter medications. This is important, because such treatment may mask the real reason for the problem and thus delay the diagnosis. The treatment for anemia may include medications, dietary supplements, or dietary restrictions.

If the anemia is due to a lack of iron, your child will be given an iron-containing medication. This comes in a drop form for infants and a liquid or tablet form for older children. To avoid giving your child too much iron, or continuing it once it is no longer needed, your pediatrician will check your child's blood hemoglobin and/or iron levels at regular intervals. Do not stop giving the medication until the physician tells you it is no longer needed.

The following are a few tips concerning iron medication:

- It is best not to give iron with milk or other dairy products because milk blocks iron absorption.
- Vitamin C may enhance iron absorption, so you might want to follow the dose of iron with a serving of fresh fruit.
- Since liquid iron tends to turn the teeth a grayish black color temporarily, have your child swallow it rapidly and then rinse their mouth with water. You also may want to brush your child's teeth after every dose of iron. Tooth-staining from iron is not permanent.
- Storing iron medication in the refrigerator can decrease the bitterness, improving palatability and increasing your child's tolerance of it. Storing the iron this way will not lessen its effectiveness.
- Iron medications cause the stools to become a dark or black color. Don't be worried by this change.

Safety precautions: Iron medications can be poisonous if taken in excessive amounts. (Iron is one of the most common causes of poisoning in children under 5 years of age.) For that reason, keep this and all medication out of reach of small children.

Arrhythmias

Your child's heart rate normally will vary to some degree. Fever, crying, exercise, or other vigorous activity makes any heart beat faster. The younger the child, the faster the normal heart rate. As your child gets older, the heart rate will slow down. A resting heart rate of 130 to 150 beats per minute is normal for a newborn infant, but it is too fast for a 5-year-old child at rest. In a very athletic teenager, a resting heart rate of 50 to 60 beats per minute may be normal.

The heart's regular rhythm or beat is maintained by a small electrical circuit that runs through nerves in the walls of the heart. When the circuit is working properly, the heartbeat is quite regular, but when there's a problem in the circuit, an irregular heartbeat, or arrhythmia, can occur. Some children are born with abnormalities in this heart circuitry, but arrhythmias also can be caused by infections or chemical imbalances in the blood. Even in healthy children, there can be other variations in the rhythm of the heartbeat, including changes that occur just as a result of breathing. Such a fluctuation is called sinus arrhythmia and requires no special evaluation or treatment because it is normal.

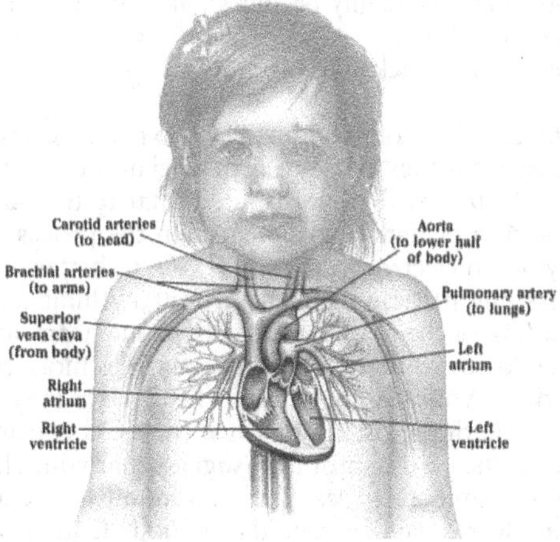

The heart

So-called premature heartbeats are another form of irregular rhythm that requires no treatment. If these occur in your child, they might say that their heart "skipped a beat" or did a "flip-flop." Usually these symptoms do not indicate the presence of significant heart disease.

If your pediatrician says that your child has a true arrhythmia, it could mean that their heart beats faster than normal (tachycardia), very fast (flutter), fast and with no regularity (fibrillation), or slower than normal (bradycardia), or that it has isolated early beats (premature beats). While true arrhythmias are not very common, when they do occur, they can be serious. On rare occasions they can cause fainting or even heart failure. Fortunately, they can be treated successfully, so it's important to detect arrhythmias as early as possible.

Signs and Symptoms

If your child has a true arrhythmia, your pediatrician may discover it during a routine visit. But should you notice any of the following warning signs between pediatric visits, notify your doctor immediately and seek emergency care:

- Your infant becomes sweaty and tired while feeding.
- Your infant suddenly becomes pale and listless; the body feels limp.
- Your infant blacks out or faints.

It's unlikely that your child will ever experience any of these symptoms, but if they do, your pediatrician (or the emergency medicine doctor) will perform additional tests and perhaps consult with a pediatric cardiologist. In the process the doctors may do an electrocardiogram (ECG) to better distinguish a normal sinus arrhythmia from a true arrhythmia. An ECG is the recording of the electrical activity of the heart, and it will allow the doctor to observe any irregularities more closely.

Sometimes your child's unusual heartbeats may occur at unpredictable times, often not when the ECG is being taken. In that case the cardiologist may suggest that your child carry a small portable recorder that continuously records their heartbeat over a one- to two-day period. During this time, you'll be asked to keep a log of your child's activities and symptoms. Comparing the ECG with your observations will help make a diagnosis. For example, if your child feels their heart "flutter" and becomes dizzy at 2:15 p.m. and the ECG shows their heart suddenly beating faster in an abnormal rhythm at the same time, the diagnosis of arrhythmia will probably be established.

Occasionally irregular heartbeats will occur only during exercise. If that's the case with your child, the cardiologist may have them ride a stationary bicycle or run on a treadmill while their heartbeat is being recorded. When your child is old enough to participate in sports, ask your pediatrician if any special tests or restrictions are necessary.

Heart Murmur

Technically, a heart murmur is simply a noise heard between the beats of the heart. When a doctor listens to the heart, they hear a sound like lub-dub, lub-dub, lub-dub. Most often, the period between the lub and the dub and between the dub and the lub is silent. If there is any sound during this period, it may be a murmur or an extra heart sound known as a gallop.

Heart murmurs are extremely common and are usually "functional" or "innocent" (that is, the sounds are caused by a healthy heart pumping blood normally). In preschool and school-age children, heart murmurs are almost never a concern. Most children with a murmur require no special care, and the sound eventually disappears.

If your child has such a murmur, the doctor will listen carefully to determine if this is a functional heart murmur or one that might indicate a problem. Usually, just by listening to its sound, the pediatrician will be able to tell if a murmur is innocent (normal blood flow through a normal heart). If necessary, they will consult a pediatric cardiologist to be certain, but additional tests are usually not needed. Sometimes a pediatrician will hear a murmur that sounds abnormal enough to indicate that something might be wrong with the heart. If the doctor suspects this, your child will be referred for an echocardiogram (ultrasound exam of the heart) or to a pediatric cardiologist to enable a precise diagnosis to be made.

Although some murmurs are normal and do not mean there is any underlying abnormality of the heart, other murmurs are more concerning. Such abnormal murmurs are not functional or innocent, and most likely they will require the attention of a pediatric cardiologist immediately. They may be due to abnormal connections between the pumping chambers (septal defects or "hole in the heart") or abnormalities in certain valves or arteries in the heart (e.g., narrowing of valves such as the aortic or pulmonary valve). Your infant will be observed for changes in skin color (turning blue), as well as breathing or feeding difficulties. They also may undergo additional tests, such as a chest X-ray, an electrocardiogram (ECG), and an ultrasound of the heart (echocardiogram). An echocardiogram creates a picture of the inside of the heart by using sound waves. The cardiologist and pediatrician together will make a decision as to next steps depending on the results of these tests. If all of these tests prove normal, then it is safe to conclude that the baby has an innocent murmur and they will not need to be seen again by a cardiologist.

When a specific condition called patent ductus arteriosus (PDA) occurs, it is often detected shortly after birth, most commonly in premature babies. In infants with PDA, blood circulates abnormally between the two major arteries that come off the heart. In most cases, the only symptom of PDA is a heart murmur until the ductus closes on its own shortly after birth, which often happens in otherwise healthy, full-term newborns. Sometimes, especially in premature babies, it may not close on its own, or it may be large and permit too much blood to pass through the lungs, which can place extra strain on the heart, forcing it to work harder and causing a rise in pressure in the arteries of the lungs.

A gallop is less common than a murmur but can indicate a more serious issue that must be evaluated right away. If your pediatrician detects a gallop, they will likely refer you to a cardiologist or an emergency department to have further testing. The most common cause of a gallop is heart failure, a condition in which the pressures inside the heart are high due to a weakness of the heart muscle. This weakness can occur due to gene mutations that may be inherited or be new (de novo), or due to the side effects of a viral infection on the heart. A gallop cannot be detected without a stethoscope. Other signs of heart failure to watch for in an infant are:

- Sweating while feeding
- Needing frequent breaks while feeding
- Vomiting and loss of appetite for more than a few days
- Difficulty breathing not explained by a respiratory infection

If your infant is displaying any of those symptoms, especially suddenly or if previously healthy, see your pediatrician or pediatric cardiologist. Heart failure can be diagnosed through testing, including a heart rhythm strip (electrocardiogram), heart ultrasound (echocardiogram), and chest X-ray showing a large heart size. A cardiologist will help determine what medications will be best for your child if they are diagnosed with heart failure, based on the result of various blood testing as well as physical examination findings.

Treatment

Functional or innocent heart murmurs are normal and therefore require no treatment. Children with this type of heart murmur do not need repeated evaluations or long-term follow-up care from cardiologists, nor do they require restrictions on sports or other physical activities. Innocent heart murmurs may be louder in situations like fever or if your child has anemia, and they generally disappear by mid-adolescence. Cardiologists don't know why they go away, any more than we know why they appear in the first place. In the meantime, don't be discouraged if the murmur is softer on one visit to the pediatrician and louder on the next. This may simply mean that your child's heart is beating at a slightly different rate each time. Most likely, this normal murmur will go away eventually.

Patent ductus arteriosus is a self-correcting problem in some cases; in others, medications can be used to close a PDA. But if the PDA remains open, it may need to be corrected surgically or with a catheter.

If other, more serious heart conditions are diagnosed from birth or shortly thereafter, and the evaluation reveals more serious defects, the pediatric cardiologist and pediatrician will consult a pediatric cardiac surgeon or a pediatric cardiac catheterization doctor, often at a children's hospital or large university hospital where complete pediatric cardiac diagnostic and intervention capabilities exist. If heart failure is diagnosed, initial management includes medications to manage the symptoms as well as diagnostic testing to try to identify the cause of the heart failure. In some cases, a heart pump or a heart transplant may be considered if medical therapies are not adequate.

Kawasaki Disease

Kawasaki disease is a rare systemic process whereby blood vessels throughout the body become inflamed. It is a potentially serious and perplexing disease, and its cause is unknown.

One sign of this disease includes fever, usually quite high, that lasts for at least five days, doesn't respond to antibiotics, and does not have an alternative cause. Fever should be present to consider a diagnosis of Kawasaki disease in the ill child; in addition, other signs must be present on examination. Most often, four of the six following signs appear in the first week of a typical case:

1. Rash over some or all of the body, often more severe in the diaper area, especially in infants under 12 months of age
2. Redness and swelling of the palms of the hands and the soles of the feet; in the later stage, peeling of the skin around the base of the nails
3. Red, swollen, and cracked lips and/or a strawberry tongue (red and bumpy)
4. Red, inflamed eyes, involving the sclerae (white part)
5. A single swollen lymph gland, or a cluster of enlarged lymph nodes, particularly on one side of the neck
6. Irritability (crankiness) or listlessness (lethargy); complaints of abdominal pain, headache, and/or joint pain

When Kawasaki-disease-associated inflammation of the blood vessels occurs, it may involve the arteries of the heart (the coronary arteries). Blood tests are used to demonstrate inflammation, and a heart ultrasound (echocardiogram) will be used to evaluate the coronary arteries in a child with Kawasaki disease. The echocardiogram can identify inflammation, which can weaken the walls of the blood vessels. In some cases, this weakening may even balloon out, causing aneurysms (blood-filled swellings of the blood vessels). In most cases the inflammation in the blood vessels appears to resolve after several months to years, but in some cases the coronary artery may become narrowed (stenotic).

Kawasaki disease occurs most frequently in Japan and Korea and in individuals of East Asian ancestry, but it can be found among all racial groups and on every continent. The exact number of cases is not known, but it is probably between 5,000 and 10,000 per year in the United States, typically occurring in infants between 18 and 24 months of age and in preschoolers. Kawasaki disease occurs rarely in infants between 6 weeks and 6 months of age; in this age group, unremitting fever may be the only sign noted. The peak age of occurrence in the United States is between 6 months and 5 years.

Kawasaki disease is not contagious. It is extremely uncommon for two children in the same household to get the disease. Likewise, it does not spread among children in childcare programs, where there is daily close contact. Although Kawasaki disease can occur in community outbreaks, particularly in the winter and early spring, no one knows the cause. Despite intensive research, no bacterium, virus, or toxin has been identified as a cause of the disease. No specific test makes the diagnosis. The diagnosis is made based on the signs of illness mentioned previously and by excluding other possible diseases.

Treatment

Kawasaki disease can be treated but not prevented. If it is diagnosed early enough, intravenous immunoglobulin (a mixture of human antibodies), also known as IVIG, can greatly reduce the risk of a child developing coronary aneurysms. If your child receives IVIG, this may impact the routine immunization schedule for so-called live virus vaccines (varicella and MMR), so you should check with your pediatrician. However, all inactivated vaccines, including influenza vaccine, should be given on schedule.

In addition to IVIG, the child with Kawasaki disease will receive aspirin, initially in high doses during the first stage of the disease and in low doses during the recovery stage, until your pediatrician tells you it is okay to stop. Aspirin can decrease the tendency of blood to clot in damaged blood vessels, and it is used to prevent clots from developing in the coronary arteries. Although it's appropriate to use aspirin to treat Kawasaki disease, aspirin should not be used to treat children with minor illnesses (e.g., a cold or influenza), as it has been linked with a serious disease called Reye syndrome. If a child is treated with aspirin for Kawasaki disease and exposed to influenza or chickenpox, the aspirin should be stopped, and parents should discuss a suitable temporary substitute medicine with their pediatrician.

Sickle Cell Disease

Sickle cell disease (SCD) is a group of chronic genetic disorders affecting the red blood cells. In children with SCD, the red cells in the blood become sickle-shaped under stresses such as low oxygen levels, cold temperatures, and infection, impacting how well the red blood cells transport oxygen around the body.

There are several types of sickle cell disease. The best-known is sickle cell anemia, or hemoglobin SS disease. Others include sickle–hemoglobin C disease and two types of sickle beta-thalassemia. All of these disorders in the SCD complex have similar symptoms, such as anemia (shortage of red blood cells), episodes of severe pain, and infections. (See Signs and Symptoms, *page 617*.)

In the United States, about 2,000 newborns each year are diagnosed with SCD. It can occur in children of any race or ethnicity, including those whose ancestors come from Africa, South and Central America, India, Saudi Arabia, Italy, Greece, or Turkey.

In healthy children, red blood cells are normally disc-shaped and flexible, and travel easily through blood vessels, transporting oxygen from the lungs to every part of the body. Children with SCD have abnormalities in hemoglobin (a component of every red blood cell) that can distort the shape of these red cells. The irregularly shaped red cells become sticky, clumping together and interfering with the flow of nourishing blood to organs and limbs, which can be painful. These cells also survive only a few days from the time they are released into the circulation, in contrast to four months for normal red blood cells. This causes ongoing anemia.

Some children do not have the disease itself, but they carry the gene responsible for causing it, and they can pass it along when they have children of their own. If a child inherits the sickle cell gene from one parent but not the other, pediatricians categorize the child as having sickle cell trait. Children with sickle cell trait do not have anemia or episodes of pain associated with sickle cell disease.

Signs and Symptoms

In most cases, infants with SCD appear healthy at birth. However, after a child is a few months old, symptoms may emerge that can range from mild to severe.

Common signs and symptoms of SCD include:

- Inflammation and swelling of the hands and/or feet (called dactylitis or hand-foot syndrome); this is commonly the first symptom of SCD
- Anemia
- Pain
- Pallor
- Jaundice (yellowing of the skin and eyes)
- Susceptibility to infections
- Delayed growth
- Enlarged spleen, which the doctor can feel in the abdomen

A sickle cell crisis may occur suddenly, with an episode of pain that typically affects the bones, joints, or abdomen. The intensity of pain can vary, and it can last from hours to many weeks. The trigger for these crises is unclear in many cases, although blocked blood flow plays a role, and in some cases so can infections. Serious SCD complications can develop, including pneumonia (called acute chest syndrome in children with SCD), stroke, and organ damage (spleen, kidney, liver, or lung).

Treatment

If your child has SCD, they should be diagnosed as early as possible so that appropriate treatment can be planned and started. Fortunately, most cases of SCD can be detected through a simple screening blood test that is universally given to newborns in all states.

Children with SCD need long-term care to minimize the risk of complications, to address problems when they occur, to prevent life-threatening infection, and to be able to access new treatments as they are developed. Commonly prescribed treatments include the following:

- Mild pain can be relieved with over-the-counter analgesic medications, such as acetaminophen or non-steroidal anti-inflammatory drugs (NSAIDs) such as ibuprofen. Heating pads also can be used for pain relief. In addition, good hydration is important.
- Antibiotics, typically a form of penicillin, should be prescribed for all children with sickle cell anemia (HbSS) and sickle beta-thalassemia (HbSS0), beginning by 2 months of age and given continuously until at least the age of 5 years. These medications are a preventive measure to reduce the risk of serious bacterial infection.
- Children with SCD should receive all childhood immunizations as recommended by the American Academy of Pediatrics (see the Appendix, *pages 696–97*) as well as some additional vaccines against meningitis and pneumonia.
- Children with sickle cell anemia or HbSS0 thalassemia should begin hydroxyurea treatment at 9 months of age. Hydroxyurea is a once-daily medication that decreases the number of pain crises, pneumonias, and blood transfusions.
- Children with sickle cell anemia or HbSS0 thalassemia should have a transcranial Doppler (TCD) every year beginning at 2 years of age. TCD is an ultrasound of the brain that helps to identify children who are at highest risk of stroke so that they can begin treatment to reduce that risk.

Your child with SCD can benefit from various lifestyle measures. They should get plenty of rest and sleep. They should drink lots of water (particularly in warm weather) and avoid becoming overly hot or cold.

If your child's pain becomes severe, or if they develop other serious symptoms or complications, your pediatrician may recommend hospitalization. While hospitalized, your child could receive:

- Morphine or other medications given intravenously (through a vein) for pain relief
- Intravenous antibiotics that can manage an infection if one develops

- Blood transfusions that can raise the number of red blood cells
- Supplemental oxygen given through a mask that can add oxygen to the blood

Because relatively mild symptoms (fever, pale skin, abdominal pain) can quickly progress to serious illness, parents should talk with their pediatrician in advance to make sure that the family has around-the-clock access to a medical facility experienced in treating SCD. If your child develops a fever, contact your pediatrician at once because of the risk of a major infection.

CHAPTER 26

IMMUNIZATIONS

Immunizations have helped children stay healthy for more than a century. Routine vaccines have become one of the best weapons available to protect your child against major childhood diseases.

Immunizations, in fact, are one of the greatest public health success stories of our times. Many diseases that were once a routine part of growing up, some of them life-threatening, are now preventable and relatively rare, thanks to improvements in sanitation, better nutrition, less crowded living conditions, antibiotics—and vaccines. At one time, most people did not reach adulthood without someone in their family or circle of friends being touched by a very serious illness or death caused by an infectious disease. But now those same diseases are at record low levels in the United States as well as many other countries in the world—and that's because immunization rates are at record highs. Routine immunization against sixteen infectious diseases is now recommended between birth and 18 years of age as well as annual immunization against influenza and COVID-19. Vaccines work extremely well—most are more than 90 percent effective in preventing diseases—so they are valuable tools for keeping children safe and healthy. When parents learn of the risks of these infections—for example, whooping cough causing seizures, brain disease, and even death—the argument in favor of childhood immunizations is persuasive. Although chickenpox, for example, is usually a mild disease, before the vaccine was available more than 11,000 children were hospitalized each year for complications from infection. Before the vaccine, about 100 people per year died of chickenpox complications, and untold numbers were scarred. But now this disease can be prevented.

Important and Safe

Because many parents (and even some doctors) have never seen a child with whooping cough, diphtheria, tetanus, polio, or measles, mothers and fathers sometimes ask their pediatrician whether their child really needs vaccines at all. But while many of the illnesses that once caused lifelong disabilities or even death are now uncommon, they haven't been wiped out completely. Yes, they are preventable, but the germs that cause many of them are still around and are regularly brought into the country by international travelers.

Just consider the case of the *Haemophilus influenzae* type b (Hib) vaccine. It protects children from serious childhood diseases like meningitis (an inflammation of the tissues that cover the brain and spinal cord) and epiglottitis (a throat infection that can block the airway). Before this vaccine became available in the 1980s, there were about 20,000 cases of Hib disease in the United States every year. *H. influenzae* type b was the most common cause of bacterial meningitis in the United States, and it was a major cause of intellectual disability and deafness. Today, because most Hib disease is prevented by immunization, there are fewer than 100 cases annually in the United States.

MORE ABOUT IMMUNIZATIONS

When you have your children immunized:

- You protect them from dangerous and potentially fatal diseases.
- You reduce the severity of the disease if your children happen to get it.
- You cut down the chances that contagious diseases will spread.
- You safeguard other people in your community who are too young to receive the vaccine or cannot receive vaccinations due to medical issues.

Also of Note

- After receiving a vaccine, some children experience mild symptoms such as a low fever and fussiness, as well as tenderness, swelling, or redness where the shot was given. They also may sleep a little longer than usual in the day or two after receiving the shot.

- On very rare occasions, children may react to a vaccine with a more concerning response, such as a seizure, rash, or high fever. Call your pediatrician if your child develops a fever over 103 degrees Fahrenheit (39.4 degrees Celsius), a rash all over the body (including hives), a large amount of swelling in the limb where the shot was given, or any other symptoms that worry you. These guidelines apply to all the immunizations described in this chapter.

At the same time, vaccines are very safe—but they're not perfect. Like medications, they can cause occasional reactions, but usually these are mild (see More About Immunizations, *page 621*). Side effects like redness or discomfort at the site of the injection can happen. They appear soon after the shot is given, and then usually go away within a day or two. Your child also may be fussy for a day or two following immunization. Although more severe reactions can occur, they are much less common. A very small number of children with certain health conditions should not receive certain vaccines. Talk to your doctor if your child had a serious reaction to a previous vaccine, is allergic to a vaccine component, has a problem fighting infections, has been diagnosed with immunodeficiency, or is sick on the day of the appointment. This type of information can help your doctor determine if your child should postpone or not receive some vaccines. In years past, some people were worried about a preservative called thimerosal, which for decades had been added to some vaccines to prevent contamination of vaccines by bacteria. Thimerosal has a small amount of organic mercury in it. Scientists wanted to investigate whether there was any link between disorders such as autism and vaccines that contain thimerosal. Numerous rigorous scientific studies in multiple countries have shown there is no causal link between thimerosal in vaccines and autism. There is no credible evidence linking vaccines, or any component of them, to autism. In addition, all vaccines now manufactured for infants and almost all for older children and adults in the United States are thimerosal-free or contain only trace amounts.

While some parents also worry that their child is receiving "too many vaccines" at one time, there is plenty of research showing that multiple childhood vaccines can be given at the same time safely. In fact, a vaccine cannot be licensed by the FDA and recommended until the manufacturers show that it can be given safely with other recommended vaccines. And although children receive more vaccines than in years past, the ones they're receiving have been improved, so children are actually receiving fewer antigens (substances that help a body build up an immunity) with each shot than in previous years. These shots are effective and safe when they're given according to the guidelines recommended by the American Academy of Pediatrics.

The important point to remember is that getting these vaccine-preventable diseases is much more dangerous than getting the vaccines. If you have questions or concerns about immunizations, talk with your pediatrician.

What Shots Does Your Child Need?

Your child should be vaccinated according to the schedule of immunizations recommended by the American Academy of Pediatrics. The entire schedule appears in the Appendix (*pages 696–97*) and includes the following immunizations for young children. Please refer to the chart often for information on the immunizations your child needs and when they should be given. Also, recommendations change as vaccines are improved and new ones are developed, so be sure to speak with your pediatrician or visit aap.org for the most current immunization schedule.

Chickenpox (Varicella)

The vaccine to protect against the varicella virus became available in 1995; it not only protects against chickenpox, but also reduces the risk of shingles in later life. Natural chickenpox infection can cause a fever and an itchy, blister-like rash all over the body. There may be as many as 250 to 500 of these blisters. Sometimes the infection causes serious complications, including skin infections, brain swelling, and pneumonia.

EASING THE HURT

Shots can hurt. When your child receives a vaccine, they can be uncomfortable and may cry for several minutes. But fortunately, any pain is very short-lived. At the moment the immunization is given, you may be able to soften the experience by distracting your child. Talk soothingly and make eye contact with them. Afterward, comfort and play with them for a while.

If your child develops side effects, you may be able to ease any fever or irritability by giving them acetaminophen or ibuprofen. The routine use of these medications prior to the child developing symptoms is not recommended. Be sure to discuss the use and proper dosage of these medicines with your pediatrician or Poison Help at 1-800-222-1222. If your child has pain at the site where the shot was given, your doctor might recommend applying cool compresses to lessen the discomfort. Certainly, if any reaction makes your child uncomfortable for more than four hours, notify your pediatrician, who will want to note it in your child's records and advise you on what to do.

Before immunizing your child, it's a good idea to talk with your doctor about what reactions could occur, if any. If unusual or severe reactions (like a fever or changes in behavior) happened in the past, you and your pediatrician should discuss the pros and cons of whether it's appropriate to give another dose of the same vaccine at the scheduled time.

As painful as it may be for you to watch your child experience the discomfort of a shot, don't lose sight of the fact that you're doing enormous good for them by making sure they are protected from the diseases that vaccines can prevent.

Varicella vaccine is safe. Reactions to the vaccine are generally mild. About 20 percent of children will develop mild pain, redness, or swelling at the injection site. If your child has a weakened immune system or is taking steroids or other drugs that can affect the immune system, check with your doctor before they get the chickenpox immunization.

Two doses of the vaccine provide more than 90 percent protection against infection. Currently if someone who has been vaccinated does get chickenpox, it is usually very mild.

They will have few spots, are less likely to have a fever or serious complications, and will recover faster.

COVID-19 (SARS-CoV-2)

COVID-19, or SARS-CoV-2, is a respiratory virus that can cause severe, life-threatening illness affecting not only the lungs, but also the brain, the heart, the kidneys, the intestines, and other organ systems. Long-term complications can include chronic tiredness/weakness and MIS-C, a serious multisystem inflammatory syndrome that can occur in children who have had COVID-19. COVID is highly contagious and especially dangerous to children with underlying conditions like heart disease, asthma, or complications of premature birth. The COVID vaccine, administered starting at 6 months of age, is safe and highly effective at preventing serious disease from COVID. Vaccinating your child can help protect every member of the family and even help safeguard your community against this infection.

Diphtheria, Tetanus, and Pertussis

The DTaP vaccine protects your child against diphtheria (D), tetanus (T), and pertussis (aP). The diphtheria portion of this vaccine guards against a throat infection that can trigger breathing difficulties, paralysis, or heart failure. The tetanus portion protects against a disease that causes the tightening or "locking" of all of the muscles in the body, especially the jaw, and is potentially fatal. The vaccine for pertussis (also called whooping cough) prevents bacteria from causing severe and violent coughing spells in infants that can make breathing and eating difficult.

What about expected side effects? Redness and tenderness may occur with the diphtheria and tetanus portions of the vaccine. Severe, but very rare, problems that have been reported after the DTaP vaccine include seizures, coma, and permanent brain damage. These are extremely rare and have occurred only in children with other underlying disorders. For the vast majority of children, the dangers of the diseases themselves far outweigh any risks of the shots. Keep in mind, for example, that 1 out of 13 people who get a tetanus infection die from it, 1 out of 100 babies under 6 months who get a pertussis infection die, and about 1 out of 10 people who get a respiratory diphtheria infection die of complications. Immunizations are very important to protect your child from these diseases. To fully protect the newborn, pregnant mothers should receive a dose of the adult version of the vaccine, Tdap, during the third trimester of pregnancy.

Hepatitis A

Like the hepatitis B vaccine (see *below*), the hepatitis A immunization protects against a common liver disease, which your child can catch by eating food or drinking water contaminated with the hepatitis A virus. This common infection can sometimes be spread in childcare settings when caregivers do not follow good handwashing procedures.

The hepatitis A vaccine is very safe. The first dose is given at 12 months of age, followed by a second dose six to twelve months later. Reactions to this vaccine are very uncommon and usually are nothing more than soreness where the shot was given.

Hepatitis B

The hepatitis B vaccine offers protection against a liver disease that can be spread by infected blood and body fluids. The infection is caused by the hepatitis B virus and can lead to cirrhosis and liver cancer. The infection can be passed from an infected mother to their baby at the time of birth, or from one household member to another.

The first hepatitis B shot should be given within twelve hours after birth, even before your baby is discharged from the hospital. A second dose should be given at 1 to 2 months of age, and a third dose when the child is 6 to 18 months old. The hepatitis B vaccine is very safe. Severe problems are rare. Possible mild reactions include soreness where the shot was given, and occasionally a fever.

Hib (*Haemophilus influenzae* Type b)

The Hib vaccine protects your child from the bacterium *Haemophilus influenzae* type b, which was the leading cause of meningitis before the vaccine became available. This serious disease occurs most often in children from ages 6 months to 5 years, leading to symptoms such as fever, seizures, vomiting, and a stiff neck. Meningitis also can cause hearing loss, brain damage, and death. These same bacteria can lead to a rare but serious inflammation of the throat called epiglottitis.

The first Hib vaccine should be given at 2 months of age, with additional doses to follow. It is important to have your child immunized with this vaccine in order to lower their risk of getting Hib diseases during the early years, when they are most vulnerable to these infections. There are no reasons to withhold this vaccine from your child unless they have had a rare life-threatening allergic reaction to a previous dose of the vaccine.

Influenza

Influenza (the flu) is a respiratory illness caused by a virus. This infection leads to symptoms such as a high fever, muscle aches, sore throat, and cough, and it may take your child several days of rest to recover. There are often two types of influenza vaccine available to protect your child:

- The inactivated (killed) vaccine, given by injection (flu shot)
- The live attenuated (weakened) vaccine, sprayed into the nostrils (flu mist)

All children 6 months of age and older—including all children, adolescents, young adults, and those caring for a child too young to receive a vaccine (such as a newborn)—should receive the annual seasonal influenza vaccine unless there is a specific and uncommon contraindication to this vaccine. Special efforts should be made to vaccinate those who have chronic medical conditions that increase their risk of severe influenza complications (such as asthma, diabetes, immunosuppression, or neurological disorders). The formulation of the influenza vaccine changes yearly, depending on the expected prevalence of the various influenza strains. This is one reason the influenza vaccine must be administered every year. It is also important to be sure that all individuals caring for young children and for children with chronic medical conditions receive an annual flu vaccine.

Measles, Mumps, and Rubella (MMR)

The measles portion of the MMR vaccine protects against an infection that causes an extensive red or brownish blotchy rash, as well as flu-like symptoms; measles can lead to severe complications such as pneumonia, seizures, and brain damage. The mumps vaccine gives your child protection against a virus that causes swollen salivary glands, a fever, and headaches, and can lead to deafness, meningitis, and painful swelling of the testicles or ovaries. The rubella (German measles) vaccine guards against an infection in which the child may have a pink rash and swollen, tender glands at the back of the neck. Being immunized is the best way to prevent rubella. The vaccine usually is administered as part of a three-in-one shot called MMR (measles, mumps, rubella) or a four-in-one shot called MMRV (measles, mumps, rubella, varicella), given when the child is 12 to 15 months old. In addition, the vaccine protects pregnant women from passing the rubella virus to the developing fetus.

There was considerable media attention in the past about a possible connection between the MMR vaccine and autism. In fact, extensive research has shown that there is no connection. There has been confusion because autism is often diagnosed at about the age at which children receive the MMR vaccine. This has led to the erroneous conclusion that the vaccine somehow causes autism. But, in fact, studies now clearly show that autism actually begins before a baby is born and vaccines play no role.

Use of the MMR vaccine was once discouraged for children who had an allergy to eggs. But because the MMR vaccine now contains only trace amounts of egg protein and research has shown that the vaccine can be safely administered to egg-allergic children without special precautions, the recommendation has been adjusted. However, if your child is taking any medication that interferes with the immune system, or if their immune system is weakened for any reason, they generally should not receive this immunization. As for side effects, sometimes, around seven to twelve days after the MMR vaccine, a child may develop mild swelling of the glands in the cheeks or neck, and a fever or mild rash. If this mild vaccine side effect does occur, it is important to note that it is not dangerous or contagious and will resolve on its own. Such side effects occur less often after the second dose. Severe problems such as seizures caused by fever occur in 1 out of 3,000 doses. Serious allergic reactions are very rare (about 1 out of 1 million doses).

Pneumococcal Vaccine

The pneumococcal conjugate vaccine protects your child from meningitis, as well as common forms of pneumonia, blood infections, and certain ear infections. Four doses are recommended starting at 2 months of age; subsequent dosages are given at 4 months, 6 months, and 12 to 18 months. A pneumococcal infection is one of the most common causes of vaccine-preventable deaths in children. Only mild reactions are associated with the vaccine. Some children become fussy or drowsy, lose their appetite, or develop a fever.

Polio

The polio vaccine provides protection from the virus that causes polio. While some infections with the virus cause no symptoms, polio can cause paralysis and death in other cases. Before the polio vaccine was available, millions of children throughout the world were left paralyzed from polio.

Today, all children need four doses of the polio vaccine before they start school, beginning with shots at 2 months of age. The inactivated polio vaccine is given as shots, and there is no risk of the vaccine causing the disease.

Rotavirus

The rotavirus vaccine protects against a potentially serious stomach virus (often referred to as "stomach flu"), which can cause vomiting, diarrhea, and related symptoms in children. Before the vaccine was available, rotavirus was the most common cause of severe diarrhea in children under the age of 2 years. In the United States before the rotavirus vaccine was given, about 50,000 children under 5 years of age were hospitalized each year because of rotavirus infection.

The rotavirus vaccine is an oral vaccine, given in a two- or three-dose series between 2 and 8 months of age. Some children may experience mild, temporary diarrhea or, rarely, vomiting within seven days of getting a dose of the rotavirus vaccine. There are no severe reactions associated with this vaccine. As with some other vaccines mentioned earlier, talk with your doctor before getting the rotavirus vaccine if your child's immune system might be weakened by conditions like HIV or steroid use. If your child has been diagnosed with severe combined immunodeficiency, they should not receive the rotavirus vaccine, as it is contraindicated in these patients or those who have a history of GI disease.

CHAPTER 27

MEDIA

Technologies such as TV, mobile devices, and internet-related games offer entertainment, culture, and education to our children. While it may offer many benefits, media use has also been associated with the risk of obesity, sleep issues, aggressive behaviors, and attention issues in preschool- and school-age children. When it comes to incorporating technology into your children's daily routine, they need your experience, judgment, and supervision.

Development and Learning

Children younger than 15 to 18 months of age may be fascinated by electronic screens. Starting as soon as their vision permits (around 6 months of age), they will stare at the colors and patterns on the screens, and they may even swipe and tap around as much as their developing motor skills allow. Parents can easily misinterpret this activity as a child understanding what they see in the way that older children and adults do. Children in this age range, however, do not yet have the mental skills to make sense of screen programming. They can be distracted by screens, but research shows they don't learn from them, no matter what the program or app suggests.

Instead, babies and toddlers learn by exploring their worlds physically, usually in the company of a parent or other caring adult. Children learn through reading, singing, rocking, clapping, and playing. Anything that distracts from these three-dimensional activities, including screen media, can interfere with learning. For this reason, the American Academy of Pediatrics strongly discourages screen time for children under 18 months of age with the exception of live video chatting in the company of a parent or caregiver, usually used to keep children in touch with distant loved ones.

Starting around 15 months of age, children may be able to learn from some screen content, but only when a parent is helping them process and understand the content. High-quality screen programming may be a limited option for children over age 18 months, but it should be used as a companion to in-person learning, not as a substitute. Children over 3 years of age can learn numbers, letters, words, and even the concept of kindness from well-crafted programming. Of the thousands of apps that promise to help teach children, very few have been rigorously studied. Before using any digital media content, parents should research whether it has any proven educational benefit. However, research shows that programming that is more interactive functions as a better teacher than programs that are passively viewed. Co-viewing with an engaged parent or caregiver helps even more, so take time to view or play with your child during digital media use.

Young children with heavy media use are at risk for delays in language development once they start school, as they may experience less "talk time" with adults when screens are on, even in the background. Research shows that this talk time is valuable for children's emerging language development. And when parents are watching their own programs and using mobile devices or computers, they may be distracted and engage in less parent-child interaction. Screen use by parents is associated with fewer parent-child verbal and non-verbal interactions, and parents may display less patience and more frustration with their children's behavior, some of which may be a plea for parental attention.

Background media may also interfere with a young child's learning from play and activities. Research shows that even when a show is not intended for a child audience, a child will glance up at the screen three times every minute. It disrupts a child's concentration when they are "at work" (playing). Children are less focused and more likely to move on to a new toy more quickly when a screen is on.

Where We Stand

Although the American Academy of Pediatrics does not hold media solely responsible for violence in our society, research shows that violence in television, movies, or video games has a clear effect on the behavior of children and contributes to the frequency with which aggression is used to resolve conflict. Entertainment media can also distort reality on matters such as drugs, alcohol, tobacco, sexuality, and family and community relations.

We encourage parents to manage both the quantity and the quality of their family's screen time. Parents can create a healthy media diet and lead by example. Children's TV programming is supported by commercial advertisers whose primary motivation is to sell products and create brand loyalty. Young children are not prepared to distinguish between programs and the commercials that interrupt them, nor do they understand that commercials are designed to sell them (and their parents) something.

Together, parents, broadcasters, programmers, and advertisers must be held responsible for the media that children consume. The American Academy of Pediatrics strongly supports legislative efforts to improve the quality of children's programming. We urge parents to limit and monitor the amount of screen time (including television, videos, computers, and video games) for their children, to monitor what their children are watching, and to watch media with them to help them learn from what they see.

Sleep

Some parents may use screen media to help their children settle down in the evening. However, screens typically emit a lot of light with wavelengths at the bluer end of the spectrum, and blue light has been proven to interfere with sleep. Screen use in early childhood contributes to delayed onset of sleep, shorter time asleep, and poorer-quality sleep. Poor sleep habits have adverse effects on mood, behavior, weight, and learning.

Ideally, screens should be off for at least sixty minutes prior to bedtime, and screen use should never interfere with or take the place of bath time, stories, puzzles, or drawing. If your child needs sound to drown out household noises, consider buying a specialized sound machine or even a box fan to create white noise. Keep the volume low, however, because young children are very susceptible to hearing loss from prolonged noise exposure.

CHAPTER 28

MUSCULOSKELETAL PROBLEMS

Arthritis

Arthritis involves inflammation of the joints that may produce swelling, stiffness, redness, heat, tenderness, and pain with motion. Although arthritis is typically thought of as a condition of the elderly, children can develop arthritis, too. The four most common forms of childhood arthritis are discussed here.

Bacterial Infection of a Joint (Septic Arthritis) or Bone (Osteomyelitis)

When a joint or bone becomes infected with bacteria, it becomes very painful, hot, swollen, and stiff. An affected child will often walk with a limp, refuse to bear weight, or have decreased movement in an arm. An affected child also will typically have a fever, and very young children may simply be irritable and refuse to walk or use an extremity. Notify your pediatrician immediately if these signs or symptoms appear, as rapid treatment can prevent further joint or bone damage. If infection involves the hip or other deep and inaccessible joints or bones, it can be difficult to diagnose, and infection of the large weight-bearing joints and bones is a very serious condition that needs to be properly diagnosed and treated by a specialist (usually an orthopedist). Treatment may include imaging such as X-ray or ultrasound, needle aspiration or surgical drainage of the infected joint or bone, and intravenous (IV) antibiotics.

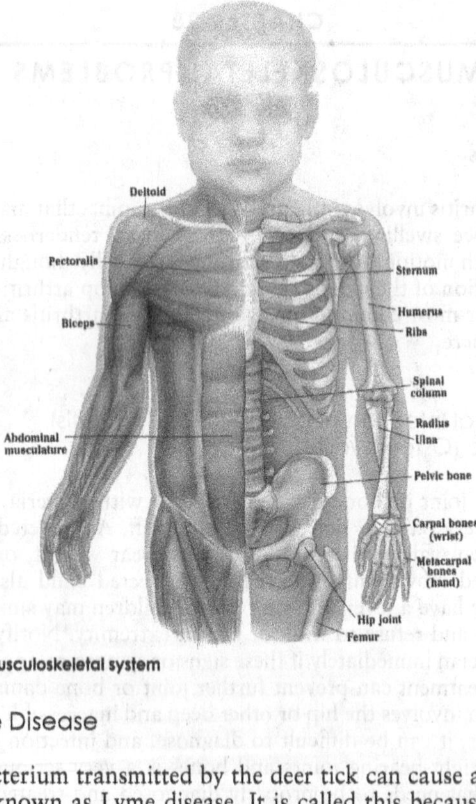

Musculoskeletal system

Lyme Disease

A bacterium transmitted by the deer tick can cause an infection known as Lyme disease. It is called this because it was first diagnosed in a child in Old Lyme, Connecticut. This infection often starts with a red mark that is surrounded by a light ring or halo (having the appearance of a red-and-white target) at the site where your child was bitten by a deer tick. Later, a similar but smaller rash may appear on other areas of the body. Your child also may develop flu-like symptoms such as headache, fever, swollen lymph nodes, fatigue, and muscle aches. More rarely, Lyme disease can cause symptoms involving the nervous system, eyes, or heart. Arthritis then typically develops weeks to months after the skin rash. If the arthritis is severe, medications can be prescribed to control inflammation and pain until the condition gradually resolves on its own.

Symptomatic Lyme disease is treated with antibiotics. However, the American Academy of Pediatrics does not recommend routinely taking antibiotics after a tick bite, for several reasons: the fact that most tick bites do not transmit the germ that causes Lyme disease, the possible side effects of antibiotics, the cost of treatment, and the risk of promoting antibiotic-resistant bacteria. The Academy also does not recommend testing your child's blood for Lyme disease shortly after a tick bite, since it takes quite a while for antibodies to show up in the blood even with an infected tick bite. To prevent Lyme disease, your child should avoid tick-infested areas such as wooded regions, high grasses, or marshes. Children also can protect themselves from ticks by wearing long-sleeved shirts, tucking their pants into their socks, and using an insect repellent that has DEET or picaridin as the active ingredient when outside. (See *pages 407, 663* for more information on DEET.) Almost all cases of Lyme disease can be readily treated with antibiotics, even if arthritis develops.

HOW TO REMOVE A TICK

1. Gently cleanse the area with an alcohol-soaked sponge or cotton ball.
2. Using forceps, tweezers, or fingers (protected by a tissue or cloth), grasp the tick as near to the mouth parts and as close to the child's skin as possible.
3. Using gentle but steady tension, pull the entire tick up and out.
4. Be sure the tick is dead before disposing of it. Removal and disposal of ticks should be done with a protective barrier (tissue or cloth) so you do not get exposed to any bacteria or infectious agents that could be spread by a tick.
5. After the tick is out, cleanse the bitten area thoroughly with alcohol or other cleansing (soap) agent.

Bowlegs and Knock-Knees

Toddlers' legs often have a bowed appearance. In fact, many children have bowing of the legs until they are about 2 years old. After this age, they often will look progressively knock-kneed until they are about 6 years of age; afterward this returns to normal. At times, children may not have straight lower legs until they are 9 or 10 years old.

Bowlegs and knock-knees usually are variations of normal and typically require no specific treatment. In most cases a child's legs will straighten naturally by the teen years, but treatment may become necessary if there is a severe deformity or the deformity occurs during the teen years. Bracing, corrective shoes, and special exercises are rarely helpful except for severe deformities, and they may hinder a child's physical development and cause unnecessary emotional stress. Rarely, bowlegs or knock-knees are the result of a disease. Arthritis, injury to the growth plate around the knee (see Fractures/Broken Bones, *page 508*), infection, tumor, Blount's disease (a growth disorder of the knee and shinbone), and rickets (caused by vitamin D deficiency) all can cause changes in the curvature of the legs.

Here are some signs that suggest a child's bowlegs or knock-knees may be caused by a serious problem:

- The curvature is extreme.
- Only one side is affected.
- The bowlegs get worse after age 2.
- The knock-knees persist after age 7.
- Your child also is unusually short for their age.
- Your child has trouble walking or running, or often stumbles and falls.

If your child shows any of these signs, talk to your pediatrician. In some cases, treatment, including referral to a pediatric orthopedist, may be needed.

Elbow Injuries

A pulled elbow (also known as nursemaid's elbow) is a common, painful injury generally among children under 4 years old. It occurs when the tissue of the outer part of the elbow slips between the bones of the joint. This happens because the child's elbow joint is loose enough to separate slightly when their arm is pulled to full length (while being lifted by the forearm, yanked, or swung by the hand or wrist). The nearby tissue slides into the space created by the stretching and becomes trapped after the joint returns to its normal position.

A nursemaid's elbow injury usually doesn't cause swelling, but the child will complain that the elbow hurts, or cry when their arm is moved. A child will typically hold their arm close to the side, with the elbow slightly bent and the palm turned toward the body. If someone tries to straighten the elbow or turn the palm upward, the child will resist because of the pain.

Treating Nursemaid's Elbow

This injury should be treated by a pediatrician or other trained healthcare provider. Since elbow pain can also be due to a fracture, especially if the child falls onto an outstretched hand, your pediatrician may need to consider this before the elbow is "reduced," or put back into place.

Your doctor will check the injured area for swelling and tenderness and any limitation of motion. If an injury other than nursemaid's elbow is suspected, X-rays may be taken. If no fracture is noted, the doctor will move and twist and flex the arm gently to release the trapped tissue and allow the elbow to return to its normal position. Once the elbow has been moved back in place, the child will generally feel immediate relief and within a few minutes should be using their arm normally without any discomfort. Occasionally the doctor may recommend a sling for comfort for two or three days, particularly if several hours have passed before the injury is treated successfully. If the injury occurred several days earlier, a hard splint or cast may be used to protect the joint for one to two weeks. Persistent pain after a reduction may mean that a fracture occurred that may not have been apparent at the time of initial X-rays.

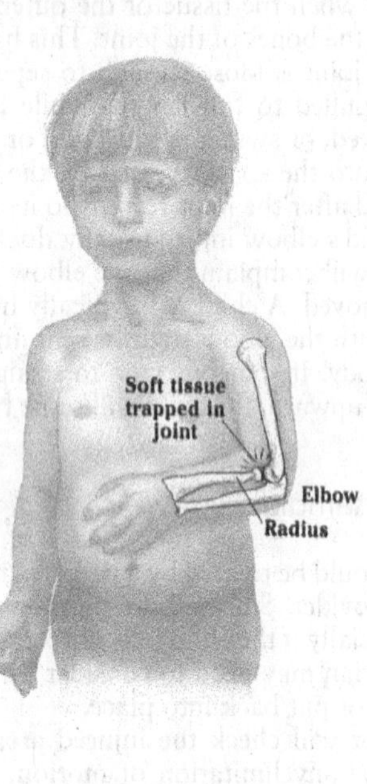

Prevention

Nursemaid's elbow can be prevented by not pulling or lifting your child by the hands or wrists or swinging them by the arms. Instead, lift your child by grasping their body under the armpit.

Flat Feet/Fallen Arches

Babies are often born with flat feet, which may persist well into childhood. This occurs because children's bones and joints are flexible, causing their feet to flatten when they stand. Young babies also have a fat pad on the inner border of their feet that hides the arch. You still can see the arch if you lift your baby up to stand on the tips of the toes, but it may disappear when they're standing normally. The foot may also turn out, increasing the weight on the inner side and making it appear even more flattened.

Normally, flat feet disappear by age 6 as the feet become less flexible and the arches develop with increased leg muscle strength. Only about one or two out of every ten children will continue to have flat feet into adulthood. For children who do not develop an arch, treatment is not recommended unless the foot is stiff or painful, which may mean that there is a connection between some of the small foot bones called a tarsal coalition (fused or connected bones), in which case an X-ray is indicated. Shoe inserts won't help your child develop an arch and may cause more problems than the flat feet themselves.

However, certain forms of flat feet may need to be treated differently. For instance, a child may have tightness of the heel cord (Achilles tendon) that limits the motion of their foot. This tightness can result in a flat foot, but it usually can be treated with special stretching exercises to lengthen the heel cord. Rarely, a child will have truly rigid flat feet due to a tarsal coalition, a condition that can cause problems. These children have difficulty moving the foot up and down or side to side at the ankle. The rigid foot can cause pain and, if left untreated, can lead to arthritis. This rigid type of flat foot is seldom seen in an infant or very young child.

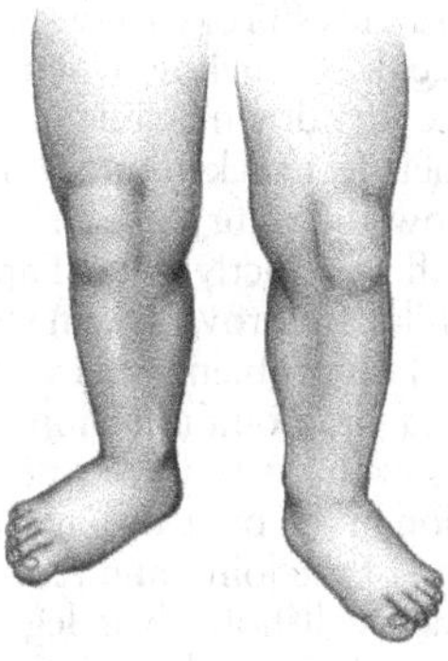

Symptoms that should be checked by a pediatrician include foot pain, sores or pressure areas on the inner side of the foot, a stiff foot, limited side-to-side foot motion, or limited up-and-down ankle motion. For further treatment you should see a pediatric orthopedic surgeon or podiatrist experienced in childhood foot conditions.

Limp

Limping can be caused by something as simple as a pebble in your child's shoe, a blister on their foot, or a pulled muscle. But a limp also can be a sign of more serious trouble, such as a broken bone, arthritis, infection, or hip dysplasia. For that reason, it's important to have your pediatrician examine a child with a limp to make sure that no serious problems exist.

Some children limp when they first learn how to walk. Early limping can be caused by neurological damage (such as cerebral palsy; see *page 443*). But any limp around the time your child begins to walk needs to be investigated as soon as possible, since the longer it goes untreated, the more difficult it may be to correct. Once walking is well established, significant sudden limping usually indicates one of several conditions:

- A "toddler fracture"
- Hip injury or inflammation (synovitis)
- Previously undiagnosed developmental dysplasia (abnormal development) of the hip
- Infection in the bone or joint
- Kohler's disease (loss of blood supply to a bone in the foot)

A "toddler fracture" is a spiral fracture of the tibia (one of the leg bones that extends from the knee to the ankle; see Fractures/Broken Bones, *page 508*). It can occur with minor accidents such as when children trip, jump, or fall, or when they go down a slide in an older child's or an adult's lap with their feet tucked under them. Sometimes children can explain how the injury occurred, but usually they have difficulty recalling exactly what happened. At times an older sibling or childcare provider can solve the mystery.

Hip problems that cause a limp at this age usually are due to a viral joint infection causing transient synovitis and should be evaluated by your pediatrician. When a child has an infection in the bone or joint, they usually experience a fever, swelling of the joint, and redness. If the infection is in the hip joint, they will hold their leg flexed or bent at the hip and be extremely irritable and unwilling to move the hip and leg in any direction, although swelling and redness may not be obvious in this deep joint.

Sometimes a child is born with a hip problem (developmental dysplasia of the hip, DDH) that may not be noticed until they start to walk. As one limb is shorter, the hip is less stable, and the buttock muscles are weaker than the other side, the child may walk with an obvious limp.

Perthes disease is another disorder that causes children to limp and that is most often not associated with any pain complaints. It is usually only a minor problem in children younger than 6 years, but in older children, usually more than 10 years of age, it can be a significantly disabling problem.

Limping is a major reason that parents of children with juvenile idiopathic arthritis seek medical care. In a typical case, a child will not complain of being in pain. But they limp nevertheless, with this limping at its worst after waking in the morning or from a nap and becoming less noticeable with activity.

Treatment

With minor injuries, such as a blister, cut, or sprain, simple first-aid treatment can be performed at home. However, if your child has just started walking and is constantly limping, your pediatrician should evaluate them. It is all right to wait twenty-four hours if your older child develops a limp, since sometimes the problem will disappear overnight. But if your child is still limping the next day or is in extreme pain or has a high fever, see your pediatrician.

X-rays of the hip or the entire leg or blood tests may be necessary to make the diagnosis. If there is an infection, antibiotics should be started, and hospitalization may be required. Intravenous (IV) antibiotics may be given in high doses to allow them to get to the joint and bone. If a bone is broken or dislocated, the limb will be placed in a splint or cast, and the child will be referred to an orthopedist for evaluation and further management. It is also advisable to see a pediatric orthopedist if DDH or Perthes disease is diagnosed.

Pigeon Toes (Intoeing)

Children who walk with their feet turned in are described as being "pigeon-toed" or having "intoeing." This is a very common condition that may involve one or both feet, and it occurs for a variety of reasons.

Intoeing During Infancy

Infants are sometimes born with their feet turning in. If this turning occurs from the front part of their foot only, it is called metatarsus adductus. Most commonly it is due to the foot being positioned in a certain way inside the uterus before the baby is born.

You can suspect that metatarsus adductus may be present if:

- At rest, the front portion of your infant's foot turns inward.
- The outer side of the child's foot is curved like a half-moon.

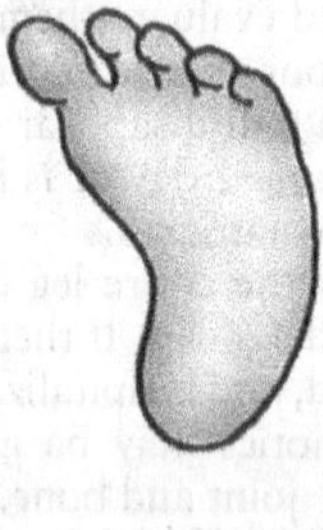

Appearance of foot in metatarsus adductus

This condition is usually mild and will resolve before your infant's first birthday. Sometimes it is more severe or accompanied by other foot deformities that result in a problem called clubfoot. This condition requires a consultation with a pediatric orthopedist, and there is extremely effective nonoperative treatment with early casting or splinting.

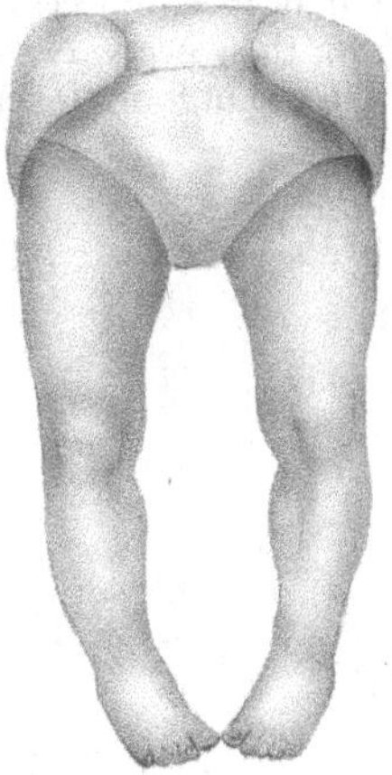

Internal tibial torsion

Treatment

Some experts feel no treatment is necessary for intoeing in an infant under 6 months of age. For severe metatarsus adductus in infancy, early casting may be useful. Studies show that most infants who have metatarsus adductus in early infancy will outgrow it with no treatment necessary. If your baby's intoeing persists after six months, or if it is rigid and difficult to straighten out, your doctor may refer you to a pediatric orthopedist, who may recommend a series of casts applied over a period of three to six weeks. The main goal is to correct the condition before your child starts walking.

Intoeing in early childhood often corrects itself over time and usually requires no treatment. But if your child has trouble walking, discuss the condition with your pediatrician, who may refer you to an orthopedist. In the past, a night brace (special shoes with connecting bars) was used for this problem, but it hasn't proven to be an effective treatment. Because intoeing often corrects itself over time, it is very important to avoid non-prescribed "treatments" such as corrective shoes, twister cables, daytime bracing, exercises, wearing the wrong shoes on each foot, shoe inserts, or back manipulations. These do not resolve the problem and may be harmful because they interfere with normal play or walking. Furthermore, a child wearing these braces may face unnecessary emotional strain because of teasing from their peers. Nevertheless, if a child's intoeing remains by the age of 9 or 10 years old, surgery may be required to correct it.

CHAPTER 29

SKIN

Skin problems in children often get the attention of parents—and sometimes raise their anxiety levels. After all, skin conditions are immediately visible, and while the overwhelming majority are not serious, they may still be a source of worry. In this chapter, you'll find an alphabetical description of common skin problems. Other skin conditions (specifically eczema, hives, and insect bites and stings) are discussed in *Chapter 13*, Asthma and Allergies.

Birthmarks and Hemangiomas

Dark-Pigmented Birthmarks (Nevi or Moles)

Nevi, or moles, are either congenital (present at birth) or acquired. Composed of so-called nevus cells, these spots range in color from light tan to dark brown or black.

Congenital Nevi

Small nevi appear at birth and are relatively common, occurring in about 1 out of every 100 newborns. They tend to grow with the child and usually don't cause any problems. Rarely, however, these moles may develop into a type of serious skin cancer (melanoma) at some later time. Therefore, while you don't have to worry about them right away, it's a good idea to watch them carefully and have them checked by your pediatrician at regular intervals or if there is any change in appearance (color, size, or shape). They may refer you to a pediatric dermatologist, who will advise you on removal and any follow-up care.

A much more serious type of nevus is a large congenital one that is over 7.9 inches (20 cm) in diameter. It might be flat or raised, may have hair growing from it (although small, insignificant nevi sometimes also have hair), and can be so large that it covers an arm or a leg. Fortunately, these nevi are very rare (occurring in 1 out of every 20,000 births). However, they are more likely than the smaller ones to develop into a melanoma (maybe up to 5 percent do), so early consultation with a pediatric dermatologist and regular mole checks are advisable.

Acquired Nevi, or Moles

Acquired nevi, or moles, usually occur after the age of 5, but sometimes develop earlier. These acquired moles are seldom a cause for worry. However, if your child develops one that's irregularly shaped (asymmetrical), has multiple colors within its structure, is larger than a pencil eraser, or is causing any symptoms, it is recommended to ask your pediatrician to examine it.

Blood Vessel Birthmarks on the Skin

Your baby may have a flat red patch on the back of the neck at birth and then at 2 to 3 weeks of age may develop a new red raised bump on the forehead. Although some of these blood vessel or vascular marks usually do not cause trouble, it's important to recognize the difference between the marks that are not concerning and those that may be associated with medical complications. Your pediatrician will also evaluate such birthmarks at each visit.

Capillary Malformations (Salmon Patches and Port-Wine Birthmarks)

Capillary malformations are recognized as flat red patches in the newborn and include salmon patches (most common) and port-wine birthmarks (less common). Nevus simplex (formerly called "salmon patches" or "stork bites") occur in more than 80 percent of infants and most commonly involve the back of the neck, the mid-forehead, the upper eyelids, the sides of the nose, and the middle of the upper lip. Although they fade during the first few years and are not associated with any serious medical problems, they may still be noticeable when children are overheated or upset or crying, because the blood vessels dilate, making the skin lesion look more prominent, especially in light-complected individuals.

Port-wine birthmarks occur in other areas of the skin, tend to be darker at birth, do not fade, and usually gradually darken with increasing age. They may be associated with other birth defects, including abnormalities of the underlying veins and arteries in the involved skin. When a port-wine birthmark involves the skin of the forehead, it may be associated with abnormalities of the eye and brain known as Sturge-Weber syndrome. Affected children should be checked for elevated intraocular (eye) pressure (glaucoma) and other eye defects as well as abnormalities of the brain. This evaluation may be performed by your pediatrician in collaboration with a pediatric neurologist, ophthalmologist, and dermatologist or in a center specializing in Sturge-Weber syndrome.

Since port-wine birthmarks usually intensify during childhood and adult life, treatment with a pulsed dye laser, which involves multiple treatments spaced six to twelve weeks apart, could be considered in infancy or early childhood if desired by the family. Special medical makeup can also be used to camouflage these marks.

Infantile Hemangioma (IH)

Infantile hemangiomas (often referred to by parents as "strawberry marks") occur in 10 percent of babies by 2 months of age, with most appearing by 2 to 3 weeks of age. They often are not present at birth or are only noted as subtle flat red spots that may be mistaken for bruises. They can involve any part of the body, but there is a predilection for the head and neck. Most children have a single IH, but in rare cases some infants have hundreds. For reasons that are not well understood, two-thirds to three-fourths occur in girls. IHs are also much more common in premature infants, especially in infants of low birth weight. IHs usually peak in size by 9 months of age, often looking reddish purplish, followed by slow but steady spontaneous regression over the next several years.

If your infant develops a hemangioma, have your pediatrician examine it so they can follow its course from the start. Newer, non-invasive treatments are available to help treat the hemangioma and prevent any future scarring. However, since the vast majority will gradually shrink without treatment, sometimes the best course of action is to leave it alone. Studies have shown that when this type of hemangioma is left untreated, few complications or cosmetic problems result.

At times, hemangiomas may need to be treated—namely, when they are large, on the face, or in an exposed area where they can be easily seen, as well as if the hemangioma occurs close to vital structures, such as the eye, throat, or mouth; when they seem to be growing much faster than usual; or when they are likely to ulcerate, which can lead to pain, infection, and scarring. Such conditions are uncommon but require careful evaluation and management by your pediatrician and pediatric dermatologist, ENT, cardiologist, or plastic surgeon. Several treatment options are available, including oral medications to help shrink the hemangioma, drops that can be placed directly on the skin, and, rarely, surgical removal.

Very rarely, IHs are found in large numbers widely scattered over the skin surface. In some of these infants, IHs may also be located on organs inside the body. If this is suspected, your pediatrician may need to conduct further tests. When large IHs are present in certain locations (such as the head and neck, the chin in a beard-type distribution, and the lower spine), they may be associated with problems in underlying bony structures and soft tissues, and may require additional evaluation by your pediatrician.

(See also How Your Newborn Looks, *page 14*.)

Chickenpox (Varicella)

Chickenpox was once one of the most common childhood illnesses. But thanks to the varicella vaccine, far fewer children now get this disease. Chickenpox is a highly contagious infection causing an itchy, blister-like rash that can cover most of the body. Children often get a mild fever along with the rash.

The chickenpox rash is usually seen approximately two weeks after exposure to the virus that causes chickenpox. Small blisters, which may have a red area around them, will begin to appear on the body and scalp, then spread to the face, arms, and legs. There may be as many as 250 to 500 of these blisters. Normally the blisters will crust over and heal, but tiny sores and possibly small scars may develop if your child scratches them and they become infected. The skin around some of the blisters may become darker or lighter, but this change in coloring will disappear gradually after the rash is gone. Blisters may also appear on the inside of your child's mouth and in the genital region or other mucosal surfaces.

Treatment

Chickenpox can be very itchy and uncomfortable, but try to discourage your child from scratching, which can lead to additional infection by bacteria. Acetaminophen or ibuprofen (in the appropriate dose for your child's age and weight) may decrease the discomfort from the rash or fever. Trimming fingernails and bathing daily with soap and water also can help prevent secondary bacterial infection. Oatmeal baths, available without prescription from your pharmacy, will ease the itch. Antihistamines can also be used to decrease the itch. (Be sure to follow the dosing instructions carefully.) A prescription medicine (acyclovir or valacyclovir) can modestly decrease the severity of the symptoms if started within twenty-four hours of the onset of the disease. This medicine should be considered for those at risk for moderate to severe disease (e.g., children with weakened immune systems or those with certain skin disorders such as eczema), but it is not recommended for healthy children younger than 12 years of age.

Do not give your child aspirin or any medication that contains aspirin or salicylates when they have chickenpox. These products increase the risk of Reye syndrome, a serious illness that involves the liver and brain. You should avoid steroids and any medicines that interfere with the immune system. If you are not sure about what medications you can safely use at this time, ask your pediatrician for advice.

Because chickenpox is now rare, doctors are likely to want to see your child and possibly do a blood test to confirm whether your child has the illness, but because it is so contagious, you should call and discuss whether your child needs to be seen before you make a trip to the doctor's office. Many times, what looks like possible chickenpox may be another virus. If your child develops a complication such as a skin infection, trouble breathing, or a fever that rises above 102 degrees Fahrenheit (38.9 degrees Celsius) or lasts longer than four days, be sure to call your pediatrician immediately. Let the pediatrician know if areas of the rash become very red, warm, or tender, as this may indicate a bacterial infection. Be sure to call your pediatrician immediately if your child develops any signs of Reye syndrome or encephalitis: vomiting, nervousness, confusion, convulsions, lack of responsiveness, increasing sleepiness, or poor balance.

If your child does have chickenpox, you should tell all parents whose children may have been exposed (especially parents of infants too young to be vaccinated), as well as any pregnant women or anyone with a compromised immune system who may have been in contact with your child. Your child is contagious one to two days before the rash starts and for twenty-four hours after the last new blister appears (usually five to seven days). In some cases, the contagious period lasts until all the blisters are dry and crusted over. After they have recovered from the chickenpox, your child usually will be immune to chickenpox for the rest of their life, but they can get shingles later on in life, since the virus stays in the nerve cells and can reactivate as shingles.

Prevention

A vaccine to protect against chickenpox is recommended for all healthy children, with the first dose given between 12 and 15 months of age, plus a second (booster) dose usually given between 4 and 6 years of age. Until your child has received this vaccine, the only sure way to protect them is to avoid exposure to the chickenpox virus. Protection from exposure is important for newborn infants, especially premature babies, in whom the disease can be more severe.

Most infants whose mothers have had chickenpox or have been vaccinated are immune to the disease for the first few months after birth, since mothers pass short-lived protective antibodies to their infants. Susceptible children who have diseases affecting the immune system (e.g., cancer) or who are using certain drugs (e.g., prednisone) should avoid being exposed to chickenpox. If these children are exposed, they may be eligible for a special medication that will provide protection against the disease for a limited period. It's important to remember that since the varicella vaccine is a live virus vaccine, children who have a weakened immune system may not have a normal response to it and may not be able to receive the vaccine.

Cradle Cap and Seborrheic Dermatitis

Your beautiful 1-month-old baby has developed a scaly rash on their scalp. You're concerned and think maybe you shouldn't shampoo as usual. You may also be concerned if you see some redness in the creases of their neck and armpits and behind their ears. What is it and what should you do?

When this rash occurs on the scalp alone, it's known as cradle cap. Although it may start as scaling and/or redness of the scalp, it also can be found later in the other areas just mentioned. It can extend to the face, body, and diaper area, too. When it extends beyond the scalp, pediatricians call it seborrheic dermatitis. Seborrheic dermatitis is a non-infectious skin condition that's very common in infants, usually beginning in the first weeks after birth and slowly disappearing over a period of weeks or months. Unlike eczema or contact dermatitis (see *page 392*), it's rarely uncomfortable or itchy.

Doctors think that seborrheic dermatitis is caused by a reaction that the skin has to certain common fungi that live on all human skin. Some doctors have speculated that it may be influenced by the mother's hormonal changes during pregnancy, which stimulate the infant's oil glands. This overproduction of oil may have some relationship to the scales and redness of the skin.

Treatment

If your baby's seborrheic dermatitis is confined to the scalp (and is therefore just cradle cap), you can treat it yourself. Don't be afraid to shampoo the hair; in fact, you should wash it (with a mild baby shampoo) more frequently than before. This, along with soft brushing, will help remove the scales. Stronger medicated shampoos (anti-dandruff or anti-seborrhea shampoos, such as those containing selenium sulfide, sulfur, salicylic acid, ketoconazole, or coal tar) may loosen the scales more quickly, but since they also can be irritating, use them only after consulting your pediatrician.

Some parents have found using petroleum jelly, ointments, or oils such as mineral oil, vegetable oil, or olive oil can help soften the scales and make them easier to remove. In some cases, especially if the seborrhea has spread to other areas of the body, your pediatrician may also recommend hydrocortisone cream or antifungal cream to help it clear. Once the condition has improved, in most cases you can prevent it from recurring by continuing with frequent hair washing with a mild baby shampoo. Fortunately, most babies' conditions clear up during the second half of the first year, so prolonged treatment is usually unnecessary.

Sometimes yeast infections occur on the affected skin, most likely in the crease areas rather than on the scalp. If this occurs, the area will become extremely reddened and quite itchy. In this case, your pediatrician might prescribe a medication such as an antifungal cream.

Rest assured that seborrheic dermatitis is not a serious condition. Nor is it an allergy to something you're using, or due to poor hygiene. It will go away without any scars.

Fifth Disease (Erythema Infectiosum)

Rosy cheeks are often considered a sign of good health, but if your child suddenly develops bright red patches on their cheeks that are also raised and warm, they may have a viral illness known as fifth disease. Like so many other childhood illnesses, this one is spread from person to person. The virus causing this disease is called a parvovirus. Once your child is exposed to the virus, it usually takes four to fourteen days for symptoms to appear.

This is a mild disease, and most children feel well even when the rash appears. However, fifth disease can occur with mild cold-like symptoms, such as sore throat, headache, pinkeye, fatigue, a mild fever, or itching. In rare cases there may be aches in the knees or wrists. The disease process may be more severe in children with abnormal hemoglobin or red blood cells, such as sickle cell anemia, and in children with cancer.

The rash usually begins on the cheeks, causing them to look as if they've been slapped. During the next few days, the arms and then the trunk, thighs, and buttocks will develop a pink, slightly raised rash that has a lacy pattern. Fever is usually absent or mild. After five to ten days the rash will fade, with the face clearing first, followed by the arms, and then the trunk and legs. Interestingly, the rash may reappear briefly weeks or months later, particularly if your child becomes hot from bathing, exercise, or sunlight, or spends time in the sun.

Treatment

For most children, fifth disease is not serious. The rash, however, may look similar to other rashes that may be more serious, as well as certain drug-related rashes; as a result, it's important to discuss the rash with your pediatrician and let them know about any medications your child may be taking. When you describe the symptoms over the phone, the doctor may suspect fifth disease, but they still may want to examine your child to be certain.

There is no specific medicine for fifth disease; treatment is geared to providing relief of the symptoms. For instance, if your child has a fever or aches and pains, you can treat them with acetaminophen or ibuprofen. If they exhibit new symptoms, feel sicker, or develop a high fever, call your pediatrician.

A child with fifth disease is contagious when they are suffering from the cold-like symptoms that precede the rash. But by the time they demonstrate a rash, they are no longer contagious. Nevertheless, as a rule, whenever your child has a rash or a fever, you should keep them away from other children until your doctor identifies the illness. As a precaution, wait until they no longer have a fever and are feeling normal before allowing them to play with other children. Also, it is important to keep your child away from pregnant women (particularly in their first trimester), since the virus that causes this disease may cause serious illness or even death in the fetus if the mother becomes infected.

Hair Loss (Alopecia)

Almost all newborns lose some amount of their hair within the first three to five months after birth. This is normal and can be expected. This loss of hair is due to the natural growth cycle that hair follicles go through in the neonatal period. This hair loss is most commonly seen on the back of the head, where the scalp rubs against the crib mattress. This hair loss occurring within the first six months is not a cause for concern, and no treatment is needed.

In very rare cases, babies may be born with alopecia (hair loss), which can occur by itself or in association with certain abnormalities of the nails and the teeth. Injury or trauma to the scalp at birth may also cause hair loss at birth, which may or may not fully resolve. There are also some birthmarks that occur on the scalp leading to hair loss in those areas. Later in childhood, hair loss may be due to other reasons, including medications, a scalp injury, or a medical or nutritional problem.

Impetigo

Impetigo is a contagious bacterial skin infection that often appears around the nose, mouth, and ears. More than 90 percent of impetigo cases are caused by staphylococcal bacteria, while the rest are caused by streptococcal bacteria (which also are responsible for strep throat and scarlet fever).

If staphylococcal bacteria are to blame, the infection may cause blisters filled with clear or yellow fluid. These can break easily, leaving a raw, glistening area that soon forms a scab with a honey-colored crust. By contrast, infections with strep bacteria usually are not associated with blisters, but they do cause crusts over larger sores and ulcers.

Treatment

Impetigo needs to be treated with antibiotics, either topically or taken by mouth. Rarely, your pediatrician may order a culture in the lab to determine which bacteria are causing the rash. Make sure your child takes the medication for the full prescribed course, or the impetigo could return.

One other important point to keep in mind is that impetigo is contagious until the rash clears, or until at least two days of antibiotics have been given and there is evidence of improvement. Your child should avoid close contact with other children during this period, and you should avoid touching the rash. If you or other family members do come in contact with it, wash your hands and the exposed site thoroughly with soap and water. Also, keep the infected child's clothing, washcloths, and towels separate from those of other family members.

Prevention

The bacteria that cause impetigo thrive in breaks in the skin. The best ways to prevent this rash are to keep your child's fingernails clipped and clean and to teach them not to scratch minor skin irritations. When they do have a scrape, cleanse it with soap and water, and apply an antibiotic cream or ointment. Be careful not to use washcloths or towels that have been used by someone else who has an active skin infection.

When certain types of streptococcal bacteria cause impetigo, a rare but serious complication called glomerulonephritis can develop. This disease injures the kidneys and may cause high blood pressure and blood in the urine. Therefore, if you notice any blood or a dark brown color in your child's urine, let your pediatrician know so they can evaluate it and order further tests if needed.

Measles

Thanks to vaccinations, cases of measles were on the decline. Unfortunately, they have been on the rise in the United States recently, with multiple outbreaks occurring in several states. The COVID-19 pandemic also led to a decline in vaccinations both in the United States and worldwide. According to the Centers for Disease Control and Prevention, eleven states reported approximately 206 measles cases in the United States from January 2019 to February 2019. Most of these cases were in people younger than 20 years old who were unvaccinated or whose vaccination status was unknown. Travelers who have not been immunized can bring measles back to the United States after traveling to a country where there is a reported outbreak. If your child has never been immunized or had the measles, they can get the disease if they are exposed. The measles virus is very contagious and passed through the air via droplets transmitted by an infected person. The virus can live up to nearly two hours in the air where an infected person coughed or sneezed. Almost everyone who breathes the droplets and is not immune to the disease will become infected.

Signs and Symptoms

For the first eight to twelve days after being exposed to the measles virus, your child will probably have no symptoms; this is called the incubation period. Then they may develop an illness that seems like a common cold, with a cough, runny nose, and pinkeye (conjunctivitis; see Eye Infections, *page 545*). The cough may be severe at times and will last for about a week, and your child probably will feel miserable.

During the first one to three days of the illness, the cold-like symptoms will become worse, and your child will develop a fever that may run as high as 103 to 105 degrees Fahrenheit (39.4–40.5 degrees Celsius). The fever will last until two to three days after the rash first appears.

After two to four days of illness, the rash will develop. It usually begins on the face and neck, then spreads down the trunk and out to the arms and legs. It starts as very fine red bumps, which may merge. If you notice tiny white spots, like grains of sand, inside their mouth next to their molars, you'll know the rash will follow soon. The rash will last five to eight days. As it fades, the skin may peel a little.

Treatment

Although there is no treatment for the disease, it is important that the pediatrician examine your child to determine that measles is, in fact, the cause of the illness. Call your doctor's office first before showing up so that they can take extra precautions not to expose others. If the illness is measles, a dose of vitamin A may be indicated, as treatment with vitamin A of children who have measles has been found to lessen the chances of the associated complications and death due to the infection. Your pediatrician will advise you on the correct dose of vitamin A.

Your child is contagious from several days before the rash breaks out until the fever and rash are gone. During this period, they should be kept at home (except for the visit to the doctor) and away from anyone who is not immune to the illness. At home, make sure your child drinks plenty of fluids, and give acetaminophen in the proper dose if your child is uncomfortable due to the fever. The conjunctivitis that accompanies measles can make it painful for the child to be in bright light or sunshine, so you may want to darken their room to a comfortable level for the first few days.

Sometimes infections develop as a complication of the measles. These most often include pneumonia (see *page 421*), middle ear infection (see *page 471*), and encephalitis (inflammation of the brain). In these cases, your child must be seen by the pediatrician, who may prescribe antibiotic treatment or admit your child to the hospital.

Prevention

Almost all children who receive two doses of the MMR (measles, mumps, rubella) vaccine after their first birthday are protected against measles for life. The first dose of the vaccine should be administered between ages 12 and 15 months, and the second one between ages 4 and 6 years old, although it can be given at a younger age as long as at least twenty-eight days have passed since the first dose. Because up to 5 percent of children may not have an adequate immune response to the initial vaccination, the second (booster) dose is recommended for all children. (See *Chapter 26*, Immunizations.)

If your unimmunized child has been exposed to someone who has the measles, or if someone in your household has the virus, notify your pediatrician at once. The following steps can help keep your child from getting sick:

1. If they are under 1 year old or have a weakened immune system, they can be given immunoglobulin up to six days following exposure. This may temporarily protect them from becoming infected, but it will not provide extended immunity.
2. An infant 6 through 11 months of age may receive the measles vaccine if they are exposed to the disease or if they are living in a community where exposure is highly likely or in an epidemic situation. If doses are given during these months, your child will still need additional doses to be fully immunized, as this dose is to address the exposure but does not count as part of the routine vaccine schedule.
3. If your child is otherwise healthy and at least 1 year old, they can be vaccinated. The vaccine may be effective if given within seventy-two hours of their exposure to an infected person and will provide extended immunity. If your child has previously received one dose of the measles vaccine and at least twenty-eight days have elapsed since that dose, they may be given a second dose after exposure.

Molluscum Contagiosum

Molluscum contagiosum is a common skin infection in young children that is caused by a virus. The small, raised lesions look like shiny flesh-colored or pinkish dome-shaped bumps or nodules on the skin with an indentation in the center. Some kids get a few, while others may get twenty or more on their body. The lesions tend to cluster and are found most often on the face, on the trunk, in body creases, and on extremities, but they may develop anywhere on the body. They are painless, harmless, non-cancerous growths in the skin's top layers, and sometimes they can itch. They can get inflamed just before they resolve, with an eczematous rash forming around lesions. The most annoying part is that they last for several months to a few years and sometimes spread to other areas of the body when children scratch lesions in one place and transmit them to another.

The disease is spread by direct contact with the skin of an infected person or sharing towels with someone who has the disease. Outbreaks have occasionally been reported in child-care centers. The incubation period varies between two and seven weeks, although it is sometimes much longer (up to six months).

Most often, molluscum lesions go away on their own without any treatment. This means that children with just one or a few widely scattered lesions do not need any special care. However, if the lesions are extensive, or if you and your child desire, your pediatrician or dermatologist may recommend topical medications to help the molluscum resolve sooner, or the bumps can be removed by a scraping procedure with a sharp instrument (curette) or by using peeling agents or freezing techniques (such as liquid nitrogen).

Mosquito-Borne Illnesses (Zika and West Nile)

There are many infections that spread to humans through the bite of an infected mosquito. Mosquitoes become carriers of the viruses by feeding on infected people or animals. Once the virus has been transmitted to a human through a bite, it can multiply in an individual's bloodstream and in some cases cause illness.

West Nile

The first outbreak of West Nile virus occurred in the United States in 1999. Although some children have become ill when infected with West Nile virus, most have mild symptoms or none at all. About one in five people with West Nile virus develop mild flu-like symptoms (fever, headaches, and body aches) and at times a skin rash. These symptoms tend to last only a few days. In fewer than 1 out of 100 infections, a severe illness can occur (West Nile encephalitis or meningitis), with symptoms such as a high fever, a stiff neck, tremors, muscle weakness, convulsions, paralysis, and loss of consciousness.

Zika

In children, Zika virus is rarely dangerous. In fact, as long as you aren't pregnant or of childbearing age, Zika is of little concern. Only one in five people infected with Zika virus have symptoms of illness. Because the disease affects people differently, some may have a rash, fever, pinkeye (conjunctivitis), joint and/or muscle pain, or headache. Symptoms usually clear up in less than a week, are mild, and rarely require hospitalization.

Zika virus is particularly dangerous, however, for women who are pregnant or who are planning to become pregnant, because the virus affects the developing fetus in the womb. Federal health officials have confirmed that Zika virus can cause microcephaly (babies born with a small head) and other brain, eye, and physical abnormalities in infants. Because Zika virus can affect the fetus's developing brain and cause long-lasting negative consequences, prevention is critical.

Prevention of Mosquito-Borne Infections

Risk of contracting Zika or West Nile virus comes mostly from mosquito bites. The disease cannot be transmitted through casual person-to-person contact. However, Zika virus can be sexually transmitted to a pregnant woman or woman of childbearing age and affect a developing or future fetus.

There is currently no vaccine available in the United States to protect from such viruses. But you can reduce the likelihood of developing the disease by taking steps to reduce the chance of a bite from a mosquito that could be carrying the virus. Here are some strategies to keep in mind (also see Insect Bites and Stings, *page 404*):

- Apply insect repellent to yourself or your child, using just enough to protect the exposed skin. (See the chart Available Insect Repellents, *page 663*.) Wash the repellent off with soap and water when it is no longer needed to protect the skin.
- Avoid products that include insect repellent and sunscreen together, because the sunscreen needs to be applied more frequently than insect repellent.
- Do not use DEET preparations on infants under 2 months of age. In older children, apply it sparingly around the ears, and don't use it on the mouth, hands, or eyes. Don't put it over cuts.
- Whenever possible, dress your child in long sleeves and long pants while they're outside. Use mosquito netting over a baby's infant carrier.
- Keep your child away from locations where mosquitoes are likely to congregate or lay their eggs, such as standing water (e.g., in birdbaths, flowerpot saucers, and pet water dishes). Remove such sources from around the outside of your home.
- Because mosquitoes are more likely to bite humans at certain times of day—most commonly at dawn, at dusk, and in the early evening—consider limiting the amount of time your child is outdoors during those hours.
- Repair any holes in your window screens.

Types of Insect Repellents

Insect repellents come in many forms, including aerosols, sprays, liquids, creams, and sticks. Some are made from synthetic chemicals, and some have natural ingredients. Insect repellents deter biting insects but not stinging insects. Biting insects include mosquitoes, ticks, fleas, chiggers, and biting flies. Stinging insects include bees, hornets, and wasps.

AVAILABLE INSECT REPELLENTS

<table>
<tr><th>What's available?</th><th>How well does it work?</th><th>How long does it protect?</th><th>Any special precautions?</th></tr>
<tr><td>Chemical repellents with DEET (N,N-diethyl-meta-toluamide)</td><td>Considered the best defense against biting insects.</td><td>Lasts about 2 to 5 hours depending on the concentration of DEET in the product.</td><td>Caution should be used when applying DEET to children. Avoid under 2 months of age.</td></tr>
<tr><td>Picaridin</td><td rowspan="2">In April 2005, the Centers for Disease Control and Prevention (CDC) recommended other repellents that may work as well as DEET: repellents with picaridin and repellents with oil of lemon eucalyptus or 2% soybean oil. Currently these products have a duration of action that is comparable to that of about 10% DEET.</td><td>Lasts about 3 to 8 hours depending on the concentration.</td><td>Although these products are considered safe when used as recommended, long-term follow-up studies are not available. Also, more studies need to be done to see how well they repel ticks.</td></tr>
<tr><td>Repellents made from essential oils found in plants such as citronella, cedar, lemon eucalyptus, and soybean</td><td>Usually lasts less than 2 hours.</td><td>Allergic reactions are rare but can occur when using repellents made from essential oils.</td></tr>
<tr><td>Chemical repellents with permethrin</td><td>These repellents kill ticks on contact.</td><td>When applied to clothing, these repellents last even after several washings.</td><td>Should only be applied to clothing, not directly to skin. May be applied to outdoor equipment such as sleeping bags and tents. Ensure that young children don't mouth or chew on treated fabrics.</td></tr>
</table>

MRSA Infections

Methicillin-resistant *Staphylococcus aureus* (MRSA) is the name of a type of staphylococcal bacterium that can cause infections not only on the surface of the skin, but also into the soft tissue, where a boil or abscess can form. In recent years, MRSA has become a major public health problem because this bacterium has become resistant to antibiotics called beta-lactams, which include methicillin and other commonly prescribed antibiotics. This resistance has made treating these infections more difficult. While MRSA was once limited to hospitals and nursing homes, it has spread into the community in schools, households, and childcare centers, among other places. It can be transmitted from person to person through skin-to-skin contact, particularly through cuts and abrasions.

If your child has a wound that appears to be infected—specifically, if it is red, swollen, hot, and oozing pus—have it checked by your pediatrician. They may drain the infection and may prescribe topical and/or oral antibiotics. The most serious MRSA infections may cause pneumonia and bloodstream infections. Even though MRSA infections are resistant to some antibiotics, they are treatable with other medications.

To prevent your child from getting MRSA at school or other public places, the following strategies can be helpful:

- Follow good hygiene practices. Your child should wash their hands frequently with soap and warm water or use alcohol-based hand sanitizers.
- Use a clean, dry bandage to cover any cuts, scrapes, or breaks in your child's skin. These bandages should be changed at least daily.
- Don't let your child share towels, washcloths, or other personal items (including clothing) with anyone else.
- Frequently clean and disinfect surfaces that your child touches.
- Use a moisturizer regularly to help keep the skin barrier intact, especially in drier climates.

Ringworm (Tinea)

If your child has a scaly round patch on their scalp or elsewhere on their skin, and they seem to be losing hair in the same area of the scalp, the problem may be a contagious infection known as ringworm.

This disorder is caused not by worms but by a fungus. It's called ringworm because the infections tend to form round or oval spots that, as they enlarge, become smooth in the center but keep an active red scaly border.

Scalp ringworm is spread from person to person, sometimes when sharing infected hats, combs, brushes, or barrettes. If ringworm appears elsewhere on your child's body, they may have the type spread by infected dogs or cats. The first signs of infection on the body are red, scaly patches. They may not look like rings until they've grown to ½ inch (1.25 cm) in diameter, and they generally stop growing at about 1 inch (2.5 cm). Your child may have just one patch or several. These lesions may be mildly itchy and uncomfortable.

Scalp ringworm starts the same way the body variety does, but as the patches grow, your child may lose some hair in the infected area. Certain types of scalp ringworm produce less obvious rings and are easily confused with dandruff or cradle cap. Cradle cap, however, occurs only during infancy. If your child's scalp is continually scaly and they're over a year old, you should suspect ringworm and notify your pediatrician.

Treatment

A single ringworm patch on the body can be treated with an over-the-counter cream recommended by your pediatrician. The most frequently used ones are clotrimazole, tolnaftate, or miconazole. A small amount is applied to the patches or rash and just beyond their borders two or three times a day for at least a week, during which time some clearing should begin. If there are any patches on the scalp or more than one on the body, or if the rash is getting worse while being treated, check with your pediatrician again. They will prescribe a stronger medication and, in the case of scalp ringworm or widespread body ringworm, will use an oral antifungal preparation. Your child will have to take medicine for several weeks, depending on the medication, to clear the infection.

You also may need to wash your child's scalp with a special shampoo when they have scalp ringworm. If there's any possibility that others in the family have caught the infection, they also should use this shampoo and be examined for possible signs of infection. Do not allow your child to share combs, brushes, hair clips, barrettes, or hats.

Prevention

You can help prevent ringworm by identifying and treating any pets with the problem. Look for scaling, itchy, hairless areas on your dogs and cats, and have them treated right away. Any family members, playmates, or schoolmates who show symptoms also should be treated.

Roseola Infantum

Your 10-month-old doesn't look or act very ill, but they suddenly develop a fever between 102 and 105 degrees Fahrenheit (38.9–40.5 degrees Celsius). The fever lasts for three to seven days, during which time your child may have less appetite, mild diarrhea, a slight cough, and a runny nose, and seems mildly irritable and a little sleepier than usual. Their upper eyelids may appear slightly swollen or droopy. Finally, after their temperature returns to normal, they get a slightly raised, spotty pink rash on their trunk, which spreads only to their upper arms and neck and fades after just twenty-four hours. What's the diagnosis? Most likely it's a disease called roseola—a contagious viral illness that's most common in children under age 2. Its incubation period is thought to be nine to ten days. The key to this diagnosis is that the rash appears after the fever is gone. We now know that specific viruses (human herpes virus types 6 and 7) cause this condition.

Treatment

Whenever your infant under 3 months of age has a fever of 100.4 degrees Fahrenheit or higher, call your pediatrician. For infants over 3 months of age, if the fever is 102 degrees Fahrenheit (38.9 degrees Celsius) or higher for more than twenty-four to seventy-two hours, call your pediatrician, especially if there are no other symptoms. If the doctor suspects the fever is caused by roseola, they may suggest ways to control the temperature and advise you to call again if your child becomes worse or the fever lasts for more than three or four days.

Since illnesses that cause fever can be contagious, it's wise to keep your child away from other children, at least until you've conferred with your pediatrician. Once their fever is gone for twenty-four hours, even if the rash has appeared, your child can return to childcare or preschool and resume normal contact with other children. While your child has a fever, dress them in lightweight clothing. If they are very uncomfortable because of the fever, you can give them acetaminophen in the appropriate dose for their age and weight. (See *Chapter* 22, Fever.) Don't worry if their appetite is decreased, and encourage them to drink extra fluids.

Although this disease rarely is serious, be aware that early in the illness, when fever climbs very quickly, there's a chance of a febrile seizure (see *page 573*). There may be a seizure regardless of how well you treat the fever, so it's important to know how to manage this, even though seizures that occur with roseola are usually quite mild and brief, if they occur at all.

Rubella (German Measles)

Although some of today's grandparents had rubella, or German measles, during their childhood, it is a rare illness now thanks to an effective vaccine. Even when it was prevalent, however, rubella was usually a mild disease—unless contracted by a pregnant woman, in whom it can cause serious illness and long-term problems in the developing baby.

Rubella is characterized by a mild fever (100–102 degrees

Fahrenheit [37.8–38.9 degrees Celsius]), swollen glands (typically on the back of the neck and at the base of the skull), and a rash. The rash, which varies from pinhead size to an irregular redness, is raised and usually begins on the face. Within two to three days, it spreads to the neck, the chest, and the rest of the body as it fades from the face.

Once exposed to rubella, a child usually will develop the disease in fourteen to twenty-one days. The contagious period for rubella begins several days before the rash appears and continues for five to seven days after it develops. Because the disease can be so mild, it goes unrecognized in about half the children who contract it.

Before the rubella vaccine was developed, this illness tended to occur in epidemics every six to nine years. Since the vaccine was introduced in 1968, there have been no significant epidemics in the United States. Even so, the disease still occurs. Each year, unvaccinated and susceptible teenagers, often in college campus settings, develop the illness. Fortunately, except for causing fever, discomfort, and occasional pain in the joints, these small epidemics are of little consequence.

What You Can Do

If your pediatrician diagnoses rubella, you may be able to make your child more comfortable by giving them extra fluids, encouraging bed rest (if they're fatigued), and giving acetaminophen if they have a fever. Keep them away from other children or adults unless you are sure that they're immunized. As a general rule, children with rubella should not be in childcare or any other group setting for seven days after the rash first appears. Pregnant women should not be exposed to rubella, as it can infect the fetus and cause serious abnormalities.

If your child is diagnosed as having the congenital form of rubella, your pediatrician can advise you on the best way to manage their complex and difficult problems. Infants born with congenital rubella are often infectious for a year after birth and therefore should be kept out of any group childcare setting, where they could expose other susceptible children or adults to the infection.

When to Call the Pediatrician

If your child has a fever and a rash and appears uncomfortable, discuss the problem with your pediatrician. If rubella is diagnosed, follow the guidelines suggested earlier for treatment and isolation.

Prevention

Being immunized is the best way to prevent rubella, or German measles. The vaccine usually is administered as part of a three-in-one shot called MMR (measles, mumps, rubella) or a four-in-one shot called MMRV (measles, mumps, rubella, varicella), given when the child is 12 to 15 months old. A booster dose needs to be given as well. (See *Chapter* 26, Immunizations.)

A child can be immunized even if their mother is pregnant at the time. However, a susceptible pregnant woman should not be immunized herself. She also should be extremely careful to avoid contact with any child or adult who may be infected with the virus. After delivery, she should be immunized immediately.

Scabies

Scabies is caused by a microscopic mite that burrows under the top layers of skin and deposits its eggs. The rash that results from scabies is a reaction to the mite's body, eggs, and excretions. Once the mite gets into the skin, it takes two to four weeks for the rash to appear.

In an older child, this rash appears as numerous itchy, fluid-filled bumps that cluster around the wrists, ankles, armpits, and genitals and between the fingers and toes. In an infant, the bumps may be more scattered over the body, varying from few to many, and often are also found on the palms and soles. Because of scratch marks, crusting, or a secondary infection, this annoying rash often is difficult to identify. Young infants may demonstrate characteristic distinct linear burrows.

According to legend, when Napoleon's troops had scabies,

one could hear the sound of scratching at night from over a mile away. A bit of exaggeration, perhaps, but it illustrates two key points to remember if you think your child has scabies: It's very itchy, and it's very contagious. Scabies is spread only by person-to-person contact, and this happens extremely easily. If one person in your family has the rash, the others may get it, too.

Treatment

If you notice that your child (and possibly others in the family) is scratching constantly, suspect scabies and call the pediatrician, who will examine the rash. The doctor may gently scrape a skin sample from the affected area and look under the microscope for evidence of the mite or its eggs. If scabies turns out to be the diagnosis, the doctor will prescribe one of several anti-scabies medications. Most are lotions that are applied over the entire body—from the scalp to the soles of the feet—and are washed off after several hours. You may need to repeat the application one week later.

Most experts feel the whole family must be treated—even those members who don't have a rash. Any live-in help, overnight visitors, or frequent babysitters also should receive care.

To prevent infection caused by scratching, cut your child's fingernails. If the itching is very severe, your pediatrician may prescribe an antihistamine or other anti-itch medication. If your child shows signs of bacterial infection in the scratched areas, notify the pediatrician. They may want to prescribe an antibiotic or another form of treatment.

Following treatment for scabies, the itching may continue for two to four weeks, because this is an allergic rash. If it persists past four weeks, call your doctor, because the scabies may have returned and need retreatment.

Incidentally, there is some controversy over the possible spread of scabies from clothing or bedding. While it is rare, clothing and bedding can host live mites, so washing everything in hot water and drying with heat can help prevent reinfection.

Scarlet Fever

When your child has strep throat (see *page 480*), there's a chance that they'll get a rash. This is known as scarlet fever. The symptoms of scarlet fever begin with a sore throat, a fever of 101 to 104 degrees Fahrenheit (38.2–40 degrees Celsius), and headache. This is followed within twenty-four hours by a red rash covering the trunk, arms, and legs. The rash is slightly raised, which makes the skin feel rough, like fine sandpaper. Your child's face may turn red, too, with a pale area around their mouth. The red rash will disappear in three to five days, leaving peeling skin in the areas where the rash was most intense (neck, underarms, groin, fingers, and toes). They may also have a white-coated, then reddened, tongue, and mild abdominal pain.

Treatment

Call your pediatrician whenever your child complains of a sore throat, especially when a rash or fever also is present. The doctor will examine them and swab their throat to check for streptococcal bacteria. If the streptococcal bacteria are found, an antibiotic (usually penicillin or amoxicillin) will be given. If your child takes the antibiotic by mouth instead of as an injection, it's extremely important to complete the entire course because shorter treatment sometimes results in a return of the disease.

Most children with streptococcal throat infections respond very quickly to antibiotics. The fever, sore throat, and headache usually are gone within twenty-four hours. The rash, however, will remain for about three to five days. If your child's condition does not seem to improve with treatment, notify your pediatrician. If other family members develop a fever or sore throat at this time—with or without a rash—they, too, should be examined and tested for strep throat.

If not treated, scarlet fever (like strep throat) can lead to ear and sinus infections, swollen neck glands, and pus around the tonsils. The most serious complication of untreated strep throat is rheumatic fever, which results in joint pain and swelling and sometimes heart damage. Very rarely, the streptococcal bacteria in the throat can lead to glomerulonephritis, or inflammation of the kidneys, causing blood in the urine and sometimes high blood pressure.

Sunburn

While those with darker skin coloring tend to be less sensitive to the sun, everyone is at risk for sunburn and the aftereffects of this skin injury. Children especially need to be protected from the sun's burning rays, since most long-term sun damage occurs in childhood. Like other burns, sunburn will leave the skin red, warm, and painful. In severe cases it may cause blistering, fever, chills, headache, and a general feeling of illness.

Your child doesn't have to be burned, however, in order to be harmed by the sun. The effects of sun exposure build over the years, so even moderate exposure during childhood can contribute to wrinkling, toughening, freckling, and even skin cancer. Also, some medications can cause a skin reaction to sunlight, and some medical conditions may make people more sensitive to the sun.

Treatment

The signs of sunburn usually appear six to twelve hours after exposure, with the greatest discomfort during the first twenty-four hours. If your child's burn is just red, warm, and painful, you can treat it yourself. Apply cool compresses to the burned areas or bathe the child in cool water. You also can give acetaminophen to help relieve the pain. (Check the package for appropriate dosage for their age and weight.)

If the sunburn causes blisters, fever, chills, headache, or a general feeling of illness, call your pediatrician. Severe sunburn must be treated like any other serious burn, and if it's very extensive, hospitalization sometimes is required. In addition, the blisters can become infected, requiring treatment with antibiotics. Sometimes extensive or severe sunburn also can lead to dehydration (see Diarrhea, *page 354*, for signs of dehydration) and, in some cases, fainting (heatstroke). Such cases need to be examined by your pediatrician or the nearest emergency facility.

Prevention

Many parents incorrectly assume that the sun is dangerous only when it's shining brightly. In fact, it's not the visible light rays but rather the invisible ultraviolet rays that are harmful. Your child may be exposed to more ultraviolet rays on foggy or hazy days because they'll feel cooler and therefore stay outside for a longer time. Exposure is also greater at higher altitudes. Even a big hat or an umbrella is not absolute protection because ultraviolet rays reflect off sand, water, snow, and many other surfaces.

Try to keep your child out of the sun when the peak ultraviolet rays occur (between 10 a.m. and 4 p.m.). In addition, follow these guidelines:

- Always use a sunscreen to block the damaging ultraviolet rays. Choose a sunscreen made for children with a sun protection factor (SPF) of 30 or higher and with broad-spectrum coverage for UVA and UVB light. (Check the label.) Apply the protection half an hour before going outside. Keep in mind that no sunscreens are truly waterproof, and thus they need to be reapplied every ninety minutes to two hours, particularly if your child spends a lot of time in the water. Consult the instructions on the bottle and choose a product that is labeled "water resistant."
- Dress your child in lightweight cotton clothing with long sleeves and long pants. SPF-rated clothing and hats are also a good idea to protect your child's skin when they're outdoors.
- Have them wear a hat with a wide brim.
- Use a beach umbrella or similar shade structure to keep them in the shade as much as possible.

- Babies under 6 months of age should be kept out of direct sunlight. If adequate clothing and shade are not available, sunscreen may be used on small areas of the body, such as the face and the backs of the hands.

(See also Burns, *page 490.*)

CHAPTER 30

YOUR CHILD'S SLEEP

Sleep is an essential, healthy part of your child's life. In the same way that good nutrition is important for the development of their body, sleep is crucial for the development of their brain. When kids don't get enough sleep, it can affect their behavior, their health, and how they learn. Good sleep in infancy is also linked with good physical health, including a lower risk for obesity later in childhood. In turn, how much your child sleeps will also affect your sleep and your health. As your young child establishes and maintains a regular sleep schedule, they are more likely to consistently sleep longer and less likely to awaken during the night, allowing them to access all the health benefits of sleep. When you provide your child's growing brain with sufficient sleep, your child will be better able to concentrate and their temperament will be more even.

(While this chapter focuses on your child's sleep needs, sleep training, implementing a sleep plan, and maintaining a bedtime routine, more detailed information and specific guidance on sleep for particular age groups, including safe sleep tips, can be found in various chapters in Part 1 of the book.)

How Much Sleep Does My Child Need?

Many parents worry about the sleep habits and behaviors of their child: "Are they getting too little sleep? Or too much? How important are naps, and how many hours of napping are enough? Should I let them cry themselves to sleep at night, or should I pick them up when they're in tears? Why do they seem to go to sleep later—or earlier—than other children of the same age?" The good news is that many of these concerns can easily be addressed.

Sleep requirements are one of the most common issues pediatricians are asked about, and while there are normal variations in sleep patterns between children, the following are specific recommendations on how many hours of sleep a child needs.

The American Society of Sleep Medicine and the AAP recommend the following amounts of sleep:

- Infants (4 months to 12 months): 12 to 16 hours per 24 hours (including naps) on a regular basis to promote optimal health.
- Children (1 year to 2 years): 11 to 14 hours per 24 hours (including naps) on a regular basis to promote optimal health.

In addition to sleep duration, another common question many parents have is "When will my baby sleep through the night?" While this is an understandable question, the answer isn't the same for all infants. After all, not all children are alike. Some babies may develop regular sleep rhythms in the first several months; others, however, may have unpredictable sleep behaviors that stay that way for many months—or longer.

SCENARIO #1

The mother of a 4-month-old baby complained to friends that while her infant had slept extremely well in the first week after birth, the baby's sleep patterns seemed to have unraveled after that. More than anything, their sleep times were erratic and unpredictable. She explained that she tried to keep her baby awake well into the evening so her husband could play with the infant upon returning home from work between 8:00 and 8:30 p.m. Before his arrival, her baby would often fuss and cry, and even though they seemed drowsy at times, she would keep them awake for a little while longer, awaiting her husband's arrival. More often than not, the infant had become so overtired that they just couldn't be consoled.

Mother and father were conflicted over what to do: Dad seemed comfortable with the baby crying until he arrived home, while Mom worried they were being heartless. Sometimes she would try putting the baby down for a brief nap in the very late afternoon, but the child would still become cranky later that night, and tension escalated between husband and wife.

They decided to ask their pediatrician for advice. The doctor explained the importance of being respectful of the child's evolving sleep schedule. For a typical 4- to 8-month-old, a healthy nightly bedtime is between 6 and 8 p.m. Keeping the child up longer to greet the father would leave the child overtired and out of sync with their own biological rhythms.

Always be mindful of your own child's sleep needs. Their biological clock is evolving, and when they feel the need to sleep, they should be allowed to do so. If their sleep-wake schedule is artificially disrupted, they will probably become moody and less attentive when they are awake. If they go to bed earlier, they may get up a little earlier, but their total night sleep will be longer. This will allow more time for a working parent to spend with their child in the morning. If any adjustments in schedules need to be made, they should begin with Mom and Dad, who should find a way to be available to their child when the child is awake and alert.

In most cases, your baby will learn to stretch out their nighttime feeds over the first few months. You can help your infant achieve this by having a consistent bedtime routine, such as bath, breast or bottle, book, and bed (placed on their back to sleep). Also, allow them to soothe themselves to sleep at night, keep the room dark and quiet, and ensure that they get plenty of time outdoors (weather permitting) and that they feed well during the day.

As an infant gets older, they will continue to stretch out their nighttime sleep, as long as you let them do so. Their distinctive temperament could be influencing their sleep behavior. Also, family circumstances can vary, affecting when, how long, and how well a child sleeps. In general, as long as you have a good sleep routine, your child will adjust on those evenings where the routine changes, such as sleeping at a different house or being woken early for a sibling playdate.

Getting Sleep in Sync

Despite parental concerns—or in some cases, perhaps because of them—moms, dads, and other caregivers sometimes unknowingly disrupt children's sleep. For example, even though parents want to do what's healthy for their child, they don't always understand the effect that their own busy schedules and family decision-making may have on their child's sleep.

Most commonly, parents may not recognize the importance of adopting a lifestyle that keeps their child in sync with their emerging biological system. When it comes to sleep, timing is everything, or nearly so. It is important to understand that when your children sleep is probably more important than how long they sleep. The quality of a child's sleep, which can restore alertness and maintain an even temperament, depends largely on when sleep occurs. That means encouraging them to sleep in rhythm with their own biological clock. A consistent bedtime that is in sync with a child's biological clock will typically result in restful and prolonged sleep.

Pay attention to your child and you'll find that, just like adults, they have drowsy times during the day. If they sleep during these drowsy periods, the quality of that sleep will be better than sleep that occurs out of phase with their biological cycles. But if you wait to place them for sleep until well after they've shown signs of drowsiness, they're likely to be overtired by then, which may make it more difficult for them to fall asleep.

The First Year

As a parent, you need to nurture and support your child's need to sleep. As much as possible, encourage them to sleep during those times of the day when they're likely to benefit the most from it. However, adopting an optimal sleep schedule won't happen overnight. Give it time, and it will develop naturally. Your challenge as a parent is to be sensitive to those moments when their body is telling them (and you) that they're ready for sleep. Otherwise, you may be placing them in their crib way too early or way too late, and the ease with which they fall asleep—and the restorative capacity of that sleep—will be affected.

Sleep Routines and Dealing with Crying

Some babies cry every night when they're placed in their crib for sleep; others almost never do. For many parents, it can be gut-wrenching when a baby cries in their crib for long periods of time. As your baby cries, your heart may be breaking, and it can be anguishing to keep your distance while you wait for them to fall asleep. Or you might feel frustration or anger at their apparent unwillingness or inability to quiet down and sleep. Even just a few minutes of tears can seem like an eternity.

Often concerned about why their baby is crying, parents may wonder whether the infant is simply letting off steam, is feeling lonely, or is really in distress. Not surprisingly, some of the most common questions asked of pediatricians are "Should I let my baby cry themselves to sleep, or should I pick them up and comfort them?" and the more fundamental question "How much sleep should they really be getting?" To a large degree, the answers to these questions depend on the age of the infant.

The First Month

During this period, your baby will spend most of their time asleep. When you place them on their back in their crib for sleep, or when they awaken, try to avoid letting them cry. Instead, respond to those tears and do whatever you can to soothe your baby, such as singing quietly, talking to them quietly, playing soft music, keeping the lights dim, and/or rocking them gently. Pick them up if necessary, placing them back in the crib again five to ten minutes later. By minimizing their discomfort in whatever way works, you'll maximize their sleep time and its quality. (For additional information about soothing a crying baby, see the information later in this section, as well as *pages 682 and 685* later in this chapter.)

When is an infant of this age ready for sleep, whether or not they're crying? In general, after they have been awake for one to two hours, they need sleep. Sometimes they may need to fall asleep even before an hour goes by, and rarely they may stay awake for three hours. If they are a little fussy or have some low-level crying, wait to see if it escalates once you place them back in the crib, and if it does, then of course pick them up. But they just might drift off to sleep.

Generally, no matter what the circumstances, they will begin to show signs of being overtired and irritable if they don't get their nap when they need it. So start soothing them to sleep. After they've been awake for an hour or two, they may need to be soothed. Place them in their crib when they're drowsy but still awake (this approach will be particularly helpful for daytime napping). If you wait too long, they're likely to become cranky and have even more difficulty falling asleep. (For more information on crying and colic, see *page 140*.)

Sharing the Bedtime Routine

During these early weeks after birth, it can help to get other adults, such as your spouse or partner, a grandparent, a sitter, or a nanny, involved in bedtime rituals. When you are the only one participating in getting your child to bed, they will associate only you with going to sleep. The more people who are involved, the less likely it is that your baby will associate a certain scenario with falling asleep.

Parent Sleep Deprivation

In your baby's first weeks after birth, another issue may surface: You may be sleep-deprived. A newborn's sleep schedule may leave either parent anxious and overwhelmed, particularly if they feel that they now have more responsibilities when they are feeling so sleep-deprived and exhausted. Support each other, and when necessary, provide the caregivers with additional periods for a break, a nap, or another way to recharge their batteries.

Planning ways to reduce caregiver exhaustion is also important to protect infants from sudden infant death syndrome (SIDS), as new research has demonstrated that parents are more likely to disregard safe sleep guidance when they are overly fatigued and desperate to get rest. Understanding your options when both caregivers are struggling with sleep and creating a plan for those times is a wise way to keep your baby safe.

Implementing a Sleep Plan

It is important that every adult who is involved with sleep time agree to a sleep plan for your child. If there is inconsistency, the plan is unlikely to succeed. Decide together whether to adopt any new steps gradually or quickly. Many pediatricians advise small, simple steps first, making it a little easier for both parent and child to adjust. A slightly earlier bedtime, for example, may improve your child's mood and lead to less disappointment.

Whenever a change is made, wait and watch for a while to see how successful it is. Do not make your evaluation on a day-by-day (or night-by-night) basis. Try a new approach for at least several days before concluding that the change is worth continuing.

- At about 6 weeks of age (counting from the baby's due date for an infant born prematurely): Your baby's sleep-wake schedule will start to settle into more of a routine at this time. They will begin to sleep longer at night, and may exhibit signs of drowsiness (and perhaps some crying) earlier in the evening. For example, while they may have once been ready for sleep between 9 and 11 p.m., they may start to need sleep somewhat earlier—perhaps between 6 and 8 p.m. Their longest sleep period will be in the late evening, lasting for three to five hours.

SCENARIO #2

A mother and father brought their 5-month-old daughter to the pediatrician and explained that her napping (or lack of it) had become a serious problem that affected the entire family. They would place her in her crib for a daytime nap, but she would awaken about thirty-five to forty minutes later, ready to continue her day, at least for a while. They agreed that their baby needed lengthier naps, but were frustrated in their attempts to make them longer. They had tried leaving the baby in her crib for twenty more minutes after awakening, but she would cry non-stop and resisted returning to sleep.

Their pediatrician explained that in infants 4 to 5 months old, it can be challenging to initiate a regular nap schedule because their biological rhythms are continuing to change and mature; nap times may not become well established for about another month or two. The doctor suggested that they could try extending the naps by responding promptly when the child first makes noises or calls out for attention. When that happens, they can try gently patting their baby or giving her a massage for a short time. With this approach, many children will fall back asleep for another twenty to thirty minutes, providing a truly restorative nap that leads to greater alertness and attention spans later in the day.

As a child becomes older, however, these particular approaches can become more stimulating than soothing in some children, and thus become counterproductive. After discussing the matter further with the parents, the pediatrician felt there were a couple of factors at play. The child's bedroom might not be dark enough and the apartment might not be quiet enough to encourage sleep. But more important, the timing of the child's naps was likely not in sync with her natural rhythms. The pediatrician recommended that they adjust the sleep environment to make it more conducive to napping, and to be patient until their child's biological rhythms made her body more agreeable to predictable daytime napping.

Variations exist, of course, so be sensitive to your own baby's needs and anticipate that they may require an earlier bedtime—no longer at 11 p.m. but rather at 8 p.m. So to minimize crying, try an earlier bedtime, spend some time soothing your baby if needed (although if they fuss a little, it won't cause any harm), and let their own biological rhythm dictate whether it will turn into a thirty-minute nap or a four-hour snooze.

As you and your baby get in tune with their rhythms, they'll gradually learn to soothe themselves to sleep when you place them in the crib. As that happens, there will be little or no crying. By about 3 months of age, some babies sleep six to eight hours in one stretch. If they awaken too early, you might be able to encourage them to go back to sleep by soothing them and keeping the lights off and the shades drawn.

- 4 to 12 months of age: With a 4-month-old, and continuing into the weeks and months ahead, keep working at being sensitive to your baby's bodily rhythms, which will minimize episodes of crying. From 4 months through the rest of the first year, most infants need at least two naps, one at midmorning and the other at midday; some children may nap a third time later in the afternoon. Try to get them on a schedule of napping at about 9 a.m., then at 1 p.m., and finally a late afternoon nap if they need it. Most parents hate to awaken a young child from a nap. Let them nap for as long as they wish unless they have difficulty falling asleep at night; in that case, talk to your pediatrician about waking them from their afternoon nap a little earlier than they might wake up on their own. If they take late and lengthy naps, it might be because their bedtime is too late, and they are partially compensating for lost sleep at night by taking long naps. Skipping the third nap and having an earlier bedtime might be warranted. By about 9 months of age, try to dispense with late afternoon naps so that they'll be ready for bedtime for the night at an earlier time than if those late afternoon naps continued.

At this age, a baby's nighttime sleep will be their longest sleep period of the day, and by about 8 months old, it should last from ten to twelve hours without them awakening for a nighttime feeding. But if a baby of this age seems overtired and they cry at the mere sight of their crib, their naps may be too short (less than thirty minutes long), their naps may not be occurring in sync with their sleep rhythms, or perhaps bedtime is too late at night. In the last case, place them in the crib much earlier, at least temporarily—perhaps at 5:30 or 6 p.m.—to respond to their excessive tiredness. If they cry, check on them and console them with a few comforting words. Change their diaper if needed, and make sure they are comfortable, but keep the lights dim and don't arouse them more fully by picking them up and walking with them. Then leave the room quietly. As the days and weeks pass, gradually give them less attention at night; this will help them stop anticipating that you'll show up whenever they cry or call out for you, and they'll be more likely to learn self-soothing techniques such as sucking on their hand, rocking their head, or rubbing the sheet.

It's important to keep in mind that there are times when you may need to let your baby cry themselves to sleep; it won't cause any harm. Remember, you have all day to show your infant how much you love them and care for them. At night, they'll get the message that nighttime is for sleeping, and on those nights when you let them cry, you're helping them learn to soothe themselves. They won't be thinking that you're abandoning them or that you don't love them anymore; they know by your daytime behaviors that this isn't the case at all. In other words, there's no need to worry.

Daytime Nap Evolution

About ages 10 to 12 months: The morning nap will begin to taper off in a few infants around 10 to 12 months. Around 12 months of age, some babies may drop their morning nap altogether. As that happens, you can start moving their nighttime bedtime somewhat earlier (perhaps by about twenty to thirty minutes); the afternoon nap can be started a little sooner, too. Your baby's bedtime may vary for a while, depending on factors such as how tired your baby seems and the quality of their daytime napping.

SCENARIO #3

Many parents recognize the importance of bedtime routines—but for some parents, these routines don't always work. One mother tried out many she had heard about, including bathing her 3-month-old baby, massaging them after the bath, singing soft lullabies, and swaddling the baby, but none was effective. In fact, her baby often became more irritable with these approaches.

When this mother expressed her frustration to her pediatrician, the pediatrician offered some pointers to make these bedtime routines more effective. They told the mother to begin using these routines early, before the baby is already overtired and becoming crabby. They also urged her to be consistent, using the same bedtime routines day after day until the baby begins to associate them with sleep. The pediatrician stressed persistence, explaining that changes don't happen overnight, and that routines need to be consistent over time to have a positive effect.

The pediatrician had another suggestion. They asked the parents to place their infant in the crib for a nap about twenty to thirty minutes before they thought the nap should actually begin. As the baby relaxed in their crib, they almost always had a bowel movement within ten to twenty minutes, which prompted them to cry. But then once their diaper was changed, they were now in the correct biological time frame for the nap to begin. The parents soothed them, and the baby fell asleep for a lengthy nap.

Getting the Most Out of Sleep

So how do you prepare and soothe your child to sleep? Soothing techniques may vary based on the age of your child. Some gentle massage can help at almost any age. For young infants, patting them, kissing their forehead, touching your cheek to theirs in a rhythmic pattern that coincides with their breathing, or encouraging sucking behavior with a pacifier or finger may be useful.

Bedtime routines can start as early as 4 to 6 months of age, which will help get your baby ready for rest, particularly as they start to associate these routines with sleep. Stop all screen time one to two hours before bedtime. Read them a story. Or give them a warm bath or a massage, sing them a lullaby, or play soothing music. Cut down on rambunctious playtime with them right before bedtime, close the curtains, dim the lights, and avoid using your mobile phone.

More important than your choice of a specific routine or ritual, you need to continue to stay in sync with your child's circadian rhythm. When it's time to sleep, keep your child away from situations where there is a lot of stimulation, which can lead to crankiness and make sleep difficult. Family activities with the baby before bedtime should be low-key, so as not to overstimulate them. Remember, timing is the key to healthy sleep. So while it's fine to sit quietly with your child for ten to twenty minutes and read them a story, what you choose to do is usually of less importance than the time you choose to do it.

SCENARIO #4

A father called the family's pediatrician with a problem that he and his wife were trying to solve. They understood the value of keeping their 9-month-old infant on a sleep schedule. At the same time, however, they had two older children with activities that didn't always fit in with the parents' commitment to be protective of their baby's need to nap.

Their pediatrician recommended that the parents work hard at finding a balance between the older children's social needs and the baby's biological requirement to nap during the day. Noting that they may not always find the perfect solution that meets the needs of everyone, the doctor added that compromises may be necessary. "Sometimes," they said, "you may have to tell an older child, 'You'll be a little late to your playdate because we're going to wait a few extra minutes until the baby finishes sleeping.' But other times, when the older child has a special event, you may decide to wake up the infant to make sure the older sibling gets to where they need to go on time."

It's true that in most cases, you should try to avoid awakening a sleeping baby. But a slightly shorter nap now and then won't cause harm, as long as it doesn't become a regular pattern.

Do you have to keep to the bedtime routine every single night? No! Once your child adopts a regular schedule in sync with their own internal clock, you can occasionally take your child out for special events without too much problem.

If your infant is in childcare during the first year, ask their caregivers to keep them on a regular napping schedule as much as possible. It should be the same schedule that you follow at home to minimize disruptions. Sometimes you may not even notice if your child is overtired because they are so excited to see you when you pick them up at the childcare facility, and you are so enthusiastic about seeing them. But pay attention to what they're experiencing. The staff's willingness to adapt to your own preferences for napping may be an important factor when you're choosing a facility.

Of course, many (but not all) childcare facilities are willing and able to make the timing of napping a priority. However, depending on where your child is being cared for, there may not be a dark, quiet room for napping, which can make sleeping difficult. Your child may be ready for a nap between 9 and 10 a.m. and then again between 1 and 3 p.m.—but the childcare environment may not be conducive to napping at those times. There might be too much light, or lots of noise (including crying) from other children. As a result, they may not get the sleep they need at the time when they most need it. When that happens, they could be overtired when you pick them up at the end of your workday, and an early bedtime may be most appropriate. If you're missing that evening bonding time, you may be able to shift some of that time to the morning, when you can spend time bathing, feeding, and dressing your baby.

Try your best to continue your child's weekday sleep schedule on the weekends and during vacations. Nevertheless, some disruptions in sleep schedules are inevitable. Holidays, vacations, or a family gathering can keep your child from napping or getting to bed on time. Because the temperament of children varies, some are much more adaptable to changes like these than others; while one child will adjust to changing circumstances very easily, others may not.

As much as possible, respect your child's nature, and try to maintain normal sleep routines. At the same time, if you know that a disruption of their sleep schedule is on the horizon, they will fare better and adapt more successfully—and have a cheerier disposition—if they are more rested ahead of time. So when you look ahead to a family party, for example, try to keep your child well rested in the preceding day or two so that this intrusion into their sleep schedule will unfold as smoothly as possible. The more rested your child is, the better their temperament and the more adaptable they will be to changes in their environment—and the better they will sleep.

How often can you disrupt your child's sleep schedule? Exceptions to sleep routines, when you can adjust naps and bedtimes, can occur once or twice a month, so you and your baby can enjoy holidays, birthdays, and other special events. Most well-rested children adapt to these occasional events.

If your baby does get off schedule—perhaps because of a grandparent's visit, or when an unexpected illness occurs—think of the notion of a "reset" that lasts just one night. For this night of readjustment, place your child in bed very early, ignoring protest crying related to the sleep debt they have accumulated. A more gradual approach often fails due to the child's overtiredness and their battle to get extra attention. It can be frustrating for parents, but a single "reset" night should resolve the problem. The key here is to get back to the normal bedtime routine.

Dealing with Other Sleep Concerns

Sometimes family issues can affect your child's sleep. For example, if you have trouble setting limits during the day, if parents (and grandparents) aren't on the same page, or if you've had an exhausting day at work, sleep in your home may be more challenging for everyone, especially your child. Dealing effectively with everyday problems can help your entire family get appropriate sleep.

Also, does your child have health or developmental issues, such as colic, autism spectrum disorder, severe eczema, or sleep apnea, that make sleeping difficult? (Colic is a frequent cause of sleep-disrupting fussiness in very young babies; see *page 140* for more information and guidance.) Or your child could have a short-term health problem like an ear infection that is causing pain and keeping them awake. Tend to their immediate needs, then talk with your pediatrician and/or pediatric specialist and follow their instructions on how to manage the problem and ease your child's discomfort.

Putting Sleep in Perspective

When it comes to your child's sleep, do the best you can, but don't feel bad if things don't always go smoothly. Make a concerted effort to get your child to bed on time for naps and at night. If your baby spends time at childcare or with a nanny and you're not present at nap time, make sure that their caregivers understand and try to be consistent with your own preferences about your child's sleep schedule. But you also need to set aside any anxiety and blame you might feel if you aren't doing everything perfectly. Inevitably, there will be days and nights when your child doesn't sleep well. Don't beat yourself up if your child goes to bed a little late for a night or two (or more). Just get back on track as soon as possible, and help them return to a normal sleeping routine. Dealing effectively with your child's sleeping problems is important, not only for your child, but also because their sleep difficulties can interfere with your own need to rest. Meeting your own sleep needs (as well as those of your partner) is important to effectively care for your baby and the rest of your family. Chronically overtired parents also have a greater risk of becoming depressed.

As we mentioned earlier, sleep is an essential, healthy part of your child's life. Helping your child sleep can be one of parenting's biggest challenges. But it can have an enormous payoff in terms of your child's health, now and in the future. Many adults are chronically poor sleepers because of patterns that may have begun during their own childhood. Sleeping poorly is a learned behavior, and when a child doesn't get quality sleep, they may not learn how to sleep well. In many cases, such sleep issues are likely to become part of their life for many years. The younger your child is when you begin to deal with their sleep problems, the more likely you are to resolve them. Remember that your pediatrician can be an ongoing source of support, advice, and reassurance. Additionally, many pediatric medical centers have individuals who specialize in helping children sleep better.

APPENDIX

American Academy of Pediatrics

DEDICATED TO THE HEALTH OF ALL CHILDREN®

Recommendations for Pre

Bright Futures/Ameri

Each child and family is unique; therefore, these Recommendations for Preventive Pediatric Health Care are designed for the care of children who are receiving nurturing parenting, have no manifestations of any important health problems, and are growing and developing in a satisfactory fashion. Developmental, psychosocial, and chronic disease issues for children and adolescents may require more frequent counseling and treatment visits separate from preventive care visits. Additional visits also may become necessary if circumstances suggest concerns.

These recommendations represent a consensus by the American Academy of Pediatrics (AAP) and Bright Futures. The AAP continues to emphasize the great importance of continuity of care in comprehensive health supervision and the need to avoid fragmentation of care.

Refer to the specific guidance by age as listed in the *Bright Futures: Guidelines for Health Supervision of Info* of Pediatrics; 2017).

The recommendations in this statement do not indic of medical care. Variations, taking into account indivi

The Bright Futures/American Academy of Pediatrics updated annually.

	INFANCY								EARLY CHILDHOOD			
AGE[1]	**Prenatal[2]**	**Newborn[3]**	**3-5 d[4]**	**By 1 mo**	**2 mo**	**4 mo**	**6 mo**	**9 mo**	**12 mo**	**15 mo**	**18 mo**	**24 mo**
HISTORY Initial/Interval	●	●	●	●	●	●	●	●	●	●	●	●
MEASUREMENTS												
Length/Height and Weight		●	●	●	●	●	●	●	●	●	●	●
Head Circumference		●	●	●	●	●	●	●	●	●	●	●
Weight for Length		●	●	●	●	●	●	●	●	●	●	
Body Mass Index[5]												●
Blood Pressure[6]		★	★	★	★	★	★	★	★	★	★	★
SENSORY SCREENING												
Vision[7]		★	★	★	★	★	★	★	★	★	★	★
Hearing		●[8]	●[9] ⟶	⟶	⟶	★	★	★	★	★	★	★
DEVELOPMENTAL/SOCIAL/BEHAVIORAL/MENTAL HEALTH												
Maternal Depression Screening[11]				●	●	●	●					
Developmental Screening[12]								●			●	
Autism Spectrum Disorder Screening[13]											●	●
Developmental Surveillance		●	●	●	●	●	●		●	●		●
Behavioral/Social/Emotional Screening[14]		●	●	●	●	●	●	●	●	●	●	●
Tobacco, Alcohol, or Drug Use Assessment[15]												
Depression and Suicide Risk Screening[16]												
PHYSICAL EXAMINATION[17]		●	●	●	●	●	●	●	●	●	●	●
PROCEDURES[18]												
Newborn Blood		●[19]	●[20] ⟶	⟶	⟶							
Newborn Bilirubin[21]		●										
Critical Congenital Heart Defect[22]		●										
Immunization[23]		●	●	●	●	●	●	●	●	●	●	●
Anemia[24]						★			●	★	★	★
Lead[25]							★	★	● or ★[26]		★	● or ★[26]
Tuberculosis[27]				★			★		★			★
Dyslipidemia[28]												★
Sexually Transmitted Infections[29]												
HIV[30]												
Hepatitis B Virus Infection[31]		★ ⟶	⟶	⟶	⟶	⟶	⟶	⟶	⟶	⟶	⟶	⟶
Hepatitis C Virus Infection[32]												
Sudden Cardiac Arrest/Death[33]												
Cervical Dysplasia[34]												
ORAL HEALTH[35]							●[36]	●[36]	★		★	★
Fluoride Varnish[37]							⟵	⟵	⟵	⟵	●	⟶
Fluoride Supplementation[38]							★	★	★		★	★
ANTICIPATORY GUIDANCE	●	●	●	●	●	●	●	●	●	●	●	●

1. If a child comes under care for the first time at any point on the schedule, or if any items are not accomplished at the suggested age, the schedule should be brought up to date at the earliest possible time.
2. A prenatal visit is recommended for parents who are at high risk, for first-time parents, and for those who request a conference. The prenatal visit should include anticipatory guidance, pertinent medical history, and a discussion of benefits of breastfeeding and planned method of feeding, per "The Prenatal Visit" (https://doi.org/10.1542/peds.2018-1218).
3. Newborns should have an evaluation after birth, and breastfeeding should be encouraged (and instruction and support should be offered).
4. Newborns should have an evaluation within 3 to 5 days of birth and within 48 to 72 hours after discharge from the hospital to include evaluation for feeding and jaundice. Breastfeeding newborns should receive formal breastfeeding evaluation, and their mothers should receive encouragement and instruction, as recommended in "Policy Statement: Breastfeeding and the Use of Human Milk" (https://doi.org/10.1542/peds.2022-057988). Newborns discharged less than 48 hours after delivery must be examined within 48 hours of discharge, per "Hospital Stay for Healthy Ter
5. Screen, per "Clinical Practice Guideline for the Evaluatio (https://doi.org/10.1542/peds.2022-060640).
6. Screening should occur per "Clinical Practice Guideline and Adolescents" (https://doi.org/10.1542/peds.2017-19 specific risk conditions should be performed at visits be
7. A visual acuity screen is recommended at ages 4 and 5 y may be used to assess risk at ages 12 and 24 months, in Assessment in Infants, Children, and Young Adults by Pe for the Evaluation of the Visual System by Pediatricians"
8. Confirm initial screen was completed, verify results, and per "Year 2007 Position Statement: Principles and Guide (https://doi.org/10.1542/peds.2007-2333).

KEY: ● = to be performed ★ = risk assessment to be performed with appropriate action to follow, if positive ⟵ ★ or ● ⟶ = range during which a service

ediatric Health Care

of Pediatrics

Bright Futures.

ines (Hagan JF, Shaw JS, Duncan PM, eds. olescents. 4th ed. American Academy

rse of treatment or serve as a standard , may be appropriate.

or Preventive Pediatric Health Care are

	MIDDLE CHILDHOOD						ADOLESCENCE										
4y	5y	6y	7y	8y	9y	10y	11y	12y	13y	14y	15y	16y	17y	18y	19y	20y	21y
●	●	●	●	●	●	●	●	●	●	●	●	●	●	●	●	●	●
●	●	●	●	●	●	●	●	●	●	●	●	●	●	●	●	●	●
●	●	●	●	●	●	●	●	●	●	●	●	●	●	●	●	●	●
●	●	●	●	●	●	●	●	●	●	●	●	●	●	●	●	●	●
●	●	●	★	●	★	●	★	●	★	★	●	★	★	★	★	★	★
●	●	●	★	●	★	●	←		●	→	←	●	→	←		●	→
●	●	●	●	●	●	●	●	●	●	●	●	●	●	●	●	●	●
●	●	●	●	●	●	●	●	●	●	●	●	●	●	●	●	●	●
							★	★	★	★	★	★	★	★	★	★	★
								●	●	●	●	●	●	●	●	●	●
●	●	●	●	●	●	●	●	●	●	●	●	●	●	●	●	●	●
●	●	●	●	●	●	●	●	●	●	●	●	●	●	●	●	●	●
★	★	★	★	★	★	★	★	★	★	★	★	★	★	★	★	★	★
★	★	★															
★	★	★	★	★	★	★	★	★	★	★	★	★	★	★	★	★	★
★		★		★	←	●	→	★	★	★	★	★	←			●	→
							★	★	★	★	★	★	★	★	★	★	★
							★	★	★	★	●						→
																	→
														●			→
							★										→
																	●
★	★	★															
	→																
★	★	★	★	★	★	★	★	★	★	★	★	★					
●	●	●	●	●	●	●	●	●	●	●	●	●	●	●	●	●	●

ttps://doi.org/10.1542/peds.2015-0699).
ldren and Adolescents with Obesity"

agement of High Blood Pressure in Children
asurement in Infants and children with

erative 3-year-olds. Instrument-based screening
ts at 3 through 5 years of age. See "Visual System
.org/10.1542/peds.2015-3596) and "Procedures
2/peds.2015-3597).
ate. Newborns should be screened,
Detection and Intervention Programs"

9. Verify results as soon as possible, and follow up, as appropriate.
10. Screen with audiometry including 6,000 and 8,000 Hz high frequencies once between 11 and 14 years, once between 15 and 17 years, and once between 18 and 21 years. See "The Sensitivity of Adolescent Hearing Screens Significantly Improves by Adding High Frequencies" (https://www.sciencedirect.com/science/article/abs/pii/S1054139X16000483).
11. Screening should occur per "Incorporating Recognition and Management of Perinatal Depression Into Pediatric Practice" (https://doi.org/10.1542/peds.2018-3259).
12. Screening should occur per "Promoting Optimal Development: Identifying Infants and Young Children With Developmental Disorders Through Developmental Surveillance and Screening" (https://doi.org/10.1542/peds.2019-3449).
13. Screening should occur per "Identification, Evaluation, and Management of Children With Autism Spectrum Disorder" (https://doi.org/10.1542/peds.2019-3447).

(continued)

(continued)

14. Screen for behavioral and social-emotional problems per "Promoting Optimal Development: Screening for Behavioral and Emotional Problems" (https://doi.org/10.1542/peds.2014-3716), "Mental Health Competencies for Pediatric Practice" (https://doi.org/10.1542/peds.2019-2757), "Clinical Practice Guideline for the Assessment and Treatment of Children and Adolescents With Anxiety Disorders" (https://pubmed.ncbi.nlm.nih.gov/32439401), "Screening for Anxiety in Adolescent and Adult Women: A Recommendation From the Women's Preventive Services Initiative" (https://pubmed.ncbi.nlm.nih.gov/32510990), and "Anxiety in Children and Adolescents: Screening" (https://www.uspreventiveservicestaskforce.org/uspstf/recommendation/screening-anxiety-children-adolescents). The screening should be family centered and may include asking about caregiver emotional and mental health concerns and social determinants of health, racism, poverty, and relational health. See "Poverty and Child Health in the United States" (https://doi.org/10.1542/peds.2016-0339), "The Impact of Racism on Child and Adolescent Health" (https://doi.org/10.1542/peds.2019-1765), and "Preventing Childhood Toxic Stress: Partnering With Families and Communities to Promote Relational Health" (https://doi.org/10.1542/peds.2021-052582).
15. A recommended tool to assess use of alcohol, tobacco and nicotine, marijuana, and other substances, including opioids is available at http://crafft.org. If there is a concern for substance or opioid use, providers should consider recommending or prescribing Naloxone (see https://www.cdc.gov/ore/search/pages/2018-evidence-based-strategies.html and https://nida.nih.gov/publications/drugfacts/naloxone).
16. Screen adolescents for depression and suicide risk, making every effort to preserve confidentiality of the adolescent. See "Guidelines for Adolescent Depression in Primary Care (GLAD-PC): Part I. Practice Preparation, Identification, Assessment, and Initial Management" (https://doi.org/10.1542/peds.2017-4081), "Mental Health Competencies for Pediatric Practice" (https://doi.org/10.1542/peds.2019-2757), "Suicide and Suicide Attempts in Adolescents" (https://doi.org/10.1542/peds.2016-1420), and "The 21st Century Cures Act & Adolescent Confidentiality" (https://adolescenthealth.org/press_release/naspag-sahm-statement-the-21st-century-cures-act-adolescent-confidentiality/).
17. At each visit, age-appropriate physical examination is essential, with infant totally unclothed and older children undressed and suitably draped. See "Use of Chaperones During the Physical Examination of the Pediatric Patient" (https://doi.org/10.1542/peds.2011-0322).
18. These may be modified, depending on entry point into schedule and individual need.
19. Confirm initial screen was accomplished, verify results, and follow up, as appropriate. The Recommended Uniform Screening Panel (https://www.hrsa.gov/advisory-committees/heritable-disorders/rusp/index.html), as determined by The Secretary's Advisory Committee on Heritable Disorders in Newborns and Children, and state newborn screening laws/regulations (https://www.babysfirsttest.org/) establish the criteria for and coverage of newborn screening procedures and programs.
20. Verify results as soon as possible, and follow up, as appropriate.
21. Confirm initial screening was accomplished, verify results, and follow up, as appropriate. See "Clinical Practice Guideline Revision: Management of Hyperbilirubinemia in the Newborn Infant 35 or More Weeks of Gestation" (https://doi.org/10.1542/peds.2022-058859).
22. Screening for critical congenital heart disease using pulse oximetry should be performed in newborns, after 24 hours of age, before discharge from the hospital, per "Endorsement of Health and Human Services Recommendation for Pulse Oximetry Screening for Critical Congenital Heart Disease" (https://doi.org/10.1542/peds.2011-3211).
23. Schedules, per the AAP Committee on Infectious Diseases, are available at https://publications.aap.org/redbook/pages/immunization-schedules. Every visit should be an opportunity to update and complete a child's immunizations.
24. Perform risk assessment or screening, as appropriate, per recommendations in the current edition of the AAP *Pediatric Nutrition: Policy of the American Academy of Pediatrics* (iron chapter).
25. For children at risk of lead exposure, see "Prevention of Childhood Lead Toxicity" (https://doi.org/10.1542/peds.2016-1493) and "Low Level Lead Exposure Harms Children: A Renewed Call for Primary Prevention" (https://stacks.cdc.gov/view/cdc/11859).
26. Perform risk assessments or screenings as appropriate, based on universal screening requirements for patients with Medicaid or in high prevalence areas.
27. Tuberculosis testing per recommendations of the AAP Committee on Infectious Diseases, published in the current edition of the AAP *Red Book: Report of the Committee on Infectious Diseases*. Testing should be performed on recognition of high-risk factors.
28. See "Integrated Guidelines for Cardiovascular Health and Risk Reduction in Children and Adolescents" (http://www.nhlbi.nih.gov/guidelines/cvd_ped/index.htm).
29. Adolescents should be screened for sexually transmitted infections (STIs) per recommendations in the current edition of the AAP *Red Book: Report of the Committee on Infectious Diseases*.
30. Screen adolescents for HIV at least once between the ages of 15 and 21, making every effort to preserve confidentiality of the adolescent, as per "Human Immunodeficiency Virus (HIV) Infection: Screening" (https://www.uspreventiveservicestaskforce.org/uspstf/recommendation/human-immunodeficiency-virus-hiv-infection-screening); after initial screening, youth at increased risk of HIV infection should be retested annually or more frequently, as per "Adolescents and Young Adults: The Pediatrician's Role in HIV Testing and Pre- and Postexposure HIV Prophylaxis" (https://doi.org/10.1542/peds.2021-055207).
31. Perform a risk assessment for hepatitis B virus (HBV) infection according to recommendations per the USPSTF (https://www.uspreventiveservicestaskforce.org/uspstf/recommendation/hepatitis-b-virus-infection-screening) and in the 2021–2024 edition of the AAP *Red Book: Report of the Committee on Infectious Diseases*, making every effort to preserve confidentiality of the patient.
32. All individuals should be screened for hepatitis C virus (HCV) infection according to the USPSTF (https://www.uspreventiveservicestaskforce.org/uspstf/recommendation/hepatitis-c-screening) and Centers for Disease Control and Prevention (CDC) recommendations (https://www.cdc.gov/mmwr/volumes/69/rr/rr6902a1.htm) at least once between the ages of 18 and 79. Those at increased risk of HCV infection, including those who are persons with past or current injection drug use, should be tested for HCV infection and reassessed annually.
33. Perform a risk assessment, as appropriate, per "Sudden Death in the Young: Information for the Primary Care Provider" (https://doi.org/10.1542/peds.2021-052044).
34. See USPSTF recommendations (https://www.uspreventiveservicestaskforce.org/uspstf/recommendation/cervical-cancer-screening). Indications for pelvic examinations prior to age 21 are noted in "Gynecologic Examination for Adolescents in the Pediatric Office Setting" (https://doi.org/10.1542/peds.2010-1564).
35. Assess whether the child has a dental home. If no dental home is identified, perform a risk assessment (https://www.aap.org/en/patient-care/oral-health/oral-health-practice-tools/) and refer to a dental home. Recommend brushing with fluoride toothpaste in the proper dosage for age. See "Maintaining and Improving the Oral Health of Young Children" (https://doi.org/10.1542/peds.2022-060417).
36. Perform a risk assessment (https://www.aap.org/en/patient-care/oral-health/oral-health-practice-tools/). See "Maintaining and Improving the Oral Health of Young Children" (https://doi.org/10.1542/peds.2022-060417).
37. The USPSTF recommends that primary care clinicians apply fluoride varnish to the primary teeth of all infants and children starting at the age of primary tooth eruption (https://www.uspreventiveservicestaskforce.org/uspstf/recommendation/prevention-of-dental-caries-in-children-younger-than-age-5-years-screening-and-interventions1). Once teeth are present, apply fluoride varnish to all children every 3 to 6 months in the primary care or dental office based on caries risk. Indications for fluoride use are noted in "Fluoride Use in Caries Prevention in the Primary Care Setting" (https://doi.org/10.1542/peds.2020-034637).
38. If primary water source is deficient in fluoride, consider oral fluoride supplementation. See "Fluoride Use in Caries Prevention in the Primary Care Setting" (https://doi.org/10.1542/peds.2020-034637).

Summary of Changes Made to the Bright Futures/AAP Recommendations for Preventive Pediatric Health Care (Periodicity Schedule)

This schedule reflects recommendations approved in December 2024 and published in February 2025. For updates and a list of previous changes made, visit www.aap.org/periodicityschedule.

RECOMMENDATIONS APPROVED IN DECEMBER 2024

No changes have been made to clinical guidance or footnotes in the recommendations published in 2025.

HRSA

Health Resources & Services Administration

This program is supported by the Health Resources and Services Administration (HRSA) of the U.S. Department of Health and Human Services (HHS) as part of an award totaling $1,966,000 with 0% financed with non-governmental sources. The contents of this document are those of the author(s) and do not necessarily represent the official views of, nor an endorsement, by HRSA, HHS, or the U.S. Government. For more information, please visit HRSA.gov.

Your child needs vaccines as they grow

2024 Recommended Immunizations for Birth Through 6 Years O

VACCINE OR PREVENTIVE ANTIBODY	BIRTH	1 MONTH	2 MONTHS	4 MONTHS	6 MONTHS	7 MONTHS	8 MON
RSV antibody	Depends on mother's RSV vaccine status						
Hepatitis B	Dose 1	Dose 2					
Rotavirus			Dose 1	Dose 2	Dose 3		
DTaP			Dose 1	Dose 2	Dose 3		
Hib			Dose 1	Dose 2	Dose 3		
Pneumococcal			Dose 1	Dose 2	Dose 3		
Polio			Dose 1	Dose 2			
COVID-19							At
Influenza/Flu							
MMR							
Chickenpox							
Hepatitis A							

KEY

- ALL children should be immunized at this age.
- SOME children should get this dose of vaccine or preventive antibody at this age

Talk to your child's health care provider for more guidance if:

1. Your child has any medical condition that puts them higher risk for infection.
2. Your child is traveling outside the United States.
3. Your child misses a vaccine recommended for their a

U.S. Department of Health and Human Services
Centers for Disease Control and Prevention

FOR MORE INFORMATION
Call toll-free: 1-800-CDC-INFO (1-800-232-4636)
Or visit: www.cdc.gov/vaccines/parents

Want to learn more?
Scan this QR code to find out which vaccines your child might need. Or visit **www.cdc.gov/vaccines/tool/child.html**

-2 NTHS	15 MONTHS	18 MONTHS	19 MONTHS	20–23 MONTHS	2–3 YEARS	4–6 YEARS
ends on child's health status						
	Dose 4					Dose 5
Dose 4						
Dose 4						
						Dose 4
of updated (2023–2024 Formula) COVID-19 vaccine						
very year. Two doses for some children						
Dose 1						Dose 2
Dose 1						Dose 2
2 doses separated by 6 months						

AAFP AMERICAN ACADEMY OF FAMILY PHYSICIANS

American Academy of Pediatrics
DEDICATED TO THE HEALTH OF ALL CHILDREN®

Birth to 24 months: Boys
Length-for-age and Weight-for-age percentiles

NAME ____________________

RECORD # ____________

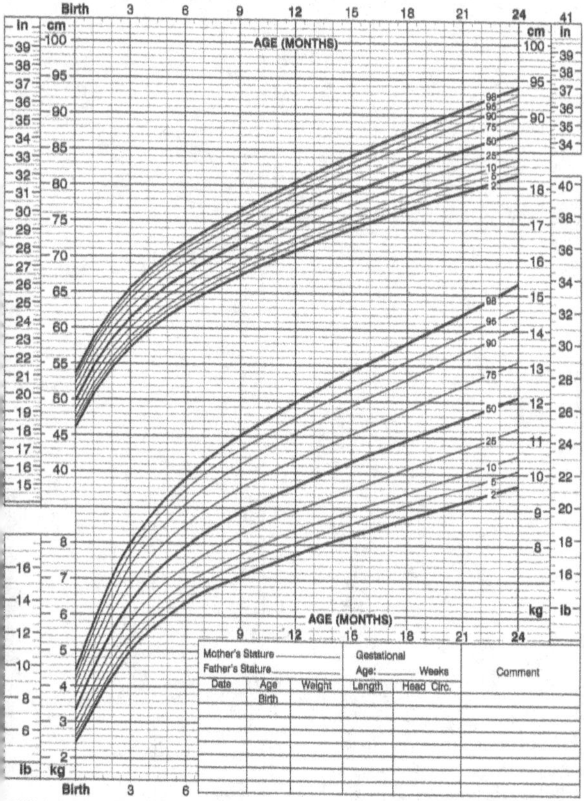

Mother's Stature ______			Gestational		Comment
Father's Stature ______			Age: ______ Weeks		
Date	Age	Weight	Length	Head Circ.	
	Birth				

Published by the Centers for Disease Control and Prevention, November 1, 2009
SOURCE: WHO Child Growth Standards (http://www.who.int/childgrowth/en)

SAFER · HEALTHIER · PEOPLE™

Reprinted by the American Academy of Pediatrics
The recommendations in this publication do not indicate an exclusive course of treatment or serve as a standard of medical care. Variations, taking into account individual circumstances, may be appropriate.
Additional copies are available for purchase in quantities of 100.
To order, contact: American Academy of Pediatrics
345 Park Blvd
Itasca, IL 60143

Website – www.aap.org
Minimum order 100

HE0510

Birth to 24 months: Girls
Length-for-age and Weight-for-age percentiles

NAME ____________________

RECORD # ____________

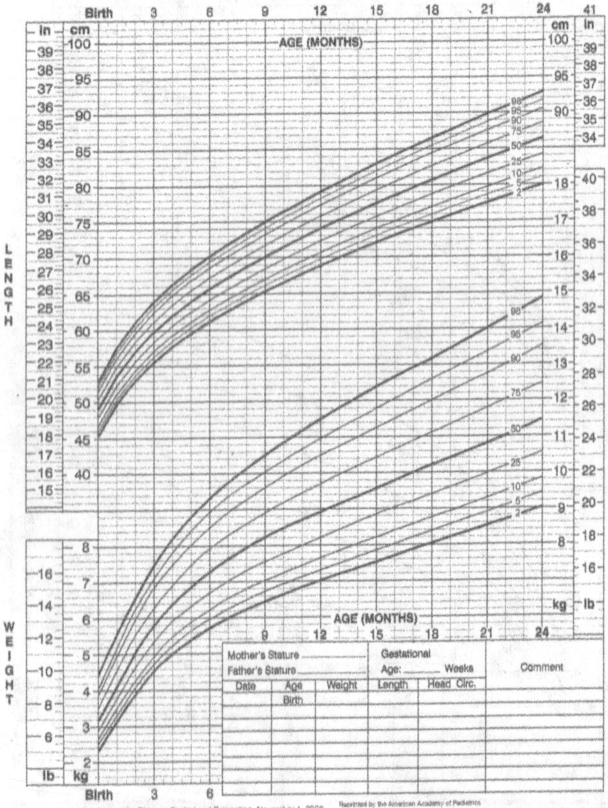

Mother's Stature ____________

Father's Stature ____________

Gestational Age: ________ Weeks

Date	Age	Weight	Length	Head Circ.	Comment
	Birth				

Published by the Centers for Disease Control and Prevention, November 1, 2009
SOURCE: WHO Child Growth Standards (http://www.who.int/childgrowth/en)

Reprinted by the American Academy of Pediatrics

The recommendations in this publication do not indicate an exclusive course of treatment or serve as a standard of medical care. Variations, taking into account individual circumstances, may be appropriate.

Additional copies are available for purchase in quantities of 100.
To order, contact: American Academy of Pediatrics
345 Park Blvd
Itasca, IL 60143

Website—www.aap.org
Minimum order 100

9-254/rep1122

HE0511

Birth to 24 months: Boys
Head circumference-for-age and Weight-for-length percentiles

NAME ____________________

RECORD # ____________

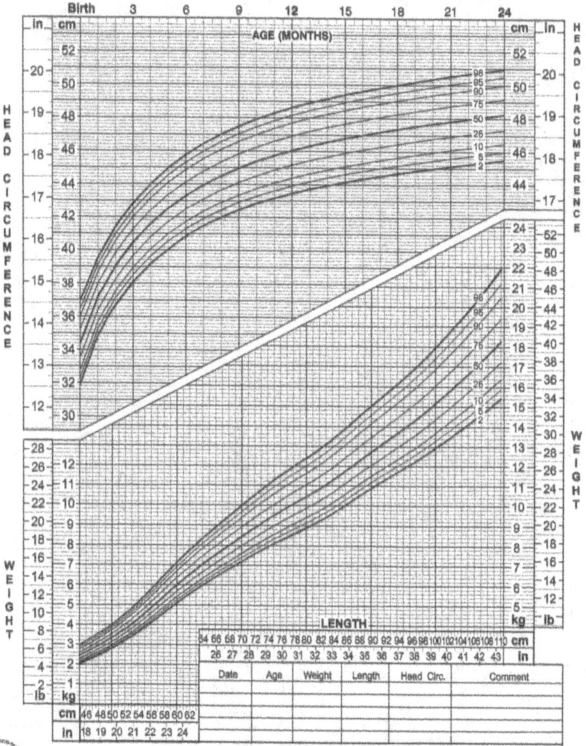

Date	Age	Weight	Length	Head Circ.	Comment

Published by the Centers for Disease Control and Prevention, November 1, 2009
SOURCE: WHO Child Growth Standards (http://www.who.int/childgrowth/en)

American Academy of Pediatrics

DEDICATED TO THE HEALTH OF ALL CHILDREN

Reprinted by the American Academy of Pediatrics

The recommendations in this publication do not indicate an exclusive course of treatment or serve as a standard of medical care. Variations, taking into account individual circumstances, may be appropriate.

Additional copies are available for purchase in quantities of 100.

To order, contact: American Academy of Pediatrics, 345 Park Blvd, Itasca, IL 60143

Website—www.aap.org
Minimum order 100

9-283/1122

HE0610

Birth to 24 months: Girls
Head circumference-for-age and Weight-for-length percentiles

NAME ______________________

RECORD # ____________

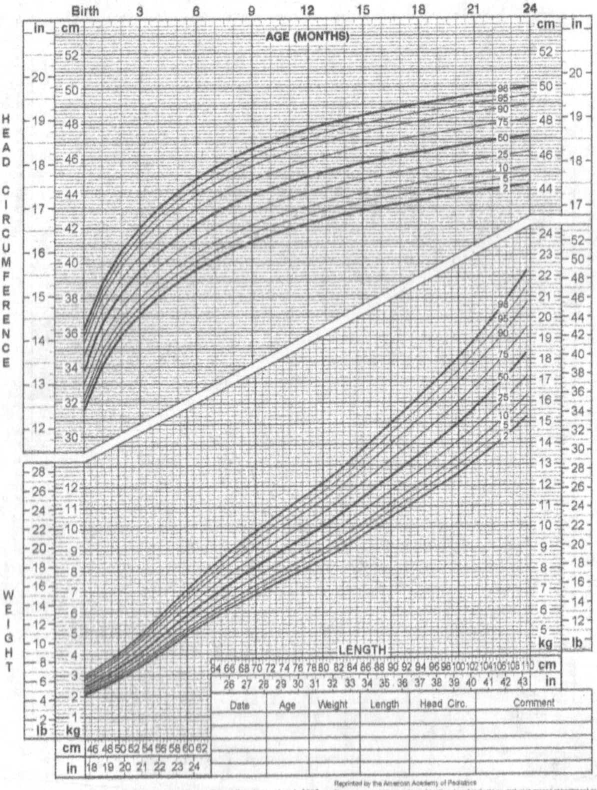

Published by the Centers for Disease Control and Prevention, November 1, 2009
SOURCE: WHO Child Growth Standards (http://www.who.int/childgrowth/en)

Reprinted by the American Academy of Pediatrics

The recommendations in this publication do not indicate an exclusive course of treatment or serve as a standard of medical care. Variations, taking into account individual circumstances, may be appropriate.

Additional copies are available for purchase in quantities of 100.
To order, contact: American Academy of Pediatrics, 345 Park Blvd, Itasca, IL 60143

Website—www.aap.org
Minimum order 100

9-284/rep1122

HE0811

CHOKING/CPR

LEARN AND PRACTICE CPR (CARDIOPULMONARY RESUSCITATION).

IF ALONE WITH A CHILD WHO IS CHOKING...

1. SHOUT FOR HELP. 2. START RESCUE EFFORTS. 3. CALL 911 OR YOUR LOCAL EMERGENCY NUMBER.

START FIRST AID FOR CHOKING IF	DO *NOT* START FIRST AID FOR CHOKING IF
• The child cannot breathe at all (the chest is not moving up and down). • The child cannot cough or talk or looks blue. • The child is found unconscious/unresponsive. (Go to CPR.)	• The child can breathe, cry, or talk. • The child can cough, sputter, or move air at all. The child's normal reflexes are working to clear the airway.

FOR INFANTS YOUNGER THAN 1 YEAR

INFANT CHOKING

If the infant is choking and is unable to breathe, cough, cry, or speak, follow these steps. Have someone call 911.

1 GIVE 5 BACK BLOWS (SLAPS).

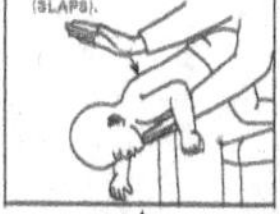

ALTERNATING WITH

2 GIVE 5 CHEST COMPRESSIONS.

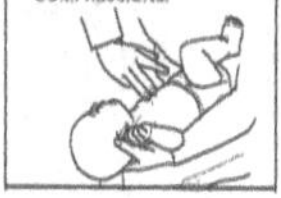

Alternate back blows (slaps) and chest compressions until the object is dislodged or the infant becomes unconscious/unresponsive. If the infant becomes unconscious/unresponsive, begin CPR.

INFANT CPR

To be used when the infant is UNCONSCIOUS/UNRESPONSIVE or when breathing stops. Place infant on flat, hard surface.

1 START CHEST COMPRESSIONS.

- Place 2 fingers of 1 hand on the breastbone just below the nipple line.
- Compress chest at least ⅓ the depth of the chest, or about 4 cm (1.5 inches).
- After each compression, allow chest to return to normal position. Compress chest at a rate of 100 to 120 times per minute.
- Do 30 compressions.

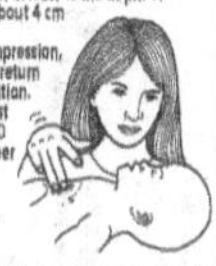

2 OPEN AIRWAY.

- Open the airway (head tilt-chin lift).
- If you see a foreign body, sweep it out with your finger. Do NOT do blind finger sweeps.

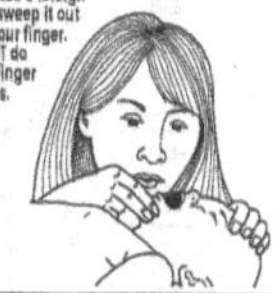

3 START RESCUE BREATHING.

- Take a normal breath.
- Cover infant's mouth and nose with your mouth.
- Give 2 breaths, each for 1 second. Each breath should make the chest rise.

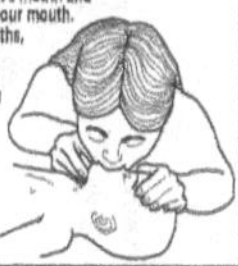

4 RESUME CHEST COMPRESSIONS.

- Continue with cycles of 30 compressions to 2 breaths.
- After 5 cycles of compressions and breaths (about 2 minutes), and if no one has called 911 or your local emergency number, call it yourself.

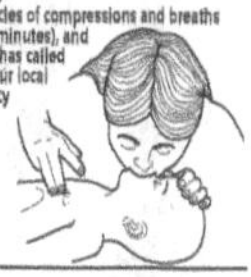

Adding Peanut Protein to Your Baby's Diet

iREACH

These are general instructions for feeding peanut-containing foods to your baby. When introducing peanut-containing foods, *pick a time when your infant is healthy and able to have your full attention for at least 2 hours* to watch for an allergic reaction.

If your baby has severe eczema or an egg allergy, please wait to give peanut-containing foods until your doctor says it is okay.

How To Introduce

Offer a small amount* of smooth peanut butter on the tip of a baby spoon.

↓

Wait 10 minutes to see how your baby responds.

↓

If there is no allergic reaction (see below), continue feeding your baby.

Allergic Reaction Signs

MILD symptoms include new rash or hives, especially around the mouth.

SEVERE symptoms include:

Lip or tongue swelling	Widespread hives
Vomiting or diarrhea	Skin color changes
Wheezing	Repetitive coughing
Difficulty breathing	Sudden fatigue

***Start with one serving containing 2g of peanut protein. Gradually increase to three servings per week, adapting to your baby's appetite and preferences.**

Recipe #1

Smooth Thinned Peanut Butter

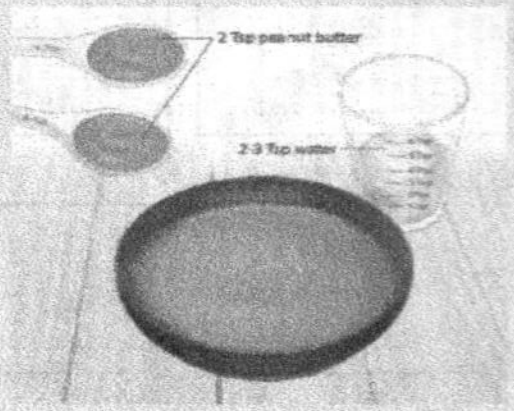

1. Measure 2 teaspoons of smooth peanut butter.
2. Add 2-3 teaspoons of hot water and stir until mixed, thinned, and blended. Let mixture cool.
3. Add water or baby cereal to make the mixture as thin or thick as your baby likes.

Contains 2g of peanut protein per serving.

Recipe #2

Smooth Peanut Butter Puree

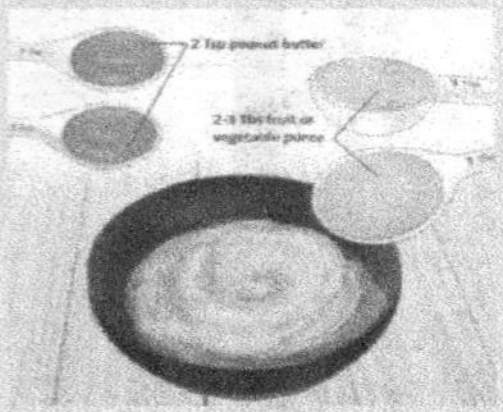

1. Measure 2 teaspoons of smooth peanut butter.
2. Add 2-3 tablespoons of a fruit or vegetable puree that your baby has eaten before. Stir until well blended.
3. Add more puree to make the mixture as thin or thick as your baby likes.

Contains 2g of peanut protein per serving.

Is This The Right Place For My Child?

(Make a copy of this checklist to use with each program you visit.)

Place a check in the box if the program meets your expectations.

Will my child be supervised?

- [ ] Are children watched at all times, including when they are sleeping?[15]
- [ ] Are adults warm and welcoming? Do they pay individual attention to each child?[40]
- [ ] Are positive guidance techniques used? Do adults avoid yelling, spanking, and other negative punishments?[16]
- [ ] Are the caregiver/teacher-to-child ratios appropriate and do they follow the recommended guidelines:
  - One caregiver per 3 or 4 infants
  - One caregiver per 3 or 4 young toddlers
  - One caregiver per 4 to 6 older toddlers
  - One caregiver per 6 to 9 preschoolers[19]

Have the adults been trained to care for children?

- [ ] If a center,
  - Does the director have a degree and some experience in caring or children? [27/28/29]
  - Do the teachers have a credential*** or Associate's degree and experience in caring for children?[27/28/29]

  If a family child care home:
  - Has the provider had specific training on children's development and experience caring for children?[30]
- [ ] Is there always someone present who has current CPR and first aid training?[32]
- [ ] Are the adults continuing to receive training on caring for children?[33]
- [ ] Have the adults been trained on child abuse prevention and how to report suspected cases?[12/13]

Will my child be able to grow and learn?

- [ ] For older children, are there specific areas for different kinds of play (books, blocks, puzzles, art, etc.)?[21]
- [ ] For infants and toddlers, are there toys that "do something" when the child plays with them?[41]
- [ ] Is the play space organized and are materials easy-to-use? Are some materials available at all times?[21]
- [ ] Are there daily or weekly activity plans available? Have the adults planned experiences for the children to enjoy? Will the activities help children learn?[22]
- [ ] Do the adults talk with the children during the day? Do they engage them in conversations? Ask questions, when appropriate?[43]
- [ ] Do the adults read to children at least twice a day or encourage them to read, if they can read?[43]

Is this a safe and healthy place for my child?

- [ ] Do adults and children wash their hands (before eating or handing food, or after using the bathroom, changing diapers, touching body fluids, eating, etc.)?[4]
- [ ] Are diaper changing surfaces cleaned and disinfected after each use?[5]
- [ ] Do all of the children enrolled have the required immunizations?[6]
- [ ] Are medicines labeled and out of children's reach?[7]
- [ ] Are adults trained to give medicines and keep records of medications?[7]

Notes:

Place a check in the box if the program meets your expectations.

Notes:

- ☐ Are cleaning supplies and other poisonous materials locked up, out of children's reach?[8]
- ☐ Is there a plan to follow if a child is injured, sick or lost?[9]
- ☐ Are first aid kits readily available?[10]
- ☐ Is there a plan for responding to disasters (fire, flood, etc.)?[11]
- ☐ Has a satisfactory criminal history background check been conducted on each adult present?
  - ➤ Was the check based on fingerprints?[14]
- ☐ Have all the adults who are left alone with children had background and criminal screenings?[13]
- ☐ Is the outdoor play area a safe place for children to play?[39]
  - ➤ Is it checked each morning for hazards before children use it?[23]
  - ➤ Is the equipment the right size and type for the age of the children who use it?[24]
  - ➤ In center-based programs, is the playground area surrounded by a fence at least 4 feet tall?[25]
  - ➤ Is the equipment placed on mulch, sand, or rubber matting?[23]
  - ➤ Is the equipment in good condition?[39]
- ☐ Is the number of children in each group limited?
  - ➤ In family child care homes and centers, children are in groups of no more than**
    - 6-8 infants
    - 6-12 younger toddlers
    - 8-12 older toddlers
    - 12-20 preschoolers
    - 20-24 school-agers[20]

Is the program well-managed?

- ☐ Does the program have the highest level of licensing offered by the state?[42]
- ☐ Are there written personnel policies and job descriptions?[17]
- ☐ Are parents and staff asked to evaluate the program?[37]
- ☐ Are staff evaluated each year; do providers do a self-assessment?[18]
- ☐ Is there a written annual training plan for staff professional development?[33]
- ☐ Is the program evaluated each year by someone outside the program?[38]
- ☐ Is the program accredited by a national organization?[36]

Does the program work with parents?

- ☐ Will I be welcome any time my child is in care?[1]
- ☐ Is parents' feedback sought and used in making program improvements?[1]
- ☐ Will I be given a copy of the program's policies?[2]
- ☐ Are annual conferences held with parents?[3]

These questions are based on research about child care; you can read the research findings on the NACCRRA website under "Questions for Parents to Ask" at http://www.naccrra.org.

* These are the adult-to-child ratios and group sizes recommended by theNational Association for the Education of Young Children. Ratios are lowered when there are one or more children who may need additional help to fully participate in a program due to a disability, or other factors.

** Group sizes are considered the maximum number of children to be in a group, regardless of the number of adult staff.

*** Individuals working in child care can earn a Child Development Associate credential.

For help finding child care in your area, contact Child Care Aware®, a Program of NACCRRA toll-free at 1-800-424-2246 or visit online at www.childcareaware.org.

For information about other AAP publications visit: www.aap.org

Endorsed by:

American Academy of Pediatrics

DEDICATED TO THE HEALTH OF ALL CHILDREN®

Office of Child Care

INDEX

Page numbers of illustrations appear in italics.

abdominal distension, 17, 40, 358
abdominal/gastrointestinal tract, 81, 84–85, 288, 347–81, *347*, *373*, *375*
  pediatrician exam of, 129
abdominal pain, 347–50
  colic, 348
  constipation, 352
  cramps, milk allergy, 349
  diarrhea, severe pain, 358
  food poisoning, 362
  gastroenteritis, 349, 355, 379
  infections, 349
  intussusception, 348
  lead poisoning, 349
  strep throat, 350
  when to call doctor, 347
acetaminophen (Tylenol), 370, 475, 479, 499, 618, 624, 655
  dosage chart, 578
  fever and, 410, 419, 469, 577–78, 604, 667
achondroplasia, 450
adenoids, 476
adenovirus, 379, 416
adoption, 77, 555–56
air pollution, 520–21
  AirNow.gov chart, 521
alcohol
  breastfeeding and, 61, 62
  poisoning danger, 313
  pregnancy and, 20, 108, 139, 451
  water safety and, 340
allergies
  "allergic shiners," 399
  animals and, 384, 391
  asthma and, 382–85
  atopic dermatitis and, 392
  "atopic march," 392
  baby formulas and, 84
  breastfeeding and, 50, 79, 399
  chronic, 400, 414, 416
  common allergens, 400
  dermatitis and, 392–94
  diarrhea and, 79
  eczema and, 79, 394
  food, 79, 200, 395–99
  hives and, 402, 404, 406
  how they develop, 396
  insect bites/stings, 404–7
  latex, 456
  milk, 79, 81, 84–85, 349, 354
  nasal allergy, 399–401
  "nasal salute," 399
  patch test for, 394
  prevention, 399
  seasonal (pollen), 399
  See also anaphylaxis
alopecia areata, 655–56
amblyopia, 543, 544, 553
American Academy of Pediatrics (AAP)
  "Car Safety Seats: Product Listing," 322
  Deployment and Military Medical Home Resources webpage, 565

American Association on Intellectual and Developmental Disabilities, 466
American Heart Association, 494
American Red Cross, 494
anaphylaxis, 396–97, 403, 406, 607–8
  food allergies, 79, 396–97
  insect bites/stings, 405
  what to do, 396, 405
anemia, 29, 532, 605–8, 616, 617, 618
animals
  allergies to pets, 400
  asthma and, 384, 391
  bites, 487–90
  flea bites, 405
  rabies, 342, 488–89
  safety, 246, 341–42, 487
  toxoplasmosis, 342, 459
antibiotic ointment/cream, 394, 498, 499, 550
  for eyes, 8, 11, 32, 160
antibiotics, 223
  for bites, 489
  diarrhea from, 354, 360
  for Lyme disease, 637
  for meningitis, 600, 604
  for MRSA infections, 664
  overuse, 473–74
  probiotics and, 360
  resistance to, 664
  for strep, 350, 481–83
  when needed, not needed, 224, 418, 428, 473–74, 550, 592, 618, 656, 659
antifungals, 162, 654, 665–66
antihistamines, 394, 402, 404, 651
antivirals, 421, 479–80, 651
Apgar scores, 8, 9–10
apnea, 26, 27, 453, 688
appetite loss, 358, *532*, *599*, 666
arrhythmias, 608–11
  bradycardia, 26, 609
  fibrillation, 609
  flutter, 609, 610
  premature beats, 609, 610
  sinus, 609, 610
  tachycardia, 609
arthritis, 635–37
  juvenile idiopathic, 642
  limping and, 641, 643
  Lyme disease, 636–37
  septic, 635, 642
asbestos/guidelines, 521–22
aspirin, 419, 475, 577, 615
asthma, 382–91, *382*, 520
  action plan, 386
  breathing tests, 385
  coping with, 430–37
  coughing and, 414, 415
  diagnosis, 382–83
  pneumonia and, 422
  prevention, 391
  smoking and, 383, 391
  treatment/medications, 387–90 *388*, *389*, *390*
  triggers, 382–85, 391
  wheezing, 382–83, 414
  when to call doctor, 385–86
atopic dermatitis, 392–94
autism spectrum disorder (ASD), 438, 440–43, 447, 622, 628
  AAP on, 442
Automotive Safety Program, 323–24

baby acne, 132
baby blues, 23
baby carriers, 334–35
baby monitor, 255
baby powder, 111, 496
babysitters. *See* childcare choices
baby talk, 39

bacterial infections, 224
  of a joint, 635, 642
  perianal strep, 350
  vomiting and, 381
baldness, 655–56
basic care
  1 month, 150–56
  2 months, 179–85
  4 months, 199–202
  6 months, 213–22
  9 months, 248–55
  day to day care, 101–26
basic healthcare, 127–30
bassinets, 34, *34*
bathing, 118–21, 164
  bath toys, 121, 246
  boys, penis care, 118–19
  caution, 121, 164, 205
  cord stump care, 119
  how to bathe your baby, 119–21, *120*
  safety check, 163–64, 205
  supplies, 118, 119
  towel with hood, 121, *121*
  water temp., 119, 164
batteries, 310–11, 320
  National Battery Ingestion Hotline, 311
  what to do if swallowed, 311, 495
bedbugs, 405
bedding, 107–8, 110, 302, 391, 400, 401
bee stings, 404–7
behavior
  autism and, 441
  discipline and, 255–58
  fears and, 247
  lead poisoning and, 532
  regressive, 562
  selective, 177
  separation anxiety, 206, *242*, 243, 244–46
  stranger anxiety, 189, 241, 242, *242*
  style and parenting, 212
  thumb sucking, 247–48
bilingual babies, 235–36
bilirubin, 28, 42–43
birth injuries, 40
birthmarks/hemangiomas, 15–16, 647–50
bisphenol A and phthalates, 89, 524–25, 526
bites
  animal or human, 487–90
  insect bites/stings, 404–7
  rabies and, 488–89
  signs of infection, 489
  tetanus shot, 488, 490
  treatment, 488–90
  when to call doctor, 489
black eye, 548
blood
  bleeding, 485, 486, 497
  desaturation, 26, 27
  hemophilia, 450
  in stool, 79, 117, 349, 352, 358
  in urine, 115–16, 581–83, 592
blood diseases. *See* anemia; leukemia; sickle cell disease; thalassemia
blood pressure, 397, 582, 592, 657
Blount's disease, 638
blue baby, 40
blue skin, lips, or nails
  emergency: lack of oxygen, 31, 40, 44, 385, 397, 415, 418, 428, 485, 603, 611
  normal: newborns or from cold, 9, 10, 40, 132–33
body temperature
  best ways to take a temperature, 127, 574–75

body temperature (*cont'd*)
  fever range, 572
  heatstroke and, 576
  normal, 572
  See also fever
bonding, 4, 24–25, 31
bones
  bacterial infection, 635, 642
  Blount's disease, 638
  fractures, 506, 508–11, 641
  Kohler's disease, 642
  rickets, 638
bottle-feeding, 80–94, 200
  amount and schedule, 90–92
  bowel movements and, 117–18, 180
  BPA in bottles, 89, 525
  breaking the bedtime bottle habit, 253
  breast milk in, 69–73, 74
  burping, 95–96, 97–98
  cleaning bottles, 87
  colic and, 141, 142
  ear infections and, 89, 253, 472, 477
  feeding cues, 142
  nipples and, 89, 99
  paced feedings, 90–91
  partner's role, *89*
  position for, 90
  rooting reflex and, 90
  self-feeding, 89
  signs of too much or too little feeding, 92–93
  spitting up and, 96, 98–99
  supplemental feedings, 94
  tooth decay and, 86, 89, 220, 253
  weaning, 215, 252–54
  where and how to bottle-feed, 90, *90*
  See also formula
botulism, 362, 367, 416
bowel movements
  age of child and, 150–51, 159, 180, 218
  blood in stool, 79, 117, 159, 349, 352, 358
  breastfed baby, 48, 68, 73–74, 116, 117, 151, 159, 180, 352
  color of stool, 116–17, 159, 218, 355
  cystic fibrosis and, 412
  formula-fed baby, 116–18
  hard/dry stools, 116, 159
  newborns, 48, 73–74, 116, 150–51, 352
  "rabbit pellets," 352
  solid foods and, 116
  spina bifida and, 457
  when to call doctor, 117, 159
bowlegs, 638
boys
  fragile X, 450–51, 467
  growth, weight, and BMI charts, *699*, *701*
  hydrocele, 17, 374–75, *375*
  inguinal hernia, 17, 372–73, *373*, 591
  middle ear infections, 472
  sex-linked genetic abnormalities, 450–51
  See also circumcision; genitals, boys
brain
  baby's states of consciousness, 139–40
  baby's versus adult's, 137
  damage, shaken baby, 104, 140, 142–43, 166, 178
  early development, 136–40
  skin-to-skin care and, 136–37
  surgery, meningitis and, 599
  whooping cough and disease of, 620

brain: stimulating development
  1 month, 137–39, 176
  2 months, 184–85
  4 months, 203–4, 213
  6 months, 220–21
  9 months, 240–41
  elements/environment for, 137, 203–4
breastfeeding, 46–80, 179–81
  AAP position on, 48, 200
  benefits, 47, 49, 50, 56, 477
  burping, 67, *67*, 95–96, *97–98*
  CDC report card, 48
  colic and, 141
  common problems, 51, 75–76
  coughing by baby, 180
  diarrhea and, 347
  distracted baby, 195, 198
  doubts or fears, 47, 74–75
  excessive crying, 78–80
  feeding cues, 135, 142, 200
  growth spurts, 78, 179–80
  help from family, 49, 50
  how much per feeding, 63
  how often, how long, 48, 50, 66–69, 74, 135, 179–81, 360
  infant fussiness, 78–80
  interrupting a feeding, *60*
  iron supplements, 605
  lactation, 52–53, 77
  lactation consultants, 6, 23–24, 51–52
  latching on, 5, *5*, 53–58, *55*, *59*
  let-down-process and tips to help, 54, 56–61
  medications and, 51
  multiples and, 65–66, *65*, 567–68
  nipples, 52–54, *54*, 56, *75*
  nursing after delivery, 4–6, *5*, 48, 66
  nursing bras, 53, 69
  overfeeding, 141
  pain, 51, 56, 62–63, 76
  partner's role, 50
  positions and holds, 57–58, *57*, *58*
  preterm babies, 23–24, 47
  recommended reading, 99
  reflux and, 79
  self-confidence, 52, 99
  signs of correct or incorrect nursing, 64–65
  signs of successful breastfeeding, 58
  signs of too much or too little feeding, 92–93
  signs of well-nourished newborn, 73–74
  skin-to-skin contact and, 49, 55
  sleeping baby and, 66–67
  special circumstances that may prevent, 50–51
  supplemental bottle, 69
  supplemental nurser, 76–77, *77*
  supplemental water, 94
  support for mothers, 48
  time spent on, 49
  traveling and, 156
  urine color, number of wet diapers, 68, 74
  vitamins and, 64–65, 248
  weaning, 215
  website for info on, 99
  weight gain, 68–69, 73, 180
  where to sit, 60–61, 195
  See also bowel movements
breast milk, 47
  benefits, 49, 213
  bottle-feeding of, 181
  colostrum, 6, 24, 52
  donated, 24

breast milk (*cont'd*)
drug warning, 61–62
expressing milk, 62, 69–73, *71*, 181
hindmilk, 58
increase in, 62–63
ingredients, 49, 84, 361
jaundice and, 43
medications or supplements and, 51, 61
mother's diet and, 79, 141
newborns' sense of smell and taste and, 30
preterm babies and, 24
smoking, marijuana, or illegal drugs, 71, 538
storing, 72–73
SUID/SIDS risk and, 107
transitional, 62
volume of, 62–63, 65, 79, 180
breast pumps, 24, 62, 70, 71–72, *72*, 181
breasts
areola, 54, *55*
cancer, 80
care of, 53
engorgement, 62–63, 75
how milk is produced, 52–53, *53*
inverted nipples, 54, *54*
lanolin/lotions on, 53, 75
mastitis, 75–76
plastic surgery, 80
sore/cracked nipples, 75
breath-holding, 603
breathing
Apgar score, 10
breaths per minute, 158
premature babies, 22–23
stridor, 158
breathing difficulties
anaphylaxis and, 396, 405, 406
asthma, 382–91, *382*
at birth, 9
chickenpox and, 651
emergencies, 485
fever and, 158
first month, 158
hives and, 403
humidifier for, 158
infection and, 27
nasal congestion, 44, 158
pneumonia and, 422
preterm babies, 22–23, 25–26
Bright Futures/AAP Preventive Pediatric Health Care, 695
bronchiolitis, 225, 408–11, *408*, 413, 414
when to call doctor, 409, 410
bronchitis, 408
bronchodilators, 387, 410, 416
bronchopulmonary dysplasia, 25–26, 409
burns, 484, 490–93
bathroom and, 307–8
categories of, 490
cigarettes and, 538
electrical or chemical, 320, 491
emergency treatment, 491–92
fireplaces, stoves, or heaters and, 312–13
hot-water heater setting, 119, 164, 202, 493
kitchen and, 305–6
precautions, 205, 320
prevention, 492–93
safety checks by age, 186, 205, 261
burping, 67, *67*, 95–96, 103
for GER, 379
how to, 96–98, *97–98*

Campylobacter, 362–63
cancer, 80, 410, 422, 647, 648

carbon monoxide poisoning, 309, 522–23
car safety, 321, 322, 331–32, 484, 487
  airbags, 325–26, 331, 333
  booster seats, 291, 322, 333
  car pools and, 290
  child in the rear seat, 321, 325–26, 331
  child left in a car, 330
  kids around cars, 332–33
  overheating deaths, 330, 576
  strangulations, 330
car safety seats, 152, 290, 321–30, *323*
  AAP on, 333
  AAP's "Car Safety Seats: Product Listing," 322
  baby sleeping in, 107, 163, 315, 330
  children with medical conditions and, 323–24
  choosing, 322–25
  emergency sticker, 487
  expiration dates, 163, 324
  forward-facing, *323*, 328
  hot weather tip, 329
  infants/toddlers, 325
  installing, 325–28
  LATCH system, 163, 205, 326–28
  multiples and, 570
  newborns and, 32, 333
  pickups or vehicles with no rear seat, 326, *326*
  preterm baby, 323, 333
  rear-facing, 322, *322*, 325, 331
  recalls, 325
  registering, 324
  safety checks, 163, 204–5, 260
  supervision and, 165
  traveling tips, 156
  types, 325–28
  used seats, warning, 324
  using, 156, 328–30
cataracts, 129, 543, *544–45*
celiac disease, 350–51
Centers for Disease Control and Prevention, 657
  breastfeeding report card, 48
  ASD resources, 443
  ASD symptoms, 441
  congenital abnormalities resources, 458
  developmental disabilities resources, 466
cereals, 82, 83, 116, 180, 215, 250, 379
cerebral palsy (CP), 27, 438, 443–49, 642
Cesarean (C-section), 6–7, 14, 21
chalazae, 550
changing tables, 164, 171, 229, 302–3, *303*
chest and lungs, 408–29, *408*
  asthma and, 382–91, *382*
  breastfeeding benefits, 50
  breathing tests, 385
  bronchi, 413
  coughs, 409, 413–16
  seasonal allergies, 399
  See also specific diseases
"chestfeeding," 46
chickenpox (varicella), 650–52
  complications, 620, 651
  shingles and, 652
  vaccine, 130, 286, 615, 623–25, 652
child abuse/neglect, 556–60
childcare, 263–96
  accreditation, 269
  acquainting baby with caregivers, 260
  attributes of a good caregiver, 264–65

childcare (*cont'd*)
building a relationship with caregivers, 279–80
child/staff ratios, 270, 274
conflict resolution, 281–82
controlling infectious diseases and, 284–89
CPR and first aid at, 155, 339, 494
guidelines for choosing, 263–65, *264*
how to find, 270, 272
injury prevention and car safety, 280, 289–91
monitoring caregivers, 221, 241, 263, 267, 270
mothers returning to work and, 167–68
naps and, 278, 686–87
newborns/first month and, 153–55
questions to ask, 274–78
safety, 266–67, 269, 342
safety checklist, 292–94
separation anxiety, 244
sick children care, 275, 282–84, 411
special-needs care, 291, 294–96
SUID/SIDS and, 278
transitioning to, 280–82
trial period, 267
Child Care Aware, 270, 272
childcare choices
babysitters, 154–55, 244–45, 342
centers, 271–78, 284
family-based programs, 268–71, 284
grandparents or other relatives, 266
Head Start, 272
in-home/nanny, 266–68
"Is This the Right Place for My Child," 705–6
Child Care Technical Assistance Network, 269
Child Passenger Safety (CPS) Technicians, 328
child-proofing, 226–27, 299–320
equipment/toys, 313–20
inside home, 300–313
outside home, 321–43
poison-proofing, 514–15
choking, 484, 494
batteries/magnets, 495
emergency treatment and CPR, 494–96, 703, *703*
foods to avoid, 200, 216, 251–52, 262, 495–96
pacifier safety and, 152
prevention, 187, 205, 261–62, 310, 495–96
sudden cough and, 415
teething necklaces, 219
chordee, 584–85
chromosome abnormalities, 449–51
chronic conditions and diseases, 430–67
coping with, 430–31
getting help for your baby, 435–47
"medical home" and, 433
navigating the health care system, 433–34
parental stressors and decisions, 432
receiving the diagnosis, 431–32
See also asthma; cystic fibrosis; developmental disabilities; IDD
circumcision, 118–19, 583
cleanliness
bedding, 391, 401
disease prevention, 420–21

hand washing, 420
humidifiers, 470
rugs, stuffed animals, 391
cleft palate, 129, 451
Clostridium perfringens, 363
clothing
dermatitis and, 393
garments that make dressing easier, 126
going outside, 153, 673–74
heatstroke and, 576
newborns/first month, 123–26
preventing insect bites/sting and, 407
safety check, 164
sleepwear, 107, 164
towel with hood, 121, *121*
clubfoot, 644
cochlear implants, 463
cognitive development, 194, 197–98, 210–11, 237–39, *239*
cold sores. *See* herpes simplex
colds, 185, 224, 286, 413, 421, 468–71
acetaminophen or ibuprofen for, 410, 469
antibiotics and, 224
asthma attacks and, 384
childcare and, 286
congested nose, 44, 410, 158, 470
cough or cold medicine caution, 416, 470
coughs and, 409, 413–16
ear infection and, 469
fever and, 468, 572
RSV and, 408
when to call doctor, 44, 469
colic, 140–41, 348
baby formula and, 84, 85
behavior/crying, 78, 104
breast milk and, 78–79, 141
non-medication options, 104, 348
when it starts, 79
color blindness, 451
colostrum, 6, 24, 52
communicating hydrocele, 374–75, *375*
complementary or alternative therapies, AAP on, 435–36
congenital abnormalities, 411, 449–58
Down syndrome, 452–54
pregnancy and, 444, 451, 454–55
rate of occurrence, 449
resources, 452, 457–58
spina bifida, 452, 454–57
conjunctivitis (pink eye), 160, 225, 287, 481, 545–46, 658
constipation, 116, 352–53
abdominal distension, 40
iron-fortified foods, 83
lead poisoning, 349, 532
newborns and first month, 116, 118, 159, 352
when to call doctor, 159
Consumer Product Safety Commission (CPSC), 294
Improvement Act of 2008, 313
label for infant seats and bouncers, 315
lead content of child products and, 349
reporting an injury or unsafe products, 321
window covering recommendation, 311
contact dermatitis, 392–94
convulsions. *See* seizures
cord blood, 11–12
corticosteroids, 387, 388, 390, 410, 418

cortisone/hydrocortisone cream, 394, 654
cough, 413–16
  allergies and, 400, 416
  bronchiolitis, 409, 410
  choking and, 415
  chronic, 414, 415
  colds/upper respiratory infections, 469
  common causes, 414
  cystic fibrosis and, 413
  issues related to, 414–15
  newborn feeding and, 41
  nighttime, 413, 414, 416
  teaching your child how to cough, 420–21
  when to call doctor, 414, 415
  See also asthma; croup; pneumonia; whooping cough
cough medicine, 410, 416, 418, 428, 470
COVID-19, 625
  MIS-C complication, 625
  vaccine, 130, 259, 620, 625
Coxsackie virus, 481
CPAP, 23, 25, 26
CPR, 155, 338, 339, 340, 486, 493–94, 502, 505
  instructions, 703, *703*
cradle cap, 161, 653–64
crawling, 229–30, *229*, 445
  injury risk and, 298
crib death. *See* SUID/SIDS
cribs
  bumpers, 300, 302
  gyms, 302
  location for, 302
  mattress for, 107, 301–2
  mobiles for, 149, 150, 172, 184, 195, 302
  for newborns, 32
  safety, 156, 164, 165, 195, 300–302, *300*
  suffocation and, 164
Cronobacter bacteria, 87
croup, 225, 413, 416–18, *417*
crying
  baby's states of consciousness and, 140
  at bedtime, 201, 218–19
  colic and, 104, 140–41
  consoling techniques to try, 103, 141–42, 254
  diaper change and, 685
  excessive, 41, 201
  fever as cause, 104
  fussiness, 78–80, 102, 140
  hunger and, 78, 92, 102
  middle-ear infection, 472
  newborns, 30, 102, 140
  pacifier for, 142
  parental coping, 140, 143, 178
  parental tension and, 104
  responding to, 102–4, *103*
  self-soothing, 104, 141, 178, 219, 254, 682
  shaken baby and, 140
  types, 102, 177–78, 189, 254, 257–58
cryptorchidism, 363, 590–91, *591*
cuts/lacerations, 497–501
  bleeding and, 497–98
  on eyelid, 548
  tetanus booster and, 499
cystic fibrosis (CF), 411–13, 450
  bronchiolitis and, 409
  centers for, 412–13
  genetic testing for, 411
  malabsorption and, 376
  newborn screening, 412
  pneumonia and, 422
  support groups, 413

Cystic Fibrosis Foundation, 413
cystitis, 592
cytomegalovirus (CMV), 286–87, 451

dactylitis or hand-foot syndrome, 617
dehydration
  diarrhea and, 355, 357
  electrolyte solution for, 347, 357, 359
  fever and, 94, 576, 580
  ibuprofen warning, 419
  signs of, 159, 357, 409
  sunburn and, 673
  vomiting and, 355, 380
  when to go to the ER or doctor, 358, 480
delirium, 576, 577
delivery and the first moments, 3–12, *3*
  birth injuries, 16, 40, 596
  bonding, 4
  breech birth, 6, 175, 596
  Cesarean birth, 6–7
  cutting the cord, 4
  delivery room procedures, 8–10
  first nursing, 4, 5–6, *5*, 55, 66
  forceps marks, 41–42
  hepatitis vaccine, 8, 626
  ID bracelet or name label, 8, 10
  leaving delivery area, 10–11
  skin-to-skin care, 4, 7, 8
  vaginal birth, 3–5
Department of Transportation's Vehicle Safety Hot Line, 325, 328
depression
  baby blues, 23
  parental, 557
  postpartum, 23, 34, 36
  SIDS death and, 219–20
dermal melanocytosis spots, 15
dermatitis
  atopic, 392
  contact, 392–93, 653
  seborrheic, 161, 653–54
dermoid cysts, 550
developmental disabilities, 438–67
  AAP on, 438–39
  brain development and, 138
  causes of developmental delays, 465, 449–58, 466–67
  conditions during pregnancy and, 451
  family support, 439–40
  information sources, 466
  learning difficulties, 438
  preterm babies, 28–29
  programs available for, 439, 465, 467
  See also specific disabilities
diabetes, 47, 50, 217, 419, 421, 430, 451, 455, 627
diapering, 111–13
  diaper types, 112, *112*
  how to diaper, 111–12, *113*
  late-night changes, 105
diaper rash, 114–15, 162
diarrhea, 185, 354–60
  bloody, 84, 349, 355, 358
  breastfeeding and reduced risk, 50, 347
  causes, 117, 218, 349, 354–55
  childcare and, 287
  chronic, 358
  dehydration and, 94, 117, 355, 357, 358
  foods/liquids to avoid, 355, 357
  Giardia lamblia and, 349
  infants and, 81, 94, 117, 159, 225
  milk allergy and, 79, 81, 84–85, 349, 354

diarrhea (*cont'd*)
prevention, 359–60
probiotics for, 356
roseola infantum and, 666
significant versus mild, 356–57
stool color and, 355
"toddler's diarrhea," 358
treatment, 355–59
when to call the doctor, 159, 358, 362, 365
diphtheria, 130, 620, 625
See also DTaP vaccine
discipline, 255–58
AAP on, 257
consistency of, 256
distraction method, 256
immediacy of, 256–57
physical punishment, 257
saying "no," 256
time-outs/time-ins, 257
what not to do, 256
divorce and separation, 560–61, 564, 567
Down syndrome (trisomy 21), 450, 452–54
AAP guidelines for, 454
resources for, 458
drooling, 96, 219, 393, 514, 517
drowning
bathing caution, 121, 307
bathrooms, 307
CPR and, 502
emergency help, 501–3
non-fatal, 484
prevention, 502–3
recovery from, 502
safety precautions, 205, 261, 338–41, 502–3
what to do, 502
DTaP vaccine, 186, 204, 225, 429, 625–26, 696
side effects/reactions, 625
dust mites
allergy to, 399, 400–401
asthma and, 384, 391
controlling, 391, 401

ear infections, 185, 224, 225, 471–78
antibiotics for, 224, 474, 475, 476
bottle-feeding and, 89, 253, 472, 477
breastfeeding and, 50, 477
fever and, 473, 572
hearing loss and, 210, 473
heredity and, 472
measles and, 658
middle ear (otitis media), 471–78, *471*, 658
nasal allergy/allergic rhinitis and, 400
scarlet fever and, 671
second-hand smoke and vape emissions, 472, 477
swimmer's ear, 473
tympanostomy tubes, 462, 477–78, *477*
when to call doctor, 476
Early Hearing Detection and Intervention (EHDI) program, 459
ears, nose, and throat, 468–83
cross section of ear, *471*
ear wax (cerumen), 459
"nasal salute," 399
otoscope for, 128
what the pediatrician checks, 128
See also colds; hearing loss; upper respiratory infections
e-cigarettes/vaping devices, 383–84, 477, 540
battery explosion, 539
Child Nicotine Poisoning

Prevention Act of 2015, 539
child safety, 539–40
dangers, 538–39
ear infection risk and, 477
E. coli bacteria, 363–64
well water testing, 529
eczema, 185, 392–94, 653
allergies and, 79, 200, 213, 383
chickenpox and, 651
dermatitis and, 392–93
infants and, 122
eggs, 248
allergy to, 395, 398
immunizations and, 420, 628
introducing in diet, 200
elbow injuries, 638–40, *640*
electric shock, 308, 320, 484, 503–5
what you should do, 504
electrolyte solution, 357
amounts, by body weight, 359
emergencies, 484–519
anaphylaxis, 396–97, 403
bites, 487–90
bleeding, 485, 486, 497–98
blue skin, lips, or nails, 31, 40, 44, 385, 397, 415, 418, 428, 485, 611
burns or smoke inhalation, 484, 490–93
choking, 415, 484, 494–96
CPR instructions, 703, *703*
croup, 417–18
cuts and scrapes, 497–501
dental trauma, 501
drowning, 484, 501–3
electric shock, 484, 503–5
eye injuries, 547, 548
falls/sudden impacts, 484
fingertip injuries, 505–6
firearms or other weapons, 484, 506–8
first-aid supplies, 499
fractures/broken bones, 506, 508–11
head injury/concussion, 485, 511–13
heatstroke, 576, 673
motor vehicle–related injuries, 484, 487
pain, 485
Poison Help line (1-800-222-1222), 337
poisoning, 484, 486, 513–19
seizure, 485, 486–87
sports accidents, 484
what to do, 486–87
encephalitis, 577, 597, 651, 658
enteritis, 355
environmental hazards, 520–40
air pollution, 520–21
asbestos, 521–22
carbon monoxide, 522–23
congenital abnormalities and, 451
drinking water, 524–29
fish contaminants, 529–30
lead poisoning, 530–35
organic foods, 534–35
pesticides/herbicides, 536
plastic bottles, 524–25
radon, 537
smoke exposure, 537–40
Environmental Protection Agency
fish advisory, 530
Radon Fix-It Hotline, 537
Safe Drinking Water Hotline, 527
epilepsy, 438, 573, 602–4
Epilepsy Foundation, 604
epinephrine, 403, 405, 418
equipment, 313–20
activity center, 232
air filter, 391, 521
baby carriers, 334–35

equipment (*cont'd*)
baby monitor, 255
carbon monoxide/smoke detectors, 309, 493, 523
car safety seats, 32, 152, 156, 163, 260, 290, 321–30, *323*
cribs and accessories, 32, 300–302, *300*
gates, room or stairs, 230, 260, 309–10, *310*
high chairs, 314, *314*
humidifiers, 410, 470
infant seats/bouncers, 315
play yards, 316–17
sound machine, 634
strollers, 335–36
toy boxes and chests, 318
See also furniture, toys
erythema toxicum, 15–16
exercise
asthma and, 385, 386
irregular heartbeats and, 610–11
parental, 36
stationary exercise saucer, 232
eyes, 541–54, *541*
amblyopia, 543, 544, 554
astigmatism, 553
birthmarks or growths on, 549–50
cataracts, 129, 543, 544–45
chemicals in, 548
congenital glaucoma, 543
conjunctivitis (pinkeye), 160, 225, 545–46, 658
droopy eyelid, 544, 549
epicanthus and, 552
eyelid problems, 549–50
eyes turning in or out, 195
farsightedness, 553–54
first exam, 541
first month health watch, 159–60
infections, 159, 160, 185, 545–46
injuries, 546–48, 554
Kawasaki disease, 613–16
leukocoria, 543
light sensitivity, 543, 658
nearsightedness, 554
newborns, 8, 11, 14, 30, 132
particle in, 548
poisoning in, 516
ROP, 26, 541–42
signs of possible problems, 543–44
strabismus, 448, 550–52, *551*
styes and chalazae, 550
tear production problems, 159–60, 552–53, *552*
vision screening, 542–43
what the pediatrician checks, 129

failure to thrive, 84
fainting (syncope), 523, 603, 610, 673
falls
bunk beds, 303–4
changing tables, 302
cribs, 300
high chairs, 314
infant seats/bouncers, 315
risks by age, 186, 205, 260
walking and, 231
while running, dental or head trauma, 311
from windows, 312
family issues, 555–71
adoption, 555–56
child abuse/neglect, 556–60
divorce/separation, 560–61
military families, 565
sibling rivalry, 561–64
single parents, 564–67

stepfamilies, *567*
twins/multiples, 567–71
See also chronic conditions and diseases
Family Voices support network, 439
febrile seizures or convulsions, 572–73, 577, 602–3, 604, 667
what to do, *573*
when to call 911, *573*
feeding, 46–100, *703*
4 months, 199–200
6 months, 213–18
9 months, 248–52, *249*
bottle-feeding, 80–94
breastfeeding, 46–80
calorie requirements, 248
demand feeding, 66, 92
ending middle of night feedings, 92
family mealtimes, 213, 249
finger foods, 216, 248, *250*, 251, 496
fluid intake daily, 359
nighttime, 105
oral health and, 85–86
responsive, and brain development, 138
routines, 200, 203
sample menu, 250–51
self-feeding, 249
signs a nursing baby is well-fed, 73–74
signs of too much or too little feeding, 92–93
soft table foods, 248
solid foods, 116, 213–16
using a spoon, 249
weight gain, newborn and first month, 162–63
See also bottle-feeding; breastfeeding
feet, *228*
arch, 228
clubfoot, 644
flat feet/fallen arches, 640–41, *641*
pigeon toes, 643–46, *644*
fever, 185, 225, 572–80
acetaminophen and ibuprofen dosage chart, 578
acetaminophen or ibuprofen for, 410, 419, 577–78
chickenpox, 651
colds/upper respiratory infections, 468
diarrhea, 358
ear infections, 472–73
eczema, 394
febrile convulsions, 572–73, 577, 602–3, 604, 629, 667
first month, 127, 160
flu, 418, 419
heat-related illness confused with, 576
home treatment, 577–80
immunizations, 622, 629
inconsolable crying, 104
Kawasaki disease, 614
keeping hydrated, 94, 580
measles, 658
medications for, 577–79
meningitis, 599
MMR vaccine, 629
newborns, 116, 160
non-drug treatment, 580
pneumonia, 423
roseola infantum, 667
sore or strep throat, 350, 481
sunburn and, 673
temperature range of, 572
when to call the doctor, 127, 158, 160, 185, 575–76, 651
See also body temperature

fifth disease (erythema infectiosum), *654–55*
finger sucking. *See* thumb sucking
fingertip injuries, 505–6
fingertips turning blue, 409, 422, 428, 469
firearms, 313, 484, 506–8
  emergency action, 506–7
fire prevention, 165, 305–6
  battery explosion, 539
  cigarettes and, 538
  smoke detectors, 309, 493
fireworks, 493
first-aid
  choking/CPR, 493–94, 703, *703*
  courses, 494
  supplies for, 499
first month, 131–66
  baby acne, 132
  baby's states of consciousness, 139–40
  basic care, 101–30, 150–56
  bathing, 118–21, 163–64
  birth injury healing, 132
  body uncurling from fetal position, 132
  bowel movements, 116–17, 150–51
  brain development, 136–40
  breathing difficulties, 158
  carrying baby, 151, *151*
  child-care help, 153–55
  clothing, 123–26
  colic, 140–41
  constipation, 159
  cow's milk caution, 116
  crying, how to respond, 102–4, *103*
  crying and consoling techniques, 140–42
  diapering, 111–13, *113*
  diarrhea and, 117, 159
  dressing/undressing baby, 123, 125–26, *126*
  excessive sleepiness, 159
  eye infections/tear duct problems, 159–60
  feeding difficulty, 158–59
  fever, 127, 160
  first babysitter, 154–55
  first movements, 144–45, *144*
  first smile, 143
  going outside, 152–53, 673–74
  growth, appearance, and development, 131–51
  growth charts, *699–702*
  hair loss or bald spot, 132
  head growth/shape, 132
  head support needed, *171*
  health watch, 158–63
  hearing, 147, 160–61
  home help, 153–55
  immunizations, 133, 696–97
  jaundice, 161, 444
  jitters, 161
  pacifiers, 108, 142, 151–52
  pediatrician visits, 20, 127–30, 133
  personality development, 148–49
  rashes and infections, 161–62
  rectal temperature, 127
  reflexes, 133–36
  safety check, 163–66
  siblings and, 156–57
  skin and nails, 122–23, *122*, 132–33
  skin-to-skin care, 136–37
  sleep, 67, 105–10, 139, 679–80
  smell and touch, 148
  supervision, 165
  swaddling, 123–25, *124*, 142
  temperament, 148–50
  thrush, 162

toys, 149
traveling with baby, 156
tummy time, 108, 110
umbilical cord stump, 133, 161
urination, 115–16
vision, 145–46, *145*, *146*
vomiting, 162
weight gain/loss, 131–32, 158–59, 162–63
when to call the doctor, 127, 150, 159, 161, 162
See also newborns

floppiness (hypotonia), 160, 444, 445

flu (influenza), 286, 418–21
antibiotics and, 224
antiviral medication, 421
avoidance, 202
children at risk, 419, 421
common cold versus, 419
cough and, 413, 419
fever and, 418, 419, 572
vaccine, 130, 224, 225, 259, 286, 384, 420, 620, 627–28
treatment, 419, 615

fluoride, 95, 216

fly bites, 405

folic acid, 451, 454–55, 606
AAP on, 455

fontanelles. *See* soft spots

food allergies, 354, 395–99
anaphylaxis, 79, 396–97
breast milk and, 79
common causes, 79, 395
eggs, 200, 395, 398, 399, 628
fish and seafood, 395
hives and, 402
introducing solid foods and, 199–200, 213, 215, 399, 704, *704*
milk/dairy products, 79, 81, 84–85, 349, 354, 395, 398
outgrowing, 398
peanuts/tree nuts, 200, 395, 398, 399, 704, *704*
sesame seeds, 395
soy, 141, 395, 398
symptoms, 79, 396
tests for, 397
wheat, 395, 398

food and nutrition
cereals, 82, 83, 116, 180, 215, 250, 379
finger foods, 215, 251, 251–52, 496
fish, 529–30
foods high in iron, 215
honey warning, 362, 367
juice, 94, 216
organic foods, 534–35
sample menu, 250–51
solid food introduction, 199–200, 213–16, 704, *705*
table foods, 216
See also breast milk; feeding; formula

food poisoning and contamination, 354, 361–68
botulism, 362, 367, 416
Campylobacter, 362–63
Clostridium perfringens, 363
cryposporidiosis, 363
E. coli, 363–64
prevention, 367–68
salmonella, 364
shigellosis, 364–65
Staphylococcus aureus, 365
treatment, 365, 366
USDA information, 368
when to call doctor, 362

formula, 81–86
"anti-reflux," 379
bowel movements and, 117–18
breast milk versus, 47

formula (*cont'd*)
colic and, 141
cost, 84
cow's milk and, 81–85
Cronobacter bacteria and powdered formula, 87
diarrhea and, 86
elemental or amino-acid-based, 84
fortification and added nutrients, 83–84
goat's milk, 84
hydrolyzed, 84
microwave warning, 73, 88, 305
oral health and, 89
preparing, sterilizing, and storing, 86–88, *87–88*
protein hydrolysate, 141
soy-based, 83, 84, 85
vitamin D in, 64
four months, 188–205
basic care, 199–202
cognitive development, 197–98
crying, 189
daily routines, 188
emerging perceptive abilities, 188
feeding routines, 188, 203
growth, appearance, and development, 189–99
health watch, 202
hearing, 197
immunizations, 204, 696–97
language development, 196–97, 203
motor abilities, 188–89
movement, 190–93, *190*, *191*, *192*
naps, 682–83
personality development, 189
play yards, 316–17
safety check, 204–5
sleep, 67, 198, 201, 203, 676, 682–83
social/emotional development, 198–99
solid foods, 199–200
stimulating brain growth, 203–4
stranger anxiety, 198
SUID alert, 201
toys, 193, 195, 203
vision, 190, 194–95, *194*
vitamin D, 200–201
working mothers and, 188
FPIAP (food protein–induced allergic proctocolitis), 79, 84–85
fractures/broken bones, 506, 508–11
limp and, 641
"toddler fracture," 642
fragile X syndrome, 450–51, 467
fruit juice, 94, 216, 360, 355, 358
furniture
bassinets/cradles, 34, *34*
changing table, 302–3, *303*
cribs, 32, 164, 300–302, *300*
crush injuries from falling furniture or TVs, 312
high chairs, 217
infant seats/bouncers, 315
safety check, 260–61
sharp edges or corners, 311–12

galactosemia, 84
gastrocolic reflex, 117, 180
gastroenteritis, 349, 355, 365, 379
gastroesophageal reflux (GER), 79, 107, 185, 378–79, 414
genital and urinary systems, 581–94
of boys, 17–18, 584–85, 589
blood in urine, 581–83

of girls, *582*, *585–86*, *586*
hydronephrosis, 583–84
posterior urethral valve and, 587–89, *588*
spina bifida and, 457
UTIs, 591–94
genitals, boys, 17
circumcision, 18, 583
collecting urine from, 593
foreskin, 18, 19, 118, 585
hydroceles, 17, 374–75, *375*
hypospadias and chordee, 584–85
inguinal hernia, 17, 372–73, *373*, 591
meatal stenosis, 587
newborns, 17
pediatrician exam, 129
penis care, newborns, 18–19, 118
testicular torsion, 17–18, 589
undescended testicles, 590–91, *591*
genitals, girls
labial adhesions, 585–86, *586*
newborns, 17
pediatrician exam, 129
German measles. *See* MMR vaccine; rubella
Giardia lamblia, 349, 529
girls
blood on newborn's diaper, 115–16
growth, weight, and BMI charts, *700*, *702*
sex-linked genetic abnormalities, 450–51
UTIs, 591–94
See also genitals, girls
glomerulonephritis, 657, 672
gluten sensitivity. *See* celiac disease
growth (physical)
1 month, 131–33
2 months, 168–69
4 months, 189
6 months, 207
9 months, 227–28
average birthweight, 20
charts, 20, 189, *699–702*
failure to thrive, 84
measuring, 128
newborn, 19–21
spurts, 78, 168
gun safety. *See* firearms

haemophilus influenzae (Hib) infections, 286, 621. *See also* Hib vaccine; meningitis
hair, 22
"baby hair," 16–17
care, 119, 161
first month loss and bald spot, 132
lanugo, 14
loss (alopecia), *655–56*
hand and finger skills
2 months, 172
4 months, 192–93
6 months, 207–8, *207*
9 months, 233–34, *233*
pincer grasp, 208, 233
using a spoon, 249
head
1 month, 132, 145
2 months, 169
4 months, 191, *192*
9 months, 228
abusive head trauma, 104, 140, 142–43, 166, 178
carrying baby and, 151, *151*
cradle cap, 161
infant, 128
injuries, 311, 511–13

head (*cont'd*)
  measurement, 20, 132, 179, 189, 228, *701–2*
  plagiocephaly, 169
  soft spots, 16, 128, 169
  swelling after birth, 16
  vaginal birth and, 16
head, neck, and nervous system, 595–604
headaches
  carbon monoxide and, 523
  emergency and, 485
  flu and, 418
  head injury and, 485, 512
  lead poisoning and, 532
  sunburn and, 673
head injury/concussion, 511–13, 599
  when to seek help, 513
head lice, 287–88
Head Start, 272
head tilt (torticollis), *595–97*, *596*
health watch
  1 month, 158–63
  2 months, 185–86
  4 months, 202
  6 months, 222–25
  newborns, 40–45
hearing
  1 month, 160–61
  2 months, 174–75, *174*
  4 months, 197
  6 months, 210
  newborns, 30, 147
  noisy toys warning, 320
  screening newborns, 32, 147, 160, 459–60
  tests, 161, 197, 210, 459–60, 692–94
hearing loss, 458–63
  causes, 458–59
  cerebral palsy and, 449
  cochlear implants, 463
  developmental delays and, 465
  diagnosis, 459–60
  ear infections and, 210, 458, 473
  hearing aids, 462–63
  language development lag and, 219, 234, 463, 458
  lead poisoning and, 532
  surgery for, 462
  tests for, 460–61
  treatment, 462–63
  tubes, 462, 477, *477*
  types: conductive and sensorineural, 459, 463
  what to look for, 461–62
heart and blood, 605–19, *609*
  Apgar scores, 10
  blue baby, 40
  changes in skin color and turning blue, 31, 40, 44, 385, 397, 415, 418, 428, 485, 611
  congenital defects, 453
  congenital disease, 409
  heart rates, normal, 608–9
  hemoglobin, 605, 606
  intraventricular hemorrhage, 26–27
  pediatrician exam of, 129
heart failure, 612–13
  "gallop" and, 612
  signs and symptoms, 612
heart murmur, 611–13
  heart abnormality and, 611–12
  narrowing of aortic or pulmonary valve, 611
  PDA and, 612, 613
  septal defects or "hole in the heart," 611
heat-related illness or heatstroke, 576, 673

hemophilia, 450
hepatitis, 368–72
A, 288, 368, 368–69
A vaccine, 130, 286, 368, 371, 626
B, 288, 368, 369
B vaccine, 8, 32, 130, 133, 186, 204, 225, 259, 368, 371, 626
C, 368, 369, 370
liver damage and, 371
prevention, 371–72
signs/symptoms, 369–70
treatment, 370–71
hernia
inguinal, 17, 372–73, *373*, 591
umbilical, 45, 373
herpes simplex (cold sores, fever blisters), 287, 478–80
HFNC (high-flow nasal cannula), 23, 25, 26
Hib vaccine, 130, 186, 204, 225, 600, 627
hiccups, 30, 96
hips and legs
bacterial infection of the joint, 635, 642
bowlegs and knock-knees, 638
first steps and, 228
hip dysplasia, 641, 642, 643
limb shortening, 448
pediatrician exam of, 129
transient synovitis of a hip, 642
HIV/AIDS, 285, 288–89
childcare centers and, 285, 288–89
hives/urticaria, 402, 404
allergies, 79, 396, 397
insect bites/stings, 406
honey, 362, 367, 416
humidifiers, cool-mist, 410, 416, 419, 428, 470–71
hydrocele/communicating hydrocele, 17, 374–75, *375*
hydrocephalus, 27, 456, 467
hydronephrosis, 583–84
hypertrophic pyloric stenosis, 378, *378*
hypospadias, 584–85

ibuprofen (Motrin, Advil), 63, 410, 469, 475, 499, 618, 624, 655
dosage chart, 578
for fever, 419, 577, 604
warning, 419, 469–70, 577
immune system, weakened
bronchiolitis and, 410
chickenpox and vaccine and, 625, 652
HIV/AIDS and, 630
MMR vaccine and, 628–29
pneumonia and, 422
steroids and, 624, 630, 651
See also HIV/AIDS
immunizations, 108, 130, 620–30
AAP position on, 623
AAP schedule, *696–97*
by age, 8, 11, 186, 204, 259
childcare and, 285–86
concerns about, 622–23
contraindications, 630
easing the hurt, 624
safety of, 620–23
side effects and reactions, 621–22, 624, 629, 630
thimerosal and, 622
when to call doctor, 622
See also specific vaccines
impetigo, 287, 550, 656–57
infections
antibiotics for, 27–28
childcare facilities and, 284–89
first month, 161–62
floppiness and, 160

infections (*cont'd*)
hydrocephalus and, 456
perianal strep, 350
preterm babies, 27–28
spina bifida and, 456
tests for, 27
injury, 297
childcare setting, 289–91
equipment and, 297
why children get injured, 297–99
See also safety; *specific injuries*
insect bites and stings, 404–7
anaphylaxis and, 405, 406
chart of types, 405–6
hives and, 402
how to remove a tick, 637
mosquito-borne illnesses, 660–63
prevention, 407, 662
treatment, 404–5
when to call doctor, 405
insect repellents/DEET, 407, 637, 662
chart of, 663
intellectual development disorder (IDD), 447, 464–67
IQ and, 464
prevention, 466–67
signs/symptoms, 464–65
when to call doctor, 465
intellectual disability, 453, 532. *See also* cerebral palsy; developmental disabilities; Down syndrome; spina bifida
intraventricular hemorrhage (IVH), 26–27
intussusception, 2, 348
iron
deficiency, 605–6, 608
foods high in, 215
-fortified foods, 83
low, symptoms of, 607
safety precautions, 608
stool color and, 117, 608
supplements, 65, 605, 608
IVIG (intravenous immunoglobulin), 615

jaundice, 28, 358, 370, 444, 607, 617
breast-fed versus bottle-fed babies, 161
first month and, 161
in newborns, 42–43
phototherapy, 28, *42*, 43
joints
bacterial infection (septic arthritis), 635, 642
joint contractures, 448
Kawasaki disease, 614

kangaroo care, 24–25, 149
Kawasaki disease, 613–16
kidneys
blood in urine, 581–83
glomerulonephritis, 657, 672
hydronephrosis, 583–84
nephritis, 581
pyelonephritis, 592
scarlet fever and, 672
stones, 582, 583
knock-knees, 638
Kohler's disease, 642

labial adhesions, 585–86, *586*
LactMed database app, 51
La Leche League, 99
language development
2 months, 168, 174–75, *174*, 176, 177, 184, 196
4 months, 196–97
6 months, 209–10
9 months, 234–37, 240
ASD and, 440, 441
"baby talk," 30, 147, 240

bilingual babies, 185, 235–36
cerebral palsy and, 444
comprehension, 235
early brain development and, 138
first conversations, 175
first words, 234, 236
hearing loss and, 210, 234, 458
IDD and delay in, 464
"smile talk," 199
waving bye-bye, 241
when to alert your pediatrician, 210
lanugo, 14, 22
laryngomalacia, 158
larynx, 158, 413, 416
See also cough; croup
lazy eye. *See* amblyopia
lead poisoning, 261, 349, 530–35
learning disabilities, 438, 457, 465
lethargy (listlessness)
as symptom, 348, 349, 423, 456, 606, 614
in newborns, 43
shaken baby syndrome and, 143
leukemia, 12, 47, 50
leukocoria, 543
lice, head, 287–88
limp/limping, 641–43
causes, 641, 642, 643
Perthes disease, 643
sign of serious trouble, 641
lips
anaphylaxis and, 396
anemia and, 607
breastfeeding and, *55*, *56*, 63
dermatitis of, 393
herpes simplex and, 478–80
insect bite/sting on, 406
Kawasaki disease and, 614
normal color, 133
poisoning and, 514
smacking, and hunger, 91
turning blue, 40, 44, 409, 422, 428, 469, 485
Lyme disease, 636–37

magnets (refrigerator or in toys), 306, 319
malabsorption, 350, 375–77
March of Dimes, 458
Marfan syndrome, 450
marijuana, 61, 108, 139, 539
edibles danger, 514
mastitis, 75–76
measles, 621, 628, 657–59
avoidance of, 202
hospitalization for, 659
immunization, 130, 659
signs/symptoms, 657–58
treatment, 658–59
vitamin A and, 658
See also MMR vaccine; rubella
meatal stenosis, 587
meconium, 41, 116, 150
melanoma, 647, 648
melanosis, pustular, 15
meningitis, 577, 597–600, *598*, 621
children at risk, 598–99
complications and fatalities, 599
seizures and, 604
signs and symptoms, 599
spinal tap, *598*, 599, 604
treatment, 599–600
vaccines, 598, 621, 627
meningococcal vaccine, 286
metabolic disorders, 466
microwave warning, 73, 88, 305
milia, 15
miliaria (heat rash, prickly heat), 15

military families, *565*
  AAP's Deployment and Military Medical Home Resources webpage, *565*
  MilitaryOneSource.mil, *565*
milk and dairy products
  AAP on, 353
  allergy to, 84–85, 349, 354, 395
  anemia and, 605–6
  constipation and, 116
  fat-content for, 82
  feeding restrictions, 216
  in formula, 81–82, 83, 84
  hives and, 402
  iron and, 605
  raw (unpasteurized), 359
mitochondrial diseases, 451
MMR vaccine, 130, 286, 600, *628–29*, *659*, *669*
MMRV vaccine, 628, 669
mold, 121, 293, 384, 391, 399, 400, 401, 470
moles or nevi, *550*, *647–50*
molluscum contagiosum, 660
mononucleosis, 481
mosquito bites, 405
mosquito-borne illnesses, 660–63
movement
  1 month and newborn, 144–45
  2 months, 169–72, *170*, *171*, *172*
  4 months, 190–93, *190*, *191*, *192*
  6 months, 207–8, *207*
  9 months, 226–33, *229*, *230*, *232*, 233
  CP and, 444–45
  IDD and, 464
MRSA infections, 664
Multiples of America, 570–71
mumps, 600–602, *601*
  vaccine, 600, 628
muscle tone and strength
  Apgar scores, 10
  floppiness, 160, 444, 445
  stiffness, 444, 445
  weakness or paralysis and spina bifida, 456
muscular dystrophy, 451
musculoskeletal system, 635–46, *636*

nails
  chicken pox itch and, 651
  fingertip injuries, 505–6
  impetigo and, 656–57
  infections, 161
  trimming, 14, 122–23, *122*
naps, 676, 681–82
  2 months, 168
  4 months, 682–83
  9 months, 685–86
  in childcare settings, 278, 686–87
  evolution of, 684
  exceptions to routines and readjusting, 687
  limiting time, 105
  for newborns, 106
  SUID/SIDS and, 278
nasal allergy/allergic rhinitis, 399–401
National Association for Family Child Care, 269, 270
National Battery Ingestion Hotline, 311
National Capital Poison Center, 310
National Center for Missing & Exploited Children, 343
National Down Syndrome Congress, 458
National Highway Traffic Safety Administration website, 325
National Smokers' Helpline, 383

necrotizing enterocolitis (NEC), 23, 26, 28, 50
neonatal intensive care unit (NICU), 9–10, 22
  baby blues/postpartum depression and, 23
  delayed development after stays in, 189
  developmental care, 149
  kangaroo care, 149
nephritis, 581
neural tube defects (NTDs), 455
newborns, 3–45, *34*
  abdominal distension or hernia, 17, 40
  antibiotic eye ointment, 8, 11, 32, 160
  Apgar scores, 8, 9–10
  appearance, 4–5, 14–18
  "baby hair," 16–17
  basic infant care, 101–30
  bathing, 11, 118–21
  behavior, 29–31
  birth injuries, 40
  birthweight and measurements, 19–21
  blue baby, 40
  bonding, 4, 11, 31
  bowel movements, 40, 41, 116
  breastfeeding, 4, 5–6, *5*, 48, *55*, 66–68, 74
  car seat for, 32
  Cesarean birth, 6–7
  coughing, 41
  crying, excessive, 41
  crying, normal, 30, 102
  diaper rash, 162
  dressing/undressing your baby, 123, 125–26, *126*
  essentials for home, 32
  examinations, 11, 20, 45
  eyes and vision, 14, 30, 145–46, *145*, *146*, 541–42
  fetal position and, 29–30
  fever and, 116, 185
  first checkup, 74
  first moments, 5
  floppiness, 160
  forceps marks, 41–42
  girls, pseudo-menses, 17
  going home from the hospital, 31–32
  head, 16
  health watch, 40–45
  hearing, 30, 147
  heart rate, 608
  how to diaper, 111–13, *113*
  immunizations, 8, 32, 130, 371, 626, 652, 696–97
  jaundice, 28, 42–43, 444
  leaving delivery area, 10–11
  lethargy/sleepiness, 43
  low birth weight, 20, 150
  nails, 14, 122–23
  natal teeth, 29
  NICU and, 9–10
  penis care, 18–19
  respiratory distress, 43–44
  screening tests, 11, 32, 459–60, 466, 588, 692–94
  senses of, 30–31, 148
  siblings and, 38–39, *38*, *39*, 156–57
  signs to watch for, 31
  size, large/small, 19–20
  skin, 5, 14
  skin care, 122
  skin color, 14, 132–33
  skin-to-skin care, 4, 7, 8, 23, 30, 54, 136–37
  sleep, 43, 66, 105–10, 106, 139
  swaddling, 123–25, *124*, 142, 144
  tummy time, 108, 110
  umbilical cord, 8, 44–45

newborns (*cont'd*)
urination and, 74, 115–16
vaginal delivery, 3–5
vitamin K, 8–9, 11, 32
weight loss, 21, 68, 73
when to call doctor, 32
New Mother's Guide to Breastfeeding (Meek and Tippins), 50, 64, 74, 99
nine months, 226–62
acquainting your baby with a sitter, 244–45
basic care, 248–55
behavior, 255–59
bilingual babies, 235–36
brain development, 240–41
calorie requirements, 248
cerebral palsy and, 445
childcare and, 241
cognitive development, 237–39, *239*
concept of object permanence, 238
crawling, 226, 229–30, *229*, 261
exercise saucer or activity center for, 232, 260
falls, 231, 260
fears of, 247
feeding, 248–52, *249*, *250*
growth, appearance, and development, 227–48
hand and finger skills, 233–34, *233*, 249
head size, 228
immunizations, 259
language development, 234–37, 240
mirror and sense of identity, 245–46
movement, 226–33, *229*, *230*, *232*
parental supervision, 226
peekaboo variations, 238–39
safety check, 260–62
sample menu, 250–51
self-esteem, 227
self-feeding, 227, 249
separation anxiety, *242*, *243*, 244–46
siblings, 258–59, *259*
sitting, 229, 233
skin-to-skin contact, 241
sleep, 254–55, 685–86
social/emotional development, 242–48
stair safety, 230, 260
standing, 230–31, *230*
stranger anxiety, 241, 242, *242*, 281
teeth, 255
thumb sucking, 248
toys, 234, 240, 241, 246
transitional objects, 247–48
turning off TV, 236, 241
walking and first steps, 228, 231, *232*, 233
weaning: introducing a cup, 252–54, *252*, *253*
weight/height, 227–38
noroviruses, 379
nose
congested, 44, 410, 158, 470
nasal allergy, 399–401
nasal aspirators, 470
saline nose drops, 44, 158, 410, 470
nursemaid's elbow, 638–40, *640*

obesity or overweight
asthma and, 382
breastfeeding and, 50
drinking juice, 94, 216
overfeeding, 217
reduced-fat milk, 82
sleep and, 675

organ transplants, 410
oxytocin, 56

pacifiers, 151–52
  bottle-feeding or breastfeeding and, 91, 108, 109
  calming crying baby, 142
  colic and, 142
  reducing SUID risk, 108, 109, 151
  safety check, 152, 166, 317–18
parainfluenza, 416
parasites, 349, 363, 529
parents/parenting
  abusive head trauma and, 142–43
  anger or loss of control, what to do, 143
  anxiety and, 34
  avoiding alcohol and drug use, 108, 139
  becoming a parent, 33–39
  bedtime routine, sharing, 680
  best response to frustration, anger, 178
  child abuse/neglect and, 556–60
  child's behavioral style and, 212
  child's brain development and, 138
  child's temperament and, 211–12
  chronic illness of a child and, 430–32
  concerns after new baby arrival, 33–36
  consistent routines, 139
  creating a "village," 139
  crying baby, coping and responding, 103–4, *103*, 140, 143
  dancing with baby, 221
  discipline and, 255–58
  emotions after birth, 33–34
  family issues, 555–71
  family mealtimes, 213, 249
  getting help with anger, anxiety, or depression, 140
  healthy diet and, 139
  helping baby sleep, 105, 110–11, 677–68
  home help, 153–55
  interacting, activities for, 139, 241 (*see also* peekaboo)
  love and attention for your child, 139
  media consumption or screen time and, 236, 338, 631–34
  multiple children, concerns, 35 (*see also* siblings)
  navigating the health care system, 433–34
  newborn and partner's feelings, 36–37, *37*
  partner's role, 36, 50, 89, 571
  positive environment, 138–39
  positive parenting, 138
  reading to baby, 139, 184, *194*, 203, 204, 221, 235, 241
  recognizing a baby's uniqueness, 206–7
  singing to baby, 184, 203, 204
  sleep deprivation and, 680
  smiles and responses, 143
  smoking and, 108, 383
  stress and, 36, 153, 180, 181, 188, 207, 212, 282, 299, 559, 560, 565
  support for, 139, 434, 559
  See also working mothers
patent ductus arteriosus (PDA), 612, 613
peanuts, 200, 398
  "Adding Peanut Protein to Your Baby's Diet," 704, *704*

peanuts (*cont'd*)
allergy, 79, 200, 395, 398, 399, 402
choking, 495, 496
pediatricians
checkup schedule, 692–94
first checkup after hospital discharge, 74
first exam, 127
immunization schedule, *696–97*
screening tests, 11, 692–94
visits to, 128–30
weight and measurements by, 20, 128, 699–702
pediatric specialties, 86, 159, 353, 386, 583, 588–89, 604, 638, 643
peekaboo, 185, 201, 211, 238–39, 241
perianal strep, 350
personality development, 13, 149–50, 168, 177, 189, 206, 211–13
Perthes disease, 643
pesticides/herbicides, 534–36
pets. *See* animals
phenylketonuria (PKU), 466
phototherapy, 42, 43
pica, 607
pigeon toes (intoeing), 643–46, *644*, *645*
pink eye. *See* conjunctivitis
plagiocephaly, 169
play yards, 221–22, 316–17
pneumococcal vaccines, 130, 186, 204, 225, 423–24, 600, 629
pneumonia, 225, 421–24
breastfeeding and, 50
cough, 413, 414, 422, 423
measles and, 658
MRSA infections and, 664
warning signs, 422
when to call doctor, 423
poisoning, 513–19
alcohol, 313
bathroom dangers, 307
emergency, 484, 486
in eye, 516
fumes, 517
garage and basement dangers, 308
kitchen dangers, 304–5
laundry room dangers, 306
lead, 261, 530–35
medication, 307–8
mushrooms, 365
nicotine, 539
plants/list of plants, 310, 337
Poison Help line (1-800-222-1222), 261
poison-proofing home and yard, 337, 514–15
prevention, 261–62, 304–5, 306, 519
signs of poisoning, 514
on skin, 516
swallowed, 517–18
treatment, 516
what *not* to do, 517–18
polio, 620
vaccine, 130, 186, 204, 225, 286, 629
port-wine stains, 16, 549–50, 648–49
posterior urethral valve, 587–89, *588*
postpartum depression, 23
posture, 27, 228, 443
premature babies, 21–29
appearance, 22
backpack warning, 334
bonding, 24–25
breastfeeding, 23–24, 47
bronchiolitis and, 409
cerebral palsy, 27, 444
chickenpox vaccine, 652

cup-feeding, 74
donor breast milk for, 24
formulas for, 85
health issues, 21–23, 25–29, 149, 541–42, 612, 613
hearing tests, 161
hospitalization of, 21
kangaroo care, 24–25, 149
lanugo and, 14
NICU and, 22, *22*, 24, 29
pediatrician visits and, 29
reaction to stimuli, 149
reflux and, 79
skin-to-skin care, 22, 23, 24
supplemental nurser, 77, *77*
temperament and, 149

Prevent Child Abuse America, 556–57
probiotics and prebiotics, 28, 83–85, 348, 356, 360–61
prolactin, 56
ptosis (droopy eyelid), 544, 549
pustular melanosis, 15
pyelonephritis, 592

rabies, 342, 488–89
Radon Fix-It Hotline, 537
Raising Twins (Flais), 66, 568
rashes
baby acne, 132
diaper rash, 114–15, 162
diarrhea and, 358
feeding allergy and, 79
hives, 402, 404
immunizations and, 629
Kawasaki disease, 614
measles, 657–59
milk allergy, 349
miliaria (heat rash, prickly heat), 15
MMR vaccine and, 629
newborn, 161–62
roseola infantum, 666–67
scarlet fever, 671
strep throat and, 350
See also eczema

reading to your baby, 139, 184, *194*, 203, 204, 221
reflexes
Apgar scores, 10
gastrocolic, 117, 180
Moro (or startle) reflex, 135, *135*, 136, 169
newborn, 133–36
pediatrician exam, 130
rooting, 55, 90, 133–34
stepping, *136*, 171
sucking, 134–35
tongue-thrust, 199
tonic neck, 135–36, *136*, 169
when to call doctor, 136

respiratory distress, 403, 405
blue skin, lips, or nails, 31, 40, 44, 385, 397, 415, 418, 428, 485, 603, 611
in newborns, 43–44
syndrome, 25, 26
when to call doctor, 44

respiratory syncytial virus (RSV), 185, 408
vaccine, 11, 411

retinopathy of prematurity (ROP), 26, 541–42
Reye syndrome, 419, 475, 577, 615
rheumatic fever, 482, 671
rickets, 638
ringworm, 289, 665–66
rolling over, 171, 191, 218, 229
roseola infantum, 666–67
rotavirus, 355, 379, 630
vaccine, 130, 186, 204, 225, 286, 355, 360, 629–30

rubella, 451, 628, 667–69
pregnancy and, 451, 667, 669
when to call doctor, 669

rubella (*cont'd*)
  See also MMR vaccine; MMRV vaccine

safety, 162–66, 260–62, 297–343
  animals, 341–42
  baby carriers, 334–35
  baby equipment, 313–20
  baby walkers, 317
  backyard, 337
  bathrooms, 306–8
  batteries, 310–11
  bunk beds, 303–4
  burns, 186, 261, 305–6, 312, 320, 484, 490–93
  carbon monoxide, 309, 523
  car seats, 321–30
  changing tables, 164, 171, 302–3
  childcare settings, 289–94
  child-proofing a home, 226–27, 300–320
  choking, 187, 251–52, 262, 306, 415, 484, 495–96, 703, *703*
  community and neighborhood, 342–43
  computers, 311–12
  CPR instructions, 703, *703*
  cribs, 165, 300–302, *300*
  cuts, 497–501
  doors/glass doors, 311
  electric shock, 308, 309, 484, 503–5
  falls, 186, 231, 260, 300, 311, 312, 314, 315
  firearms, 313
  fire, 165, 305–6, 309, 492–93, 523
  furniture and, 311–12
  garage/basement, 308–9
  heat sources, 312–13
  kidnapping and abduction, 342–43
  kids around cars, 332–33
  kitchen, 304–6
  laundry room, 306
  magnets, 306, 319
  necklaces and cords, 151, 165–66, 311
  nursery, 300–304
  outside the home, 321–43
  reporting unsafe products, 320
  shopping carts, 336
  situations associated with injuries, 299
  stair gate, 230, 260, 310, *310*
  strollers, 335–36, *335*
  toys, 318–20
  water, 338–41
  why children get injured, 297–99
  See also car seats; poisoning
saline nasal drops, 44, 158, 470
salmonella bacteria, 264
salmon patches (stork bites), 15, 648
scabies, 287, 669–70
scarlet fever, 671–72
scoliosis, 448
screens and media devices, 203, 236, 631–34
  AAP on, 633
security blankets or bottle, 247–48
seizures, 380, 438, 485, 602–4
  cerebral palsy and, 447
  febrile convulsions, 572–73, 577, 604, 667
  head trauma and, 511, 513
  medications for, 604
  meningitis and, 599, 604
  poisoning and, 514
  Reye syndrome and, 651
  seizure-like episodes, 603

types of, *599*, 602
what to do, 486–87, *573*
when to seek help, 603
whooping cough and, 620
See also epilepsy
self-esteem, 143, 150, 177, 446
separation anxiety, 206, *242*, 243, 244–46, *254*
tips for transitioning to childcare, 281
shaken baby syndrome (abusive head trauma), 104, 140, 142–43, 166, 178
shigella infections, 364–65
shock, circulatory, 79, 339
shock, electric, 484, 503–4
shoes, 393, 645
first pair, 232
shy child, 212
sibling rivalry, 561–64, 569
siblings
baby's age and, 182–84, *183*, 202, *202*, 222, 258–59, *259*
multiples and, 569
newborns and, 38–39, *38*, *39*, 156–57
sickle cell disease (SCD), 606, 616–19
complications, 617, 618
fifth disease and, 654
newborn screenings, 606
pain and, 616, 617, 618
types of, 616
when to call doctor, 619
single-parent families, 564–67
sinus infections, 224, 400, 414, *478*, 598, 671
sippy cups, 74, 216, 252, *252*
sitting up, 191, *191*, 195, 208, 214, 229, 233
six months, 206–25, *206*
appearance/growth, 207
basic care, 213–22
behavioral style and parenting, 212
bowel movements, 216
choking prevention, 216
cognitive development, 210–11
common illnesses, 225
feeding and food choices, 213–18
health watch, 222–25
immunizations, 225, 696–97
language development, 209–10
liquids for, 216
movement, 207–8, *207*
overweight concerns, 217
personality development, 211–12
practice "walking," 208
rolling over, 218
safety check, 225
self-feeding, 215
separation anxiety, 206
siblings, 222
skin-to-skin care, 220
sleeping, 218–19, 221
social/emotional development, 211–13
stimulating brain growth, 220–21
stranger anxiety, 206
teething, 216, 219–20
temperament, 211–12
toys and equipment, 208, 220–22
vision, 209
skin, 647–74
Apgar scores, 9, 10
baby acne,132
birthmarks and hemangiomas, 15–16, 549–50, 647–50
changes in color (turning blue), 31, 40, 44, 385, 397, 415, 418, 428, 485, 603, 611

skin (*cont'd*)
- chickenpox, 650–52
- cold sores, 287
- common infections, 287, 289
- cradle cap, 161, 653–54
- dermatitis, 392–94
- eczema, 79, 122, 185, 200, 392–94, 651, 653
- fifth disease, 654–55
- freckles, 15
- hair loss, 655–56
- hives, 402, 404
- impetigo, 287, 550, 656–57
- insect bites/stings, 404–7
- jaundice and, 42, 161
- Kawasaki disease, 614
- measles, 657–59
- molluscum contagiosum, 660
- MRSA infections, 664
- newborns, 5, 14, 40, 122, 132–33, 152
- poison on, 516
- preterm babies, 22
- ringworm (tinea), 665–66
- roseola infantum, 666–67
- rubella, 667–69
- scabies, 287, 669–70
- scarlet fever, 671–72
- seborrheic dermatitis, 161, 653–54
- sunburn, 152, 672–74
- yeast infection, 654

sleep, 675–89
- 1 month and newborns, 43, 66, 105–10, 139, 679–80
- 2 months, 180–82, *181*, 681–82
- 4 months, 201, 676, 677, 682–83
- 6 months, 218–19, 221, 677
- 9 months, 254–55, 685–86
- adequate amount, 675–79
- allergies and, 400
- apnea and, 26
- avoiding overheating, 108
- baby monitor and, 255
- baby's states of consciousness and, 139
- bedtime routines, 86, 105, 201, 203, 218, 684–85, 687
- breastfeeding and, 66–67
- child's bedroom and, 682
- clothing for, 107, 164
- crib/bedding, 107–8, 110
- crying at bedtime, 201, 676–79
- daytime drowsiness, 678
- disorders, 603
- environment for, 201
- excessive sleepiness, 159
- getting sleep in sync, 677–78
- getting the most out of sleep, 685–88
- health issues and, 688
- helping baby sleep, 105, 110–11, 624
- how baby sleeps, 105–6
- naps, 105, 106, 168, 278, 676, 681–87
- nighttime feedings and, 201, 677
- pacifier and, 108, 109
- parental sleep deprivation, 680, 688–89
- perspective on, 688–89
- positioning for, 106–7, 164–66
- safety and, 107–8
- Scenario #1, 676–67
- Scenario #2, 681–82
- Scenario #3, 684–85
- schedule for, 675
- screens and media devices and, 633–34
- separation anxiety and, 254
- sharing the bedtime routine, 680

sleeping through the night, 676–67
sleep plan, 680–81
sleep position, 106–7, 109–10, 181, *181*
sleep wraps, 34
suffocation risk, 107–8, 164–65
swaddling and, 34
temperament and, 148–49, 676, 678
waking and length of sleep periods, 110
where babies should not sleep, 107, 108, 109, 163, 201, 315, 330
where to put a crib or bassinet, 66, 109, 110
See also SUID/SIDS
smell, sense of, 30, 148
smiles, 143, 167, 168, 173, *174*, 175, 176, *176*
"smile talk," 199
smoking, 108, *539*
risks to baby, 383, 391, 472, 477, 538
safety and, 539–40
secondhand and thirdhand smoke, 472, 537, 538
social/emotional development
by age, 175–79, 198–99, 211–13, 242–48
ASD and, 440, 441
transitional objects, 247–48
when to alert your pediatrician, 212–13
soft spots (fontanelles), 16, 169
sore throat, 480–83, 572
See also strep throat
special-needs children, 291, 432. *See also specific conditions*
spina bifida, 450, 452, 454–58
Spina Bifida Association, 458
spinal tap (lumbar puncture), *598*, *599*, 604
spine, curvature of, 448
spitting up, 41, 79, 96, 98–99
vomiting versus, 377–78
"spoiling a child," 179, 242, 257
Staphylococcus aureus (Staph), 365, 664
stepfamilies, 567
strabismus, 448, 550–51, *551*
stranger anxiety, 189, 198, 206, 241, 281
strep throat, 350, 480–83
scarlet fever and, 671
when to call doctor, 482
Streptococcus pyogenes, 350, 480–83, 671, 657
stress, 36, 254–55, 299, 688
accidents and injuries associated with, 299
baby's temperament and, 212
help at home to reduce, 153–55
overwhelming, getting help for, 188
premature birth and, 23
sibling behavior and, 39
sick child and, 282
TV shows or news programs and, 241
stridor, 158, 418
strollers, 107, 335–36, *335*
Sturge-Weber syndrome, 649
styes (hordeola), 550
SUID/SIDS (sudden unexpected infant death)
breastfeeding and reduced risk, 50, 107
in childcare settings, 278
cigarette smoke and, 538
pacifiers to reduce risk, 108, 109, 151, 317
peak occurrence, 201

SUID/SIDS (*cont'd*)
sleep position and, 106–7
swaddling and, 109
sunburn, 152, *672–74*
sunscreens, 152, 673
swaddling, 103, 109, 123–25, *124*, 142, 144
swimming, 338–40
swollen glands, 425, 469, 479, 481, 489, 614, 668, 671. *See also* mumps

tachycardia, 609
Tay-Sachs disease, 450
teeth
breastfeeding and, 85
cavities, prevention, 86, 89, 220, 253, 255
cerebral palsy and, 448–49
cleaning for baby, 219–20
emergencies, 485, 501
falls and injury to, 311
feeding and, 85–86
first, 219–20
first dentist visit, 255
fluoride and, 95, 216, 526
natal teeth, 29
nighttime "brush, book, bed" routine, 86
teaching baby to brush, 255
teething, 219–20, 320
temperament, 148–50, 211–12
sleep behaviors and, 148–49, 676, 678
tetanus, 488, 490, 499, 620, 625–26
thalassemia, 606
thermometers
AAP on, 574
best ways to take a temperature, 574–75
types of, 127, 574
thrush, 162
thumb sucking, 57, 248
ticks, 406, 637
tonsillectomy, 483
tonsillitis, 480–83, *481*
torticollis, 169, *596*
touch, sense of, 30–31, 148
toxoplasmosis, 342, 549, 617
toy boxes or chests, 318
toys
1 month, 150
2 months, 184
4 months, 193, 195, 203
6 months, 208
9 months, 234, 236, 240, 241, 246
activity center, 232
balloons, 320, 496
balls, 193, *233*, 234, 246
bathtub toys, 121, 246
blocks, 234
books, 184, 193, 194, 208, 235, 246
cars, trucks, trains, 246
chewable toys, 184
dolls, 246, 319
household objects, 235, 241
kiddie push cars, 232
mirror, 193, 195, 245, 246
mobiles, 149, 150, 172, 184, 195, 302
musical toys, 208
music boxes, CDs, iPods, or tapes, 149, 184, 246
push-pull, 246
rattles, 184, 193, 208, 319
soft or textured, that make sounds, 149, 193
squeeze toys, 246, 319
stacking toys, 246
stationary exercise center, 232
stuffed animals, 319
telephones, 246
wagon, 232

toy safety, 318–20
  balloons, 320, 496
  button and coin battery dangers, 310–11, 320
  lead poisoning and, 349
  magnets' danger, 319
  most dangerous toys, 319–20
  recalls, 320, 349
  reporting unsafe toys, 321
trachea (windpipe), 413, 415–17, *417*
transient synovitis of a hip, 642
transitional objects, 247–48
traveling safety, 156. *See also* car safety
tuberculosis, 415, 424–26
  TB tests, 425–26
tummy time, 108, 110, 169, 190
tumors, 591, 551, 638
twins/multiples, 567–71
  breastfeeding, 65–66, *65*, 567–78
  connecting with other families, 570–71
  extra help and, 571
  financial pressures, 568
  NICU and, 567
  partner's role, 571
  recommended reading, 66, 568
  transporting, 570
  in vitro fertilization, 568
twitching, 573, 603
two months, 167–87
  basic care, 179–85
  bowel movements, 180
  cerebral palsy and, 445
  emotional and social development, 175–79
  feeding, 179–81
  fever and, 175
  fussiness, 178
  growth, appearance, and development, 168–79
  growth spurt, 179–80
  health watch, 185–86
  hearing, making sounds, 168, 174–76, *174*, 196
  immunizations, 184, 186, 696–97
  meningitis and, 598, 599
  movement, 169–72, *170*, *171*, *172*
  neck strength, 169–70, *170*, *172*
  neediness levels, 177–79
  preventing torticollis and plagiocephaly, 169
  reflexes, 169
  rolling over, 171
  safety check, 186–87
  self-esteem, 177
  siblings, 182–84, *183*
  skin-to-skin care, 184
  sleeping, 177–78, 180–82, *181*, 219, 221, 681–82
  smiles, 167, *174*, 175, *176*
  social/emotional development, 175–79
  stimulating brain growth, 184–85
  toys for, 184
  tummy time, 169
  vision, 172–74, *173*, *174*
  working mothers and, 167–68, 181
tympanostomy tubes, 462, 477–78, *477*

umbilical cord, 8, 17
  bathing and, 119
  care of the stump, 44, 133
  delayed or timed cord clamping, 4
  infections, 44, 161–62

umbilical cord (*cont'd*)
  storing cord blood, 11–12
  when to call doctor, 44
umbilical granuloma, 44–45
umbilical hernia, 17, 45, 373
United Cerebral Palsy, 447, 458
upper respiratory infections (URIs), 185, 408, 468–71
urethritis, 582, 592
urinary tract infections (UTIs), 591–94
  cystitis, 592
  fever and, 572
  posterior urethral valve and, 588
  pyelonephritis, 592
  spina bifida and, 457
  urethritis, 592
urination/urine
  blood in urine, 115–16, 581–83, 592, 657
  breastfeeding and, 68, 74
  color of urine, 115, 581, 582, 657
  newborns and, 115–16
  posterior urethral valve and, 587–89, *588*
US Department of Agriculture
  food poisoning information, 368
  organic food certification program, 534
  pamphlets and newsletters on food preparation, 368
  website, 368

vegetarian or vegan diet, 65
  baby formula choices, 85
vernix, 5, 22
viruses/viral infections, 224, 349, 355, 422
  antiviral medication, 421
  hives and, 402
  prevention, 420
vision
  1 month and newborns, 30, 145–46
  2 months, 172–74, *173*, *174*
  4 months, 194–95, *194*
  6 months, 209
  cerebral palsy and, 448
  corrective lenses, 553–54
  developmental delays and, 465
  first eye exam, 541
  photoscreening, 543
  signs of problems, 195, 209
  testing, 129, 692–94
vitamin A, 658
vitamin B12, 65
vitamin C, 608
vitamin D, 64–65, 91, 248
  AAP on, 64, 201
  deficiency (rickets), 638
vitamin K, 8–9, 11, 32
vitamin supplements, 248
  for baby, 64–65, 91–92, 200–201
  for premature babies, 65
  prenatal, 139, 451
vomiting, 225, 377–81
  allergies and, 79
  blood in, 358
  causes, 349, 378–81, *378*
  from coughing, 414
  dehydration and, 380, 381
  diarrhea and, 358
  first month, 162
  meningitis and, 599
  poisoning and, 517–18
  reflex trigger and, 277
  Reye syndrome and encephalitis, 651
  spitting up, 96, 98–99, 377–78
  when to call doctor, 380

walking, *136*, 171, 228, 231–33, *232*
  baby walker, 231, 260
  shoes, 232
water
  bottle-feeding and supplemental, 94
  contaminants, 524–29
  filters, 527
  fluoride in, 216, 526
  sippy cup and, 216
  well water testing, 216–17, 527–29
water safety, 205, 261, 338–41, 502–3
  AAP on, 338
  bathrooms and, 307
  boating, 340
  hot-water heater setting, 119, 164, 202, 307, 493
  pools, spas, hot tubs, 339–40
  swim lessons, 338, 339
  "water watcher," 341
weaning, 252–54, *252*, *253*
  baby-led, 215
weight
  at birth, 21
  by age, 162–63, 168, 217
  charts, *699–702*
  loss, 68, 73, 78
West Nile virus, 660–63
wheezing, 79, 414. *See also* asthma
whooping cough (pertussis), 427–29, 620, *625*, 626
  "100-day cough," 427
  when to call doctor, 428
  See also DTaP vaccine
Women, Infants, and Children (WIC) program, 72, 181
working mothers
  added stress and, 188
  breastfeeding, 48–49, 181
  childcare, 167–68, 181
  expressed milk, 181
  help for housework, 181
  milk supply and, 180, 181
  returning to work, 167–68, 181, 188
  sick child and, 282–84
wryneck. *See* head tilt

yeast infections, 114, 654

Zika, 451, 660–63